DVT	deep venous thrombosis	IAT	indirect antiglobulin test
EACA	epsilon aminocaproic acid	IBC	intraoperative blood collection
EDTA	ethylenediaminetetraacetic acid		
EIA	enzyme immunoassay	IgA	immunoglobulin A
ELAT	enzyme-linked antiglobulin test	IgE	immunoglobulin E
		IgG	immunoglobulin G
ELISA	enzyme-linked immunosorbent assay	IgM	immunoglobulin M
		IH	intraoperative hemodilution
EPA	Environmental Protection Agency	IHA	immune hemolytic anemia
EXP	expiration	IS	immediate spin
FDA	Food and Drug Administration	ITP	idiopathic thrombocytopenic purpura
FFP	Fresh Frozen Plasma	IUT	intrauterine transfusion
FMH	fetomaternal hemorrhage	JCAHO	Joint Commission on Accreditation of Healthcare Organizations
FNH	febrile nonhemolytic		
F-RBCs	frozen Red Blood Cells		
FTA-ABS	fluorescent Treponemal antibody absorption test	LDH	lactate dehydrogenase
		LISS	low ionic strength saline
GC	granulocyte concentrate	LR	leukocyte-reduced
GVHD	graft-vs-host disease	LR-RBCs	leukocyte-reduced Red Blood Cells
Gy	Gray (1 Gy = 100 rads = 1 Joule/kg)		
		MF	mixed field
Hb	hemoglobin	MLC	mixed lymphocyte (leukocyte) culture
HBc	hepatitis B core antigen		
HBIG	hepatitis B immunoglobulin	MLR	mixed lymphocyte (leukocyte) reaction
HBsAg	hepatitis B surface antigen	MNC	mononuclear cells
		MoAb	monoclonal antibody
HCFA	Health Care Financing Administration	MOD	modified
		MSBOS	maximum surgical blood order schedule
Hct	hematocrit		
HCV	hepatitis C virus	MSDS	material safety data sheets
HDN	hemolytic disease of the newborn		
		NA	no activity
HIV	human immunodeficiency virus	NAIT	neonatal alloimmune thrombocytopenia
HSA	human serum albumin	NCCLS	
HTLV-I	human T-cell lymphotropic virus type 1		
HTR	hemolytic transfusion reaction	NRC	
HUS	hemolytic uremic syndrome	NS	nonspecific
		NT	not tested

OSHA	Occupational Safety and Health Administration	RR	repeatedly reactive or relative response
p	probability	RT	room temperature
PBC	postoperative blood collection	SD-APC	single donor apheresis platelet concentrate
PBS	phosphate-buffered saline	SGP	sialoglycoprotein
PBPC	peripheral blood progenitor cell	SOP	standard operating procedure
PBSC	peripheral blood stem cell	SSO	sequence-specific oligonucleotide
PC	platelet concentrate		
PCH	paroxysmal cold hemoglobinuria	STS	serologic test for syphilis
		TA	transfusion-associated
PCR	polymerase chain reaction	TPE	therapeutic plasma exchange
PEG	polyethylene glycol		
PI	paternity index	TQM	total quality management
PLT	primed lymphocyte typing	TTP	thrombotic thrombocytopenic purpura
PPF	plasma protein fraction		
PRA	panel reactive antibody	VDRL	Venereal Disease Research Laboratory
PRDPC	pooled random donor platelet concentrate		
		VEC	vascular endothelial cell
PT	prothrombin time	v	volume
PUBS	percutaneous umbilical blood sampling	vWD	von Willebrand's disease
		vWF	von Willebrand factor
PW	prewarmed	WAIHA	warm autoimmune hemolytic anemia
QA	quality assessment		
QACI	quality assessment and continuous improvement	WB	Whole Blood
		W-RBCs	washed Red Blood Cells
QC	quality control	w	weight
RBCs	Red Blood Cells (blood donor unit)	XM	crossmatch
		4+	One solid agglutinate
rbcs	red blood cells	3+	Several large agglutinates in a clear background
RD-PC	random donor platelets or platelet concentrate		
RES	reticuloendothelial system	2+	Many medium size agglutinates in a clear background
RFLP	restriction fragment length polymorphism		
		1+	Many small agglutinates in a turbid background
Rh	Rhesus factor		
Rh+	Rh positive	0	No agglutination seen macroscopically
Rh−	Rh negative		
RhIG	Rh Immune Globulin		
RPR	rapid plasma reagin (serologic test for syphilis)		

TECHNICAL MANUAL

aa
BB

AMERICAN
ASSOCIATION
OF BLOOD BANKS

11TH EDITION

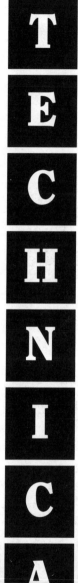

aa
BB

**AMERICAN
ASSOCIATION
OF BLOOD BANKS**

8101 GLENBROOK ROAD
BETHESDA, MARYLAND 20814

**11TH EDITION
1993**

Text paper meets EPA guidelines for minimum recovered material content (50% recycled fiber, including 10% postconsumer waste).

American Association of Blood Banks
8101 Glenbrook Road
Bethesda, MD 20814-2749

Library of Congress Cataloging-in-Publication Data

Technical manual—11th ed.
     p.   cm.
   Editor-in-chief: Richard H. Walker.
   Includes bibliographical references and index.
   ISBN 1-56395-019-7
   1. Blood banks. 2. Blood banks—Quality control.
3. Blood collection and preservation. 4. Blood—Trans-
portation.
I. Walker, Richard H. II. American Association of
Blood Banks.
[DNLM: 1. Blood banks—laboratory manuals. WH 25
T2548 1993]
RM172.T43   1993
615' .39—dc20
DNLM/DLC
for Library of Congress   93-998
                                    CIP

Editor-in-Chief
Richard H. Walker, MD

Editors

Donald R. Branch, PhD
Walter H. Dzik, MD
W. John Judd, FIMLS, MIBiol
Ram Kakaiya, MD
Ann McMican, MS, MT(ASCP)SBB
Paul Ness, MD
Herbert F. Polesky, MD
Susan D. Rolih, MS, MT(ASCP)SBB
Virginia Vengelen-Tyler, MBA, MT(ASCP)SBB

Technical Manual Committee Liaisons

P. Ann Hoppe, *Food and Drug Administration*

Lt. Col. Michael J. Ward, USAF, BSC,
MS, MT(ASCP)SBB
Department of Defense

Acknowledgments

The Technical Manual Committee extends special thanks to those volunteers who reviewed the manuscripts and made other contributions:

Frances K. Widmann, MD and the members of the AABB Standards Committee
Herbert Silver, MD and members of the Inspection and Accreditation Committee
Eugene Berkman, MD
Robin Biswas, MD
Joyce Blank, MT(ASCP)SBB
Joseph R. Bove, MD
Stephen Brzica, Jr., MD
Suzanne H. Butch, MT(ASCP)SBB
Frances E. Butler, RN, BSN, MBA
Marjana F. Callery, RN, MS, MT(ASCP)
Pamela Campbell-Knafl, MT(ASCP)
John Case, FIMLS
Jeanne Dahl, MT(ASCP)SBB
Geoffrey Daniels, BS, PhD
Victoria Davis
E. Nicole DeLong, MS, MT(ASCP)SBB
Mary Ann Denham, MBA, MT(ASCP)SBB
Dana V. Devine, PhD
R. Diane Earp, BS, MT(ASCP)SBB
Louise Eisenbrey, MT(ASCP)
Jay S. Epstein, MD
Martin Favero, PhD
Susan Frantz-Bohn
Jane Fry
George Garratty, PhD, FIMLS, FRCPath
Lani Gerber, RN

Margaret Hanson, MT(ASCP)SBB
Patricia Headley
Nancy Heddle
Nora V. Hirschler, MD
Paul Holland, MD
LCDR Jerry Holmberg, PhD, MT(ASCP)SBB
Michelle Horan, MT(ASCP)
Douglas Huestis, MD
Peter Issitt, PhD
Linda Issitt, MT(ASCP)SBB
Christina Kasprisin, MS, RN
John G. Kelton, FRCP(C)
William Kline, MS, MT(ASCP)SBB
Jerry Kolins, MD
Mary Kowalski, MT(ASCP)BB
Eileen Kreiner, MT(ASCP)
Margot Kruskall, MD
Sanford R. Kurtz, MD
William Leach, PhD
Betty Ann Leaman
Susan F. Leitman, MD
Elizabeth R. Malynn, RN
Paul McCurdy, MD
Locksley McGann, PhD
Jay E. Menitove, MD
Paul Mintz, MD
Mitchell Moheng, MT(ASCP)SBB
Gary Moroff, PhD
Marilyn Moulds, MT(ASCP)SBB
Sandra J. Nance, MS, MT(ASCP)SBB
Afzal Nikaein, PhD
Samuel Pepkowitz, MD
Sylvia Phillips, BSc
Mark A. Popovsky, MD
Harry E. Prince, PhD
Emily Reisner, PhD

Joseph G. Ridley
Stanley C. Roberts, SBB(ASCP)
Jenni Lee Robins
David Rohrkemper, MT(ASCP)
Ronald A. Sacher, MD
Concepcion Samia, MT(ASCP)SBB
S. Gerald Sandler, MD, FACP
Christine Santos, MT(ASCP)SBB
Patricia A. Sataro, RN, MS, CNA
Paul J. Schmidt, MD
Leslie E. Silberstein, MD
Arthur J. Silvergleid, MD
Marcus B. Simpson, Jr., MD
Susan South, MT(ASCP)SBB
Susan Steane, MS, MT(ASCP)SBB
Linda Stehling, MD
John F. Stone, MT(ASCP)
Ronald Strauss, MD
Pearl T.C.Y. Toy, MD
Pam Troyer, MSA, MT(ASCP)SBB
Marjory Stroup Walters, MT(ASCP)SBB
Martha A. Wells, MPH
Robert G. Wenk, MD, MF(HumGenet)
Susan Wilkinson, EdD, MT(ASCP)SBB
Kenneth R. Williamson, MD
Janet Wilson, MT(ASCP)SBB
Leonard Wilson
Chester Zmijewski, PhD

The Committee is grateful to Ruth Mougey, MT(ASCP)SBB, for preparing the index. Special thanks are due to Laurie Munk, Janet McGrath and Brenda George of the AABB National Office who provided invaluable editorial and administrative support to the Committee during preparation of this edition.

Introduction

In the 3 years that have elapsed since the last edition of the *Technical Manual*, there has been change, but more importantly, an adjustment to change. We are experiencing an enhanced awareness of our need to develop programs that will enable us to monitor performance in terms of the expectations of our users. These new programs in quality assessment and the application of continuous improvement should result in better patient care and increased safety for our patients and donors. Emphasis continues on more careful donor screening and better laboratory tests to detect disease markers in donor blood. Relevance and streamlining in red cell serology are increasingly evident as Laboratory Information Systems are becoming more widely used to store information, track components/bone/tissues and assist the user to meet the complex requirements that exist today in blood centers and hospital transfusion services.

Transfusion practice is dynamic and is being modified as new information and methods become available. This edition of the *Technical Manual*, the 11th, contains the same chapters found in the 10th edition. However, the material has been extensively updated and revised, and some sections have been rewritten. Any edition of the *Technical Manual* is a snapshot in time of this evolving theory and practice. The editors, contributors and reviewers have attempted to capture this snapshot, as reflected by the 15th edition of *Standards for Blood Banks and Transfusion Services* in the Spring of 1993.

The editors are especially grateful to all of the contributors and reviewers of this edition for their assistance. Their comments, suggestions and critiques have been most valuable and greatly appreciated. The review process has strengthened the value of this book.

Richard H. Walker, MD
Editor-in-Chief

Contents

Blood Groups

Application of Serologic Principles of Transfusion Practice

Clinical Considerations in Transfusion Practices

Other Considerations

Methods

Appendices   763

Index   775

Technical Manual

1

Blood Collection

Blood Donors

Blood centers and transfusion services depend on voluntary donors to provide the blood necessary to meet the needs of the patients they serve. To attract volunteer donors initially and to encourage their continued participation, it is essential that conditions surrounding blood donation be as pleasant, safe and convenient as possible.[1]

The donor area should be attractive, well-lighted, comfortably ventilated, clean and open at convenient hours for donors. Personnel should be friendly and understanding, as well as professional and well-trained. Whether blood is collected at the blood center or on mobile units, every effort should be made to make the donation a safe and pleasant experience.

Each blood bank must have a manual detailing its standard operating procedures (SOPs). The SOP manual should indicate actual practices and cover all phases of activity in the donor area. The procedures must meet the requirements of the AABB *Standards for Blood Banks and Transfusion Services*[2] for AABB accreditation. The manual should reflect local, state and federal regulations pertaining to blood bank operation. The SOP manual must be reviewed annually by the medical director of the blood bank, and should be available at all times to blood bank personnel.[2,3] The SOP manual should include descriptions of:

1. Criteria used to determine donor suitability.
2. Methods of performing tests to qualify donors (minimum and maximum acceptable values should be documented).
3. Solutions and methods used to prepare the phlebotomy site.
4. The method of relating the components collected to the donor.
5. Procedures for drawing blood including precautions taken to ensure that only an appropriate volume is removed.
6. Quality control procedures for supplies, reagents and equipment used in blood collection.[3]

Registration

The information obtained from the donor during registration must make it possible to identify and, if necessary, notify or recall that individual. Current information must be obtained and recorded for each donation; single-use or multiple-donation forms may be used. This record must be kept indefinitely.[2] The following information should be included:

1. Date of donation.
2. Name: Last, first and middle initial.
3. Address: Residence and/or business.
4. Telephone: Residence and/or business.
5. Sex.
6. Age and/or date of birth: Blood donors must be at least 17 years of age with the following exceptions:

a. Donors who are considered minors under applicable law may be accepted only if written consent to donate blood has been obtained in accordance with applicable law. Since these laws vary among jurisdictions, local legal opinion should be obtained and a copy of the state law should be readily available.

b. Elderly prospective donors may be accepted at the discretion of the blood bank physician. Many blood centers safely involve their senior citizen population in the donation process.[4] The decision to accept these donors may be made on a case-by-case basis or there may be general policy statements embodied in the SOP manual.

c. Autologous collection. There are no age limits for drawing blood for autologous use, although each donor-patient must be evaluated to determine if collecting blood will be safe.

7. A record of reasons for previous deferrals, if any.[2]

a. Persons who have been placed on indefinite deferral or surveillance must be identified before components are available for release and/or shipment. Blood may be collected from unsuitable donors (individuals with repeatably reactive tests for viral agents, needing specified testing for reentry, or with a medical history that would preclude donation); however, a system must be present to prevent the distribution of components from these donors.[5] Ideally, a donor deferral registry will be available to identify these donors prior to drawing blood. If such a registry is not available at a mobile or fixed site, a procedure shall be available to review prior donation records and/or deferral registries before labeling of the components.[6]

The following information may also be useful:

1. Additional identification such as social security or driver's license number, and/or other name used by the donor on a previous donation. This information may be necessary for information retrieval in some computerized systems and provides additional identifying information.

2. Name of patient or group to be credited, if a credit system is used. Even if the donor is deferred, a record of these donors may be useful to those concerned with donor recruitment or credit accounts.

3. Race. This information may be particularly useful when blood of a specific phenotype is needed for patients who have unexpected antibodies. Care should be taken to be sure that minority populations understand the medical importance and scientific applications of this information.[7,8]

4. Unique characteristics of the donor. Certain information about the donor may enable the blood bank to make optimal use of the donation. For example, blood from donors who are seronegative for cytomegalovirus (CMV), or who are group O, Rh−, is often designated for neonatal patients. The blood center may wish to specify that blood from these individuals be drawn routinely into special bags for pediatric transfusion. Individuals known to have circulating antibodies may be identified so that their blood can be processed into components that contain only minimal amounts of plasma.

5. A record of special communications to a donor, special drawing of blood samples for studies, etc may be useful.

6. If the donation is directed to a specific patient, information about when and where the intended recipient will be hospitalized, date of birth, social security number or other identifiers may be required by the transfusion service. If the donor is related to the intended recipient, the type of relationship should be noted. The AABB's National Blood Exchange has developed a protocol and form to be used when shipping autologous and directed donor units to another facility.

Information Provided to the Prospective Donor

All donors must be given educational materials informing them of the clinical signs and symptoms associated with HIV infection and AIDS, of high risk activities for HIV transmission, and of the importance of refraining from donating blood if they have engaged in these activities or experienced these signs or symptoms. A suitably qualified person should question prospective donors about risk behaviors and indicate whether satisfactory responses are received. The interviewer should evaluate all responses to decide suitability for donation, and document in the record the decision concerning donor suitability. This material should include a list of activities that increase the risk of exposure to the human immunodeficiency virus (HIV). A description of HIV-associated clinical signs and symptoms including the following should be provided[9]:

1. Unexplained weight loss.
2. Night sweats.
3. Blue or purple spots typical of Kaposi's sarcoma on or under the skin, or on mucous membranes.
4. Swollen lymph nodes lasting more than 1 month.
5. Persistent white spots or unusual blemishes in the mouth.

6. Temperature greater than 100.5 F for more than 10 days.
7. Persistent cough and shortness of breath.
8. Persistent diarrhea.

Information on the tests to be done on the donor's blood, the people who will be notified of abnormal results and the possible inclusion on a registry of ineligible donors should be provided. The possibility that testing may fail to identify an individual who might transmit disease because the donor is in an early stage of infection should be included in the information provided.[9] The same educational material can also be used to warn the prospective donor of possible reactions and provide suggestions for postphlebotomy care. It is very important that this information be presented in a way that the donor will read and understand it.[9,10] In some locations it may be necessary to have brochures in more than one language. It is also helpful to provide more extensive information for first-time donors. Information as to alternative sites and or mechanisms to obtain HIV antibody tests should be available to all prospective donors.

Donor Selection

The suitability of donors must be determined by a qualified physician or persons under his/her direction.[2,11]

Donor selection is based on a limited physical examination and a medical history done on the day of donation to determine whether giving blood will harm the donor or if transfusion of the unit will harm the recipient.[2,11,12] Careful donor selection contributes vitally to the safety of both donor and recipient.

Volunteer donors come to the collection site because they want to give blood. Deferring or rejecting potential donors often leaves those persons with negative feelings about themselves as well as the system. Donor deferral rates should be closely monitored by the blood bank physician to ensure they are within a reasonable range.[13] Donors who are deferred should be given a full explanation and be informed whether and when they can return.[14]

The medical history questions may be asked by a qualified interviewer or donors may complete their own record, which must then be reviewed with the donor and initialed by a trained, knowledgeable individual responsible to the blood bank.

The interview and physical examination should be performed in a manner that ensures adequate auditory and visual privacy, allays apprehensions and allows time for any necessary discussion or explanation. Answers to questions must be recorded "yes" or "no" with details explaining "yes" answers inscribed as indicated. Results of all tests must be recorded.

Medical History

During the medical history, some very specific questions will be necessary to ensure, to the extent possible, that it is safe for the donor to donate and for the blood to be transfused. To be sure that all the appropriate questions are asked and that donors are given a consistent message, use of a uniform donor medical history questionnaire has been suggested.[15] (See Appendix 1-1.) A great deal of pertinent information can be obtained by using some general or leading questions that are phrased in simple language that the donor can understand. The examples given below include all current requirements and are followed by suggested or required responses to information received.

Questions To Protect the Donor

1. *Blood donation: Have you ever donated blood, platelets or plasma?*

Have you donated blood or plasma in the last 8 weeks?

Donors should not be bled of >525 mL of whole blood, including samples for testing, within an 8-week period. In unusual circumstances more frequent donation is permissible. These donors must have the written permission of the blood bank physician after examination. At least 48 hours must elapse before whole blood donation in an individual who has undergone hemapheresis. At the request of the recipient's physician and with the approval of the blood bank physician, consenting individuals may donate more frequently if they are in a program to provide components from a single donor for a specific recipient.[2] Except for donation interval, these donors must meet all the usual criteria for allogeneic donors.

2. *Deferral as a donor: Have you ever been deferred as a blood donor, told not to donate blood or notified of an abnormal result after donation? When? Why?*

Information regarding prior donations and deferrals should be considered when evaluating current eligibility.

3. *Surgical procedures or major illnesses: Have you had surgery or a major illness in the last 12 months? When? What type? Are you under the care of a doctor for any reason? Why?*

Donors who have undergone operations should be deferred for at least 12 months if they received blood components or derivatives known to transmit disease. Uncomplicated surgery is disqualifying only until healing is complete and full activity has been resumed. Questionable answers that might indicate the donor is not in good health should be referred to the blood bank physician for further evaluation.

4. *Heart, lung and liver diseases: Have you ever had heart disease? When? What type? Do you ever suffer from chest pain? Shortness of breath? Explain. Have you had any serious lung disease? Explain. Have you had any type of liver disease? Explain.*

A history of coronary heart disease or rheumatic heart disease with known residual damage is cause for deferral unless evaluated and approved by the blood bank physician. A single episode of rheumatic fever or pericarditis, a heart murmur or successful repair of a congenital defect does not necessarily disqualify a donor.

Active pulmonary tuberculosis, or any active pulmonary disease, is cause for deferral. Previous tuberculosis, successfully treated and no longer active, need not disqualify a donor. Donors with a history of a reactive tuberculin skin test may be accepted.

An active inflammatory or chronic disease of the liver or one that might impair organ function is cause for deferral of the donor. Chronic conditions must be evaluated by a physician.

5. *Drugs and medications: Are you taking any drugs or medications? Why? What?*

In general, medications taken by a donor are not harmful to the recipient. Most donors taking medications, even prescription medications, are acceptable blood donors.

Deferral for most drugs is based on the nature of the disease process, not for properties of the drug itself. This is true of most donors requiring antibiotics, anticonvulsants, anticoagulants, digitalis, insulin, systemic corticosteroids, vasodilators and antiarrhythmic or anti-inflam-

matory drugs. Isotretinoin (Accutane®), a drug used to treat acne, disqualifies a donor for 30 days, as it may be a teratogen. Etretinate (Tegison®), a drug used to treat psoriasis, may be present in the blood for up to 3 years after its last use.[5]

Use of drugs and medication should be evaluated by the blood bank physician. Listed below are some drugs and medical conditions that are often permitted in blood donors, at the discretion of the individual facility's medical director.[16,17] The approval to draw these donors may be: 1) a general approval included in the facility SOP manual or 2) an approval given individually as each problem arises, providing verbal approval is documented on the donor's record.

a. Tetracyclines and other antibiotics for acne.

b. Topical steroid preparations for skin lesions not at the venipuncture site.

c. Blood pressure medications, taken chronically and successfully so that pressure is at or below allowable limits. The prospective donor taking antihypertensives should be free from side effects of the drug, especially episodes of postural hypotension, and should be free of any cardiovascular symptoms.

d. Isoniazid given because the tuberculin skin test has converted but without evidence of active tuberculosis.

e. Over-the-counter bronchodilators and decongestants.

f. Oral hypoglycemic agents in well-controlled diabetics without any vascular complications of the disease.

g. Tranquilizers, under most conditions. A physician should evaluate the donor to distinguish between tranquilizers and antipsychotic medications.

h. Hypnotics used at bedtime.

i. Marijuana (unless currently under the influence), oral contraceptives, mild analgesics, vitamins, replacement hormones or weight reduction pills.

j. Aspirin or aspirin-containing compounds depress platelet function for 1-5 days. Platelets from a donor who has taken these drugs within 3 days should not be the only source of platelets for a patient.

6. *Unexplained weight loss: Have you lost weight recently? How much? Why?*

Unexplained excessive weight loss, defined as 10 pounds (4.5 kg) or more, could indicate an undiagnosed serious illness including AIDS, and should be investigated further and evaluated by a physician.

7. *Cancer: Have you ever had cancer? What type? Have you ever had any form of blood disease? What type?*

Prospective donors who have had cancer, other than localized skin cancer, or carcinoma-in-situ of the cervix should be evaluated by a qualified physician before being accepted as a blood donor. Individuals who have definitive therapy and are free of disease for at least 5 years may be acceptable donors. Donors who have or have had leukemia or lymphoma must be permanently deferred. If the donor has another blood disease, it should be evaluated by the blood bank physician.

8. *Abnormal bleeding tendencies: Do you bleed a long time when you have a cut or a tooth pulled? After surgery? After childbirth?*

An abnormal bleeding tendency may be cause for deferral subject to evaluation by the blood bank physician. Individuals with such a history may experience excessive bleeding at the site of venipuncture and require special care following donation. Plasma from a donor deficient in coagulation factors would not confer expected therapeutic benefits if given to a recipient who needed these factors.

9. *Pregnancy: Are you pregnant? Have you been pregnant during the last 6 weeks?*

Defer during pregnancy and for 6 weeks following conclusion of pregnancy. Exception may be made by the blood bank physician if the woman's blood is intended for transfusion of her infant. Pregnancy is not an absolute contraindication for autologous collection (see Chapter 20).

10. *General health: Do you feel well now? Do you have other health problems?*

The donor should appear to be in good health. Pain, persistent cough, sore throat, cold or influenza symptoms, headache, nausea, dizziness or extreme nervousness may be cause for deferral.

Questions To Protect the Recipient

1. *Hepatitis: Have you ever had hepatitis or yellow jaundice? Have you had a reactive test for hepatitis (HBsAg)? Have you had intimate contact with a person with hepatitis? When? Have you received injections of hepatitis B immune globulin (HBIG)? When? Have you been transfused with blood or blood components? When? Have you had a tattoo? When? Have you ever injected drugs?*

Donors should be questioned about ear piercing, skin piercing, electrolysis and acupuncture to make sure that single-use equipment, disposable or properly sterilized needles were used.[2,5,18] Health-care workers should be carefully evaluated to determine if they have had needlestick injuries or exposure to blood from an unknown source and/or patients suspected to have had hepatitis during the past 12 months.

The presence of hepatitis virus cannot be detected with certainty by any presently available means including history, physical examination or laboratory tests, including those for HBsAg, anti-HCV and anti-HBc; therefore, strict regulations for donor acceptability must be established and followed (see also Chapter 4). Defer indefinitely prospective donors who:

a. Have a history of viral hepatitis after their 11th birthday. (Note: In 21 *CFR* 640.3(c)(1) and 640.63(c)(11) no age is specified in the requirement to reject donors with a history of hepatitis; however, the FDA's Center for Biologics Evaluation and Research has issued a memorandum indicating that individuals with a history of viral hepatitis prior to age 11 are acceptable as donors of Whole Blood and Source Plasma.[19]) Liver inflammation associated with well-documented infectious mononucleosis, CMV infection or use of a therapeutic drug is not a cause for permanent deferral.

b. Have a history of hepatitis B or a confirmed positive test for HBsAg or who have had a repeatedly reactive test for anti-HBc on more than one occasion.

c. Have present or past clinical or laboratory evidence of infection with hepatitis C, HTLV-I/II or HIV viruses.

d. Have a high (more than twice the highest acceptable value) alanine aminotransferase (ALT) level on one occasion or ALT levels above the highest acceptable values for blood release on more than one occasion.

e. Have used intravenous drugs. Check both arms for evidence of needle use.

f. Have donated the only unit of blood or blood component transfused to a patient who developed clinical or laboratory evidence of transfusion-associated hepatitis or infection with HIV or HTLV-I/II, and who received no other blood component or derivative known to transmit these infections and had no other probable cause of infection.

g. Whose involvement in two or more transfusion-associated hepatitis cases results in a cumulative probability value greater than 0.4 (see Chapter 4).[20,21]

Defer for at least 12 months:

a. Recipients of blood, blood components or clotting factor concentrate. This includes donors who are in blood immunization programs. Receipt of other FDA-licensed plasma derivatives such as albumin (human) or immunoglobulins does not specifically require a deferral.

b. Recipients of a skin allograft or tattoo. Persons undergoing ear piercing, skin piercing, depilation or acupuncture where the sterility of the equipment used cannot be verified.[2,5,18]

c. Donors who share living quarters or are a sexual partner of a person with viral hepatitis or AIDS.

The type of contact that hospital personnel and physicians encounter in their work is not always considered close contact and may not be cause for deferral. Personnel with blood and body fluid contact have high potential exposure to patients at risk of HBsAg and/or

HIV positivity.[22] Donors with unprotected or accidental exposure to blood and body fluids in a healthcare setting or other job should be deferred.[9] Percutaneous exposures (ie, needlesticks or mucous membrane splashes of potentially infectious materials) should result in donor deferral. Note: feces, nasal secretions, sputum, sweat, tears, urine or vomitus are not known to be infectious for HIV or HBV unless visibly contaminated with blood.[23] The medical director of the blood drawing facility should establish a policy for such potential donors.

d. Inmates of penal or mental institutions, since the likelihood of exposure to transfusion-transmissible agents is very high among such individuals.

e. Prospective donors who have received HBIG, since this is given only to individuals with especially close contact with hepatitis B. HBIG may prolong the incubation period of hepatitis B beyond the usual 6-month period.

2. *Malaria: Have you ever had malaria? When? Have you been out of the US in the past 3 years? When? Where? Have you taken any medication to prevent malaria?*

Travelers who have been in areas considered endemic for malaria by the Malaria Program, Centers for Disease Control and Prevention (CDC), US Department of Health and Human Services, may be accepted as regular blood donors 6 months after return to the nonendemic area, providing they have been free of unexplained febrile illnesses and have not taken antimalarial drugs. The CDC's "Health Information for International Travel" [HHS Publication No. (CDC) 92-8280] should be available to the interviewing personnel to determine which areas are considered endemic.[5] (See p 768.) Periodic updates can be purchased from the Superintendent of Documents, US Government Printing Office, PO Box 371954, Pittsburgh, PA 15250-7954, (202) 783-3238. Prospective donors (travelers, immigrants, refugees, citizens or residents) following a visit to or coming from an endemic area who have had malaria or taken antimalarial prophylaxis must be deferred for 3 years after cessation of therapy, or after departure from the malarial area, if they have been asymptomatic in the interim. Donations to be used for the preparation of plasma, plasma components or fractions devoid of intact red blood cells are exempt from these restrictions.

It is helpful to have a recent world map available to personnel interviewing donors to locate areas where travelers or immigrants have been.

3. *Babesiosis or Chagas' disease[2,24]: Have you ever been bitten by a tick? When? Where? Have you ever visited or lived in rural parts of Latin America? When? Where?*

More detailed follow-up questions as to the exact circumstances of possible exposure to these diseases may be necessary. Donors with a history of disease caused by either *Babesia* species or *Trypanosoma cruzi* must be indefinitely deferred. Persons who originate from endemic areas such as rural parts of Latin America may have chronic Chagas' disease without evidence of an acute episode in the past.

4. *Acquired immune deficiency syndrome (AIDS)[2,9]: Have you ever had night sweats, unexplained fevers, unexpected weight loss, persistent diarrhea, generalized lymph node enlargement or unusual skin le-*

sions, especially purple bumps under the skin that seem to spread locally or to be present in widely separated areas? Have you had intimate or sexual contact with an individual at increased risk for AIDS?

Donors must be given educational material informing them of high risk activities for AIDS and the necessity of refraining from donating blood if at risk. Direct oral or written questioning in a setting that affords privacy must be done on each donation. Questions and subsequent deferral should be based on the following criteria:

a. Persons with clinical or laboratory evidence of HIV infection.

b. Men who have had sex with another man even one time since 1977.

c. Past or present IV drug users.

d. Persons with hemophilia or related clotting factor disorders who have received clotting factor concentrates.

e. Men and women who have engaged in sex for money or drugs since 1977.

f. Persons who have had sex with any person meeting the above descriptions (items a through e) during the preceding 12 months.

g. Persons with a history of or treatment for syphilis or gonorrhea in the preceding 12 months. The deferral should be from the date of cessation of treatment for either of these sexually transmitted diseases. Slang terms for these diseases used by the local population should be included in the questioning.[25] Donors responding positively to this question may have risk behaviors that make it more likely they could be exposed to hepatitis or AIDS viruses.

h. Transfusion of blood and components or clotting factor concentrate in the past 12 months.

i. Contact with blood and or body fluids (also see section above on hepatitis deferrals) through percutaneous inoculation or an open wound during the past 12 months.

j. Persons who volunteer they have been a victim of rape in the past 12 months.

If possible, direct questions designed to elicit information about items a through h above should be presented orally to each prospective donor. An FDA-sponsored field trial found that providing an illustrated answer sheet for use by the donor was an effective way to obtain information during the interview process. It is not necessary for the donor record to include the answer to each of the direct questions about risk behavior; however, deferral based on risk behavior history should be documented.

Prior to the requirement for routine testing of blood for anti-HIV-2 (June 1, 1992), donors emigrating from countries where heterosexual activity is thought to play a major role in the transmission of HIV-2 infection were deferred based on geographic origin.[9]

Donors should be informed that there is a time early after exposure to HIV during which the test for antibodies, done on all donations, may not detect infection. Information should be provided about donor deferral registries maintained for individuals with repeatedly reactive tests for anti-HIV-1 or anti-HIV-2. Persons who are not suitable as donors but desire to learn their antibody status should be given instructions about alternate mechanisms to obtain testing. All donors must be asked if they have read and understood the educational material informing potential donors that persons at increased risk of AIDS should refrain from donating blood. Donors must also sign a consent equivalent in meaning to the following:

"I have reviewed and understand the information provided to me regarding the spread of AIDS virus (HIV) by blood and plasma. If I am potentially at risk for spreading the virus known to cause AIDS, I agree not to donate blood or plasma for transfusion to another person or for further manufacture. I understand that my blood will be tested for antibodies to HIV and other disease markers. If this testing indicates that I should no longer donate blood or plasma because of a risk of transmitting the AIDS virus, my name will be entered on a list of permanently deferred donors. I understand that I will be notified of a positive result. If, instead, the result of the testing is not clearly negative or positive, my blood will not be used and my name may be placed on a deferral list without my being informed, until the results are further clarified."[9]

All donors, including autologous donors whose blood might be used for others, should be given the opportunity to indicate confidentially whether their unit of blood *is* or *is not* suitable for transfusion. Confidential unit exclusion (CUE) can be accomplished by having a detachable "ballot" as part of the educational material given the donor. At the time of drawing the phlebotomist can attach a bar-coded number to the ballot and ask the donor to mark the appropriate response. The "ballots" can then be deposited in a box when the donor leaves the donor room. Another method is to provide the donor with a sheet having a bar-coded *yes* or

no sticker. Each donor is asked to choose the desired sticker and place it on the blood bag or donor card. If the bar-coded response is placed directly on the unit (an ideal location is the area to be covered by the ABO group label) the whole blood unit can then be scanned and discarded if need be before any further processing is carried out. A procedure must be developed to ensure that no unit of blood or components is released unless an "*OK to use*" is obtained. All units lacking a ballot or marked "*do not use for transfusion*" must be discarded.

If an opportunity is provided to the donor to indicate that blood collected should not be used for transfusion, the donor should be assured that the blood will be subjected to testing, that there will be notification of any positive results and that counseling or referral will be provided for positive HIV antibody results. If such an opportunity for CUE is provided, it may be either in a private interview with a suitably trained person, or in a manner that provides strict confidentiality of the decision and privacy in which to make it.

Since CUE procedures do not preclude donation, an alternate method to augment self-exclusion may be used. A private interview conducted by a trained and competent healthcare professional may include orally presenting the option for self-exclusion along with other AIDS-related educational material. This early assessment of donor suitability may lead to deferral before a procedure such as apheresis is started.[9]

5. *Injections with human pituitary-derived growth hormone (pit-hGH): Have you ever been injected with growth hormone?*

Note: From 1958-1986 pit-hGH was used to treat children of short stature and was taken by some individuals during rigorous physical training. Several cases of Creutzfeldt-Jakob disease (CJD) have been found in persons given pit-hGH.[26] Since the virus causing this disease might be transmissible by transfusion, donors who have received pit-hGH must be permanently deferred. Deferral is not necessary if the donor has only been given recombinant growth hormone.

6. *Vaccinations, inoculations: Have you been vaccinated or had any shots in the past 12 months? What? When?*

   a. Symptom-free donors who recently have been immunized with toxoids or killed vaccines need not be deferred. Included in this group of immunizations are those for anthrax, cholera, diphtheria, influenza, paratyphoid, pertussis, plague, polio (injection, Salk), Rocky Mountain spotted fever, tetanus, typhoid and typhus.

   b. Measles (rubeola), mumps, yellow fever, oral polio vaccine (Sabin): Donors are acceptable 2 weeks after their last immunization.

   c. German measles (rubella): Donors are acceptable 4 weeks after their last injection.

   d. Rabies: No deferral is needed unless vaccination is given following an animal bite; then defer for 1 year.

   e. Hepatitis B vaccine: Prospective donors are acceptable provided they would not otherwise be disqualified.

   f. Immune serum globulin: Deferral not necessary if otherwise acceptable. Note: HBIG—1 year deferral (see p 83). If donor has been given IVIG, defer based on underlying condition.

7. *Dental procedures: Have you had any recent dental work?*
   Routine dental exams, filling of cavities and cleaning usually do not require deferral of the donor. If more extensive work such as a root canal or an extraction has been done, deferral for at least 72 hours should be considered because of the possibility of a bacteremia associated with the procedure.[5]

Physical Examination

Exceptions to the following guidelines must be evaluated individually by the blood bank physician.

1. General appearance: If the donor looks ill, appears to be under the influence of drugs or alcohol, or is excessively nervous, it is best to defer. This should, if possible, be done in a way that does not antagonize the donor and, if appropriate, encourages donation at a future time.

2. Weight: Donors weighing 50 kg (110 lb) or more may ordinarily give 525 mL (450 ± 45 mL of blood as well as up to 30 mL for processing tubes). For donors weighing less than 50 kg (110 lb), as little as 300 mL may be drawn *without reducing the amount of anticoagulant in the primary bag.* Units with 300-405 mL must be labeled as "Low Volume Unit: _____ mL." These units should only be used as RBCs. If it is necessary to draw less than 300 mL, the amount of anticoagulant must be reduced proportionally by expressing the excess into an integrally attached satellite bag and sealing the tubing. The volume of blood drawn must be measured carefully and accurately. To determine the amount of anticoagulant to remove, the following formula may be used:
   Calculation for drawing donors weighing less than 50 kg (110 lb):

a. Volume of blood to draw (approximately 12% of blood volume) = (Donor's weight in kg/50) × 450 mL

b. Amount of anticoagulant (CPD or CPDA-1) needed = (a./100) × 14

c. Amount of anticoagulant to remove from a 450 mL bag = 63 − (b.)

3. Temperature: The oral temperature must not exceed 37.5 C (99.5 F). Lower than normal temperatures are usually of no significance in healthy individuals. Caution: If a glass thermometer is used, it should not be in the donor's mouth during puncture to obtain blood for hematocrit or hemoglobin determination. The use of thermometer covers is advised.

4. Pulse: The pulse should be counted for at least 15 seconds. It should ordinarily exhibit no pathologic irregularity, and should be between 50 and 100 beats per minute. If a prospective donor is an athlete with high exercise tolerance, a lower pulse rate may be acceptable. A blood bank physician should evaluate marked abnormalities of pulse and recommend acceptance, deferral or referral for additional evaluation.

5. Blood pressure: The blood pressure should be no higher than 180 mm Hg systolic and 100 mm Hg diastolic. Prospective donors whose blood pressure is above these values should not be drawn without individual evaluation by a qualified physician. (Note: The FDA suggests upper and lower limits be defined in the SOPs.[5])

6. Hemoglobin or packed cell volume (hematocrit): Prior to donation the hemoglobin or packed cell volume must be determined from a sample of blood obtained by fingerstick, earlobe puncture or venipuncture. This screening test is designed to prevent taking blood from a donor with anemia; however, it does not ensure that the donor has an adequate store of iron.[27,28] The lower limits for accepting an allogeneic or autologous donor are shown for various commonly used methods in Table 1-1. Individuals with hemoglobin >175 g/L (17.5 g/dL) or hematocrit >0.52 (52%) may need to be evaluated by a physician.[29] Screening methods include specific gravity determined by copper sulfate (see Method 10.1), spectrophotometric measurement of hemoglobin and determination of the hematocrit (packed cell volume).

7. Skin lesions: The skin at the site of venipuncture must be free of lesions. Both arms must be examined for signs

Table 1-1. Minimum Levels of Hemoglobin (Hb) and Hematocrit (Hct) for Accepting a Blood Donor

Type of Donor	Test Method	Acceptable Value
Allogeneic	Hb	125 g/L (12.5 g/dL)
	Hct	0.38 (38%)
	Copper sulfate	1.053 (sp gr)
Autologous	Hb	110 g/L (11 g/dL)
	Hct	0.33 (33%)
	Copper sulfate	1.049 (sp gr)

of intravenous drug abuse, especially multiple needle puncture marks and/or sclerotic veins. Stigmata of parenteral drug use and/or alcohol intoxication are reasons to exclude a prospective donor. Mild skin disorders such as acne (unless under treatment with Accutane®), psoriasis (unless treated with Tegison®) or the rash of poison ivy should not be cause for deferral unless unusually extensive and/or present in the antecubital area. Donors with boils, purulent wounds or severe skin infections anywhere on the body should be deferred, as should anyone with purplish-red or hemorrhagic nodules or indurated plaques suggestive of Kaposi's sarcoma (see above).

The record of physical examination and medical history must be identified with the examiner by initials or signature. Any reasons for deferral must be recorded and explained to the donor. A mechanism should exist to notify the donor of clinically significant abnormal findings in the physical examination, medical history or postdonation laboratory testing (especially a positive test for HBsAg or anti-HIV). Predonation abnormalities may be explained verbally by qualified personnel. Abnormalities found in testing of the sample from the donor that preclude further donation may be reported by telephone or letter.

Prior to obtaining consent for donation, donors should be informed of the testing to be done on their blood and to whom abnormal results will be reported. Donors who are accepted should be made aware that recipients are at risk of being infected by a transfusion and that donor blood can test negative early in infection with some viruses; they should be asked to report any illness developing within a few days of donation and especially to report hepatitis, a positive HIV test or AIDS that develops within 12 months.

Written informed consent that allows blood center personnel to take and use blood from the prospective donor is required. The consent form is part of the donor record, to be completed prior to donation. The procedure must be explained in terms the donors can understand, and they must have an opportunity to ask questions and to indicate their decision to give consent by signing the form. The signed donor card or consent should also indicate that the donor has read and understood the information about infectious diseases transmissible by transfusion and has given accurate and truthful answers to the medical history questions. (See p 28 for the recommended language on a donor release form.)

Special Donor Categories

Exceptions to the usual requirements may be made for special donor categories:
1. Therapeutic bleeding: This term is used when phlebotomy is done as treatment for a medical indication. The records must include the request of the patient's physician and specify the amount of blood to be drawn, the frequency of bleeding and/or a hemoglobin or hematocrit level at which the patient should be bled. The record may be a written request or documentation by blood bank personnel of a telephoned request. The blood bank physician must decide whether to accept responsibility for having these patients bled in the donor area. If the patient is clinically unstable, phle-

botomy should be performed in a hospital setting.

If the patient's blood is unsuitable for allogeneic transfusion, it must be labeled "Not for Transfusion" and either discarded or used for research purposes. If the unit is suitable for allogeneic transfusion, as determined by the blood bank physician, it may be transfused after the usual processing, provided that the label indicates a therapeutic bleeding and specifies the donor's disease. The recipient's physician must agree to use the blood for transfusion and a record must be made of this agreement.

2. Autologous donors: The indications and variations from usual procedures for autologous collection are discussed in Chapter 20.
3. Hemapheresis: Special requirements and recommendations for cytapheresis donors or for donors in a plasmapheresis program are detailed in Chapter 2.
4. Recipient-specific designated donations: There are certain situations in which it may be appropriate for blood collection facilities to draw, process and store allogeneic blood intended for a specific recipient. One such situation is for the patient anticipating a kidney transplant from a living (usually related) donor. For these patients, protocols have been developed[30] whereby the intended recipient is transfused prior to transplantation with blood from the intended donor. Donor-specific transfusions (DSTs) have been shown to improve graft survival, especially when lymphocytotoxicity testing performed after transfusion but before transplantation reveals absence of antibody formation.[31] Medically designated donors (from a rare donor file or family members) may be required when a patient has an antibody to a high-incidence antigen or a combination of antibodies

that makes it difficult to find compatible blood from random donors. The mother selected to provide platelets for her newborn with neonatal thrombocytopenia or a family member used as a source of cytapheresis components are other examples of designated donors.

AABB *Standards* allows for use of a single donor to supply components needed for a single patient provided this is requested by the patient's physician and approved by the blood bank physician. The donor must meet all the usual requirements for donation, except that the frequency of donation can be as often as every 3 days as long as the predonation hemoglobin level is above the minimum value for normal donors.

In this situation, as in programs of autologous transfusion, collected blood must be processed according to AABB *Standards*. Special tags identifying the donor and the intended recipient must be affixed to the blood or component bag, and all such units must be segregated from the normal inventory. A protocol for the handling of such units must be developed and made a part of the SOP manual.

5. Directed donors: The public's fear about AIDS and the safety of transfusion has led to demands from potential blood component recipients that they be allowed to choose the donors to be used for their transfusions. In several states, laws have been passed establishing this as a procedure that must be followed in nonemergency situations if requested by a potential blood recipient or blood donor. There are several logistical and philosophical problems associated with directed donations. However, most blood centers and hospitals provide this ser-

vice. The selection and testing of directed donors must be the same as for other allogeneic donors. To avoid problems it is important that procedures be established covering the time interval required between drawing the donor and availability to the recipient, whether donors will be pregrouped, and when and if units can be released for other patients.[32]

Collection of Blood

Blood is to be collected only by trained personnel working under the direction of a qualified, licensed physician. Blood collection must be by aseptic methods, using a sterile, closed system. The phlebotomist may wear gloves during the procedure.[22,23] If more than one skin puncture is needed, a new container and donor set must be used for each additional venipuncture. If an FDA-approved sterile connection device is used to connect a new needle to the container before phlebotomy, shelf life of the component is limited to 24 hours.[2] The phlebotomist must sign or initial the donor record, whether or not the phlebotomy resulted in collection of a full unit.

Materials and Instruments

Many items used for phlebotomy are available in sterile, single-use, disposable form. If these leak or the paper envelope becomes wet, the contents must not be used. Items such as gauze, cotton balls, applicators, forceps and forceps holders may be adequately sterilized by steam under pressure for at least 30 minutes at 121.5 C, by dry heat for at least 2 hours at 170 C or by gas sterilization. Containers of bulk-sterilized items should be labeled and dated as to when they were sterilized and when opened. Transfer forceps should have at least the lower third immersed in an effective antiseptic solution (eg, 70% alcohol) and should be resterilized after 1

week. Unopened sterilized containers may be stored for 2-3 weeks if the container closure ensures sterility of the contents. Open containers may be used for 1 week if the lids are replaced after removal of contents and contents are removed with aseptic technique.

Blood Containers

Blood must be collected into an FDA-approved container that is pyrogen-free, sterile and contains sufficient anticoagulant for the quantity of blood to be collected. The container label must state the kind and amount of anticoagulant, and the approximate amount of blood collected.

Blood bags may be supplied in containers holding more than one bag. The manufacturer's directions should be followed for the length of time unused bags may be stored in containers that have been opened and resealed.

Identification

Identification is important in each step from donor to final disposition. A numeric or alphanumeric system must be used to identify and relate the donor record, the processing tubes and the containers to the donor. Extreme caution is necessary to avoid any mix-up or duplication of numbers. All cards and labels should be checked for printing errors. Duplicate numbers must be discarded. It is good practice to record voided numbers.

Before starting the phlebotomy:
1. Identify donor record, at least by name, with the donor.
2. Attach identically numbered labels to donor record, blood collection container and attached satellite bags and test tubes for donor blood samples. Attaching the numbers at the donor chair, rather than during the examination procedures, helps reduce the likelihood of identification errors.

3. Be sure that the processing tubes are correctly numbered and that they accompany the container during the collection of blood. These may be attached in any convenient manner to the primary bag or integral tubing.
4. Recheck all numbers.

Preparing Venipuncture Site

Blood should be drawn from a large, firm vein in an area (usually the antecubital space) that is free of skin lesions. It is often helpful to inspect both arms and, to make the veins more prominent, to use either a tourniquet or a blood pressure cuff inflated to 40-60 mm Hg. Having the donor open and close the hand a few times is also helpful. Once the vein is selected, the pressure cuff should be released before the skin site is prepared.

There is no way to prepare a completely aseptic site for venipuncture, but surgical cleanliness can be achieved to provide maximal assurance of a sterile unit. Several acceptable procedures exist. (See Method 10.2.)

After the skin has been prepared, it must not be touched again. Do not re-palpate the vein. If this is done the entire preparation of the site must be repeated.

For the infrequent donor who may be sensitive to the iodine commonly used in venipuncture site preparation, another method, such as green soap scrub followed by acetone-alcohol, should be designated by the blood bank physician.[33]

Phlebotomy and Collection of Samples

A technique for the drawing of a donor unit and the collection of samples appears in Method 10.3. The donor unit should be collected by a single venipuncture. During collection the blood should be mixed with the anticoagulant. The amount of blood collected should be carefully monitored so as not to exceed 525 mL including samples. When the appropriate amount has been collected, pilot tubes and segments must be filled, and the needle and any blood-contaminated waste disposed of safely. A check should be made to ensure that the identification of the unit, the donor history and the tubes are the same.

Gloves must be available for use during phlebotomy and must be worn if the phlebotomist has cuts, scratches or other breaks in the skin.[22,23] Gloves must also be worn by individuals who are in training as phlebotomists and are required when collecting blood from an autologous or uncooperative individual. At the completion of the collection, the needle must not be recapped and must be disposed of in a puncture-proof container.

Care of the Donor After Phlebotomy

1. Check arm and apply bandage after bleeding stops.
2. Have donor remain reclining on bed or in donor chair for a few minutes under close observation by staff.
3. Allow donor to sit up when his/her condition appears satisfactory. Someone should monitor the donor as the donor assumes an upright position and walks to an observation area. The period of observation and provision of refreshment should be designated in the SOP manual.
4. Give donor instructions about postphlebotomy care. The medical director may wish to include some of the following suggestions:
   a. Eat and drink something before leaving.
   b. Do not leave until released by staff member.
   c. Drink more fluids than usual in next 4 hours.

d. It is probably better not to have any alcohol until you have eaten.
e. Do not smoke for a half-hour.
f. If there is bleeding from the phlebotomy site, raise arm and apply pressure.
g. If you feel faint or dizzy, either lie down or sit down with your head between your knees.
h. If any symptoms persist, either call or return to blood bank or see a doctor.
i. You may resume all normal activities after about a half-hour if you feel well. Donors who work in certain occupations (ie, construction workers, operators of machinery) or persons working at heights should be cautioned of possible dangers if they return to work immediately after giving blood.
j. Remove bandage after a few hours.
k. Your blood volume rapidly returns to the normal level, usually 4000-5500 mL or 8-11 pints, depending on size and weight. With adequate fluid intake, complete blood volume restoration should take less than 72 hours.

5. Thank the donor for an important contribution, encourage repeat donation after proper interval (56 days) and offer refreshments to the donor. The personnel on duty throughout the donor area should be friendly and qualified to observe for signs of impending reaction such as lack of concentration, pallor, rapid breathing or excessive perspiration. They should be competent to interpret instructions and answer questions, and to accept responsibility for releasing the donor in good condition.

6. Note on the donor record any adverse reactions that occurred and, if the donor leaves the area before being released, note this on the record.

Adverse Donor Reactions

Most donors tolerate giving blood very well, but occasionally adverse reactions may occur.[34] Personnel must be trained to recognize reactions and to provide initial treatment. In many blood banks, donor room personnel are required to have training in cardiopulmonary resuscitation (CPR).

Syncope (fainting or vasovagal syndrome) may be caused by the sight of blood, by watching others give blood, by individual or group excitement or for unexplained reasons. Whether caused by psychologic factors or by neurophysiologic response to blood donation, the symptoms may include weakness, sweating, dizziness, pallor, loss of consciousness, convulsions and involuntary passage of feces or urine. The skin feels cold and blood pressure falls. Sometimes the systolic levels are as low as 50 mm Hg or cannot be heard with the stethoscope. The pulse rate often slows significantly, occasionally a useful sign in distinguishing between vasovagal attack and severe cardiogenic or hypovolemic shock, in which pulse rates rise.[35] This distinction, although characteristic, is far from absolute. Deep breathing or hyperventilation may cause the anxious or excited donor to lose an excess of CO_2, resulting in alkalosis and hyperventilation tetany, characterized by spontaneous muscular contractions or spasm.

The blood bank physician must provide written instructions for handling donor reactions. This must include a procedure for obtaining emergency medical help.

1. General.
   a. Remove the tourniquet and withdraw the needle from the arm at the first sign of reaction during the phlebotomy.
   b. If possible, remove any donor who experiences an adverse reaction to

an area where he/she can be attended in privacy.

c. Call the blood bank physician or the physician designated for such purposes if the measures given below do not lead to rapid recovery.

2. Fainting.

a. Place the donor on his/her back and raise the feet above the level of the donor's head.

b. Loosen tight clothing.

c. Be sure the donor has an adequate airway.

d. Apply cold compresses to the donor's forehead or the back of the neck.

e. In some situations administering aromatic spirits of ammonia by inhalation may be useful. Test the ammonia on yourself before passing it under the donor's nose, as it may be too strong or too weak. Strong ammonia may injure the nasal membranes; weak ammonia is not effective. The donor should respond by coughing, which elevates the blood pressure.

f. Check and record the blood pressure, pulse and respiration periodically until the donor recovers. Note: Some donors who experience prolonged hypotension may respond to an infusion of normal saline. The decision to initiate such therapy should be made by the blood bank physician either on a case-by-case basis or in a policy stated in the facility SOP manual.

3. Nausea and vomiting.

a. Make the donor as comfortable as possible.

b. Instruct the donor who is nauseated to breathe slowly and deeply.

c. Apply cold compresses to the donor's forehead and/or back of neck.

d. Turn donor's head to the side.

e. Provide a suitable receptacle if the donor vomits, and have cleansing tissues or a damp towel ready. Be sure the donor's head is turned to the side because of the danger of aspiration.

f. Give the donor a paper cup of water to rinse out his/her mouth.

4. Twitching or muscular spasms. The most common cause of twitching or muscular spasms occurs with loss of consciousness. Almost one-half of unconscious donors have brief, weak, convulsion-like movements of one or more extremities. Extremely nervous donors may hyperventilate, causing faint muscular twitching or tetanic spasm of their hands or face. Donor room personnel should watch closely for these symptoms during the phlebotomy. Diverting the donor's attention by engaging in conversation can interrupt the hyperventilation pattern. However, if symptoms are apparent, having the donor rebreathe into a paper bag will usually bring prompt relief. **Do not give oxygen.**

5. True convulsions are rare.

a. Call someone to help you immediately. Prevent the donor from injuring him/herself. During severe seizures, some people exhibit great muscular power and are difficult to restrain. If possible, hold the donor on the chair or bed; if not possible, place the donor on the floor. Try to prevent injury to the donor and to yourself.

b. Be sure the donor has an adequate airway.

c. Notify the blood bank physician.

6. Hematoma.

a. Remove the tourniquet and the needle from the donor's arm.

b. Place three or four sterile gauze squares over the hematoma and apply firm digital pressure for 7-10 minutes with the donor's arm held above the heart level. An alternative procedure is to apply a tight bandage to occlude the venipuncture site.

c. Apply ice to the area for 5 minutes, if desired.

d. Should an arterial puncture be suspected, immediately withdraw needle and apply firm pressure for 10 minutes. Apply pressure dressing afterwards. Check for the presence of a radial pulse. If pulse is not palpable or is weak call blood bank physician.

7. Serious cardiac difficulties are exceedingly rare.

a. Call for medical aid and/or an emergency care unit immediately.

b. If the donor is in cardiac arrest, begin CPR immediately and continue until medical aid and/or an emergency care unit arrives.

The nature and treatment of all reactions should be recorded on the donor record or a special incident report form. This should include a notation as to whether or not the donor should be accepted for future donations.

The medical director should decide what supplies and drugs should be in the donor bleeding area, readily available to personnel. The distance to the nearest emergency room or emergency care unit heavily influences decisions about necessary supplies and drugs. Most blood banks maintain some or all of the following:

1. Emesis basin or equivalent.
2. Towels.
3. Sterile needles (both 20-gauge, 2-inch and 25-gauge, 3/4-inch).
4. Sterile hypodermic syringes, 1 or 2 mL.
5. Administration sets.
   a. Intravenous fluids.
   b. Blood.
6. Sodium chloride injection USP (normal saline).
7. Oropharyngeal airway, plastic or hard rubber.
8. Oxygen and mask.
9. Emergency drugs: Drugs are seldom required to treat a donor who has had a reaction. If the blood bank physician wishes to have any drugs available, the kind and amount to be kept on hand must be specified in writing. In addition, the medical director must provide written policies as to when and by whom any of the above may be used.

Processing Donor Blood

All reagents used for required tests must meet or exceed appropriate FDA regulations. All procedures must have been tested in parallel with reference methods and/or reagents.

Previous records of a donor's ABO and Rh group must not be used for labeling a unit of blood. Every unit intended for allogeneic use must undergo complete testing. The results of all tests must be recorded immediately after observation, and the interpretation recorded upon completion of testing. The record system must be such that any unit of blood and any component can be traced from its source to its disposition. All laboratory records pertaining to an individual unit must be retrievable, including investigations of reported adverse reactions. For a drawing facility, the source would be the donor; for a transfusion service it could be the donor or another blood provider. Disposition could be transfusion to a named patient; shipment to a named receiving facility; or discarding in a manner specified by the local SOP manual. Records of the source of blood and components and their final disposition should be retained indefinitely.[2]

Details of testing procedures, storage and shipping requirements and inspection criteria appear in subsequent chapters of this manual. The current edition of *Standards* should be consulted for requirements of preparation, testing and labeling. General considerations in processing donor blood are as follows:

1. Numbers on blood bag, processing tubes and donor record should be rechecked prior to processing.
2. ABO group must be determined by testing the red blood cells with anti-A and anti-B sera and by testing the serum or plasma with A_1 and B cells. Blood must not be released until any discrepancies are resolved. Accurate ABO testing and labeling assume even greater importance in areas where the conventional crossmatch is abbreviated or eliminated.
3. The Rh type must be determined with anti-D serum. Units found to be D− in direct agglutination tests shall be tested by a method designed to detect weak D (D^u). Units that are reactive by either test must be labeled Rh+. Routine testing for additional red cell antigens is not required.
4. Blood from donors with a history of prior transfusion or pregnancy should be tested for unexpected antibodies before the crossmatch, preferably at the time of processing. Most blood banks test all donor blood for unexpected antibodies, because of the difficulty determining donors' past histories and/or attempting to segregate those to be tested from those not to be tested.

    Methods for testing for unexpected antibodies must be those that will demonstrate clinically significant antibodies. Blood in which such antibodies are found should be processed into components that contain only minimal amounts of plasma. In processing donor blood, it is permissible to pool serum from several donors or to use pooled reagent red cells; pooled reagents must not be used in pretransfusion testing of patient blood samples.

5. All donor blood must be tested to detect units that might transmit disease (see Chapter 4). Currently required tests include HBsAg, anti-HIV-1, anti-HIV-2 (or a combination anti-HIV-1/2), anti-HTLV-I, anti-HCV, anti-HBc, ALT and a serologic test for syphilis (STS). The blood component or unit of whole blood must not be used for transfusion unless the tests are nonreactive, negative or in the normal range. In an emergency, blood may be transfused before all testing is complete, but this fact must appear conspicuously on a label or tag attached to the unit. If a test is subsequently found to be reactive, the recipient's physician must be notified.
6. Prior to issue each unit must be appropriately labeled. As a minimum each unit should include the proper name of the component; the unique donor number; the kind and amount of anticoagulant (except for components prepared by hemapheresis and frozen, deglycerolized, rejuvenated or washed red cells); the volume of the unit; the required storage temperature; the statement "Caution: Federal law prohibits dispensing without prescription"; the name and address of the collecting facility (the National Drug Center Labeler Code and FDA license number, if appropriate, should be shown); a reference to the *Circular of Information*; whether the donor is volunteer, autologous or paid; and the expiration date. Also required are statements indicating "this product may transmit infectious agents" and "properly identify intended recipient." Depending on the component, various test results such as ABO, Rh and antibody screening are required. Autologous units that are reactive for anti-HCV, anti-HIV-1 or -2, HBsAg, or have a positive STS require the use of biohazard la-

bels (see p 494). Uniform guidelines for labeling should be used.

The facility performing the compatibility testing must do confirmatory tests on a sample obtained from an originally attached segment of all units of WB or RBCs. This must include, for all units containing significant amounts of red cells, confirmation of ABO group on all units, and the Rh type of units labeled as Rh--. Confirmatory testing for weak D (D^u) is *not* required. Discrepancies must be reported to the collecting facility and must be resolved before issue of the blood for transfusion purposes. Routine repetition of other tests on donor units is not required or recommended.

7. A stoppered or sealed sample of each donor's blood must be stored in the transfusion service at 1-6 C for at least 7 days after transfusion. Many workers prefer storage for longer periods, up to 14 days.

References

1. Piliavin JA. Why do they give the gift of life? A review of research on blood donors since 1977. Transfusion 1990;30:444-59.
2. Widmann FK, ed. Standards for blood banks and transfusion services. 15th ed. Bethesda, MD: American Association of Blood Banks, 1993.
3. US Department of Health and Human Services, Food and Drug Administration. The code of federal regulations, 21 CFR 606.100 (b). Washington, DC: US Government Printing Office, 1992. (Revised annually.)
4. Pindyck J, Avorn J, Kuriyan M, et al. Blood donation by the elderly. Clinical and policy considerations. JAMA 1987;257:1186-8.
5. Instruction booklet for blood bank inspection checklist and report. Form FDA-2609. May 1991.
6. US Department of Health and Human Services, Food and Drug Administration. The code of federal regulations, 21 CFR 606.160 (e). Washington, DC: US Government Printing Office, 1992. (Revised annually.)
7. Beattie KM, Shafer AW. Broadening the base of a rare donor program by targeting minority populations. Transfusion 1986;26:401-4.
8. Vichinsky EP, Earles A, Johnson RA, et al. Alloimmunization in sickle cell anemia and transfusion of racially unmatched blood. N Engl J Med 1990;322:1617-21.
9. Recommendations for the prevention of human immunodeficiency virus (HIV) transmission by blood and blood products. Washington, DC: Center for Biologics Evaluation and Research, Revised April 1992.
10. Mayo DJ, Rose AM, Matchett SE, et al. Screening potential blood donors at risk for human immunodeficiency virus. Transfusion 1991; 31:466-74.
11. US Department of Health and Human Services, Food and Drug Administration. The code of federal regulations, 21 CFR 640.3 (a). Washington, DC: US Government Printing Office, 1992. (Revised annually.)
12. Mollison PL, Engelfriet CP, Contreras M. Blood transfusion in clinical medicine. 9th ed. Oxford: Blackwell Scientific Publications, 1993.
13. Tomasulo PA, Anderson AJ, Paluso MB, et al. A study of criteria for blood donor deferral. Transfusion 1980;20:511-18.
14. Piliavan JA. Temporary deferral and donor return. Transfusion 1987;27:199-200.
15. Kolins J, Silvergleid AJ. Creating a uniform donor medical history questionnaire. Transfusion 1991;31:349-54.
16. Widmann FK. Questions and answers. AABB News Briefs 1978;8(4):41-3.
17. Guernsey BG, Patton E, Fuchs JE, et al. Drug use and blood donor acceptability guide. Berkeley, CA: Cutter Biological, 1983.
18. Bond WW. Risk of infection from electrolysis. JAMA 1988;260:99.
19. Zoon KC. Exemptions to permit persons with a history of viral hepatitis before the age of eleven years to serve as donors of Whole Blood and Plasma: Alternate procedures. 21 CFR 640.120. Bethesda, MD: FDA, April 23, 1992.
20. Hanson M, Polesky HF. A method for calculating the risk of donors implicated in transfusion-associated hepatitis. Paper presented at 2nd International Workshop on Viral Hepatitis. Sterling, Scotland, 1982.
21. Ladd DJ, Hillis A. A new method for evaluating the hepatitis risk of the multiply-implicated donor. Transfusion 1984;24:80-2.
22. Centers for Disease Control. Update: Universal precautions for prevention of transmission of human immunodeficiency virus, hepatitis B virus, and other bloodborne pathogens in health-care settings. MMWR 1988;37:377-82, 387-88. (Also in JAMA 1988;260:528-31.)
23. Enforcement procedures for occupational exposure to hepatitis B virus (HBV) and human

immunodeficiency virus (HIV). OSHA Instruction CPL 2-2.44B. Washington, DC: US Department of Labor, February 27, 1990.

24. Schmuñis GA. *Trypanosoma cruzi*, the etiologic agent of Chagas' disease: Status in the blood supply in endemic and nonendemic countries. Transfusion 1991;31:547-57.

25. Revised recommendations for the prevention of human immunodeficiency virus (HIV) transmission by blood and blood products—section I, parts A & B only. Washington, DC: FDA Center for Biologics Evaluation and Research, December 5, 1990.

26. Holland PV. Why a new standard to prevent Creutzfeldt-Jakob disease? Transfusion 1988; 28:293-4.

27. Milman N, Sondergaard M. Iron stores in male blood donors evaluated by serum ferritin. Transfusion 1984;24:464-8.

28. Morse EE, Cable R, Pisciotto P, et al. Evaluation of iron status in women identified by copper sulfate screening as ineligible to donate blood. Transfusion 1987;27:238-41.

29. Zanella A, Silvani C, Banfi B, et al. Screening and evaluation of blood donors with upper-limit hematocrit levels. Transfusion 1987;27: 485-7.

30. Carpenter CB. Deliberate transfusion of potential renal transplant recipients with specific donor blood. Am J Kidney Dis 1981;1:116-8.

31. Salvatierra O, Iwaki Y, Vincenti F, et al. Incidence, characteristics, and outcome of recipients sensitized after donor-specific blood transfusions. Transplantation 1981;32:528-31.

32. Pura LS, Smith LE, Goldfinger D. Establishment of a directed donor blood program in a hospital-based blood bank. In: Garner RJ, Silvergleid AJ, eds. Autologous and directed blood programs. Arlington, VA: American Association of Blood Banks, 1987:31-45.

33. Smith LG. Blood collection. In: Green TS, Steckler D, eds. Donor room policies and procedures. Arlington, VA: American Association of Blood Banks, 1985:23-7.

34. Rutman RC, Di Pascuale-Barrios S. Donor reactions. In: Green TS, Steckler D, eds. Donor room policies and procedures. Arlington, VA: American Association of Blood Banks, 1985: 81-9.

35. Roekel IE. Donor reactions. In: Donor room procedures. Washington, DC: American Association of Blood Banks, 1977:23-7.

Appendix 1-1. Uniform Donor History Questionnaire

Donor History Questions	American Association of Blood Banks (AABB)	Food and Drug Administration (FDA)
1. Have you ever given blood under a different name?	No specific requirement.	A record shall be available from which unsuitable donors may be identified so that products from such individuals will not be distributed. (21 CFR 606.160(e) April 1992)
2. In the past 8 weeks, have you given blood, plasma or platelets?	Frequency of blood donation is every 8 weeks. (Standard B1.130*)	Frequency of blood donation is every 8 weeks unless otherwise approved by the medical director. (21 CFR 640.3(f) April 1992)
3. Have you ever been refused as a blood donor or told not to donate blood?	No specific requirement.	No specific requirement.
4. Have you ever had chest pain, heart disease or lung disease?	Prospective donors with diseases of the heart or lungs shall be excluded subject to evaluation by a qualified physician. (Standard B1.110)	Donor must be free of acute respiratory disease. (21 CFR 640.3(b)(4) April 1992)
5. Have you ever had cancer, a blood disease or a bleeding problem?	Prospective donors with a history of cancer or abnormal bleeding tendency shall be excluded subject to evaluation by a qualified physician. (Standard B1.110)	Persons with hemophilia or related clotting disorders who have received clotting factor concentrates must not donate blood or blood components. (FDA Memo 4/23/92†)
6. Have you ever had yellow jaundice, liver disease, hepatitis or a positive test for hepatitis?	Prospective donors with diseases of the liver shall be excluded subject to evaluation by a qualified physician. (Standard B1.110) Donors with a history of hepatitis after their 11th birthday or a confirmed test for HBsAg are permanently deferred. (Standard B1.261)	No individual with a history of hepatitis shall be a source of whole blood donation. (21 CFR 640.3(c) April 1992) Exemptions for history of hepatitis before age 11. (FDA Memo 4/23/92‡)

Appendix 1-1. Uniform Donor History Questionnaire (continued)

Donor History Questions	American Association of Blood Banks (AABB)	Food and Drug Administration (FDA)
7. Have you ever had Chagas' disease or babesiosis?	A history of babesiosis or Chagas' disease shall be cause for permanent deferral. (Standard B1.266)	No specific requirement.
8. Have you ever been given growth hormone?	Individuals who have received pituitary growth hormone of human origin must not be accepted for donation of blood, tissue or organs. (Standard B1.265)	(FDA Memo 11/25/87)
9. Have you ever taken Tegison® for psoriasis?	No specific requirement.	No specific requirement. Instruction Booklet for Blood Bank Inspection Checklist and Report recommends that donors taking Tegison® should be deferred for 3 years after receipt of the last dose.
10. Are you feeling well and healthy today?	The prospective donor shall appear in good health. (Standard B1.210)	Donor must be determined to be in general good health. (21 CFR 640.3(b) April 1992)
11. In the past 3 years, have you been outside the US or Canada?	Travelers to areas considered endemic for malaria may be accepted for red cell donation 6 months after return. (Standard B1.263)	Donor must be free of any disease transmissible by blood transfusion based on history and examinations. (21 CFR 640.3(b)(6) April 1992)
12. In the past 3 years, have you had malaria or take antimalarial drugs?	Donors who have had malaria, taken antimalarial prophylaxis or immigrated from endemic countries are deferred for 3 years. (Standard B1.263)	Donor must be free of any disease transmissible by blood transfusion based on history and examinations. (21 CFR 640.3(b)(6) April 1992)
13. In the past 12 months, have you been under a doctor's care or had a major illness or surgery?	No specific requirements.	Persons who have received a transfusion of whole blood or a blood component within the past 12 months should not donate blood or blood components. (FDA Memo 4/23/92†)

Appendix 1-1. Uniform Donor History Questionnaire (continued)

Donor History Questions	American Association of Blood Banks (AABB)	Food and Drug Administration (FDA)
14. In the past 12 months, have you received blood or had an organ or tissue transplant?	History of blood transfusion is cause for 12-month deferral. (Standard B1.250)	Persons who have received a transfusion of whole blood or a blood component within the past 12 months should not donate blood or blood components. (FDA Memo 4/23/92[†])
15. In the past 12 months, have you had a tattoo, ear or skin piercing, acupuncture or an accidental needle-stick?	Donor must be specifically queried about history of tattoo or other parenteral exposure to blood within 12 months. (Standard B1.262)	Persons who have had contact with blood and body fluids through percutaneous inoculation (such as needlestick) during the preceding 12 months should be deferred (FDA Memo 4/23/92[†])
16. In the past 12 months, have you had close contact with a person with yellow jaundice or hepatitis, or have you been given Hepatitis B Immune Globulin (HBIG)?	Close contact with person who has viral hepatitis is cause for 12-month deferral.	Close contact with person who has viral hepatitis is cause for 12-month deferral. (FDA Memo 4/23/92[§])
17. In the past 12 months, have you been given rabies shots?	Donor is deferred for 12 months after vaccine treatment for rabies. (Standard B1.232)	No specific requirement.
18. A. In the past 12 months, have you had a positive test for syphilis? B. In the past 12 months, have you had or been treated for syphilis or gonorrhea?	A history of syphilis or gonorrhea, or treatment for either, shall be cause for deferral for 12 months after completion of therapy. (Standard B1.273)	Persons who have had, or have been treated for, syphilis or gonorrhea during the preceding 12 months should not donate blood or blood components. Persons with a positive serologic test for syphilis should be deferred for 12 months. (FDA Memo 12/12/91)
19. In the past 12 months, have you given money or drugs to anyone to have sex with you?	Donor must be given educational material on AIDS high risk activity, and such at risk persons should refrain from donating blood. (Standard B1.264)	Men and women who have engaged in sex for money or drugs since 1977 and persons who have engaged in sex with such people during the preceding 12 months should not donate blood or blood components. (FDA Memo 4/23/92[†])

Appendix 1-1. Uniform Donor History Questionnaire (continued)

Donor History Questions	American Association of Blood Banks (AABB)	Food and Drug Administration (FDA)
20. Female Donors: In the past 6 weeks, have you been pregnant or are you pregnant now?	Existing pregnancy or pregnancy in past 6 weeks is cause for deferral. (Standard B1.180)	No specific requirement.
21. In the past 4 weeks, have you had any shots or vaccinations?	Donors must be queried about vaccines and immunizations. (Standard B1.230)	No specific requirement.
22. In the past 4 weeks, have you taken any pills, medication or Accutane®?	Drug therapy needs to be evaluated by medical director. (Standard B1.120)	21 CFR 640.3(b) (April 1992) and query donor regarding use of Accutane® within the last 30 days. (FDA Memo 2/28/84)
23. In the past 3 days, have you taken aspirin or anything that has aspirin in it?	Aspirin within 3 days precludes use of donor as sole source of platelets. (Standard B1.280)	No specific requirement for whole blood donation. Donors who have recently taken medication containing aspirin, especially within 36 hours, may not be suitable donors for plateletpheresis. (FDA Guidelines 10/7/88)
24. A. Have you ever used a needle, even once, to take any drug (including steroids)? B. In the past 12 months, have you had sex, even once, with anyone who has?	A. Stigma of narcotic habituation is cause for permanent deferral. (Standard B1.271) B. Refer to question #19.	A. Donor must be free from skin punctures or scars indicative of addiction to self-injected narcotics. (21 CFR 640.3(b)(7) April 1992) Past or present intravenous drug users should not donate blood or blood components. (FDA Memo 4/23/92[†]) B. Persons who have had sex with any person who is a past or present intravenous drug user should not donate blood or blood components for 12 months. (FDA Memo 4/23/92[†])
25. A. At any time since 1977, have you taken money or drugs for sex? B. In the past 12 months, have you had sex, even once, with anyone who has?	Refer to question #19.	Men and women who have engaged in sex for money or drugs since 1977 and persons who have engaged in sex with such people during the preceding 12 months should not donate blood or blood components. (FDA Memo 4/23/92[†])

Appendix 1-1. Uniform Donor History Questionnaire (continued)

Donor History Questions	American Association of Blood Banks (AABB)	Food and Drug Administration (FDA)
26. Male Donors: Have you had sex with another male, even once since 1977?	Refer to question #19.	Men who have had sex with another man even one time since 1977 should not donate blood or blood components permanently. (FDA Memo 4/23/92[†])
27. Female Donors: In the past 12 months, have you had sex with a male who has had sex, even once since 1977, with another male?	Refer to question #19.	Persons who have had sex with men who have had sex with another man even one time since 1977 should not donate blood or blood components for 12 months. (FDA Memo 4/23/92[†])
28. A. Have you ever taken clotting factor concentrates for a bleeding problem, such as hemophilia? B. In the past 12 months, have you had sex, even once, with anyone who has?	No specific requirement.	A. Persons with hemophilia or related clotting disorders who have received clotting factor concentrates should not donate blood or blood components. (FDA Memo 4/23/92[†]) B. Persons who have had sex with any person with hemophilia or related clotting disorders who has received clotting factor concentrates should not donate blood or blood components for 12 months. (FDA Memo 4/23/92[†])
29. A. Do you have AIDS or have you had a positive test for the AIDS virus? B. In the past 12 months, have you had sex, even once, with anyone who has?	Refer to question #19.	A. Persons with clinical or laboratory evidence of HIV infection must not donate blood or blood components. (FDA Memo 4/23/92[†]) B. Persons who have had sex with persons with clinical or laboratory evidence of HIV infection should not donate blood or blood components for 12 months. (FDA Memo 4/23/92[†])
30. Are you giving blood to be tested for AIDS?	No specific requirement.	No specific requirement.

Appendix 1-1. Uniform Donor History Questionnaire (continued)

Donor History Questions	American Association of Blood Banks (AABB)	Food and Drug Administration (FDA)
31. Do you understand that if you have the AIDS virus, you can give it to someone else even though you may feel well and have a negative AIDS test?	No specific requirement.	Donors should be informed that there is an interval during early infection when the HIV antibody test may be negative although the infection may still be transmitted. (FDA Memo 4/23/92[†])
32. Have you read and understood all the donor information presented to you, and have all your questions been answered?	No specific requirement.	Information should be written in language that ensures that the donor understands the definition of high-risk behavior and the importance of self-exclusion. Donors should not be considered suitable unless information about risks can be communicated in the language appropriate to each donor and is constructed to be culturally sensitive to promote comprehension. (FDA Memo 4/23/92[†])

[*]Standards referred to are from the 15th edition of *Standards for Blood Banks and Transfusion Services.*

[†]FDA Memorandum, April 23, 1992: Revised Recommendations for the Prevention of HIV Transmission by Blood and Blood Products.

[‡]FDA Memorandum, April 23, 1992: Exemptions To Permit Persons With a History of Viral Hepatitis Before the Age of 11 Years To Serve as Donors of Whole Blood and Plasma: Alternative Procedures, 21 CFR 640.120.

[§]FDA Memorandum, April 23, 1992: Revised Recommendations for Testing Whole Blood, Blood Components, Source Plasma and Source Leukocytes for Antibody to Hepatitis C Virus Encoded Antigen (Anti-HCV).

2

Hemapheresis

Hemapheresis (apheresis) is the removal of whole blood (WB) from a donor or patient, followed by its separation into components, retention of the desired component and return of the recombined remaining elements to the donor or patient. Hemapheresis can be used to collect a component intended for transfusion or to remove a pathologic component in order to treat a patient's disease. This procedure, when limited to removal of less than 10% of the individual's intravascular volume, usually does not require infusion of fluids or blood components. This chapter devotes separate sections to component preparation and therapeutic applications. Cell separators that separate components by centrifugal force can be used for either application. Instruments that apply other approaches to separation are available for use in therapeutic or plasma collection applications.

Cytapheresis, the collection of cells, requires an instrument capable of processing sufficiently large volumes of whole blood for a satisfactory yield of the desired component. Plasmapheresis, in contrast, can be accomplished using either a manual multiple-bag system or automated equipment. The manual system, which utilizes a refrigerated centrifuge and multiple bags joined by tubing, is simple and inexpensive, but time-consuming. It also carries a risk that red cells could be returned to the wrong

donor. The manual procedure is described in detail in Method 10.18.

Both AABB *Standards for Blood Banks and Transfusion Services*[1] and the *Code of Federal Regulations*[2] contain sections concerned with hemapheresis. All personnel involved in performing hemapheresis procedures should be thoroughly familiar with these regulations and qualified by training and/or experience to perform apheresis.

Component Preparation

Apheresis machines that use centrifugal force depend on the different densities of various blood components to achieve separation of the desired fraction. The remainder of the blood is returned to the donor by either intermittent or continuous flow. All such systems require prepackaged sets of sterile bags, tubing and centrifugal devices unique to the machine. Each machine has a mechanism to allow the separation device to rotate without twisting the attached tubing.[3] Both rotating seals and a "lariat" design have been used. Intermittent flow machines, in which the centrifuge bowl is alternately filled and emptied, require only a single venipuncture because drawing blood and returning it to the donor can be accomplished through the same line. Continuous flow equipment requires two venipunctures, one for removal and the other for return. Some instruments have protocols for use in either a continuous or discontinuous mode. The latter use has the advantage of only requiring a single venipuncture.

The anticoagulant solution is added in a metered quantity to the whole blood as it enters the tubing. The blood is pumped into a spinning centrifugal container (bowl, chamber or tubular rotor) wherein separation of components occurs. This process is similar to the operation of a dairy cream separator, with less dense elements layered above the densest constituents—in this case, the red blood cells. After the desired component(s) are harvested, the remaining elements are recombined and returned to the donor. Donation may require about 2 hours. Each manufacturer supplies detailed information and operational protocols for the various apheresis machines. Each facility must have, in a manual readily available to nursing and technical personnel, detailed descriptions of all procedures performed, specific for each type of cell separator.

Donors

Plasmapheresis and cytapheresis donors must meet the criteria applicable to donors of WB. Donors who do not meet these requirements may be drawn if a physician certifies in writing that the donor's health permits the hemapheresis and the component will be of special value to the intended recipient, such as HLA-matched platelets. If the exception imposes an element of risk to the recipient, the recipient's physician should be notified.[1]

During thrombocytapheresis, the donor's platelet count decreases about 30%; although this usually has little clinical significance, the count may require up to 72 hours to return to normal.[4,5] It is unlikely this drop could harm a donor;

however, plateletpheresis donors should be carefully evaluated for a personal and family history of excessive bleeding. In addition, a drug history should be obtained. Donors who have taken aspirin or aspirin-containing medications within 3 days of donation should ordinarily be deferred, because the platelet concentrates (PCs) obtained by apheresis are often the single source of platelets given to a patient.[1] Evidence exists that platelets collected 36 hours after aspirin ingestion may function satisfactorily.[6]

Leukapheresis donors who will receive predonation corticosteroid stimulation to increase granulocyte yields should be carefully questioned about hypertension, diabetes and peptic ulcer history or symptoms. Donors with previous or current disease that might be exacerbated by steroids should not receive them. The consent must include specific permission for use of steroids and hydroxyethyl starch (HES).

Laboratory Monitoring

Before initiation of any apheresis procedure, the hemoglobin or hematocrit must be measured. It is desirable to evaluate the platelet count, white blood cell count and differential. A platelet count below 150×10^9/L (150,000/µL) is a contraindication to platelet donation. Although a platelet count is not required before the initial apheresis procedure, it is required if a subsequent procedure is done at an interval of less than 8 weeks. The result of a pre- or postdonation count can be used to determine eligibility for a subsequent procedure.[1(p 20)] The quantity of granulocytes harvested in leukapheresis is directly related to the absolute granulocyte count in the peripheral blood. For satisfactory yields the donor's absolute granulocyte count should be greater than 4×10^9/L (4000/µL). Coagulation profiles are not needed for most donors. A congenital or acquired bleeding tendency usually disqualifies a donor. If multiple frequent donations are anticipated, serum protein concentration must be above 60 g/L (6.0 g/dL) and levels of IgG and IgM normal. Other laboratory studies increase costs and are rarely indicated.

Frequency of Donation

Frequency of donation is limited by the following[2]:

1. RBC loss incidental to the procedure, including samples collected for testing, should not exceed 25 mL per week. No more than 200 mL of red cells should be removed per 8 weeks. If it is not possible to return the donor's red cells during an apheresis procedure, the donor should be deferred for 8 weeks.

2. The amount of whole blood, not including anticoagulant, that was removed for processing. During a manual procedure this should not be more than 500 mL at one time for donors weighing less than 80 kg (176 lbs); or 600 mL for donors weighing more than 80 kg. Twice these volumes may be processed in a single session, but within a 7-day period shall not exceed 2000-2400 mL based on the donor's weight.

3. For manual apheresis procedures, the volume of the blood components (ie, plasma and platelets, etc) retained per procedure should not exceed 500 mL [600 mL for donors weighing more than 80 kg (176 lbs)].[6] For automated procedures, the volume is determined by the FDA approval for the instrument.

4. A serum protein electrophoresis or quantitative determination of IgG and IgM must be determined at 4-month intervals for donors undergoing plasmapheresis more often than once

every 8 weeks and must be within normal limits. This requirement also applies to donors undergoing plateletpheresis if plasma by-products are also collected.[6]

5. At least 48 hours must elapse between successive procedures. Donors should not undergo more than two procedures within a 7-day period. A donor should not have more than 24 plateletpheresis procedures in a calendar year.[6] Exceptions to these limits require a physician's approval as described above.

6. Plateletpheresis donors must have a platelet count of at least 150×10^9/L (150,000/μL) if less than 8 weeks has elapsed since the prior procedure.[1]

Records

There must be records of donor consent, identification, anticoagulants given, drugs used, duration of the procedure, volumes of all components and lot numbers of disposables and solutions. The average red cell loss for each type of procedure should be calculated. All adverse reactions during and following the procedure must be recorded. For donors undergoing repeated (more than once every 8 weeks) hemapheresis procedures, records of all laboratory findings and collection data must be reviewed and found to be within acceptable limits by a knowledgeable physician at least once every 4 months.

Donor Care

Apheresis, particularly when techniques using on-line blood separation are used, is more complex than ordinary blood donation. The apheresis facility must make provision to care for unusual reactions. This should include equipment, medications, personnel training and prompt physician coverage for serious problems.

Drugs Administered for Leukapheresis

Hydroxyethyl Starch

Rouleaux-promoting agents are used in leukapheresis to produce aggregates of red cells, which sediment in the centrifugation phase more effectively than single cells, producing a sharply defined interface between red cells and buffy coat. This enhances granulocyte harvest and minimizes red cell contamination of the product. HES is a synthetic analog of naturally occurring starch. Its intravascular half-life is 24-29 hours. Macrophages clear some from the circulation, but residual colloid can be detected in blood for as long as a year after injection.[7] Because HES is cleared only gradually, decreasing sequential doses may be utilized during intensive leukapheresis (eg, for three successive donations 48 hours apart, doses might be 500 mL, 300 mL and 200 mL of a 6% HES solution). The erythrocyte sedimentation rate (ESR) has been reported to correlate with residual HES.[8]

A low-molecular-weight HES (Pentastarch) has been evaluated for use in granulocyte collection.[9] This material gives similar yields to regular HES (6%) and seems to be cleared from the circulation within 24-96 hours.

Since HES is a colloid, it acts as a volume expander. Leukapheresis donors who have received frequent doses of HES may experience headaches or peripheral edema as a result of their expanded circulatory volume. Rare anaphylactoid reactions have occurred when HES is used.[10]

In therapeutic procedures used to reduce leukocytes (to be discussed later in this chapter) HES is not often needed since abnormal leukocytes are often less dense than normal cells and good separation from the patient's red cells can usually be achieved without a sedimenting agent.

Corticosteroids

Oral administration of corticosteroid preparations (hydrocortisone, prednisone, methylprednisolone or dexamethasone) are often used to increase the donor's granulocyte count. Since granulocyte yields depend upon the level of cells circulating at the time of leukapheresis, raising the circulating cell count increases the number of cells collected. Corticosteroids cause the granulocytes in the bone marrow storage pool to leave the marrow and also decrease egress of granulocytes from the peripheral blood. Corticosteroids can double the number of circulating granulocytes, but dosage, timing and route of administration affect the increment in granulocyte harvest. A protocol using 20 mg of oral prednisone at 17, 12 and 2 hours before donation gives superior granulocyte harvests with minimal systemic steroid activity.[11,12] Protocols using hematopoietic growth factors to increase the number of granulocytes collected are under investigation.

Platelet Concentrates

Cytapheresis is done to obtain Platelets, Pheresis from random volunteer donors, family members or donors selected on the basis of their HLA phenotype. An ever-increasing demand for this component has been observed with attempts to limit the number of random-donor exposures. Some patients who are thrombocytopenic from bone marrow failure or suppression become refractory to transfusions of random-donor platelet concentrates. (See Chapters 13 and 17.) Such patients may respond with better platelet count increments when transfused with platelets obtained from a donor selected on the basis of HLA antigens and/or after a compatible platelet crossmatch.[13,14]

Platelet Content

The commonly used cell separators consistently produce platelet harvests of at least 3×10^{11} platelets.[6,15] See Table 2-1. Various methods, including centrifugation, filtration and surge protocols may be used to remove red cells and leukocytes contaminating the platelets.[16,17] In some methods this may be at the expense of 20-30% of the final platelet yield. Other methods to reduce white cells below 10^6 may be required to decrease immunization and delay the onset of the refractory state in platelet recipients.[18] *Standards* requires 3.0×10^{11} platelets in at least 75% of the units tested.

In addition to platelets, it is also possible to collect plasma from the same donor. The procedure needs to be carried out using a closed system and the total volume removed is limited to the quantities described above.

Platelet concentrates intended for transfusion to bone marrow transplant recipients, to immunodeficient or severely immunosuppressed patients, or to recipients who are blood relatives of the donor must be irradiated to avoid the risk of graft-vs-host disease (GVHD).[19] Irradiation has also been suggested for HLA-matched components and for PCs intended for patients with Hodgkin's disease. Since viable lymphocytes (the cause of GVHD) contaminate many other blood components, not only should PCs be irradiated, but also all lymphocyte-containing components should be similarly irradiated with at least 25 Gy.

Table 2-1. Currently Approved Instruments for Automated Plateletpheresis and Plasmapheresis*

Manufacturer	Instrument	Minimal Platelet Concentration Per Unit	Maximal Storage
Plateletpheresis			
Haemonetics	H-30, H-30S	3.0×10^{11}	24 hours
Haemonetics	V-50 (without surge)	2.0×10^{11}	24 hours
Haemonetics	V-50 (with surge)	3.0×10^{11}	24 hours
Haemonetics	V-50 (with surge)	3.0×10^{11}	5 days in functionally closed system using CLX
Baxter	Fenwal CS-3000	3.0×10^{11}	24 hours
Baxter	Fenwal CS-3000	3.0×10^{11}	5 days in functionally closed system using PL-732
COBE/IBM	IBM-2997 (dual/stage)	3.0×10^{11}	24 hours
COBE/IBM	Spectra	3.0×10^{11}	5 days in functionally closed system
Dideco	Progress 790/A	3.0×10^{11}	24 hours
Plasmapheresis			
Haemonetics	V-50		
Haemonetics	PCS		
Baxter	Autopheresis C		
Baxter	Fenwal CS-3000		

*Used with permission from the FDA Center for Biologics Evaluation and Research (HFB-480).

Laboratory Testing

ABO and Rh typing, antibody screening and required testing for transfusion-transmitted diseases must be done by the collecting facility in a manner similar to that for other blood components. Testing must be done on each collection unless the donor component is dedicated to the support of a single patient. Under these circumstances repeat testing for disease markers need only be done at 10-day intervals.[1(p 21)] (Note: The FDA requires that testing be done only once if a dedicated or family donor is collected repeatedly during a period not to exceed 30 days.[6]) A blood specimen tube may be attached to the primary container so that the transfusion service can perform indicated pretransfusion testing.

Platelet concentrates prepared by hemapheresis need not be crossmatched if prepared by a method expected to cause contamination with less than 5 mL red cells.[1] If a cytapheresis concentrate contains more than 5 mL red cells, there should be compatibility with the recipient's serum. (Note: FDA guidelines state that a sample of donor blood should be attached to the component container for compatibility testing if the final component contains more than 2 mL of rbcs as determined by a hematocrit, which is to be done on all units containing visibly apparent rbcs.[6]) If the recipient has a negative antibody screening test, only ABO compatibility must be demonstrated. If the recipient has a clinically significant red cell antibody, an antiglobulin crossmatch must be done and the donor red cells shown to lack the corresponding antigen(s).[1] The donor plasma should be ABO-compatible with the recipient's red cells, especially when the recipient is a newborn. When the recipient does not show expected platelet increments after transfusion and is thought to be alloimmunized, or when febrile transfusion reactions are fre-

quent, leukocytes may be removed by one of the methods described above, a soft spin technique described in Method 10.15 or at the time of administration using a special filter.

Storage

Platelets prepared as described should be stored at 20-24 C with continuous gentle agitation. Platelets, Pheresis units that have been prepared in an open system may be stored for no longer than 24 hours. Those prepared in a closed system may be stored for 5 days. The pH must be 6.0 or higher at the end of allowable storage in all units tested.

Quality Control

During establishment of the procedure, it is advisable to test every unit of Platelets, Pheresis for red cell content, leukocyte count, pH, volume, platelet count and sterility (this can be done on 20 mL separated from the unit at the time of collection and stored at 20-24 C for the intended dating period of the unit). This makes it possible to calculate the total number of platelets and red cells in the unit and to estimate loss of donor's erythrocytes. Once the procedure is operating satisfactorily, fewer concentrates need to be extensively tested. However, FDA guidelines require that the actual platelet content (volume × platelet count) be determined on each unit.[6] This information need not be on the unit at the time of issue, but should be part of the issue records. A method for collecting a representative specimen is given in Method 11.9.

Granulocyte Concentrates

The therapeutic efficacy and indications for granulocyte transfusion are not well-defined. Many controlled studies support the conclusion that, for properly selected patients, transfusions of concentrates containing adequate numbers of granulocytes are effective in clearing the bloodstream of bacteria and achieving short-term control of infection.[20,21] Unless the patient subsequently experiences bone marrow recovery, granulocyte transfusions eventually become futile because of immunization to leukocyte antigens or infection with virulent organisms. One reason for the lack of therapeutic efficacy is that, in some studies, suboptimal numbers of granulocytes were infused.[22,23] A daily dose of at least 10^{10} functional granulocytes seems to be an essential minimum to achieve a therapeutic effect. To achieve this dose, the method used will have to achieve a mean yield of about 2×10^{10} granulocytes. With most available equipment, consistent harvests of more than 1×10^{10} granulocytes require that donors be pretreated with corticosteroids.

Granulocyte concentrates are often given to patients with thrombocytopenia. On some occasions platelet concentrates are also ordered for the same patient. Before giving a component from another donor, it is worth evaluating the effect of the granulocyte concentrate on the recipient's platelet count since the usual granulocyte concentrate also contains more than 3×10^{11} platelets. Protocols are also available to harvest adequate doses of both platelets and granulocytes from the same donor.

Storage and Infusion

Granulocyte function changes on storage. Thus, concentrates should be transfused as soon as possible after donation.[24,25] *Standards* allows storage at 20-24 C, for no longer than 24 hours. The use of gentle agitation during storage is probably undesirable. Irradiation before infusion should be considered for clinical situations similar to those described above for platelets. Infusion through microaggregate filters may impair clinical efficacy.

Laboratory Testing

ABO and Rh typing, antibody screening and all required testing for infectious disease markers are required. If possible, these should be accomplished before or during donation so that transfusion of the granulocyte concentrate is not delayed. Because red cell contamination in granulocyte concentrates is usually significant, the red cells should be ABO-compatible with the recipient's plasma. D– recipients should receive granulocyte concentrates from D– donors. If it is necessary to use a D+ donor for a D– recipient, the administration of RhIG should be considered. If more than 5 mL of red cells contaminate the unit, the red cells must be compatible with the recipient's serum.

Quality Control

Concentrate volume, white blood cell count with leukocyte differential and calculation of total number of granulocytes harvested should be recorded. The donor's red cell loss and the amount of HES given at each donation should be documented in records of both the apheresis procedure and of the individual donor. *Standards* requires at least 1×10^{10} granulocytes in 75% of the units tested.

Peripheral Blood Progenitor Cells

Cytapheresis techniques can be used to collect lymphohematopoietic progenitor cells.[26] (See Chapter 6.) The primary use of this procedure is to obtain autologous cells to reconstitute the bone marrow of patients with cancer, leukemia in remission and various lymphomas. Generally, multiple collections are done before treatment with intensive chemotherapy and/or irradiation. The use of granulocyte-macrophage colony-stimulating factor may improve the yield of hematopoietic stem cells.[27] The number and frequency of the apheresis procedures are determined for each donor-patient based on the yield of cells obtained and the anticipated recovery after frozen storage. Procedures must be available to ensure informed consent and appropriate care of the donor-patient during the apheresis procedure. Protocols should be defined in the facilities procedure manual for the manipulation, storage and quality control testing including viability and sterility tests of the peripheral blood progenitor cells collected.[1] A system for labeling, storage and record-keeping consistent with *Standards* should be used.

Therapeutic Hemapheresis

Hemapheresis has been used to treat patients with many different diseases. Cells, plasma or plasma components may be removed from the circulation, to be replaced by normal plasma or solutions of electrolytes or albumin. The theoretical basis for

benefit from hemapheresis is the reduction in the patient's blood of a pathologic substance to levels that will allow improvement in the course of the disease. In some conditions the replacement plasma may supply an essential substance that is absent. Other possible effects of plasma exchange include alteration of the antigen-to-antibody ratio, alteration of mediators of inflammation or immunity, improved clearance of immune complexes and a placebo effect.[28]

Physiology

Removal of Material

During plasma exchange, plasma that contains the pathologic substance is continuously being removed while replacement fluid is infused. The efficiency of removal of the pathologic substance during an exchange can be estimated by calculating the patient's plasma volume and using Fig 2-1.

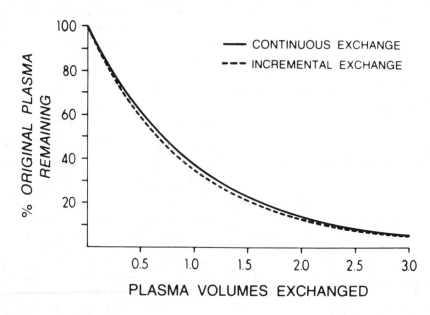

Figure 2-1. The relationship between the volume of plasma exchange and the patient's original plasma remaining.

Use of these estimates depends on the following assumptions: 1) the patient's blood volume does not change, 2) mixing occurs immediately and 3) the pathologic substance undergoes neither increased production nor mobilization from the extravascular into the vascular compartment.[29] The same information can be used to estimate the effect of an exchange transfusion or the amount of donor blood present in a patient given a massive transfusion.

As seen in Fig 2-1, efficiency of removal is greatest early in the procedure and diminishes progressively during the exchange. Exchanges are usually limited to about one plasma volume (ie, approximately 40 mL plasma exchanged per kg of body weight, depending upon the hematocrit). This minimizes the time required for each procedure but may necessitate more frequent procedures. Occasionaly, two or three plasma volumes are exchanged, resulting in greater initial diminution of the pathologic substance. These procedures are less efficient and require considerably more time to complete.[30] During the initial phases of the plasma exchange, the removed plasma may be replaced with less expensive crystalloid solution, but as the exchange reaches one-third to one-half plasma volume, colloid fluids (ie, albumin) are generally used to avoid an excessive drop in the patient's colloid osmotic pressure.[31] Following removal of several plasma volumes, FFP may be required to maintain normal coagulation mechanisms. The acute phase of a life-threatening disease usually requires a series of one-volume plasma exchanges. For maintenance therapy of chronic diseases, smaller volumes are appropriate. The optimal schedule has not been determined for most diseases.

Effects on Normal Constituents

The plasma volume of an average-sized adult is 2.5-3.0 L. With currently available equipment, it is possible to exchange 2 L of plasma in 1 hour and 4 L in 2 hours. The rate of plasma exchange should be individualized for each patient; smaller patients may not tolerate exchanges of 2 L/hour. When plasma exchange exceeds 1.5 times the plasma volume, various blood components manifest different rates of removal and restitution.[32] Depletion is more efficient than predicted for fibrinogen, the third component of complement (C3) and immune complexes, when present, with 75-85% of the original substance actually removed following a one-volume plasma procedure. Immunoglobulins are removed as expected, about 65% per plasma volume. Electrolytes, uric acid and some proteins, including Factor VIII, are removed at less-than-expected rates. Erythrocyte loss is about 30 mL and a 25-30% drop in platelet count generally occurs. Three to 4 days are required for fibrinogen and C3 to return to normal levels. Platelets reach preexchange values in 2-4 days and coagulation factors (except fibrinogen) achieve preapheresis levels within hours. Recovery patterns for immunoglobulins vary, because IgM is predominantly (75%) intravascular, but only about 45% of total body IgG is intravascular. See Table 7-3. Thus, IgG levels return to 40% of the pretreatment level within 48 hours because of reequilibration. Their rate of synthesis becomes the rate-determining factor and recovery to 80% of normal requires about 2 weeks. These facts are important when considering frequency of therapeutic procedures. Weekly procedures permit rapid recovery of normal plasma components, while daily procedures will deplete most normal, as well as abnormal, constituents.

The rate at which the pathologic substance is synthesized and its relative distribution between intravascular and extravascular fluid may determine success or failure in application of therapeutic plasmapheresis. For example, the abnormal IgM of Waldenstrom's macroglobulinemia is mostly intravascular and is synthesized slowly, making apheresis an effective mode of treatment, particularly when hyperviscosity is present.[33] In contrast, anti-D antibody is IgG; efforts to prevent hydrops fetalis by lowering maternal IgG levels with intensive plasmapheresis have been less successful and require a more intensive regimen than that necessary for treating macroglobulinemia.[34,35] When IgG antibody levels are rapidly and massively decreased by plasmapheresis, antibody synthesis increases rapidly and may even overshoot the pretreatment levels. This rebound response complicates treatment of autoimmune diseases. Immunosuppressive regimens blunt the IgG rebound response to apheresis.

Indications for Cytapheresis

Therapeutic cytapheresis is usually only indicated for very high cell counts as occasionally encountered in patients with thrombocythemia (platelets $>1500 \times 10^9$/L) or leukocytosis (white cells $>100 \times 10^9$/L).[28] Reduction of the platelet count is indicated in patients with evidence of hemorrhage or thrombosis thought to be secondary to the high count.[36] Apheresis has also been effective in reducing platelet counts in patients with idiopathic thrombocytosis who require surgery.[37] Leukapheresis is indicated in patients with acute leukemia when there is evidence of leukostasis causing cerebral or pulmonary symptoms. In some situations this may be required as an emergency procedure.[38] Reducing the tumor burden prior to initiation of definitive treatment can reduce spleen size and prevent hemorrhage and signs of vascular insufficiency. Apheresis is not indicated in chronic lymphocytic leukemia, which can be controlled by chemotherapy.

Evaluating Efficacy

Controlled Studies

Therapeutic hemapheresis has been applied to many different diseases, but many publications are case reports and small series that quote historical controls. The evidence of efficacy is often insufficient and unreliable.[28,39] Controlled studies of therapeutic apheresis are few because, among other problems, they require use of sham treatments as a control. Sham procedures have two major drawbacks: they are expensive, because personnel and equipment costs are the same as for a therapeutic procedure, and they do carry some risk and morbidity without providing any benefit to the individual serving as a control.[40] Using sham treatment as a control process requires patients to be screened from view of the apheresis equipment. The separated plasma and cells are recombined before reinfusion to the sham group, while plasma is exchanged with 5% albumin or FFP for the treatment group. Evaluation before and after therapy must be performed by personnel blinded to mode of therapy. The complexity and problems of such controlled double-blind investigations are illustrated by the ambiguous results of three studies of rheumatoid arthritis treated with hemapheresis.[41-43]

Placebo Effect

When new therapies are first used, 30-40% of patients appear to respond simply as a result of a placebo effect.[44] The complicated apheresis machines and associated intensive attention from nursing and medical personnel may well amplify the placebo effect and bias evaluation of clinical improvement. For many of the diseases being treated, the etiology, pathogenesis and natural history are incompletely understood and changes in the measured variables, such as decrease in complement components, rheumatoid factor or immune complexes, cannot reliably be correlated with changes in disease activity. For example, the ESR is a commonly used index of rheumatoid activity. The ESR invariably decreases during intensive plasmapheresis, but this reflects decreases in fibrinogen, not necessarily in disease activity.

Conclusions

Despite the difficulties in documenting its effects, there is general agreement that hemapheresis is effective treatment for some conditions.[45,46] See Tables 2-2 and 2-3. When the pathologic substance is identifiable (such as the IgM causing hyperviscosity in Waldenstrom's macroglobulinemia) and the treatment clearly reduces the level of a known pathogenic factor, treatment can be followed by appropriate laboratory tests. Unfortunately, this is not the case for most diseases treated by therapeutic hemapheresis and controversy is likely to continue. For conditions being treated by cytotoxic or immunosuppressive therapy, reducing autoantibodies, circulating immune complexes, plasma proteins and decreasing the number of circulating lymphocytes probably augments therapeutic benefits. Apheresis seems to be useful chiefly as adjunctive or palliative therapy. Its effects are usually short-term and not curative,[47,48] although lengthy remissions may occur.

Peer Review

A group of responsible physicians (such as the Hospital Transfusion Committee) may help to establish and monitor all policies relating to therapeutic apheresis; review the indications for, and effectiveness of, each procedure or series of procedures; and maintain surveillance of all adverse effects.[49] This committee could establish a list of conditions for which therapeutic apheresis is appropriate and evaluate all unusual requests. For a regional blood center, a Medical Advisory Committee could serve the same function.

Patient Care Considerations

Informed Consent

The informed consent of a prospective patient should be obtained and documented in writing after a qualified person explains the procedure, the risks and possible alternative therapy.[49] The patient or the legal guardian must have an opportunity to ask questions and to refuse consent. The patient's personal physician should certify in writing that the possible benefit warrants the risk.

The Patient's Condition

Evaluation of the patient's general condition is the responsibility of both the personal physician and the physician in charge of the apheresis facility. Close consultation between these physicians is important, especially when the patient is small or elderly, or has cardiovascular instability or poor vascular access. The physician in charge of the apheresis facility has final responsibility to determine that the procedure is indicated and the patient is a suitable candidate.[1,49] A treatment plan including dose, timing and duration of therapy should be established in advance. Adequate means to care for untoward reactions in patients must be readily available. This should include equipment, medications, personnel training and prompt medical coverage for serious problems.

Laboratory Tests

When specific tests are available and there are explicit indications, the following occasionally may be helpful to monitor patients:

Table 2-2. Indications for Use of Hemapheresis in Selected Diseases[46]

Plasma Exchange	Cytapheresis
Category I—Standard and acceptable under certain circumstances, including primary therapy	
Coagulation factor inhibitors	Leukemia with hyperleukocytosis syndrome
Cryoglobulinemia	Sickle cell syndromes (also see Category III)
Goodpasture's syndrome	Thrombocytosis, symptomatic
Guillain-Barré syndrome	
Homozygous familial hypercholesterolemia	
Hyperviscosity syndrome	
Myasthenia gravis	
Posttransfusion purpura	
Refsum's disease	
Thrombotic thrombocytopenic purpura (TTP)	
Category II—Sufficient evidence to suggest efficacy; acceptable therapy on an adjunctive basis	
Chronic inflammatory demyelinating polyneuropathy	Cutaneous T-cell lymphoma (cytoreduction or
Cold agglutinin disease	photopheresis)
Drug overdose and poisoning (protein bound toxins)	Hairy cell leukemia
Hemolytic uremic syndrome (HUS)	Hyperparasitemia (eg, malaria)
Pemphigus vulgaris	Peripheral blood stem cell collections for hematopoietic
Rapidly progressive glomerulonephritis	reconstitution
Systemic vasculitis (1° or 2° to RA or SLE)	Rheumatoid arthritis

Category III—Inconclusive evidence for efficacy; uncertain benefit/risk ratio

ABO-incompatible organ or marrow transplantation
Maternal treatment of maternal-fetal incompatibility (HDN)
Thyroid storm
Multiple sclerosis
Progressive systemic sclerosis
Pure red cell aplasia
Transfusion refractoriness due to alloantibodies (red cell, platelet, HLA)
Warm autoimmune hemolytic anemia

Life-threatening hemolytic transfusion reactions
Multiple sclerosis
Organ transplant rejection (also photopheresis)
Sickle cell disease (prophylactic use in pregnancy)

Category IV—Lack of efficacy in controlled trials

AIDS (for symptoms of immunodeficiency)
Amyotrophic lateral sclerosis
Aplastic anemia
Fulminant hepatic failure
ITP (chronic)
Lupus nephritis
Polymyositis/dermatomyositis
Psoriasis
Renal transplant rejection
Rheumatoid arthritis
Schizophrenia

Leukemia without hyperleukocytosis syndromes
Hypereosinophilia
Polymyositis/dermatomyositis

Table 2-3. Conditions for Which Apheresis Is Reimbursable (Not Considered Investigative)*

Leukemia (acute debulking or blast crisis)
Leukemia (chronic myelogenous)
Hairy-cell leukemia (for maintenance)
Thrombocytosis (symptomatic or presurgical)
Sickle-cell disease

Acquired myasthenia gravis
Guillain-Barré syndrome
Chronic inflammatory demyelinating polyradiculoneuropathy (CIDP)
Eaton-Lambert syndrome
Progressive systemic sclerosis (scleroderma): refractory

Waldenstrom's (primary) macroglobulinemia
Myeloma with renal failure
Hyperviscosity syndrome
Cryoglobulinemia (refractory)
Vasculitis: life-threatening or organ-threatening

Overdose with certain drugs
Thyroid storm or thyroid hormone overdose
Cholestasis with intractable pruritus
Familial homozygous hyperlipidemia, type II A
Refsum's disease

Goodpasture's syndrome (without anuria or with pulmonary hemorrhage)
Glomerulonephritis (rapidly progressive secondary to vasculitis or idiopathic, rapidly progressive type)
Rheumatoid vasculitis, with neuropathy
Progressive systemic sclerosis (scleroderma), when refractory
Polymyositis (refractory to corticosteroids)
Dermatomyositis (refractory to corticosteroids)

Posttransfusion purpura
Thrombotic thrombocytopenic purpura
Maternal-fetal incompatibility (high risk of fetal death—early delivery or IUT not possible)
Coagulation factor inhibitors (conventional therapy has failed, significant bleeding requiring medication or elective surgery is planned)
ABO-incompatible bone marrow transplantation
Pemphigus vulgaris: refractory

*Blue Cross and Blue Shield of Minnesota. Provider letter. March 1992.

Table 2-4. Comparison of Replacement Fluids

Replacement Solution	Advantages	Disadvantages
Crystalloids	Low cost Hypoallergenic No hepatitis risk	2-3 volumes required Hypo-oncotic No coagulation factors No immunoglobulins
Albumin	Iso-oncotic No contaminating "inflammatory mediators" No hepatitis risk	High cost No coagulation factors No immunoglobulins

Plasma Protein Fraction	Slightly less expensive than
	  albumin
		Possible induction of
		  hypotensive
		  reactions

Fresh Frozen Plasma	Maintains normal levels of:
	  immunoglobulins
	  complement
	  AT III
	  other proteins
		Hepatitis, HIV risk
		Citrate load
		ABO incompatibility
		Allergic reactions
		Sensitization

1. Viscosity, for hyperviscosity syndromes.
2. Platelet count and lactic dehydrogenase, for thrombotic thrombocytopenic purpura.
3. Anti-acetylcholine receptor, for myasthenia gravis.
4. Antiglomerular basement membrane antibody, for glomerulonephritis.
5. Low density lipoproteins, for familial hypercholesterolemia.

Replacement Fluids

The choice of replacement fluids varies. The responsible physician should prescribe fluids to be given, and the records must note the nature and volume of the replacement fluids as well as the volume of plasma or cells removed. The selection significantly affects the total cost of the procedure. The three commonly used replacement solutions are: crystalloids, albumin solutions and, if indicated, FFP. There are advantages and disadvantages to each (see Table 2-4). A combination is usually used, the relative proportions being determined by the patient's physical condition, the disease, the planned frequency of procedures and cost.

Plasma that has been removed during a therapeutic procedure should be handled carefully and disposed of properly. Therapeutically removed plasma must not be shipped interstate for further manufacture without an FDA license.

Complications of Hemapheresis

Death

Patients undergoing therapeutic apheresis are often critically ill, having failed more traditional therapies. Manipulation during apheresis of their intravascular fluid volumes and the associated movement of electrolytes, globulins and other substances from one physiologic compartment to another can stress the patient's already compromised homeostatic mechanisms. Worldwide, more than 50 deaths have been associated with therapeutic hemapheresis.[50] The estimated case fatality rate is about 3 in 10,000 procedures.[51] The two most common mechanisms of death are cardiovascular (characterized by cardiac arrhythmias or arrest during or shortly after the procedure) and respiratory (characterized by acute pulmonary edema or adult respiratory distress syndrome occurring during a procedure). Other complications that, on occasion, lead to death are anaphylaxis, vascular perforation, hepatitis, sepsis, thrombosis and hemorrhage.

Vascular Access

Patients referred for therapeutic apheresis often have received intensive medical care that has included repeated venipunctures. As a result, vascular access often is difficult. Special venous access devices, such as an indwelling double-lumen catheter, requiring surgical techniques for placement may be required. These devices may produce more vascular damage or inflict infrequent, but severe, complications such as perforation of the great vessels or heart, thrombosis or septicemia.[52] Arterial puncture, dissecting deep hematomas and arteriovenous fistula formation have been reported.[51]

Alteration of Pharmacodynamics

Plasmapheresis can precipitously lower blood levels of drugs. Plasma levels of antibiotics, anticonvulsants and digitalis are decreased by apheresis. Drugs that bind to albumin will be significantly decreased. The pharmacokinetics of all drugs used to treat patients undergoing apheresis should be considered before

starting therapy, and dosage schedules adjusted appropriately.

Effects of Citrate

Most patients with normal parathyroid function maintain calcium homeostasis during therapeutic plasma exchange.[53] Perioral paresthesia resulting from reduced serum levels of ionized calcium can occur and is related to the rate at which citrate anticoagulant is returned to the patient. The use of FFP as a replacement solution exacerbates citrate toxicity. Hyperventilation may also contribute to hypocalcemic reactions. Perioral paresthesia, when it occurs, can usually be controlled by reducing the proportion of citrate or slowing the reinfusion rate. Symptoms can become more severe if untreated, progressing to twitching of muscles of the extremities, chills, pressure in the chest, nausea, vomiting and, finally, tetany. Asking the patient to report any vibrations or tingling sensations can help determine the correct reinfusion rate. Extra precautions must be taken in patients who are unable to respond during therapy. In patients with low calcium levels because of their underlying disease, symptoms of hypocalcemia are more likely to occur during plasma exchange.

When central catheters are used for reinfusion, arrhythmias may result from direct perfusion of the cardiac conduction system with citrated fluid and/or cold fluids. Blood warming devices can be useful in selected patients. Electrocardiographic changes have been noted to remit upon partial withdrawal of central catheters.

Circulatory Effects

Intermittent-flow cell separators that require large extracorporeal volumes increase the risk of hypotensive reactions. Use of a large centrifuge bowl makes hypovolemia more likely. Such reactions occur more frequently if the volume of extracorporeal blood exceeds 15% of total blood volume. Hypotension is more common in children and the elderly. Hypotensive medications also aggravate hypovolemic reactions. Slow infusion and rapid withdrawal may produce hypovolemia in the patient and excessive volume in the cell separator. In patients with severe anemia, care must be taken not to remove excess volume before initiating the reinfusion process. Some centers routinely use a double line setup to facilitate rapid infusion of fluids when using intermittent-flow procedures. Continuous-flow machines are less likely to produce large extracorporeal volumes. Hypovolemic reactions can occur with continuous-flow machines if return flow is accidentally diverted to a waste collection bag, either through operator oversight or mechanical failure of a switch. During all procedures it is essential to maintain careful and continuous records of the volumes removed and returned.

Mechanical Hemolysis and Equipment Failures

Kinked plastic tubing, malfunctioning pinch valves or improperly threaded tubing may damage the red cells in the extracorporeal circuit. In a survey reporting 12,658 therapeutic procedures, eight (0.06%) equipment-related hemolytic episodes were reported.[54] A similar percent (0.07%) of machine-related hemolysis was observed in 195,372 apheresis procedures done on volunteer donors in the UK.[55] Although the patient is usually asymptomatic, in all apheresis procedures the operator should carefully observe the plasma collection lines for the pink discoloration of traumatic hemolysis. Other types of equipment failure such as problems with the rotating seal, leaks in the plasticware, roller pump failure, etc, are infrequent.[5]

Respiratory Distress

The differential diagnosis for respiratory embarrassment during or immediately following apheresis includes: pulmonary edema, massive pulmonary embolus, pulmonary microvascular obstruction and anaphylactic reactions. Pulmonary edema resulting from volume overload or cardiac failure is usually indicated by an increase of more than 50 mm Hg in the diastolic blood pressure. Acute pulmonary edema secondary to alveolar capillary membrane damage may be the result of an immune reaction or the presence of a vasoactive substance in FFP or other colloidal solutions. Massive pulmonary embolus associated with apheresis could be due to inadequate anticoagulation of the withdrawn blood.

Minor allergic reactions with urticaria and bronchospasm are fairly common during apheresis and usually respond to antihistamines and/or steroids.[56,57] Generalized urticarial reactions have occurred in some donors who are sensitized to the ethylene oxide gas used to sterilize disposable plastic apheresis kits.[58] Complement activation has been detected during some of these urticarial reactions when FFP was being used as the replacement solution.[56] Complement activation may also be mediated by granulocyte aggregation induced by apheresis. High dose steroids may prevent the phenomenon.[59]

Infections

Among the commonly used replacement solutions, only FFP is capable of transmitting infectious viruses. Other potential sources of contamination or infection could be leakage of the centrifuge seal or plastic harness, defects in the prepackaged software, or bacterial sepsis from indwelling catheters. Intensive apheresis procedures decrease immunoglobulin levels and the opsonic components of complement. In addition, immunosuppressive drugs may have been prescribed to prevent rebound increases in antibody levels after apheresis therapy. This induced immunocompromised state might be expected to result in increased susceptibility to infections. Indeed, a high incidence of complicating infections has been reported in patients treated for glomerulonephritis.[60] In contrast, neurological patients treated with apheresis have a much lower frequency of infections.[61] This suggests the basic disease process is an important factor in determining susceptibility to infection.

Newer Developments

The equipment used for therapeutic and donor hemapheresis has evolved from the instruments that were originally developed to collect plasma, platelets and granulocytes. Currently available instruments are more sophisticated. They include such features as automated monitoring devices and computer programming. Other instruments designed specifically for therapeutic use bear only slight resemblance to their predecessors and make it possible to reduce the need for replacement solutions and shorten the time for completing the procedure.

Membrane Filtration

Instruments that filter plasma through a membrane have been developed for therapeutic uses and for collection of plasma from healthy donors.[62,63] In these instruments whole blood, containing all protein and cellular elements, flows across a membrane. Higher pressure in the blood phase than in the filtrate pushes plasma constituents smaller than the membrane pores through the membrane into the filtrate. Most instruments have the membranes arranged as hollow fibers, although there are several flat plate devices. As blood crosses the membrane in a laminar flow, repulsive forces intrinsic to material of the wall keep cellular elements away from the membrane. Thus, platelets are not activated and red cell survival is not shortened. Plasma permeates the matrix of the membrane and escapes at right angles to the stream of flow. Varying membrane pore size permits some degree of selection in the removal of plasma proteins while the remainder are returned to the patient. Devices that combine filtration and centrifugation are also available.[3]

Adsorption

Specific removal of a pathologic material has many advantages over the removal of all plasma constituents. Membrane or centrifugal devices can be used in protocols modified for selective removal of specific soluble plasma constituents. Most of these methods are based on the principles of affinity chromatography.[64] Selective removal of low density lipoproteins (LDLs) has been accomplished using both immunoaffinity (anti-LDL) and chemical affinity (dextran sulfate) columns in patients with familial hypercholesterolemia.[65] Extraction of antibodies, antigens and immune complexes has been performed using sorbents such as staph protein A, monoclonal antibodies, blood group substances, DNA-collodion, polymers with aggregated immunoglobulin G attached, etc.[66] The treated plasma can be returned with the cellular components to the patient, eliminating the need for replacement fluids. In some protocols the immunoadsorption is performed in-line with the patient, while in others the plasma separated from the cellular components is passed through an off-line column and then reinfused. Immunoadsorbent procedures have been reported to be effective in uncontrolled studies in the treatment of acute and chronic immune thrombocytopenic purpura, thrombocytopenia associated with HIV infection, hemolytic uremic syndrome, and in selected malignancies such as Kaposi's sarcoma and breast cancer.[67] Many of these protocols are still experimental and have had only limited clinical trials. In evaluating the success of these techniques as with many of the other applications of therapeutic apheresis it is difficult to separate the effect of the apheresis from the other therapies (ie, immunosuppression, antiplatelet drugs, fresh frozen plasma, intravenous immunoglobulin, etc) used to treat patients who are desperately ill.[68]

Cryofiltration

Cold temperatures cause polymerization of many macromolecular substances, including IgM autoantibodies, immune complexes and lipids. These polymers then precipitate or gel.[69] In a two-step hemapheresis process, plasma is filtered and then cooled so that the large molecular substances gel and can be removed by a second macromolecular filter. The plasma is then rewarmed, united with the cellular elements and returned to the patient. In studies on patients with rheumatoid arthritis, this process effectively removed circulating immune complexes and rheumatoid factor, an IgM autoantibody.[69] However, this procedure did not produce significant clinical changes.

New Approaches in Cytapheresis

Several other new uses for cytapheresis have been developed by investigators searching for better methods to treat cancer. Adoptive immunotherapy by ex vivo activation of autologous leukapheresis-harvested lymphocytes in culture is one of these new techniques.[70] The apheresis-collected cells are treated with a lymphokine, interleukin-2, increasing the number of lymphocyte-activated killer

cells, which on reinfusion will destroy the tumor. Several other therapeutic approaches using various methods such as UV irradiation or photoactive chemicals to modify tumor or immune cells during apheresis are currently under study.[71]

References

1. Widmann FK, ed. Standards for blood banks and transfusion services. 15th ed. Bethesda, MD: American Association of Blood Banks, 1993.

2. Code of federal regulations. 21 CFR 640. Washington, DC: US Government Printing Office, 1992. (Revised annually.)

3. Ciavarella D. Blood processors and cell separators. Transfus Sci 1989;10:165-84.

4. Chopek M, McCullough J. Protein and biomedical changes during plasma exchange. In: Berkman EM, Umlas J, eds. Therapeutic hemapheresis. Washington, DC: American Association of Blood Banks, 1980:24-7.

5. Westphal RG. Complications of hemapheresis. In: Westphal RG, Kasprisin DO, eds. Current status of hemapheresis: Indications, technology and complications. Arlington, VA: American Association of Blood Banks, 1987:87-104.

6. Guideline for the collection of Platelets, Pheresis prepared by automated methods. Bethesda, MD: FDA Center for Biologics Evaluation and Research, 1988.

7. Boon JC, Jesch F, Ring J, Messmer K. Intravascular persistence of hydroxyethyl starch in man. Eur Surg Res 1977;8:497.

8. Mishler JM. New dosage regimens for HES during intensive leukapheresis. Transfusion 1978;18:126-7.

9. Strauss RG, Villhauer KM, Imig I, et al. Selecting the optimal dose of low-molecular weight hydroxyethyl starch (Pentastarch) for granulocyte collection. Transfusion 1987;27:350-2.

10. Ring J, Messmer K. Incidence and severity of anaphylactoid reactions of colloid volume substitutes. Lancet 1977;1:466-9.

11. Hinckley ME, Huestis DW. Premedication for optimal granulocyte collection. Plasma Therapy 1981;2:149-52.

12. Barnes A, DeRoos A. Increased granulocyte yields obtained with an oral three dose prednisone premedication schedule. Am J Clin Pathol 1982;78:267.

13. Slichter SJ. Mechanisms and management of platelet refractoriness. In: Nance SJ, ed. Transfusion medicine in the 1990's. Arlington, VA: American Association of Blood Banks, 1990: 95-179.

14. Schiffer CA. Prevention of alloimmunization against platelets. Blood 1991;77:1-4.
15. Kurtz SR, McMican A, Carciero R, et al. Plateletpheresis experience with the Haemonetics Blood Processor 30, the IBM Blood Processor 2997 and the Fenwal CS 3000 Blood Processor. Vox Sang 1981;41:212-8.
16. Dzik WH. Leukocyte-poor platelet products. In: McCarthy LJ, Baldwin ML, eds. Controversies of leukocyte-poor blood and components. Arlington, VA: American Association of Blood Banks, 1989:49-80.
17. Anderson KC, Gorgone BC, Wahlers E, et al. Preparation and utilization of leukocyte poor apheresis platelets. Transfus Sci 1991;12:163-70.
18. Sniecinski I, O'Donnell MR, Nowicki B, Hill LR. Prevention of refractoriness and HLA-alloimmunization using filtered blood products. Blood 1988;71:1402-7.
19. Holland PV. Prevention of transfusion-associated graft-vs-host disease. Arch Pathol Lab Med 1989;113:285-91.
20. Herzig RH. Granulocyte transfusion therapy: Past, present and future. In: Garratty G, ed. Current concepts in transfusion therapy. Arlington, VA: American Association of Blood Banks, 1985:267-94.
21. Cairo MS. The use of granulocyte transfusions in neonatal sepsis. Transfus Med Rev 1990; 4:14-22.
22. Schiffer CA. Granulocyte transfusions: An overlooked therapeutic modality. Transfus Med Rev 1990;4:2-7.
23. Strauss RG. Granulocyte transfusions: Uses, abuses and indications. In: Kolins J, McCarthy LJ, eds. Arlington, VA: American Association of Blood Banks, 1987:65-83.
24. McCullough J. The clinical significance of granulocyte antibodies and in vivo studies of the fate of granulocytes. In: Garratty G, ed. Current concepts in transfusion therapy. Arlington, VA: American Association of Blood Banks, 1985:125-81.
25. Lane TA. Granulocyte storage. Transfus Med Rev 1990;4:23-34.
26. Lasky LD, Smith JA, McCullough J, Zanjani ED. Three-hour collection of committed and multipotent hematopoietic progenitor cells by apheresis. Transfusion 1987;27:276-8.
27. Gianni AM, Siena S, Bregni M, et al. Granulocyte-macrophage colony-stimulating factor to harvest circulating haemopoietic stem cells for autotransplantation. Lancet 1989;2:580-5.
28. Huestis DW, Bove JR, Case J. Practical blood transfusion. 4th ed. Boston: Little Brown, 1988:367-89.
29. Collins JA. Problems associated with massive transfusion of stored blood. Surgery 1974;75:274-95.
30. Nusbacher J. Therapeutic hemapheresis. In: Myhre BA, ed. Clinics in laboratory medicine. Philadelphia: WB Saunders, 1982:87-106.
31. Lasky LC, Finnerty EP, Genis L, Polesky HF. Protein and colloid osmotic pressure changes with albumin and/or saline replacement during plasma exchange. Transfusion 1984;24:256-9.
32. Orlin JB, Berkman EM. Partial plasma replacement: Removal and recovery of normal plasma constituents. Blood 1980;56:1055-9.
33. Berkman EM, Hillyer CD. Plasma exchange in dysproteinemias. In: Rossi EC, Simon TL, Moss GS, eds. Principles of transfusion medicine. Baltimore, MD: Williams and Wilkins, 1991: 543-49.
34. Williamson LM, James V, Duncan SLB, Smith MF. Plasma exchange for Rhesus haemolytic disease: Outcome and follow-up of pregnancies over a 10-year period. Transfus Sci 1989;10:337-47.
35. Williams WJ, Katz VL, Bowes WA. Plasmapheresis during pregnancy. Obstet Gynecol 1990; 76:451-57.
36. Younger J, Umlas J. Rapid reduction of platelet count in essential hemorrhagic thrombocythemia by discontinuous flow plateletpheresis. Am J Med 1978;64:659-61.
37. Pineda AA, Brzica SM, Taswell HF. Continuous semicontinuous-flow blood centrifugation systems: Therapeutic applications with plasma, platelet and eosin-apheresis. Transfusion 1977; 17:407-16.
38. Taft EG, Sullivan SA. Leukapheresis in acute leukemia—is it necessary? In: Vogler WR, ed. Cytapheresis and plasma exchange: Clinical indications. New York: Alan R. Liss, Inc, 1982: 189-205.
39. Sloand EM, Klein HG. Therapeutic apheresis. In: Westphal RG, Kasprisin DO, eds. Current status of hemapheresis: Indications, technology and complications. Arlington, VA: American Association of Blood Banks, 1987:9-48.
40. Berkman E. Issues in therapeutic apheresis. N Engl J Med 1982;306:1418-20.
41. Karsh J, Klippel JH, Plotz PH, et al. Lymphapheresis in rheumatoid arthritis: A randomized trial. Arthritis Rheum 1981; 24:867-73.
42. Wallace D, Goldfinger D, Lowe C, et al. A double-blind, controlled study of lymphoplasmapheresis versus sham apheresis in rheumatoid arthritis. N Engl J Med 1982;306:1406-10.
43. Dwosh IL, Giles AR, Ford PM, et al. Plasmapheresis therapy in rheumatoid arthritis, a controlled, double-blind, crossover trial. N Engl J Med 1983;308:1124-9.
44. Beecher HK. The powerful placebo. JAMA 1955;159:1602-6.

45. AMA Panel on Therapeutic Plasmapheresis. Current status of therapeutic plasmapheresis and related techniques. JAMA 1985;253:819-25.
46. AABB Extracorporeal Therapy Committee. Guidelines for therapeutic hemapheresis. Bethesda, MD: American Association of Blood Banks, 1992.
47. Taft EG. Therapeutic apheresis. Hum Pathol 1983;14:235-40.
48. NIH Consensus Conference. The utility of therapeutic plasmapheresis for neurological disorders. JAMA 1986;256:1333-7.
49. AABB Hemapheresis Committee. Guidelines for transfusion review committees regarding hemapheresis procedures. Arlington, VA: American Association of Blood Banks, 1991.
50. Huestis DW. Risks and safety practices in hemapheresis procedures. Arch Pathol Lab Med 1989;113:273-8.
51. Huestis DW. Mortality in therapeutic haemapheresis (letter). Lancet 1983;1:1043.
52. Sutton DMC, Cardella CJ, Uldall PR, Deveber GA. Complications of intensive plasma exchange. Plasma Therapy 1981;2:19-24.
53. Silberstein LE, Naryshkin S, Haddad JJ, Strauss JF. Calcium homeostasis during therapeutic plasma exchange. Transfusion 1986;26: 151-5.
54. Barnes A, Taft EG. Therapeutic apheresis activities of AABB members. AABB News Briefs 1983;6:5-6.
55. Robinson A. Untoward reactions and incidents in machine donor apheresis. Transfusion Today 1990;7:7-8.
56. Rosenkvist J, Berkowitz A, Holsoe E, et al. Plasma exchange in myasthenia gravis complicated with complement activation and urticarial reactions using fresh frozen plasma as replacement solution. Vox Sang 1984;46:13-8.
57. Rubenstein MD, Wall RT, Wood GS, Edwards MA. Complications of therapeutic apheresis, including a fatal case with vascular occlusion. Am J Med 1983;75:171-4.
58. Leitman SF, Boltansky H, Alter HJ, et al. Allergic reactions in healthy platelepheresis donors caused by sensitization to ethylene oxide gas. N Engl J Med 1986;315:1192-6.
59. Boogaerts MA, Roelant C, Goossens W, Verwilghen RL. Complement activation and adult respiratory distress syndrome during intermittent flow apheresis procedures. Transfusion 1986;26:82-7.
60. Wing EJ, Bruns FJ, Fraley DC, et al. Infectious complications with plasmapheresis in rapidly progressive glomerulonephritis. JAMA 1980; 244:2423-6.
61. Rodnitzky RL, Goeken JA. Complications of plasma exchange in neurologic patients. Arch Neurol 1982;39:350-4.
62. Buchholz DH, Lin A, Snyder E, et al. Plasma separation using a hollow fiber membrane device. Transfusion 1986;26:145-50.
63. Rock G, Tittley P, McCombie N. Plasma collection using an automated membrane device. Transfusion 1986;26:269-71.
64. Pineda AA. New apheresis technologies. In: Westphal RG, Kasprisin DO, eds. Current status of hemapheresis: Indications, technology and complications. Arlington, VA: American Association of Blood Banks, 1987:71-86.
65. Berger GM, Firth JC, Jacobs P, et al. Three different schedules of low-density lipoprotein apheresis compared with plasmapheresis in patients with homozygous familial hypercholesterolemia. Am J Med 1990;88:94-100.
66. Lazarus HM, Cohen SB, Clegg DO, et al. Selective in vivo removal of rheumatoid factor by an extracorporeal treatment device in rheumatoid arthritis patients. Transfusion 1991;31: 122-128.
67. Handelsman H. Office of health technology assessment report, No. 7. Protein A columns for the treatment of patients with idiopathic thrombocytopenic purpura and other indications. Rockville, MD: DHHS, PHS, Agency for Health Care Policy and Research, 1991:1-8.
68. Moake JL. TTP—desperation, empiricism, progress. N Engl J Med 1991;325:426-8.
69. Krakauer RS, Asanuma Y, Zawicki I, et al. Circulating immune complexes in rheumatoid arthritis: Selective removal by cryogelation with membrane filtration. Arch Intern Med 1982;142:395-7.
70. Leitman SF. The role of apheresis in the adoptive immunotherapy of cancer. In: Westphal RG, Kasprisin DO, eds. Current status of hemapheresis: Indications, technology and complications. Arlington, VA: American Association of Blood Banks, 1987:105-24.
71. Koh HL. Extracorporeal photopheresis. In: Sacher RA, Brubaker DB, Kasprisin DO, McCarthy LJ, eds. Cellular and humoral immunotherapy and apheresis. Arlington, VA: American Association of Blood Banks, 1991:87-97.

3

Blood Components: Preparation, Storage and Shipment

The primary goals of procedures for the collection, preparation, storage and shipment of blood components are to: 1) maintain viability and function of each relevant constituent; 2) prevent physical and chemical changes detrimental to the constituents; and 3) minimize bacterial proliferation.

The anticoagulant-preservative solution prevents clotting and provides proper nutrients for continued metabolism and stabilization of cells during storage. As with other living systems, blood cells depend on a delicate biochemical balance of many materials for their integrity during storage, especially glucose, hydrogen ion (pH) and adenosine triphosphate (ATP). For rbcs, this balance is best preserved by storing at temperatures between 1-6 C and shipping at 1-10 C, whereas platelets and granulocytes retain better function when stored at room temperature (20-24 C). Labile coagulation factors in plasma are maintained at temperatures of –18 C or lower. Refrigeration or freezing also minimizes proliferation of bacteria that might have entered the unit during venipuncture or were present in the circulation of the donor.

Anticoagulation and Preservation

CPD, CP2D and CPDA-1

CPD and CP2D are anticoagulant-preservatives approved by the FDA for 21-day storage of RBCs maintained at 1-6 C.[1-3] Blood collected in CPDA-1 may be stored for up to 35 days at 1-6 C.[4,5]

Maintenance of ATP levels during storage correlates with posttransfusion viability in the recipient. The low storage temperature, 1-6 C, slows glycolytic activity. Dextrose is present in sufficient quantity to support continuing ATP generation by glycolytic pathways. CPD and CPDA-1 contain about 25 g/L of dextrose. CP2D contains twice this amount.[6] (See Table 3-1.) The added adenine in CPDA-1 provides a substrate from which rbcs can synthesize ATP, resulting in improved viability when compared to CPD without adenine.

The quantity of citric acid and sodium citrate in CPD, CP2D and CPDA-1 solutions is similar and sufficient to bind most of the ionized calcium present in the volume of whole blood for which the bag is designed.[6] Citrate prevents coag-

Table 3-1. Content of Anticoagulant-Preservative Solutions (g/L)[6, 31]

	ACD-A	CPD	CP2D	CPDA-1
Trisodium citrate	22.00	26.30	26.30	26.30
Citric acid	8.00	3.27	3.27	3.27
Dextrose	24.50	25.50	51.10	31.90
Monobasic sodium phosphate		2.22	2.22	2.22
Adenine				0.275

ulation by inhibiting the several calcium-dependent steps of the coagulation cascade. Additionally, it retards glycolysis. These anticoagulant-preservative solutions also contain sodium biphosphate to maintain a higher pH during storage. The ratio of anticoagulant-preservative in commercially available containers is 1.4 mL to 10 mL of blood.[6] The 63 mL volume in standard collection bags is suitable for 450 mL ± 10% of blood (ie, 405-495 mL). If lesser amounts are collected (300-404 mL) the RBCs can be used if the unit is labeled as "Low Volume Unit __mL Red Blood Cells."[7] Other components are not to be made from these units. When a donor's weight is less than the 50 kg (110 lb) minimum required or in other special circumstances, units with a volume less than 300 mL may be drawn if the anticoagulant solution is appropriately reduced prior to the collection procedure. (See p 11.)

Additive Systems

Currently approved by the FDA for extended storage of RBCs are systems in which a preservative solution to be added to the red cells for storage is present in addition to the anticoagulant-preservative solution used for whole blood collection. If components are prepared from the Whole Blood (WB) using additive systems or CPDA-1, the plasma or platelet-rich plasma must be separated from the rbcs within 8 hours of collection. If other components (FFP, PCs,

CRYO) are not made from the WB and it is refrigerated immediately after collection, RBCs with extended dating can be prepared if the additive solution is combined with the red cells as soon as possible but no later than 72 hours after phlebotomy.[3]

These additive systems consist of a primary collection bag containing an anticoagulant-preservative such as CPD or CP2D. To this bag are attached at least two satellite bags, one of which is empty and one of which contains the additive solution. FDA-approved additives include AS-1 (Adsol®), AS-3 (Nutricel®) and AS-5 (Optisol®). The additive is 100 mL of solution consisting of saline, glucose, adenine and other additives designed to enhance rbc survival and function.[6,8,9] (See Table 3-2.) When using additive solutions, maximum amounts of plasma can be recovered from WB, and RBCs with a hematocrit of about 0.60 (60%) are produced. Outside the US, other formulations (BAGPM, SAG, SAGMAN) of additive solutions have been used.[10]

Shelf Life

Maximum allowable storage time for RBCs, referred to as shelf life, has been defined by the requirement for 70% recovery at 24 hours [ie, at least 70% of the transfused cells (usually measured by a radiolabel) must remain in the recipient's circulation 24 hours after transfusion].[11] The FDA evaluates collection systems and anticoagulant-preservative solutions using 75% recovery at 24 hours

Table 3-2. Content of Additive Solutions (mM)[6]

	AS-1 (Adsol®)	AS-3 (Nutricel®)	AS-5 (Optisol®)
Dextrose	111.00	55.50	45.40
Adenine	2.00	2.22	2.22
Monobasic sodium phosphate	0	23.00	0
Mannitol	41.20	0	45.40
Sodium chloride	154.00	70.00	150.00

as the criterion for acceptability. Transfused rbcs that circulate after 24 hours will have a normal survival curve in the recipient.[12] Blood collected in ACD, CPD or CP2D may be stored for 21 days, although 24-hour recovery of rbcs is usually well over 70% at 21 days.[13] Blood collected in CPDA-1 may be stored up to 35 days. The additive solution systems approved for RBC storage permit a 42-day dating period.

Certain measurable biochemical changes occur when blood is stored at 1-6 C. These changes, some of which are reversible, are known as the "storage lesion" of blood. Changes for CPD and CPDA-1 stored blood are listed in Table 3-3 and those for additive systems are listed in Table 3-4. Except for oxygen-transporting functions, discussed below, these changes rarely have clinical significance and often they are reversed by the recipient's compensatory homeostatic mechanisms. Even in massive transfusion, the adverse effects of the rbc storage lesion are usually inconsequential unless the recipient is already severely compromised.

Oxygen Dissociation

The primary function of rbcs is to deliver oxygen from the lungs to the tissues. This function is mediated by a reversible

Table 3-3. Biochemical Changes of Blood Stored in CPD and CPDA-1

	CPD		CPD		CPDA-1	
Variable	Whole Blood		Whole Blood	Red Blood Cells	Whole Blood	Red Blood Cells
Days of Storage	0	21	0	0	35	35
% Viable Cells (24 hours post-transfusion)	100.00	80.00	100.00	100.00	79.00	71.00
pH (measured at 37 C)	7.20	6.84	7.60	7.55	6.98	6.71
ATP (% of initial value)	100.00	86.00	100.00	100.00	56.00 (±16)	45.00 (±12)
2,3-DPG (% of initial value)	100.00	44.00	100.00	100.00	<10.00	<10.00
Plasma K+ mmol/L	3.90	21.00	4.20	5.10	27.30	78.50*
Plasma Na+ mmol/L	168.00	156.00	169.00	169.00	155.00	111.00
Plasma hemoglobin mg/L	17.00	191.00	82.00	78.00	461.00	658.0*

*Values for plasma hemoglobin and potassium concentrations may appear somewhat high in 35-day stored RBC units; the total plasma in these units is only about 70 mL.

Table 3-4. Biochemical Changes of Red Blood Cells Stored in Additive Solutions (AS)

Variable	AS-3*		AS-1**
Days of storage	42	49	49
% Viable cells			
(24 hours posttransfusion)	83 ± 10	72 ± 9	76 (64-85)
ATP (% of initial value)	58.0	45.0	64.0
2,3-DPG (% of initial value)	<10.0	<15.0	<5.0
Plasma K+ (mmol/L)	NA	NA	6.5
pH	6.5	6.4	6.6
Glucose (mmol/L)	28.0	27.0	31.0
% hemolysis	0.8	0.9	0.5

*From Simon TL.[9]
**Based on manufacturer's submission to FDA (1983).

hemoglobin-oxygen equilibrium. In the lungs, where oxygen partial pressure (PO_2) is high, hemoglobin takes up oxygen to form oxyhemoglobin. In the tissues, where PO_2 is lower, hemoglobin releases oxygen. Hemoglobin may achieve 100% oxygen saturation in the lungs, and characteristically releases only some of the oxygen at the lower PO_2 of normal tissues. Oxygen saturation of hemoglobin varies at various PO_2 levels, a relationship that can be plotted as the oxygen dissociation curve. (See Fig 3-1.) Although the shape remains fixed, the position may shift to the right or left, depending on such variables as the presence or absence of rbc 2,3-diphosphoglycerate (2,3-DPG), pH and other factors. The degree of shift to the right or left can be determined by the P_{50} value, which is the partial pressure of oxygen at which hemoglobin is 50% saturated. A

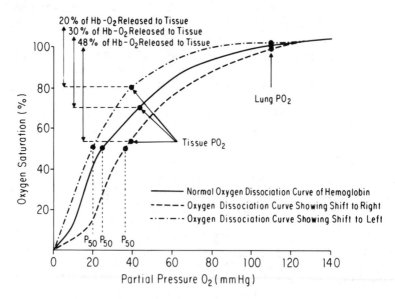

Figure 3-1. Oxygen dissociation curves under different conditions.

high P_{50} value means the curve has shifted to the right and more oxygen can be released at any given PO_2. A left shift means that the P_{50} is lower and less oxygen than normal is released at any given PO_2.[14]

In red cell storage and preservation it is important to minimize the rate of loss of oxygen-carrying and oxygen-releasing capacities of hemoglobin. The concentration of rbc 2,3-DPG influences the release of oxygen to the tissues. If 2,3-DPG levels are high, more oxygen is released at a given PO_2. Lower rbc levels of 2,3-DPG cause greater affinity of hemoglobin for oxygen so that less oxygen is released at the same PO_2. Concentrations of 2,3-DPG are affected by pH. The initial pH of blood collected in CPD and measured at the temperature of storage is approximately 7.4-7.5. As stored rbcs metabolize glucose to lactate, hydrogen ions accumulate, pH falls and 2,3-DPG declines. Table 3-3 tabulates these changes for CPD and CPDA-1. During the second week of storage, the pH of CPD-stored blood falls below 7.0. As pH drops, there is a fall in rbc 2,3-DPG. Concentrations of 2,3-DPG are normal in CPD-stored blood for about 10 days. When blood is stored in CPDA-1, 2,3-DPG levels initially fall slightly more rapidly than in CPD, but near normal levels are maintained for 12-14 days.[15,16]

Restoration of Function

Following transfusion, stored donor rbcs regenerate ATP and 2,3-DPG, resuming normal energy metabolism and hemoglobin function as they circulate in the recipient. It usually takes 3-8 hours for severely depleted cells to regenerate half of their 2,3-DPG levels and approximately 24 hours for complete restoration of 2,3-DPG and normal hemoglobin function.[17,18] In rbc storage, maintaining cell viability (ATP levels) is clearly a critical consideration, but the importance of maintaining levels of 2,3-DPG is less clear. On theoretical grounds, recipients likely to be most affected by low 2,3-DPG levels in transfused blood are those receiving massive quantities of stored blood in a short time, and those particularly vulnerable to the effects of tissue hypoxia; examples include newborns undergoing exchange transfusion and patients with small blood volume who receive large volumes of blood. Such patients usually receive "fresher" blood (less than 7 days old). Use of fresher blood with higher ATP levels and hence longer survival should be considered when transfusing patients who are likely to need repeated transfusions (ie, aplastic anemia, thalassemia, etc).

Stored red cells collected in CPD or CPDA-1 solutions, including those 3 days past the end of their allowable shelf life, can be rejuvenated with FDA-approved solutions containing pyruvate, inosine, phosphate and adenine (Rejuvesol®). Rejuvenated rbcs have increased levels of 2,3-DPG and ATP,[19] and can be gly-cerolized and frozen in the same manner as fresh rbcs. If rejuvenated rbcs are to be used within 24 hours they can be stored at 1-6 C; however, they must be washed before use to remove the inosine, which might be toxic to the recipient. These rbcs demonstrate normal oxygen transport when transfused.[20] (See p 58 for further discussion.)

Heparin

Heparin exerts its anticoagulant effect by potentiating the action of the endogenous plasma protein, antithrombin III (AT III). Synthesized in the liver, AT III is an inhibitor of most serine esterase clotting factors. Because it lacks dextrose, heparin serves only as an anticoagulant, not as a preservative. Heparinized blood must be transfused within 48 hours, preferably within 8 hours. Heparin is not recommended for routine blood collection. When blood collected in citrate is to be added to a heart/lung machine it first may be converted to heparinized blood by the addition of heparin followed by large amounts of calcium to neutralize the citrate and restore the concentration of ionized calcium to homeostatic levels.

Preparation of Components

Table 3-5 lists the proper names, commonly used terms and abbreviations for blood and components frequently used in transfusion practice.

Donor blood collected in plastic bags with integral tubing and attached satellite containers is usually processed to yield one or more of the following single-donor components: RBCs, PCs, FFP and CRYO. Multidonor pools of plasma harvested from whole blood or obtained by apheresis can be processed to yield derivatives such as albumin, plasma protein fraction, Factor VIII concentrate, immune serum globulin preparations and concentrates of Factor IX and Factor IX complex (II, VII, IX and X). Appropriate blood component therapy expands

Table 3-5. Blood and Blood Components

Proper Name*	Commonly Used Names	Abbreviation
(anticoagulant-preservative)		
Whole Blood	Whole blood	WB
Whole Blood Leukocytes Removed	Modified whole blood	
(anticoagulant-preservative)		
Red Blood Cells	Red blood cells, packed cells, red cell concentrates	RBCs
(additive designation)		
Red Blood Cells Adenine-Saline Added	Red blood cells	
Red Blood Cells Deglycerolized	Deglycerolized red blood cells, thawed red blood cells	D-RBCs
Red Blood Cells Rejuvenated Deglycerolized		
Red Blood Cells Leukocytes Removed by Filtration	Leukocyte-reduced red blood cells	LR-RBCs
Red Blood Cells Leukocytes Removed by Washing	Washed red blood cells	W-RBCs
Fresh Frozen Plasma	Fresh frozen plasma	FFP
Cryoprecipitated AHF	Cryoprecipitate, cryo, AHG	CRYO
Platelet-Rich Plasma	Platelet-rich plasma	PRP
Platelets	Platelet concentrate	PC
Platelets, Pheresis	Single-donor platelets, apheresis platelet concentrate	SD-PCs
Granulocytes, Pheresis	Granulocyte concentrate	GC
Granulocyte-Platelets Pheresis	Granulocyte-platelet concentrate	

*Terms used in Guidelines for the Uniform Labeling of Blood and Blood Components prepared by the AABB, CCBC, ABC and FDA-CBER, Draft: August, 1989.

the number of patients who can achieve therapeutic benefits from what is still a limited resource—human blood.

Blood Collection

To prevent activation of the coagulation system during collection, blood should be collected rapidly (4-7 minutes) and with minimal trauma to tissues. Ideally, there should be a single venipuncture and frequent, gentle mixing of the blood with the anticoagulant. Blood collection lasting longer than 10 minutes usually results from a poor venipuncture and slow blood flow.

Blood destined for component preparation should be drawn into bags with integrally attached satellite bags ("closed system") to avoid breaking the hermetic seal when separating components. If it is necessary to break the hermetic seal ("open system"), aseptic techniques and pyrogen-free equipment must be used. Breaking the hermetic seal is sometimes unavoidable—eg, in pooling PCs or CRYO prior to transfusion. When the hermetic seal has been broken, the resulting components must be used within 24 hours if stored at 1-6 C or within 4 hours if stored at 20-24 C.[21] If the resulting pool or component is to be stored frozen the dating is not affected.

When the final container is not the container used for collection, the source of the contents (original unit identification) must be on the final container. This applies to plasma and PCs as well as RBCs transferred to washing or freezing containers. Records must indicate that the transfer has been made. Secondary containers must be labeled while still attached to the primary container, either with the original unit number or by another means to relate it to the original unit number.

Sterile connecting (docking) devices make it possible to perform pooling and other manipulations of components using bags that were not part of the original container while maintaining the integrity of the system. The dating period of the components is the same as those prepared in a closed system except for platelets, which expire 4 hours after pooling.[3]

Centrifugation

Using large centrifuges requires caution. At high speeds, heavy rotor heads and cups develop a gravity force (g) of thousands of pounds. Contents in opposing cups must be equal in weight; eccentric loads cause impaired efficiency in centrifugation and irregular wear on the rotor. Swinging cups offer better cell-liquid interfaces for maximal removal of plasma than do fixed-angle cups. Blood bags sometimes have imperfections through which centrifuge pressures may force blood. Occasionally bags may rupture or the seals between tubing segments may leak during centrifugation. Overwrapping the bags with plastic prevents leakage into the cup if the blood or component bag breaks. The bag should be placed so that a broad side faces the outside wall of the centrifuge to reduce centrifugal force on the sealed margins.

Balancing material should be dry. Weighted rubber discs and large rubber bands are excellent, and are available in several thicknesses to provide flexibility in balancing without the need to cut discs.

Rotor size, speed and duration of spin are the critical variables in preparing components by centrifugation. Method 11.5 contains a guide for centrifugation, but these g values and spin times are approximations. *Each* centrifuge must be calibrated for optimal speeds and times of spin for each component prepared. The times listed include only the time of acceleration and "at speed," not the deceleration time. The automatic electronic braking devices on most centrifuges can decrease the deceleration time with minimal resuspension of centrifuged elements. Rapid manual braking can cause unacceptable resuspension of cells. The cover *must never be opened* until the machine has stopped.

Quality Control

Optimal conditions of speed and time for component preparation must be determined for each centrifuge in each laboratory and should be checked periodically. The most practical way to evaluate centrifugation is to scrutinize quality control data on components prepared in each centrifuge. For an example, see Method 11.5 for calculating yield in preparing PCs. If platelet concentrates give inconsistent yields, variables to examine include calibration of the centrifuge (see Method 11.5); the initial platelet count in the donors; storage time and conditions between blood collection and platelet preparation; or other parameters such as sampling technique and counting method. Records should be maintained that identify the individuals performing significant steps in the preparation of components. This may also be useful in evaluating erratic yields.

Red Blood Cells

Preparation

Most RBCs are prepared shortly after collection of whole blood. Blood collection containers with integrally attached transfer bags and/or additive solutions are usually used. RBCs may be allowed to sediment during refrigerated storage of the WB, or the cells and plasma may be separated by centrifugation at any time up to the date of expiration of the WB. A procedure for the preparation of RBCs is found in Method 10.4.

Expiration Date

After the plasma has been removed, RBCs must be refrigerated at 1-6 C. RBCs, without additive solutions, separated in a closed system and properly refrigerated, have the same expiration date as the WB from which they were separated, provided the hematocrit does not exceed 0.80 (80%). A red cell preparation with less than 20% plasma and anticoagulant-preservative solution undergoes accelerated aging during storage and the rbcs survive poorly when transfused.[22] It is important to verify that the method of preparing RBCs does not usually result in a hematocrit above 0.80 (80%). This can be done by measuring the hematocrit of units that have outdated. If additive solutions are used, the appropriate expiration date and the volume and nature of the additive must be noted on the label. If the hermetic seal was broken during processing, the RBCs must be transfused within 24 hours, and the new date and time of expiration must be noted on the label and in the records.

RBCs show a significant decrease in 2,3-DPG and ATP after storage at 1-6 C for several weeks. These depleted substances can be restored to normal levels by incubating the stored RBCs for 1 hour at 37 C with a rejuvenating solution. Rejuvenated RBCs regain normal characteristics of oxygen transport and delivery and improved posttransfusion survival.[19,20] It has been reported that rejuvenation of "fresh" blood can produce "super rbcs" with twice normal levels of 2,3-DPG.[23]

Rejuvenation may be performed up to 3 days after RBCs expire, provided they have been stored continuously at 1-6 C. After rejuvenation, the rbcs may be either: 1) washed, reconcentrated and transfused within 24 hours or 2) glycerolized and frozen.

Leukocyte-Reduced Red Blood Cells

Patients with severe and/or repeated febrile, nonhemolytic transfusion reactions often remain asymptomatic when transfused with LR-RBCs.[24] The designation "Leukocyte-Reduced Red Blood Cells" applies to those RBCs prepared by a method known to reduce the leukocyte number in the final component to less than 5×10^8 and to retain at least 80% of the original rbcs. This component is intended to prevent nonhemolytic febrile transfusion reactions. If LR-RBCs are intended for other purposes such as preventing CMV infection or alloimmunization, the method should reduce the leukocytes in the final component to less than 5×10^6.[21] The proper name for the component is "Red Blood Cells Leukocytes Removed by (method used)." Methods to remove leukocytes include filtration, centrifugation and washing.

Most reactions due to antileukocyte antibodies are dose-dependent. Thus in many cases a 50% reduction of the wbcs usually in a unit of RBCs (3.0×10^9) will prevent the reaction. However, in some patients even removal of 95% of the wbcs may not eliminate the febrile response. Methods for separating and removing the leukocytes from a donor unit can give variable results.[25] The method chosen must be appropriate for the anticoagulant and additive solution used as well as the age of the unit. The type of cells remaining after processing (ie, polymorphonuclear cells or lymphocytes) varies with each method.

Filtration Methods

A high efficiency (99%) of leukocyte removal can be achieved using commercially available polyester or cotton/wool filters. In most cases the filters need to be primed with saline and some pressure is needed to achieve reasonable flow rates. Multiple bag systems with additive solution and in-line filters for removing leukocytes prior to storage of the RBCs provide a method to obtain multiple components from the donor including LR-RBCs that can be stored for up to 42 days. Another approach to preparing LR-RBCs is to use a sterile connecting device to add a filter to the storage bag after testing has been completed. Studies have shown that early removal of leukocytes can minimize some of the storage lesions observed when rbcs are stored with leukocytes remaining.[26] Bacterial growth does not seem to be enhanced by early removal of wbcs.

Transfusion Through Microaggregate Blood Filters

Microaggregate blood filters capable of over 99% leukocyte removal have been effectively used to filter units just prior to transfusion or at the bedside. Studies have shown that bedside filtration of RBCs using nonwoven polyester in an acrylonitrate copolymer container is effective in preventing reactions in multitransfused patients with thalassemia.[27]

Preparation by Freezing and Deglycerolizing

Previously frozen, D-RBCs are leukocyte-reduced. See Chapter 5 for discussion of preparation of this leukocyte-reduced component, which has low levels of residual leukocytes and platelets and less plasma than any other leukocyte-reduced red cell component. AABB *Standards for Blood Banks and Transfusion Services*[21] requires that at least 80% of the original rbcs be recovered.

Washed Red Blood Cells

Washing RBCs is not the most efficient way to remove leukocytes[25] but it does remove most of the plasma. Febrile, nonhemolytic transfusion reactions may occur with transfusion of any component containing leukocytes. Patients who are IgA-deficient and have anti-IgA antibodies may have anaphylactic reactions following transfusion of blood or blood components containing IgA. Transfusing W-RBCs reduces the incidence of febrile, urticarial and, possibly, anaphylactic reactions.[28] Patients with anti-IgA may require blood from IgA-deficient donors, but rbcs washed at least five times with saline or D-RBCs may be satisfactory.

W-RBCs are prepared with the same kind of automated or semiautomated equipment used to deglycerolize Red Blood Cells, Frozen. Automated cell washers are more efficient than manual centrifugation techniques but they are more expensive. The washing process removes most of the plasma proteins and microaggregates. Variable amounts of platelets and leukocytes are removed by overriding the photo cell on automated machines or being sure to remove the buffy coat when doing a manual wash procedure. Red cells stored in CPDA-1 up to 35 days as WB or RBCs have been shown to have a normal survival after washing. W-RBCs must be used within 24 hours because preparation is in an open system.

Neocytes

Neocytes are relatively young red cells that may be desirable for transfusion to patients with thalassemia major or other conditions requiring chronic transfusion that may lead to transfusion-induced iron overload.[29] Several methods have been described for preparing neocyte-enriched units; however, in practice the theoretical advantages of providing longer lived rbcs have not been achieved.[30]

Plasma

Along with water and electrolytes, plasma contains albumin, globulins, coagulation factors and other proteins. Al-though it is not indicated as a replacement fluid in volume-depleted patients, plasma is sometimes appropriate for replacement of coagulation factors. Most of the coagulation factors are stable at refrigerator temperatures, except for Factor VIII and, to a lesser extent, Factor V. To maintain adequate levels of Factors V and VIII, freshly collected plasma must be stored frozen. (For further discussion of coagulation factors, see Chapter 17.)

Plasma is usually prepared from WB during the preparation of other components, such as RBCs and PCs. As a by-product of component preparation, plasma is separated according to the techniques described for these components (see below).

Plasma should be frozen in a manner that makes thawing and subsequent refreezing apparent. Some methods to accomplish this are:

1. Press a tube into the bag during freezing to leave an impression that disappears if the unit thaws.
2. Freeze plasma flat (horizontally) in the freezer but store it upright (vertically). An air bubble formed on the side of the bag during freezing will move to the top of the bag if thawing has occurred.
3. Place a rubber band around the middle of the bag of plasma prior to freezing, but cut it off after the unit is frozen, leaving an indentation that disappears with thawing.

The intended thawing procedure should be considered in developing a protocol for freezing since the configuration of the frozen unit may be critical for use of some of the available equipment (ie, the thickness of the frozen unit restricts use in some microwave thawing devices).

Fresh Frozen Plasma

To be labeled "Fresh Frozen Plasma," plasma must be separated from the red cells and placed at –18 C or below within 8 hours after collection. FFP can be obtained from a single unit of WB or from an apheresis donor. Using a closed system it is also possible to obtain approximately 400 mL of FFP "Jumbo Unit" from a plateletpheresis donor. *Standards* requires that FFP be stored at –18 C or lower, preferably –30 C or below. Stored at or below these temperatures, FFP has a dating period of 12 months after donation of the original unit of blood. Beyond this period, the Factor VIII may have decreased in some units to such an extent that the plasma is not optimal for treating patients deficient in this labile coagulation factor.

If many units of liquid plasma are placed in a mechanical freezer at the same time, freezing may be delayed. Rapid freezing can be accomplished by placing units in a dry ice-ethanol or dry ice-antifreeze bath; in layers between blocks of dry ice; in a blast freezer; or in a mechanical freezer maintained at –65 C or lower. If plasma is frozen in a liquid freezing bath, the plasma container must be overwrapped for protection from chemical alteration.

A procedure for the preparation of FFP appears in Method 10.8.

Liquid Plasma, Plasma (Formerly Called Single-Donor Plasma)

Plasma from a single donor may be prepared by separation from the red cells on or before the 5th day after the expiration date of the WB. If not frozen, Liquid Plasma must be stored at 1-6 C and may be kept for no more than 26 days from phlebotomy for CPD anticoagulant or 40 days for CPDA-1. When stored frozen at –18 C or lower this component is known as Plasma and may be kept up to 5 years.[31] The separation technique for these components is the same as for FFP.

If FFP has not been used after 1 year of storage at –18 C or colder it may be redesignated and relabeled "Plasma." Thus redesignated, Plasma has 4 more years of shelf life at –18 C or colder.

Plasma prepared from outdated whole blood is somewhat different from plasma originally prepared as FFP, the major changes being high levels of potassium and ammonia in plasma prepared after long contact with red cells. See Table 3-3 for storage changes in refrigerated blood.

If cryoprecipitate has been removed from WB or Plasma, this must be stated on the plasma label. Plasma from which cryoprecipitate has been removed must not be designated as FFP because it has been depleted of Factor VIII and fibrinogen.

In general there are very few, if any, clinical indications for the use of Liquid Plasma or Plasma. Most blood centers convert Liquid Plasma and Plasma to an unlicensed component, Recovered Plasma. This material is usually shipped to a fractionator for further manufacture (ie, production of albumin, coagulation concentrates and/or immune globulins). In order to ship Recovered Plasma it is necessary for the collection agency to have a "short supply agreement" with the manufacturer.[3,31] Since Recovered Plasma has no outdate, records for this component must be maintained indefinitely. Plasma collected from donors by plasmapheresis and intended for further manufacturing use is Source Plasma.

Cryoprecipitated AHF

CRYO is the cold-insoluble portion of plasma remaining after FFP has been thawed between 1-6 C. It contains approximately 50% of the Factor VIII (AHF), 20-40% of the fibrinogen and some of the Factor XIII originally present in the fresh plasma. CRYO contains both Factor VIII:C (the procoagulant activity) and Factor VIII:vWF (von Willebrand factor).

Standards requires that at least 75% of the bags of CRYO tested contain a minimum of 80 IU of Factor VIII. The *Code of Federal Regulations* (21 CFR 640.56) requires that there be an average of 80 IU of Factor VIII per final container and that a sample from at least four donor units be tested per month from units collected within the previous 30 days to determine the average (note: the units may be pooled before testing).[3,21] Each unit contains a variable amount of fibrinogen, usually 100-350 mg.[32] The amount present depends, in part, on the volume of residual plasma.[33] Testing for fibrinogen content is not required but is recommended if CRYO is used for fibrinogen replacement.

Use for von Willebrand's Disease or Hypofibrinogenemia

No components are available specifically for treating either von Willebrand's disease or hypofibrinogenemia. Although FFP can be used for temporary replacement therapy in both conditions, CRYO is a more suitable component because of its smaller volume. The cryoprecipitation process concentrates not only Factor VIII but also fibrinogen (Factor I) and von Willebrand factor.[34,35] In von Willebrand's disease, there is abnormal platelet function as well as deficiency of Factor VIII coagulation activity. Commercial Factor VIII concentrates have coagulation activity but do not reliably contain[35] von Willebrand factor needed for normal platelet function. CRYO may also be used to improve platelet function in uremic patients.

Fibronectin, an opsonic protein believed to participate in phagocytosis, is present in CRYO and other plasma components.[36] Because of its small volume, CRYO would be preferred over FFP should fibronectin therapy prove to be clinically useful.

CRYO has been found to be useful as part of the preparation of fibrin glue. When mixed with thrombin and calcium, CRYO applied topically stops bleeding. In some cases autologous plasma is collected preoperatively and CRYO is prepared for use as fibrin glue.[37]

Other uses for fibrin glue include the removal of kidney stones and stabilization of auditory ossicles.

Although some of the above described uses of CRYO do not involve intravenous infusion, each unit will still have a risk of transmitting disease (see Chapter 4).

Preparation

CPDA-1, CPD and ACD are suitable anticoagulants. The plasma may be obtained by apheresis or from whole blood units. A procedure for preparation of CRYO appears in Method 10.9.

Cryoprecipitated AHF Pooled

Units of CRYO can be pooled prior to labeling and storage. They should be pooled promptly after preparation, using an aseptic technique, and then be refrozen immediately to prevent possible bacterial growth and loss of labile coagulation factors.

Quality control procedures should ensure a minimum of 80 × "X" ("X" equals number of donor units in the pool) units of Factor VIII in the final pool container.

The component is to be labeled "Cryoprecipitated AHF Pooled" and the number of units pooled stated on the label. If saline has been added to facilitate pooling, the volume must appear on the label. The instruction "Use Within 4 Hours After Thawing" must be included on the label unless uniform labeling is used. In this case, the statement should appear in the *Circular of Information* rather than on the container label. The facility preparing the pool must maintain records of each individual donor traceable to the unique identifier used for the pooled component.[3,21]

Whole Blood Cryoprecipitate Removed

In the rare event WB is the desired component, it can be reconstituted after removal of the CRYO or platelets.

Aseptic removal of the platelets or CRYO requires that the blood be collected in a multibag collecting system or that a sterile connecting device be used. If the plasma is added back to the rbcs the blood must be labeled "Whole Blood Cryoprecipitate Removed"; platelet removal need not be noted on the label. Since WB stored more than 48 hours has few functional platelets and an unpredictably reduced level of Factor VIII, a unit modified by removing platelets and cryoprecipitate is functionally the same as stored Whole Blood.

Platelets

The concentrate of platelets prepared from a single unit of whole blood can temporarily elevate the platelet count by approximately $5\text{-}10 \times 10^9$/L in a 75-kg patient with thrombocytopenia.[38] Platelet transfusions are used to prevent spontaneous bleeding or stop established bleeding in patients with hypoplastic anemia, marrow failure, malignancies or chemotherapy-induced marrow suppression.

Platelet-rich plasma must be separated from Whole Blood by centrifugation within 8 hours after phlebotomy. Whole Blood intended for processing into PCs should not be cooled below 20-24 C prior to the harvest of the platelet-rich plasma. The platelets may then be concentrated by additional centrifugation and removal of most of the supernatant plasma. A procedure for preparation of PCs from single units of WB appears in Method 10.12. (A procedure for calibrating a centrifuge for optimal platelet yield is detailed in Method 11.5.)

Platelet concentrates prepared by hemapheresis are discussed in Chapter 2.

Aspirin in Donors

Aspirin-containing drugs irreversibly inhibit both in vitro and in vivo platelet activity. The effect is presumably caused by acetylation of platelet cyclo-oxygenase, which leads to reduced capacity to generate thromboxane A_2. Thus, platelets released when there is circulating salicylic acid are hemostatically ineffective. A donor who has taken a drug containing aspirin within 72 hours should not be the sole source of platelets for a single patient.[21,39] Since most adults receive multiple units, this becomes a consideration only when large numbers of platelets are collected from a single donor by apheresis or when the patient is an infant or small child who requires only one unit of PCs. Units of PCs prepared from donors who have ingested aspirin within 3 days of blood donation should be labeled so that the transfusion facility is aware that the donor has ingested aspirin and that platelet function may be impaired. In contrast to *Standards*, guidelines from the FDA for collection of Platelets, Pheresis state that platelets drawn from a donor 36 hours after ingestion of aspirin will have satisfactory function.[40]

Evaluating Platelet Concentrates

Evaluating the clinical response to transfusions of platelets can be an important part of quality assurance, but does not replace in vitro evaluation of the prepared concentrates. There must be at least 5.5×10^{10} platelets per bag in at least 75% of the units tested and the pH must be 6.0 or higher at the end of the allowable storage period. The FDA (CFR 640.25 b) requires that four units from individual donors be tested each month. Prior to issue, PCs should be inspected and units with grossly visible platelet aggregates after storage should not be used for transfusion.[21]

Leukocytes in Platelets

Many patients receiving PCs over a prolonged period of time develop a refractory state and do not get expected increments following transfusion. It has been shown that using HLA-matched donors or a platelet crossmatch test may lead to improved response in some patients who are refractory to ordinary platelets.[38,41,42] There are some studies that suggest manipulations of platelets, including leukocyte depletion, prevent the development of refractoriness. Leukocytes remaining in PC preparations may be responsible for the chills and fever that occur in many patients during a PC transfusion.[26,43,44]

Several methods have been developed to reduce the leukocyte content of PCs. These include filtration at the time of infusion or in the process of pooling,[45-47] washing and centrifugation.[48,49] Careful attention to detail in the preparation of PCs is important in minimizing the number of leukocytes remaining.[50] Quality control of PCs should include evaluation of residual leukocyte and red cell content. A procedure to remove leukocytes from apheresis platelets is detailed in Method 10.15.

Granulocytes

Granulocytes are usually prepared by leukapheresis as described in Chapter 2. They usually contain 1.0×10^{10} granulocytes per unit. They may be harvested prior to refrigeration from a freshly drawn donor unit for the treatment of a neonate; however, this component has a small number of granulocytes and may not be clinically effective.[51] Granulocytes may be stored at 20-24 C for up to 24 hours, though it is best to transfuse them as soon as possible after collection.

Storage of Blood and Components

It is permissible to store blood components, blood derivatives, blood samples from patients and donors, and reagents for blood bank tests in a refrigerator used for storing blood. Separate well-demarcated compartments must be available for anything other than blood or components when the refrigerator is used. The temperature in all areas of the refrigerator must be maintained between 1 and 6 C. The refrigerator must have a fan or be of capacity and design to ensure that the designated temperature is maintained throughout. The interior should be clean and adequately lighted, and there should be clearly apparent organization of storage areas labeled or designated for: 1) unprocessed blood, 2) labeled blood suitable for transfusion (autologous and allogeneic) and 3) rejected, outdated or quarantined blood.

Blood kept in sites outside the blood bank, such as surgical or obstetric suites, must be stored in refrigerators that meet the same standards. Temperature records are required for such refrigerators during periods of blood storage. Blood must never be stored in unmonitored refrigerators. It is best for the blood bank to assume responsibility for monitoring these refrigerators in the same way that blood bank refrigerators are monitored.

Monitoring Temperature

Recording thermometers and audible alarms are required for all blood storage refrigerators. The sensor for the temperature systems should be on a high shelf and must be in a liquid-filled container. Glass bottles or standard blood bags are generally used. These should contain water or other fluids to a volume no greater than the volume of the smallest component stored. RBCs usually have 250-350 mL volume, but if split units or pediatric units are stored, the sensors should be kept in a smaller volume. The alarm signal must be activated at a temperature that allows personnel to take proper action before the stored blood reaches undesirable temperatures. An acceptable range is 1-6 C. The electrical source for the alarm system must be separate from that of the refrigerator; either a continuously rechargeable battery or an independent electrical circuit served by an emergency generator is suitable.

In large refrigerators it is advisable to have at least two independent thermometers, one immersed with the continuous sensor and the other in a similar container on the lowest shelf on which blood is stored. The temperatures of the refrigerator determined by both these thermometers must be between 1 and 6 C at all times. These thermometers should be checked periodically and there must be a method to record the temperatures at least every 4 hours. If the thermometer immersed with the recorder sensor does not agree within 1 C with that shown on the automatic recorder, both should be checked against a National Institute of Standards and Technology certified thermometer, and suitable corrective action taken. It is desirable to record the temperatures from the two independent thermometers on the recorder chart when it is changed regularly. In large walk-in refrigerators, several thermometers should be used and placed in areas determined to reflect the possible range of temperature fluctuations.

Sophisticated automated monitoring systems are increasingly in use. Some refrigerators have automatic temperature monitor and digital readout systems as well as automatic alarms, with continuous temperature surveillance at various preset areas within the refrigerator. Another system is a central monitor and alarm system capable of monitoring numerous refrigerators simultaneously. This system has a visual alarm light, audible alarm, high and low activation temperature indicators and actual temperature display for all equipment connected with the system.

At the end of each time period, temperature charts from mechanical recording devices should be changed, dated inclusively and labeled to identify the refrigerator and the person changing the charts as well as the name of the facility. Any departure from normal temperature should be explained in writing on the chart beside the tracing. A chart that habitually traces a perfect circle suggests that the recorder is not functioning properly, because slight variations occur in any refrigerator that is actively used. Temperature records are retained as part of the blood bank records for at least 5 years to comply with *Standards* and requirements in the *CFR*.

Refrigerator and Freezer Alarms

Refrigerator and freezer thermometers and alarms should be checked periodically to ascertain that they are functioning properly. The temperatures of activation in refrigerators may be checked by following the procedure in Method 11.1.

Freezers must be equipped with a continuously recording thermometer and an audible alarm. The alarm should be checked periodically. Ideally, the alarm sensor should be accessible near the door of the freezer, but in some older units it is placed between the inner and outer freezer walls and its location is not apparent or accessible. In these cases, the site of the sensor can be determined from the manufacturer and a permanent mark placed on the wall at that location. The temperature of activation can be tested approximately by placing a flexible container (ie, water bottle) filled with cold tap water against the inner freezer wall where the sensor is located. When the alarm goes off, usually in a short time, the recording chart should be checked immediately to determine the temperature of activation. More details about checking freezer alarms are in Method 11.2. A useful way to measure the temperature of freezers that are at <–65 C is to obtain a thermocouple that responds at the desired temperature range. The output from the thermocouple can be easily read using a digital recording device that measures the difference in potential generated by the thermocouple. This difference can then be converted to temperature.

Freezers and refrigerators must have a source of electricity that operates independently of standard house circuits in case of a power failure, and it is extremely important that the alarms have a continuous power source. This should be tested periodically to ensure proper function. There must be written instructions for personnel to follow when the alarm sounds. These should include steps to determine the immediate cause of the temperature change and ways to handle temporary malfunctions, as well as steps to take in the event of prolonged power failure. It is important to list the names of key people to be notified and what steps should be taken to ensure that proper storage temperature is maintained for all blood, components and reagents.

Platelet Storage

PCs are to be stored at 20-24 C with continuous gentle agitation.[21] Shelf life and storage conditions may vary depending on the collection system used and the type of plastic bag used to store the component. The FDA (CFR 640.25 a) allows PC storage at 1-6 C for 72 hours with agitation optional. Refrigerated PCs do not maintain either function or viability as well as PCs stored at room temperature.[52]

Continuous gentle agitation is essential when platelets are stored at 20-24 C. Elliptical, circular and flat-bed agitators are available. The type of agitator and the type of plastic used for storing the platelets affect preservation of platelet function.[53] The types of platelet storage bags and the agitators giving best in vitro results[54,55] are:

1. Polyolefin without plasticizer (PL-732) for 5-day platelet storage on a circular rotator or flat-bed agitator. Elliptical rotators are not recommended.
2. Polyvinyl chloride with tri(2-ethylhexyl)trimellitate plasticizer (CLX) and PL-1240 for 5-day platelet storage on circular or elliptical agitators.

If the hermetic seal of any bag is broken, PCs should be used as soon as possible but must be transfused within 24 hours if stored at 1-6 C or within 4 hours if stored at 20-24 C.

Platelets collected using open-system procedures may be stored up to 24 hours at 20-24 C; those collected using closed-system apheresis procedures may be stored up to 5 days. Both must be stored using gentle agitation. As with PCs prepared from single units of WB, the type of agitation depends on the type of plastic used for the storage bag.

The temperature in the immediate vicinity of the platelet storage area must be monitored and recorded to ensure that the storage temperature is within the proper range (20-24 C).

Donor Blood Inspection

All stored WB and RBC units must be periodically examined, and it is required that each unit be inspected immediately before issue for transfusion or shipment to other facilities. Preissue inspections must be recorded and include the date, donor number and description of any abnormal units, the action taken and the identity of personnel involved. WB or RBC units with abnormal color or other appearance should be rejected for transfusion. Contamination should be suspected if the red cell mass looks purple, if a zone of hemolysis is observed just above the cell mass, if clots are visible or if the plasma or supernatant is murky. Purple, brown or red plasma can alert one to the possibility that blood is unsuitable for transfusion. A green hue in plasma, which is due to changes in bilirubin pigments caused by exposure to light, need not cause the unit to be rejected. The presence of blood or plasma at sealing sites in the tubing or in the ports may indicate inadequate sealing or closure, and renders the unit suspect and possibly unsuitable for transfusion. One should remember, however, that inspection of units will not always make it possible to detect contamination or other changes making the component unsuitable for transfusion.

Disposition

Blood units that are questionable for any reason should be quarantined until the responsible person decides their disposition. Evaluation of a questionable unit should include inverting it gently a few times to mix the cells and plasma. A great deal of undetected hemolysis, clotting or other alterations may have occurred in the undisturbed red cell mass. If, after sedimentation, the blood no longer appears abnormal, it may be returned to the available blood supply. Appropriate records should be completed by the responsible person.

Abnormal blood that cannot be released for transfusion should be returned to the provider or investigated to delineate the problem and the results of the investigation reported to the blood supplier. The findings may indicate the need for improvement in donor techniques, screening of donors or handling of blood units during processing. Disposal procedures must conform to the local public health codes for biohazardous waste. Autoclaving and/or incineration is recommended. If disposal is carried out off site, a contract with the waste disposal firm must be available and should specify that appropriate Environmental Protection Agency, state and local regulations are followed.[3]

Bacteriologic Examination

Routine sterility testing of blood or components is not required by the FDA or the AABB. Culturing may be desirable if inspection reveals abnormal appearance of blood or components, or if a patient has an adverse reaction clinically thought related to contaminated donor blood. A Gram's-stained smear of supernatant plasma should be made. If sealed segments remain, these should be carefully examined and cultured. Note: if a culture is taken from a segment, the volume of medium used will have to be adjusted appropriately.

If the sterility studies are done in another laboratory or institution, the director of the blood bank must ascertain that they have been done properly and reported to the blood bank adequately. Positive cultures should arouse suspicion of inadequate donor arm preparation or improper pooling technique. The health of the blood donor should be evaluated; also, if one component is contaminated, other components prepared from the same donor unit should be checked.

Reissuing Blood

Blood that has been returned to the blood bank must not be reissued for transfusion until the following conditions have been met:

1. The container closure must not have been penetrated or entered in any manner. This is to be certain that sterility is maintained.
2. The blood must have been maintained continuously between 1 and 10 C, preferably 1-6 C. Warming the blood beyond these limits, even with subsequent cooling, tends to accelerate red cell metabolism, produce hemolysis and may permit bacterial growth in the unit. Most transfusion services will not reissue a unit of blood that has remained out of a monitored refrigerator longer than 30 minutes.
3. At least one sealed segment of integral donor tubing must remain attached to the container if the blood has left the premises of the issuing facility.
4. Records must indicate that the blood has been reissued and has been inspected prior to reissue.

Inspection of Other Components

Platelets: Prior to issue or pooling, PCs should be inspected for the presence of grossly visible aggregates. If these are present the component should not be used for transfusion.

Fresh Frozen Plasma: When removed from frozen storage, each unit should be inspected to determine that thawing has not occurred.

Transportation of Blood Components

Whole Blood and Red Blood Cell Components

The temperature of WB and RBC components must be kept at 1-10 C during transport. Sturdy, well-insulated cardboard and/or styrofoam shipping containers maintain these temperatures if they contain adequate cooling material. The refrigerant recommended for most shipments is wet ice in leakproof containers such as plastic bags. Wet ice from commercial ice-making machines is satisfactory. Super-cooled cubed ice or canned ice and dry ice should not be used for shipping or storing WB or RBCs because they can cause local temperatures low enough that red cells in their immediate vicinity may undergo hemolysis. Blood shipped by air may freeze if transported in an unpressurized storage compartment. The cargo compartments of buses and trucks often reach temperatures above 100 F. The temperature of the blood or components should be monitored closely upon receipt.

Ice should be placed above the blood because cool air moves downward. During long hot trips, separation between the ice and the blood bag should be minimal; a layer of cardboard or an air space between ice and blood may act as internal insulation, preventing the ice from adequately protecting the blood from high environmental temperatures. In very hot weather and during trips of several hours, placing wet ice under as well as above the blood is necessary. Cubed wet ice may be better than chipped or broken ice for long distance shipments of blood because it melts slowly. In boxes shipped long distances or at high environmental temperatures, the volume of ice should at least equal that of the blood. In an insulated container, the temperature will usually be in the 1-6 C range as long as unmelted ice remains in the box and is in contact with the blood.

Monitoring shipping temperatures (see Method 11.3) of WB and RBCs may uncover a need for better insulated containers or larger amounts of ice. Record forms, periodically placed in shipping cartons for completion and return by blood bank personnel receiving blood shipments, provide written evidence of sufficient ice and insulation. It is the responsibility of the shipping or issuing facility to ascertain that shipping practices satisfactorily maintain the temperature below 10 C during transportation.

Follow-Up Actions

Blood exposed to temperatures above 10 C is not necessarily unsuitable for transfusion. The disposition of the unit is best decided by experienced personnel. Factors such as the length of time in shipment, mode of transportation, magnitude of variance over 10 C, presence of residual ice in the shipping box and the presence of hemolysis should be taken into account. One should also consider the age of the unit and how much longer it is likely to be stored before use. Units that have exceeded the usual limits of storage should be placed in quarantine and carefully reinspected before issue. The shipping facility should be notified whenever unacceptably high temperatures are noted.

Mobile Collection Facilities

When blood is shipped from a mobile collection facility to the component preparation laboratory for processing, cooling must be as outlined above, except that those units destined for platelet separation must not be chilled below 20 C because platelets are best separated from WB at room temperature. Such units should be transported from collection site to component preparation laboratory

as soon as possible, but elapsed time between collection and centrifugation for platelet harvest must not exceed 8 hours.

In-House Transport

Issue of WB or RBCs from the blood bank to other parts of the hospital must be controlled so that unused blood is returned within a set period of time. Because blood at 1-6 C warms to 10 C or above in approximately 30 minutes at room temperature, transfusion should ordinarily be started or the unit returned to the blood bank within 30 minutes. If a slightly longer time must elapse before transfusion, individual units may be placed in an insulated paper bag precooled to 1-6 C. Picnic chests or insulated plastic buckets with lids are useful for issuing blood to operating rooms. The insulated container maintains the appropriate temperature and conveniently segregates blood for the individual patient in the operating room.

Frozen Components

During transport, frozen components must be maintained at or below the required storage temperature. This can be achieved with a suitable quantity of dry ice in well-insulated containers or standard shipping cartons lined with insulating material such as plastic air bubble packaging or dry packaging fragments. The dry ice, obtained as sheets, should be layered at the bottom of the container, between each layer of frozen components, and on top. The use of dry ice "snow" (delivered by spray from a CO_2 tank) is useful for filling the nooks and crannies between components. This not only provides some physical cushioning that helps prevent breakage, but it also establishes a freezing temperature. Each shipping facility must determine optimal conditions for shipping frozen components depending on the temperature requirements of the component, the distance to be shipped, the shipping container used and the ambient temperature encountered. On receipt, the shipment temperature should be taken and deviations from the expected temperature should be reported to the shipping facility.

Platelets and Granulocytes

Every reasonable effort must be made to ensure that platelets and granulocytes are maintained at temperatures about 20-24 C during shipment. A well-insulated container without added ice is often sufficient. If outdoor temperatures are extreme and the distance is great, these components should not be shipped in luggage or freight compartments without heating or air conditioning (depending on the time of year). If outdoor temperatures are extremely high, special chemical coolant pouches are available that may be shipped with the components and will maintain temperatures of approximately 20-24 C for up to 12 hours. Also available are containers with a power source that maintains temperatures between 20 and 24 C.

Special Considerations

Thawing Fresh Frozen Plasma for Transfusion

FFP must be thawed at temperatures between 30 and 37 C. If a waterbath is used, it is important to prevent water from contaminating the entry port.[56] This can be accomplished by wrapping the container in a plastic overwrap, or by maintaining the container in an upright position with entry ports above the water level. Microwave warmers that have been demonstrated not to exceed acceptable temperature limits and that do not damage the plasma proteins are acceptable

for thawing FFP. Warning devices that indicate when the temperature exceeds acceptable limits must be present. As with any device, SOPs for quality control of the indicated function must be established. *Standards* requires that thawed FFP used for correction of labile coagulation factor deficiencies be stored at 1-6 C and be infused within 24 hours after thawing. FFP unused within the allowable time after thawing should not be used to correct deficiencies of labile coagulation factors.

Thawing Cryoprecipitated AHF

CRYO must be thawed at temperatures between 30-37 C. After thawing it should be transfused within 6 hours if it is being used as a source of Factor VIII.

Handling Donor Units

Blood should not remain at room temperature unnecessarily. It is desirable to monitor routine handling procedures to ensure that personnel do not keep blood out of the refrigerator too long. When units are removed from the refrigerator for testing or labeling, a fluid-filled container with a thermometer may be removed from the blood refrigerator along with the units to be labeled. The temperature in this container should be observed, and if it rises to near 6 C, the blood should be returned to the refrigerator without delay.

When blood is issued for transfusion, it should not be allowed to remain unnecessarily long at room temperature. Delayed delivery to the patient, delayed arrival of equipment or personnel to begin transfusion and delays during infusion are all undesirable. Transfusion therapy teams trained in handling and infusing blood and components have been effective in reducing mishandling of donor blood.

Labels

The following information is required in clear, readable letters on a label firmly attached to all blood and blood component containers:

1. The proper name of the component, in a prominent position.
2. ABO and Rh type (not required for CRYO) and interpretation of unexpected antibody tests when positive (not required for D-RBCs, rejuvenated or washed RBCs).
3. The name and address of the blood bank that collected the blood and/or prepared the component; if FDA licensed, its license number. For components, the label must include the name and location of all facilities performing any part of component preparation.
4. A unique numeric or alphanumeric identification relating the unit to the donor. If the component is a pool of donor units, the identification of the individual donor units in the pool must be maintained by the facility preparing the pool and should not be on the label.
5. The expiration date, including the date and year, and when applicable, the hour.
6. Essential instructions or precautions for use, including a warning that the "product may transmit infectious agents," a statement "Caution: federal law prohibits dispensing without a prescription" and "Properly Identify Intended Recipient".[3]
7. Recommended storage temperature.
8. Reference to the *Circular of Information* that shall be available for distribution, containing dosage information, adequate directions for use, route of administration, contraindications and other directions if component is not intended for further manufacturing.
9. Quantity of component in container, which shall be accurate within ± 10%, except that the quantity of cryoprecipitate need not be stated on the label.
10. The amount of blood collected and the kind and quantity of anticoagulant (not required for CRYO).
11. Additives, sedimenting agents and cryoprotective agents added to the component that may still be present in the component.
12. Results of unusual tests or procedures performed when necessary for safe and effective use. Routine tests done to ensure the safety of the unit need not be on the label if they are listed in the *Circular of Information*.
13. The appropriate donor classification statement, "autologous donor," "paid donor" or "volunteer donor" in no less prominence than the proper name of the component.
14. If intended for autologous use, the statement "For Autologous Use Only" if the donor or donor unit fails to meet all usual criteria for acceptability.
15. Pooled components must include the name and final volume of the component and a unique identification of the pool. The number of units in the pool, ABO and Rh type (not required for CRYO) of all units in the pool must be on the label or an attached tie tag.

Records

Records must be made concurrently with each step of component preparation, must be legible and indelible, must identify the person immediately responsible, must include dates of various steps and must be as detailed as necessary for clear understanding. For specific records to be kept for each component, see Chapter 23.

References

1. Gibson JG, Gregory CB, Button LN. Citrate-phosphate-dextrose solutions for preservation of human blood: A further report. Transfusion 1961;1:280-7.

2. Bailey DN, Bove JR. Chemical and hematological changes in stored CPD blood. Transfusion 1975;15:244-9.

3. Instruction booklet for blood bank inspection checklist and report. Form FDA-2690. Washington, DC: US Government Printing Office, May 1991.

4. Zuck TF, Bensinger TA, Peck CC, et al. The in vivo survival of red blood cells stored in modified CPD with adenine: Report of a multi-institutional cooperative effort. Transfusion 1977;17:374-82.

5. Valeri CR, Valeri DA, Gray A, et al. Viability and function of red blood cell concentrates stored at 4 C for 35 days in CPDA-1, CPDA-2 or CPDA-3. Transfusion 1982;22:210-6.

6. Beutler E. Preservation of liquid red cells. In: Rossi EC, Simon TL, Moss GS, eds. Principles of transfusion medicine. Baltimore, MD: Williams and Wilkins, 1991:47-56.

7. Davey RJ, Lenes BL, Casper AJ, Demets DL. Adequate survival of red cells from units "undercollected" in citrate-phosphate-dextrose-adenine-one. Transfusion 1984;24:319-22.

8. Heaton A, Miripol J, Aster R, et al. Use of Adsol® preservative solution for prolonged storage of low viscosity AS-1 red blood cells. Br J Haematol 1984;57:467-78.

9. Simon TL, Marcus CS, Myhre BA, Nelson EJ. Effects of AS-3 nutrient-additive solution on 42 and 49 days of storage of red cells. Transfusion 1987;27:178-82.

10. Högman CF. Liquid storage of human erythrocytes. In: Harris JR, ed. Blood separation and plasma fractionation. New York, NY: Wiley-Liss, 1991:63-97.

11. Mollison PL. Methods of determining the post-transfusion survival of stored red cells. Transfusion 1984;24:93-6.

12. Valeri CR. Viability and function of preserved rbcs. N Engl J Med 1971;284:81-8.

13. Bowman HS. Red cell preservation in citrate-phosphate-dextrose and in acid-citrate-dextrose. Transfusion 1963;3:364-7.

14. Huestis DW, Bove JR, Case J. Practical blood transfusion. 4th edition. Boston: Little, Brown and Company, 1988.

15. Simon ET. Adenine in blood banking. Transfusion 1977;17:317-25.

16. Åkerblom OCH, Kreuger A. Studies on citrate-phosphate-dextrose (CPD) blood supplemented with adenine. Vox Sang 1975;29:90-100.

17. Beutler E, Wood L. The in vivo regeneration of red cell 2,3-diphosphoglyceric acid (DPG) after

18. transfusion of stored blood. J Lab Clin Med 1969;74:300-4.

18. Collins JA. Abnormal hemoglobin-oxygen affinity and surgical hemotherapy. In: Collins JA, Lundsgaard-Hansen P, eds. Surgical hemotherapy. Basel: S Karger, 1980.

19. Valeri CR, Gray AD, Cassidy GP, et al. The 24-hour posttransfusion survival, oxygen transport function, and residual hemolysis of human outdated-rejuvenated red cell concentrates after washing and storage at 4 C for 24 to 72 hours. Transfusion 1984;24:323-6.

20. Valeri CR, Zaroulis CG, Vecchione JJ, et al. Therapeutic effectiveness and safety of outdated human red blood cells rejuvenated to restore oxygen transport function to normal, frozen for 3 to 4 years at −80 C, washed, and stored at 4 C for 24 hours prior to rapid infusion. Transfusion 1980;20:159-70.

21. Widmann FK, ed. Standards for blood banks and transfusion services. 15th ed. Bethesda, MD: American Association of Blood Banks, 1993.

22. Beutler E, West C. The storage of hard-packed red blood cells in citrate-phosphate-dextrose (CPD) and CPD-adenine (CPDA-1). Blood 1979;54:280-4.

23. Valeri CR, Yarnoz M, Vecchione JJ, et al. Improved oxygen delivery to the myocardium during hypothermia by perfusion with 2,3-DPG-enriched red blood cells. Ann Thorac Surg 1980;30:527-35.

24. Perkins HA, Payne R, Ferguson J, Wood M. Nonhemolytic febrile transfusion reactions: Quantitative effects of blood components with emphasis on isoantigenic incompatibility of leukocytes. Vox Sang 1966;11:578-600.

25. Wenz B. Clinical and laboratory precautions that reduce the adverse reactions, alloimmunization, infectivity, and possible immunomodulation associated with homologous transfusions. Transfus Med Rev 1990;4(Suppl 1):3-7.

26. Brecher ME, Pineda AA, Torloni AS, et al. Prestorage leukocyte depletion: Effects on leukocyte and platelet metabolites, erythrocyte lysis, metabolism, and in vivo survival. Semin Hematol 1991;28(Suppl 5):3-9.

27. Sirchia G, Rebulla A, Parravicini V, et al. Leukocyte depletion of red cell units at the bedside by transfusion through a new filter. Transfusion 1987;27:402-5.

28. Goldfinger D, Lowe C. Prevention of adverse reactions to blood transfusion by the administration of saline-washed red blood cells. Transfusion 1981;21:277-80.

29. Corash L, Klein H, Deisseroth A, et al. Selective isolation of young erythrocytes for transfusion support of thalassemia major patients. Blood 1981;57:599-606.

30. Menitove JE. Transfusion in hypoproliferative anemias. In: Rossi EC, Simon TL, Moss GS,

eds. Principles of transfusion medicine. Baltimore, MD: Williams and Wilkins, 1991:151-6.

31. US Department of Health and Human Services, Food and Drug Administration. The code of federal regulations, 21 CFR (see 640.30, 601.22). Washington, DC: US Government Printing Office, 1992. (Revised annually.)

32. Ness PM, Perkins HA. Cryoprecipitate as a reliable source of fibrinogen replacement. JAMA 1979;241:1690-1.

33. Hoffman M, Koepke JA, Widmann FK. Fibrinogen content of low-volume cryoprecipitate. Transfusion 1987;27:356-8.

34. Burka ET, Harker LA, Kasper CK, et al. A protocol for cryoprecipitate production. Transfusion 1975;15:307-11.

35. Weinstein M, Deykin D. Comparison of Factor VIII-related von Willebrand factor proteins prepared from human cryoprecipitate and Factor VIII concentrate. Blood 1979;53:1095-105.

36. Snyder EL, Ferri PM, Mosher DF. Fibronectin in liquid and frozen stored blood components. Transfusion 1984;24:53-6.

37. Gibble JW, Ness PM. Fibrin glue: The perfect operative sealant?. Transfusion 1990;30:741-7.

38. Slichter SJ. Mechanisms and management of platelet refractoriness. In: Nance SJ, ed. Transfusion medicine in the 1990's. Arlington, VA: American Association of Blood Banks 1990:95-179.

39. Stuart MJ, Murphy S, Oski FA, et al. Platelet function in recipients of platelets from donors ingesting aspirin. N Engl J Med 1972;287: 1105-9.

40. Parkman PD. Guideline for the collection of platelets, pheresis prepared by automated methods. Bethesda, MD: FDA Center for Biologics Evaluation and Research, Oct. 7, 1988.

41. Schiffer CA. Prevention of alloimmunization against platelets. Blood 1991;77:1-4.

42. Kooy MvM, van Prooijen HC, Moes M, et al. Use of leukocyte-depleted platelet concentrates for prevention of refractoriness and primary HLA alloimmunization: A prospective, randomized trial. Blood 1991;77:201-5.

43. Anderson KC, Gorgone BC, Wahlers E, et al. Preparation and utilization of leukocyte poor apheresis platelets. Transfus Sci 1991;12:163-70.

44. Mangano MM, Chambers LA, Kruskall MS. Limited efficacy of leukopoor platelets for prevention of febrile transfusion reactions. Am J Clin Pathol 1991;95:733-8.

45. Brubaker DB, Romine CM. The in vitro evaluation of two filters (Erypur and Imugard IG 500) for white-cell-poor platelet concentrates. Transfusion 1988;28:383-5.

46. Sirchia G, Parravicini A, Rebulla P, et al. Preparation of leukocyte-free platelets for transfusion by filtration through cotton wool. Vox Sang 1983;44:115-20.

47. Sniecinski I, O'Donnell MR, Nowicki B, Hill LR. Prevention of refractoriness and HLA-alloimmunization using filtered blood products. Blood 1988;71:1402-7.

48. Mintz PD, Cullis HM, Pearson TH. A technique to reduce lymphocyte contamination of plateletapheresis products collected with a centrifugal blood cell separator. Transfusion 1987;27: 159-61.

49. Schiffer CA, Patten E, Reilly J, Patel S. Effective leukocyte removal from platelet preparations by centrifugation in a new pooling bag. Transfusion 1987;27:162-4.

50. Champion AB, Carmen RA. Factors affecting white cell content in platelet concentrates. Transfusion 1985;25:334-8.

51. Cairo MS. The use of granulocyte transfusions in neonatal sepsis. Transfus Med Rev 1990;4: 14-22.

52. Slichter SJ. Controversies in platelet transfusion therapy. Annu Rev Med 1980;31:509-40.

53. Moroff G, Holme S. Concepts about current conditions for the preparation and storage of platelets. Transfus Med Rev 1991;5:48-59.

54. Snyder EL, Koerner TAW Jr, Kakaiya R, et al. Effect of mode of agitation on storage of platelet concentrates in PL-732 containers for 5 days. Vox Sang 1983;44:300-4.

55. Snyder EL, Bookbinder M, Kakaiya R, et al. 5-day storage of platelet concentrates in CLX containers: Effect of type of agitation. Vox Sang 1983;45:432-7.

56. Rhame FS, McCullough JJ. Follow-up on nosocomial Pseudomonas cepacia infection. MMWR 1979;28:409.

4

Transfusion-Transmitted Viruses

Hepatitis

Hepatitis is an inflammatory condition of the liver often caused by viral infection. The hepatitis acquired during epidemics in the United States is usually due to the hepatitis A virus (HAV), although sporadic HAV cases may also occur. Formerly called infectious hepatitis, hepatitis A is usually spread by the fecal-oral route and is very rarely transmitted by blood components.[1] Hepatitis acquired after parenteral exposure to infected blood or body fluids, or to needles or equipment contaminated with infected blood, is usually due to the hepatitis B virus (HBV) or hepatitis C virus (HCV). Until recently, HCV was usually referred to as one of the undefined agents that cause non-A,non-B (NANB) hepatitis.[2] It is becoming increasingly clear that HCV is responsible for almost all transfusion-transmitted NANB hepatitis cases as well as the majority of sporadic NANB hepatitis cases.3 There may be additional agents (non-A,non-B,non-C) that cause cases of parenteral and sporadic hepatitis. Another virus, hepatitis E virus (HEV), has been identified as the cause of an epidemic enteric form of disease.[4] Hepatitis delta virus (HDV) can also result in infection after parenteral exposure. HDV is a defective RNA virus that requires HBV to infect the host.[5] Table 4-1 lists the serologic tests used in the diagnosis of hepatitis and includes terms and abbreviations in current use.

Hepatitis B (formerly called serum hepatitis) and hepatitis C (previously called NANB hepatitis) can occur after transfusion of blood components and derivatives. However, injection of intramuscular immune serum globulin preparations licensed by the Food and Drug Administration (FDA) has never been implicated in the transmission of viral hepatitis. Monoclonal affinity purified heat-treated Factor VIII and properly heat-treated albumin or plasma protein solutions rarely, if ever, transmit viral hepatitis.[6,7] Acute liver dysfunction with or without jaundice developing up to 1 year after transfusion may be from a hepatitis virus transmitted by the blood or blood components. Cases of suspected transfusion-transmitted disease must be investigated and reported to the facility collecting the blood.[8]

Serologic Markers of Hepatitis

Healthy individuals with a negative history can be carriers of one or more hepatitis viruses. For two of the viruses that cause posttransfusion hepatitis (HBV and HCV) laboratory tests are available to identify markers of infectivity (viral antigens and antibodies) and/or evidence of prior exposure to the viruses (viral antibodies). (See Table 4-1.)

Blood from individuals with proven circulating HBsAg may infect others.[9] An asymptomatic HBsAg-positive individual may be a chronic carrier of HBV or may be in the incubation phase of

Table 4-1. Serologic Tests in the Diagnosis of Viral Hepatitis

Agent			Test Reactivity				Interpretation
B Virus	HBsAg	Anti-HBc		Anti-HBs	HBeAg	Anti-HBe	
		Tot.	IgM				
	+	+/−*	+/−	−	+/−	−	Early acute HBV before symptoms
	+	+	+	−	+	−	Acute HBV
	−	+	+	−	+/−	+/−	Convales. HBV or possible chronic carrier
	+	+	−	−	+/−	+/−	Chronic carrier[†]
	−	+	−	+	−	+	Recovered HBV
	−	−	−	+	−	−	Vaccinated or recovered HBV
	−	+	−	−	−	−	? Recovered HBV
D Virus	HBsAg	Anti-HBc		Anti-HBs		Anti-delta	
	+	+		−		+	Acute HDV or chronic HDV
	−	+		+		+	Recovered HDV
A Virus	Anti-HAV						
	Tot.	IgM					
	+	+					Acute HAV
	+	−					Recovered HAV or vaccinated
C Virus	Anti-HCV (Screen)		Recombinant Antigens				
		C-100-3	5-1-1	C22-3	C33-c		
	+	Not Available					Possible acute or chronic HCV
	+	+	+	+	+		Probable chronic HCV
	+	+	+	+	−		? acute
	+	+	+	−	−		HCV
	+	−	−	+	+		
	+	−	−	−	−		? false positive
E Virus	Anti-HEV[‡]						
	Tot.	IgM					
	+	+					Acute HEV
	+	−					Recovered HEV

Abbreviations used include: HBsAg (hepatitis B surface antigen), anti-HBc (antibody to hepatitis B core antigen), anti-HBs (antibody to HBsAg), HBeAg (hepatitis B antigen), anti-HBe (antibody to HBeAg), anti-delta (antibody to delta antigen), anti-HAV (antibody to hepatitis A virus), anti-HCV (antibody to hepatitis C virus) and anti-HEV (antibody to hepatitis E virus).

*May be either positive or negative.

†Those with HBeAg are more infectious and likely to transmit vertically.

‡Not commercially available as of 9/92.

acute hepatitis B. Testing of blood can detect as little as one nanogram of HBsAg per mL; however, a viral inoculum containing as little as one picogram per mL may transmit hepatitis.[10] Data on the infectivity of blood from individuals with reactive tests for anti-HCV are less certain. In the absence of a confirmatory test the reported rate of infectivity with first-generation tests is 30-90%.[11-14] A comparison of samples collected during the 1976-1979 Transfusion-Transmitted Virus Study (TTVS) showed that of patients with NANB hepatitis, 46 and 60% were detected by first- and second-generation anti-HCV tests, respectively.[15] If the donor is shown to be positive with a supplemental assay, infectivity rates of 80-90% have been reported.[16,17]

Figure 4-1 illustrates the usual sequence of laboratory findings in an individual with acute HBV infection that resolves. Individuals with circulating HBsAg usually have simultaneous presence of antibody to anti-HBc and either of two additional HBV markers, HBeAg or its antibody (anti-HBe). Anti-HBc without detectable HBsAg or anti-HBs may, in rare individuals, indicate the presence of hepatitis B virus in the liver or the blood.[9,18] The time when anti-HBc is circulating after the disappearance of HBsAg and before the appearance of anti-HBs is called the core antibody window. The observation that some donors suspected to be infectious have only anti-HBc suggests that testing of donor blood for this marker as well as for HBsAg might reduce the incidence of transfusion-associated HBV infection.[19,20] The simultaneous presence of HBeAg and HBsAg may indicate that a person is especially infectious for HBV, while the presence of anti-HBe in an individual with HBsAg usually indicates a lower level of infectivity.[20-22]

Anti-HCV has been detected in 60-70% of samples from recipients who developed NANB transfusion-associated hepatitis and other patients with a diag-

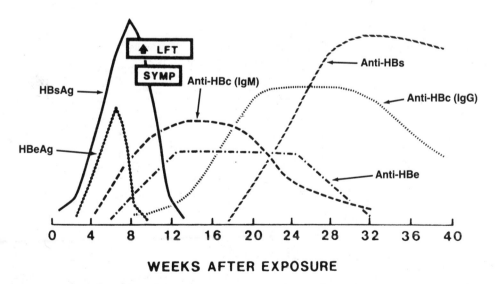

WEEKS AFTER EXPOSURE

Figure 4-1. Serologic markers in hepatitis B virus (HBV) infection. In the acute phase markers appear before onset of liver function (LFT) abnormalities and symptoms (SYMP). Numerous markers persist after recovery.

nosis of NANB hepatitis. The detection of antibody depends on the stage of the disease at the time of testing. The first-generation test licensed May 2, 1990, and the second-generation multi-antigen test (HCV-2) licensed March 13, 1992, are enzyme immunoassays (EIAs) using recombinant antigens of HCV coated on a solid phase.[23,24] The screening test may fail to detect anti-HCV in the acute stage of disease; however, it does appear that a large percent of carriers have detectable anti-HCV. Figure 4-2 shows the proposed structure of the genome of HCV and the specificity of the first- and second-generation test reagents.

The clinical significance of finding anti-HCV in healthy blood donors is unclear. In US blood donors the rate of repeatedly reactive donors is between 0.4 and 1.0%.[25] The test may identify some individuals who have asymptomatic chronic HCV infection, may be reactive in individuals with prior exposure to HCV who have developed immunity or may be falsely reactive. Studies using unlicensed tests based on recombinant immunoblot assays (RIBA) or neutralization indicate that 20-60% of screening test positive donors are nonreactive in the supplemental tests. Nevertheless, all reactive units are considered unsuitable for transfusion. The FDA recommends that only anti-HCV negative plasma be fractionated.[26]

Clinical Manifestations of Hepatitis

Many individuals who acquire viral hepatitis (whether type A, B or C) have a subclinical infection without obvious symptoms or physical evidence of disease.[27] In asymptomatic patients, as well as in patients with clinically evident hepatitis, serologic studies are the only way to discriminate between the different types of viral hepatitis. Clinically, pathologically and biochemically, the acute effects of these viruses are similar. In general, hepatitis A is less clinically severe than hepatitis C, which tends, in

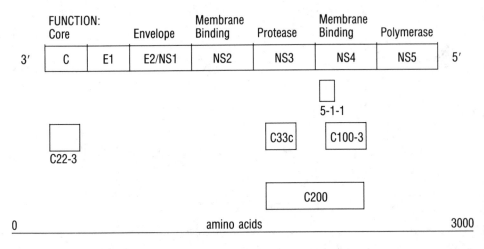

Figure 4-2. Proposed HCV genome and recombinant proteins used in testing.[24] HCV-1 test detects antibody to C100-3. HCV-2 test detects antibody to C200 (including C33c and C100-3) and C22-3. Supplementary tests detect antibody to specific gene products including C22-3, C33c, C100-3 and 5-1-1.

turn, to be milder than hepatitis B. This generalization, based on clinical observations, cannot be applied to all cases.

Infection with a hepatitis virus typically occurs in three phases: an incubation period, an acute phase and a convalescent phase. The clinical course may be additionally complicated by such sequelae as fulminant hepatitis, relapsing or recrudescent illness, chronic hepatitis or hepatocellular carcinoma.[27] A brief description of the typical clinical picture of infection with hepatitis B virus and hepatitis C virus is given below. Hepatitis A, because it so rarely follows transfusion, is not described in detail.

Patients who recover from hepatitis A infection develop anti-HAV (IgG), which makes them immune to further infection with the HAV. Similarly, all but 7-10% of persons with acute HBV infection develop protective immunity (demonstrated by finding anti-HBs). Some patients who recover from hepatitis C appear to become reinfected. Whether this is due to a different virus, relapse of a clinically asymptomatic chronic HCV infection or failure to develop immunity is unknown. Immunity to one hepatitis virus does not protect an individual from infection with another.

Incubation Period

The incubation period is the interval between exposure and either the onset of symptoms (clinical hepatitis) or the first appearance of liver function abnormalities (subclinical hepatitis). The incubation period for hepatitis A is about 30 days, with a range of 15-60 days. The incubation period for hepatitis C is approximately 50 days, with a range of 15-180 days. For hepatitis B, the mean incubation period is 90 days, with a range of 30-180 days. In hepatitis A, B and C, the length of the incubation period may be related to the number of hepatitis virus particles to which the individual is exposed and the route of exposure.

Acute Phase

In patients who develop jaundice (icterus), the acute phase can be subdivided into a prodromal or preicteric stage and an icteric stage. Probably less than 10% of patients with hepatitis B or C develop jaundice.[9,27] In a prospective study of transfusion recipients, 30% of patients with HBV infection had elevated bilirubin values compared to 5% of patients with NANB hepatitis.[28]

The earliest prodromal symptoms are nonspecific and similar to those of influenza—prominent complaints include anorexia, nausea, fatigue, severe weakness, abdominal discomfort and headache. Some patients with hepatitis B may have a prodrome that resembles serum sickness, characterized variously by skin rash including urticaria, angioneurotic edema, arthralgia or arthritis. This syndrome presumably results from the circulation and deposition of immune complexes in the skin and joints. During the prodromal stage there are relatively few physical findings. A tender and enlarged liver may be detected in 10-15% of patients. A precise diagnosis during this stage can be made only on the basis of elevated levels of aspartate aminotransferase (ASAT, AST or SGOT) and/or alanine aminotransferase (ALAT, ALT or SGPT) and positive serologic tests for viral markers.

The icteric stage is heralded by the retention of the bile pigment, bilirubin, which is usually first manifested by a dark coloration of the urine. Clinical jaundice develops soon thereafter, usually visible first in the sclerae and subsequently the skin. With the onset of jaundice, the constitutional symptoms of the prodromal stage usually diminish, although anorexia and weakness may linger. During this stage, patients may experience intense itching from retention of bile salts. The feces frequently lack bile pigment; these whitish-grey stools are described as acholic. Physical examination is remarkable only for jaundice and tender hepatomegaly. Many patients develop anorexia and lose weight during this time.

Laboratory studies during the icteric stage reveal a gradual decrease in aminotransferase levels, which generally peak just before jaundice begins, followed by a similar decline in the serum bilirubin. The duration of this phase is variable, generally lasting 1-6 weeks.

Convalescent Phase

This phase begins when the patient demonstrates sustained clinical improvement. The patient's appetite improves, weight is regained, strength and energy return to normal, jaundice is no longer evident and hepatomegaly resolves. In uncomplicated cases the convalescent phase ends with complete clinical recovery and resolution of liver function abnormalities. Convalescence is generally complete within 4 months of the onset of illness, although it may be delayed 6 months or longer. Morbidity and mortality depend to some degree on the age of the patient and may be exacerbated by pregnancy. (See Table 4-2.)

Clinical Variants

Fulminant Hepatitis. This complication is rare, occurring in approximately 1% of patients hospitalized with HBV infection. Some cases have resulted from HDV superinfection with acute or chronic HBV infection. The incidence of fulminant hepatitis following HCV infection is unknown. Clinical manifestations, which begin early in the acute phase, include mental confusion, deepening jaundice, fluid retention, coagulation disturbances, severe abdominal pain and coma. In some populations, the mortality rate among patients who develop fulminant hepatitis is 75-95%. In some populations, the mortality rate re-

Table 4-2. Morbidity and Mortality of Acute Hepatitis[29]*

Virus	Clinical Severity	Percent of Patients by Age		
		<1–14	15–39	40+
HAV		N=3188	N=8785	N=2233
	Jaundice	80.1	88.3	83.7
	Hospitalized	9.3	17.6	19.1
	Death	0.1	0.4	1.1
HBV[†]		N=136	N=7440	N=1733
	Jaundice	61.1	81.9	71.2
	Hospitalized	25.0	27.1	40.6
	Death	1.5	0.7	2.8
NANB[‡]		N=96	N=1413	N=574
	Jaundice	73.3	80.9	72.4
	Hospitalized	28.7	29.4	44.3
	Death	2.3	1.5	5.6

*Serologically defined cases with discrete date of onset of illness and jaundice or ALT >2.5 times upper limit of normal.
†Blood transfusion was implicated in 1.2% of 9410 patients of all ages and 4% of those over 40.
‡Blood transfusion was implicated in 7.7% of 2109 patients of all ages and 20.8% of those over 40.

sulting from fulminant HCV infection may be higher than that due to HBV.[30] Younger patients usually fare somewhat better than older or debilitated individuals.

Relapsing Hepatitis. This pattern of infection is common in, and thought to be characteristic of, posttransfusion hepatitis C. It consists of one or more distinct clinical or biochemical flares of hepatitis before complete recovery from the primary infection. Neither the cause nor the precipitating factors for the recrudescence are understood.

Chronic Hepatitis. Chronic hepatitis exists when laboratory evidence of hepatic inflammation persists for more than 6 months. This complication is seen in approximately 5-10% of patients with hepatitis B[31] and in perhaps as many as 40-60% of patients with posttransfusion hepatitis C.[32] Chronic hepatitis may assume either a nonprogressive form, called *chronic persistent hepatitis* or a progressive form, called *chronic active hepatitis*. Chronic persistent hepatitis, characterized by minimal clinical symptoms and mild biochemical alterations, rarely progresses to cirrhosis. Chronic active hepatitis often leads to increasing liver cell necrosis and fibrosis, and in perhaps 20-30% of cases, ultimately to cirrhosis. Liver biopsy is required to distinguish between persistent and active hepatitis.

There is increasing evidence that hepatocellular carcinoma (hepatoma) is causally related to chronic hepatitis B and chronic hepatitis C infection.[33] Hepatoma, a rare malignancy in North America and Western Europe, is the most common malignancy in Asia and sub-Saharan Africa, where carrier rates for hepatitis B virus approximate 5-15%.

Chronic HBsAg Carrier State. Individuals whose serum remains HBsAg-positive for more than 6 months following infection by HBV are considered to be chronic carriers. Some carriers have chronic hepatitis, either persistent or active, but most lack evidence of ongoing inflammation. Epidemiologic evidence suggests that there are 300 million HBsAg carriers worldwide.[34] In the United States the carrier prevalence, calculated from results of donor blood screening in the late 1970's, was estimated between 0.1 to 0.5%[35] or approximately 500,000-800,000 carriers. Recent studies indicate the rate to be 0.09% in first-time donors and 0.03-0.04% in the total allogeneic donor population.[36,37] Higher prevalence rates may be found in certain groups, including Asian immigrants, gay men, parenteral drug abusers, dialysis patients and institutionalized individuals with Down syndrome. The factors that predispose to a carrier state include: exposure early in life, male gender, impaired immunological responsiveness[9] and a postulated genetic susceptibility.[38]

Chronic HCV Carriers. It is estimated that a significant number of patients infected with HCV by blood transfusion will become chronic carriers of the virus. Some patients will have intermittent bouts of liver disease while others will remain asymptomatic for 20 or more years before they develop liver disease. Patients developing cirrhosis and hepatocellular carcinoma years after having transfusion-associated hepatitis (TAH) have been documented.[13,39]

Risk From Transfusion

The incidence of TAH is difficult to determine. Depending on whether patients are studied prospectively with biochemical monitoring or are detected retrospectively by reporting of clinical hepatitis, it has been estimated in the past that TAH occurs in less than 0.1% to as many as 10% of recipients.[40] Variation in its clinical manifestations and mortality and morbidity from the recipient's primary disease are some of the factors that lead to underreporting or failure to recognize TAH.

Mandatory screening of all donors for HBsAg and the use of volunteer donors have significantly decreased, but not eliminated, the risk of HBV infection after transfusion. This virus accounts for 10-20% of the reported cases of TAH.[41] Most are clinically recognized. The Centers for Disease Control and Prevention (CDC) has estimated the current risk at 1 in 50,000 transfused recipients or about 1 per 200,000 transfused units.[13]

The majority of TAH cases are due to HCV. Many of these infections will be asymptomatic and detected only if the patient undergoes liver function studies. Current tests for HCV screening are not as effective for detecting acute HCV as they are for chronic HCV disease and the diagnosis in some cases continues to be based on the exclusion of other agents [ie, HAV, HBV, cytomegalovirus (CMV), Epstein-Barr virus (EBV)] and observation of seroconversion during the course of the infection.[14,42-46]

In the years prior to implementation of anti-HCV testing several studies[47-49] evaluated surrogate tests of donor blood as a means to reduce NANB hepatitis following transfusion. Initially it was suggested that transfusion of donor blood with an elevated ALT level was more likely to transmit NANB hepatitis (defined by liver function abnormalities) than when the units were from donors with normal ALT levels. Subsequent data suggested that the presence of anti-HBc in the donor was also predictive of NANB infection in some recipients. These tests appear to detect different populations of donors potentially capable of transmitting NANB hepatitis. Thus in 1987, in the absence of specific tests for the NANB agents, testing for both ALT and anti-HBc were mandated by the AABB as an interim measure to reduce the risk of hepatitis transmission.[50,51]

The impact of surrogate testing on the safety of transfusion has been difficult to evaluate. Prior to the implementation of surrogate tests for NANB, more stringent criteria for donor selection were introduced in response to reports of transfusion recipients developing AIDS. Since NANB and HBV infection occur in some of the same populations at risk for human immunodeficiency virus (HIV) infection, the changes in donor eligibility also reduced the risk of TAH. Studies have shown that there was a decrease in TAH following implementation of surrogate testing. In one report there was a drop in the incidence of hepatitis in the general population; however, TAH cases fell at rates of 50% (NANB) and 35% (HBV) greater than could be accounted for by the change in background rates.[52] A comparison of samples collected prior to and 6 months after cardiac surgery showed that seroconversion to anti-HCV (first generation) was 3.84% prior to surrogate testing, 1.54% when donors were anti-HBc nonreactive and had a normal ALT, and 0.57% when donor blood was also anti-HCV nonreactive.[53]

The impact of surrogate tests on the donor population depends on the geographic area and the incidence of prior HBV infection. The incidence of anti-HBc reactivity varies from 1-10% of the general population.[54] This marker, together with anti-HBs, is found in most individuals who have developed postinfection immunity to HBV infection. It may be the only marker present in some donors carrying HBV. Approximately 2-3% of healthy donors are likely to have ALT levels greater than twice the log mean normal value of the population. The elevated level, which can reflect mild liver inflammation in carriers of HCV, can also be a physiologic response to many common hepatotoxins such as alcohol and some prescription medications. Elevated ALT levels can also be caused by biliary tract disease, hemochromatosis, Wilson's disease, alpha-1-antitrypsin deficiency, autoimmune disorders, hypothyroidism, psoriasis and obesity. Several reports have shown that there is a higher incidence of anti-HCV in donors with elevated ALT than in those with a normal level.[14,55] Some of these studies fail to show a correlation between anti-HCV and anti-HBc.[14]

Selection of Prospective Blood Donors

History

A review of some of the donor selection criteria given in Chapter 1 is presented below. Specific questions asked should detect a history of past or present viral hepatitis. Donors must be asked specifically if they have ever had a positive test for HBsAg, as well as a history of illness diagnosed as, or thought to be, viral hepatitis after reaching the age of 11. While a history of hepatitis is reason for permanent deferral, liver inflammation associated with infectious mononucleosis, CMV or drug therapy is not. To assist in identifying those individuals who may be in the incubation phase of hepatitis, donors are questioned about transfusion and direct exposure within the past 12 months to tissue grafts, to potentially contaminated needles or other equipment, and to blood, including components and derivatives known to transmit the disease. Donors with such exposure are temporarily deferred.

Contact With Patients

Although the usual incubation period of hepatitis is less than 6 months, prospective donors in close contact with individuals with viral hepatitis (eg, their spouses, or others with whom they regularly share kitchen and bathroom facilities) must be deferred from donating blood until 12 months after the last exposure. The type of patient contact most physicians, nurses and technical personnel have in their routine work is not considered close contact and such work has not been a cause for donor exclusion. Health-care workers should be questioned about unprotected blood and body fluid exposure, accidental needlesticks and vaccination. Administration of Hepatitis B Immune Globulin (HBIG) may delay the onset of manifest infection.[56] Persons who have received HBIG must not donate blood until 12 months have passed since their last injection.[8] Individuals who have been, or are in the process of being, vaccinated need not be deferred from donating, provided the vaccine was not given because of a suspected specific exposure to hepatitis B virus.

Physical Findings

Physical examination of donors must include inspection of both forearms for evidence of needle tracks or sclerotic veins suggestive of intravenous drug abuse, as this is associated with an increased incidence of HBV, HCV and HIV infection. Such evidence permanently excludes a prospective donor. Tattooing within 12 months is cause for deferral because of the risk of hepatitis infection from blood-contaminated tattoo needles.[57] Ear piercing or acupuncture within 12 months is a reason to consider deferral of the donor unless sterilized or disposable single-use instruments were used.[58,59]

Payment of Blood Donors

The risk of posttransfusion hepatitis is clearly higher in recipients of blood obtained from commercial sources as compared to blood from voluntary donors.[60,61] Payment, per se, does not affect the safety of the blood, but it can attract donors who may not give a reliable history and in whom there is increased risk of viral hepatitis, either HBV or HCV. Testing for HBsAg, anti-HBc, anti-HCV and ALT reduces, but does not eliminate, the risk of hepatitis.

Blood Derivatives With a High Hepatitis Risk

Historically, certain blood derivatives from pooled human plasma have had an especially high risk of transmitting hepatitis. These include Factor IX Complex (prothrombin-complex concentrates, Factors II, VII, IX, X), Antihemophilic Factor (Human) [AHF concentrates, Factor VIII] and specifically activated factor concentrates designed to bypass Factor VIII inhibitor activity. These and other pooled derivatives should be used only in patients with specific indications for their use. The safety of some of these coagulation concentrates has been greatly increased by newer methods of preparation that include monoclonal antibody purification steps, heat and chemical treatment.[6,7,62] (See Table 4-3.)

Tests Intended To Prevent Disease Transmission

The AABB *Standards for Blood Banks and Transfusion Services* states that: "A sample of blood from each donation shall be tested for HBsAg, anti HBc, anti-HTLV-I/II, anti-HIV-1, anti-HIV-2, anti-HCV and with a serologic test for syphilis. Whole Blood and blood components shall not be used for transfusion unless the results of these tests are negative" (B5.510).[8(p 12)] In an emergency, blood may be transfused before completion of the tests, but that information shall appear conspicuously on an attached label or tag. If a test is subsequently positive, the recipient's physician must be notified. "Alanine aminotransferase (ALT) testing shall be performed on a sample

Table 4-3. Methods of Factor Purification and Virus Inactivation for Factor VIII Concentrates Currently Available in the United States, June 1992

	Treatment Method				
Purification Method	**Aqueous Heating**		**Solvent/Detergent**		
Non-Affinity Column					
Conditions	60 C, 10 hours		TNBP*/Tween 80		
Company	Behringwerke†	: Miles	: Alpha	: Miles	: NYBC‡
Product	Humate-P™	: Koāte®-HS	: Profilate® OSD	: Koāte®-HP	: Melate
Affinity Column					
Conditions	60 C, 30 hours		TNBP/Triton X-100		
Company	Armour		Baxter-Hyland (ARC)		
Product	Monoclate-P®		Hemofil® M, AHF-M		

*Tri-n-butyl phosphate
†Distributed by Armour
‡New York Blood Center

of blood from each donation. Blood and components shall not be used for transfusion if the results are outside established limits"(B5.520).[8(p 12)]

Both *Standards*[8] and the FDA require that HBsAg, anti-HBc,[19] anti-HCV and anti-HIV-1/2 testing be performed using reagents and techniques licensed by the FDA.[62] The *Code of Federal Regulations* (21 *CFR* 610.40a and 610.45a) allows the use of certain less sensitive hepatitis tests [eg, the abbreviated radioimmunoassay (RIA)] in emergency situations and allows transfusion before completion of testing in dire emergencies. The requirement for HBsAg, anti-HCV and anti-HIV-1/2 testing applies to blood and plasma collected for any purpose: for transfusion, for processing of derivatives for transfusion, for stimulation of antibody(ies) in donors, for use in the manufacture of reagents for technical procedures or for sale to others for any purpose. Additionally, there must be a statement on the label that "This product may transmit infectious agents" [21 *CFR* 606.121(c)(9)].

Each unit of blood or blood component for transfusion or further processing must be tested by the collecting facility or by an approved laboratory and test negative before the unit is released for routine transfusion. Transfusion services that obtain blood from another facility need not do repeat testing for HBsAg, anti-HBc, anti-HCV, ALT, anti-HIV-1/2, anti-HTLV-I/II or a serologic test for syphilis.

Transfusion-Associated Disease (Hepatitis, AIDS)

All unexplained cases of acute liver dysfunction occurring 2 weeks to 6 months following transfusion of blood or blood components must be investigated as possible posttransfusion hepatitis.[8] The

source donor center should be notified of these patients.[13] Recipients, their families and their physicians often fail to report the occurrence of viral hepatitis. All patients with AIDS, AIDS-related complex or anti-HIV seroconversion thought to be due to transfusion should also be reported to the source donor center. In the case of HIV, the time between infection and the recognition of symptoms may be several years.[63] Some individuals who are asymptomatic will be discovered to be anti-HIV positive and transfusion will be the only risk factor identified. These individuals should be reported so that donor tracing can be initiated. (See p 93.) Useful sources about possible cases of posttransfusion disease include[64]:

1. The hospital's infection control officer.
2. Laboratory records, especially the hepatitis testing and chemistry laboratories.
3. The hospital's medical records, especially discharge diagnosis.
4. Gastroenterology and infectious disease services records.
5. The hospital's attorney or risk management team.
6. The hospital's social service and business office personnel.
7. The local public health service director.

Necessary Records

A system for recording and reporting all cases of known or suspected transfusion-associated disease is required by AABB *Standards*. When a case of posttransfusion hepatitis or AIDS is confirmed, the donors of blood or components given to the patient must be identified. Any components still in storage from these donors must be located and quarantined until the donor's status is decided. It must be possible to trace a unit of blood and its components from final disposition (transfused to specific recipient, shipped, processed or discarded) back to the donor source and to recheck all laboratory records applying to each component of the unit. Blood collecting facilities must have a system to record and retrieve reports on donors implicated in hepatitis and AIDS cases.

The *Code of Federal Regulations* (21 *CFR* 606.170b) requires that fatalities attributed to transfusion complications (eg, hepatitis, AIDS and hemolytic reactions) be reported to the FDA by telephone or telegraph as soon as possible and in writing within 7 days. Transfusion services and collecting facilities must keep records of reported transfusion-associated disease.

All facilities must record the number of donors found to have positive tests for anti-HIV, HBsAg and anti-HCV, and must keep a permanent record of their identity. Records should be maintained of donors who are confirmed positive for HBsAg or anti-HIV, of donors with only repeatedly reactive screening tests who may be considered for reentry, and of donors permanently deferred based on ALT or anti-HBc tests. Records must be available to determine if a donor with an ALT value above the established cutoff has had an elevated ALT result on a previous donation. It must also be possible to determine if a donor's anti-HBc test was reactive on a prior donation. Record and reporting systems must be designed to maintain donor and patient confidentiality. State and local regulations on reporting should be considered in setting up these procedures.

Donors Whose Blood or Component Was Given to Patients Who Developed Transfusion-Associated Disease

If clinical or laboratory evidence of transfusion-associated hepatitis, or infection with HIV or HTLV-I/II occurs in a recipient of a single unit of blood or blood component, the donor must be permanently excluded from giving blood. This should be noted in the donor's record and his or her name placed in a file of donors who have been permanently deferred. If a patient develops disease after exposure to multiple units of blood components, it is not necessary to defer all of the involved donors. A note should be made in the donor's file that the individual was one of several donors (specify the number) involved in a case of transfusion-associated disease. The names should be placed in a special file for implicated donors. The blood bank director may want to evaluate such donors for an interim history of hepatitis, AIDS, etc and/or a change in serologic status. A donor implicated for the first time need not be deferred as a future blood donor if there were two or more donors.[8] If, on the other hand, a donor is found to have been implicated in one or more other cases of transfusion-associated hepatitis, the blood bank physician should decide if permanent deferral is warranted.

Some blood centers routinely exclude donors implicated in two cases of transfusion-associated hepatitis[65]; other centers prefer a policy of calculating probability values.[66] The probability value for a donor who has been implicated more than once can be simply calculated as the sum of the fraction of the total donor pool he or she represents for each hepatitis case. For example, if a donor is 1 of 12 donors in one case (1/12 or 0.08), and 1 of 9 donors in another (1/9 or 0.11), the probability value is 0.19. When pooled concentrates known to be a possible source of infection (eg, Factor VIII) are administered along with other blood components, at least 10,000 donors may be implicated, but an arbitrary figure of 100 donors is assigned for including the pool in the calculation. Permanent exclusion would occur only when a donor reaches a probability value determined by the medical director of the facility (eg, 0.2 or 0.3). The probability approach avoids automatic exclusion of frequent donors, who by chance alone are likely to become implicated in more than one case. A modification of this approach has been described,[67] in which consideration of the specific history of each repeatedly implicated donor permits more accurate estimation of possible donor infectivity.

Notifying the Donor

If an individual is to be excluded as a donor, there must be notification of the exclusion and its cause. The donor must be told clearly that he/she is precluded from all future blood donations. Ideally, follow-up of an abnormal test should be done by the donor's own physician. Written consent to release information to a designated health-care provider should be obtained. If the donor does not have a physician, the donor center staff should provide initial counseling and appropriate referral. The notification process and counseling must be done with tact and understanding. The fears and concerns of the donor should be addressed. The donor should be told clearly why he or she is deferred and about the possibility of being infectious to others.

Use of Immunoglobulin With Transfusion

It is not recommended that either Immune Serum Globulin (Human) (ISG) or HBIG be given to transfusion recipients to prevent viral hepatitis.[68,69] ISG and HBIG have not been shown to prevent posttransfusion hepatitis B. The available evidence is conflicting as to whether ISG or HBIG can reduce the frequency or severity of hepatitis C.[70-72]

Preventing Viral Hepatitis

Guidelines for the immunoprophylaxis of viral hepatitis are prepared by the Public Health Service (PHS) Advisory Committee on Immunization Practices.[73] The PHS recommendations for the use of ISG and HBIG to prevent or modify viral hepatitis are summarized below.

Hepatitis A Prophylaxis

1. For a person who has had close personal contact with an individual with hepatitis A, give 0.02 mL/kg of body weight of ISG intramuscularly.
2. For foreign travel to areas endemic for hepatitis A, give 0.02 mL/kg of ISG. Travelers planning to stay more than 3 months should receive 0.06 mL/kg of ISG every 5 months.
3. Administer inactivated, purified hepatitis A virus vaccine derived from cell culture.[74] Note: As of August, 1992 this was an investigational new drug.

Hepatitis B Prophylaxis

1. Health-care workers employed in occupations that are likely to result in exposure to blood and body fluids from patients with hepatitis should be offered hepatitis B vaccine.[75]
2. For accidental needlestick exposure or contamination of mucosal surfaces or open cuts with HBsAg-positive blood, give HBIG in a dose of 0.06 mL/kg of body weight or 5 mL as soon as possible within 7 days of exposure. In another site, preferably the deltoid muscle, give the initial dose of vaccine. One month and 6 months later, follow-up injections of vaccine (but not HBIG) will be needed. (Note: individuals given this course of treatment will be ineligible as blood donors for 1 year.) Individuals who are already HBsAg-positive or

who have anti-HBs need not be given HBIG or vaccine; but, if these tests cannot be performed within the 7 days after exposure, draw a blood sample for the tests and give HBIG.

3. It is recommended that all newborns should be given hepatitis B vaccine.[76] A second dose is given at 1-2 months of age and a third at 6-18 months.

4. For infants born to mothers with acute hepatitis B in the third trimester or who are HBsAg reactive at the time of delivery, give 0.5 mL HBIG intramuscularly as soon after birth as possible.[73,77] These infants should also be given vaccine in another intramuscular site (5 μg recombinant or 10 μg plasma-derived material). Subsequent injections should be given at 1 and 6 months of age.

Hepatitis B Vaccine

In 1981 the first vaccine against hepatitis B was licensed and marketed. This vaccine was prepared from isolated and concentrated HBsAg particles that were inactivated with formalin, pepsin and urea. Such a treatment effectively inactivates hepatitis B virus as well as viruses from every known group, including agents of human NANB hepatitis and AIDS.[78] In large clinical trials the vaccine was 95% successful in stimulating antibodies to HBsAg.[79] [Responses 10 mIU/mL (anti-hepatitis B immunoglobulin - 1st Reference Preparation 1977, WHO) were found to be consistent with immunity to hepatitis B virus infection.] The vaccine must be given intramuscularly (preferably in the deltoid region) on three separate occasions; initial dose is 20 μg, followed by 20 μg at 1 month and 6 months after the primary injection. Side effects are rare and mild, and include fever, tenderness over the injection site, arthralgia and rare cases of Guillain-Barré syndrome.

In 1986 a recombinant form of the vaccine was licensed. This recombinant vaccine is produced by introducing a plasmid containing the gene for hepatitis B surface antigen into *Saccharomyces cerevisiae* (common baker's yeast). This vaccine appears to be as effective as the plasma-derived vaccine.[80] The dose for recombinant vaccine is 10 μg in an adult. The route of administration and injection schedule are the same as with the human-derived vaccine.[73]

At present, evidence suggests that the protective effect of vaccination is at least 5 years.[81] No recommendations for routine revaccination have been made. In health-care workers who have been vaccinated, it is useful to determine if they have adequate levels of circulating anti-HBs before giving a booster injection when the individual is re-exposed to HBsAg-positive blood.

Individuals at high risk of exposure to hepatitis B include technologists and pathologists who handle large numbers of patient specimens.[75,82] Studies have shown that donor center personnel are not at increased risk unless they are exposed to patient, as well as donor, blood specimens.[83,84]

Disease Prevention by Processing Blood and Blood Derivatives

Transfusion of RBCs that have been frozen, thawed and deglycerolized has been suggested as a possible means to reduce the risk of posttransfusion hepatitis.[85] An experimental study in chimpanzees did not substantiate this claim for HBV.[86] A subsequent clinical study similarly failed to justify the use of frozen or washed RBCs to reduce the risk of NANB hepatitis.[87] Data on the effects of freezing and washing blood on transmission of HIV are not available.

Heat and other treatments of blood derivatives are effective in reducing the risk of hepatitis and HIV infection.[2,6,7] Derivatives such as albumin and plasma protein fraction are routinely heated to 60 C for 10 hours. These derivatives have only rarely been associated with transfusion-associated disease. In those rare instances where infections have occurred, the processing was not proper. Since 1985, heat-treated coagulation concentrates have been available. These materials have a much lower risk of transmitting HIV; however, the effect of this heat process on HBV and HCV transmission is incompletely known and varies with the specific process. The combination of heat, chemicals and monoclonal antibody purification steps makes it possible to provide coagulation concentrates with greatly reduced hepatitis and HIV risk.[6,7,62,88,89] (See Table 4-3.)

Immunoglobulin preparations fractionated by cold-alcohol processes have been extremely safe. Cases of hepatitis infection following intramuscular administration of immunoglobulin almost never occur and no cases of HIV infection have been reported.[90,91] Intravenous immunoglobulin (IVIG) preparations also appear to be free of disease transmission, except for a few cases of NANB hepatitis that occurred during clinical trials.[92] US licensed IVIG preparations have not been implicated in the transmission of viral hepatitis.

Acquired Immunodeficiency Syndrome

AIDS is characterized by a diverse group of clinical manifestations resulting from loss of immune function and regulation following infection by the human immunodeficiency virus. This syndrome was first recognized in 1981 when a cluster of gay men were noted to have *Pneumocystis carinii* pneumonia, an opportunistic protozoan infection.[93] At about the same time, cases of Kaposi's sarcoma were identified in gay males and drug addicts.[94] Unlike the slow growing skin tumor found in Africa and in elderly males from the Mediterranean region, these tumors were more aggressive, involved visceral organs and were often associated with opportunistic infections.

It is now recognized that the mean period from infection to the diagnosis of AIDS is 8 or more years.[95,96] Once infected, asymptomatic individuals are at risk of infecting others through vertical or horizontal transmission. As the infection progresses, various manifestations may be recognized including neurologic changes, generalized lymphadenopathy, weight loss, fatigue, night sweats and increasing bouts of opportunistic infection. Of the 230,179 cases reported to the CDC through June 1992, more than 66% have died.

In July of 1982, AIDS was reported in three hemophiliacs.[97] These individuals did not have any of the risk factors associated with gay men or drug addicts. In December of 1982 the death of a 17-month-old infant who had received multiple transfusions at birth including a unit of platelets from an individual who subsequently developed AIDS was reported.[98] The clinical course of the child included numerous opportunistic infections and thrombocytopenia.

Although the cause of AIDS was unknown and the mode of transmission uncertain, in March of 1983 changes in donor selection criteria were introduced to defer blood donation by individuals at high risk for AIDS.[99] In January of 1984, the publication of a collection of cases documented that AIDS occurred in recipients of blood from healthy donors who subsequently developed the disease and/or who had a history of high risk behavior (ie, males with multiple sexual partners of the same sex).[100]

In April of 1984, Montagnier[101] and Gallo[102] identified a cytopathic retrovirus that was called lymphadenopathy associated virus (LAV) or human T-cell lymphotropic virus, type III (HTLV-III). This 100 nm RNA virus, now called HIV, preferentially infects T-helper (T4) lymphocytes, but also infects other cells such as monocytes or macrophages. The core of the virus contains an enzyme, reverse transcriptase, that enables the virus to copy its single-stranded RNA into double-stranded DNA. The genome of the virus is then integrated into host DNA. The provirus can, through transcription, produce both viral genomic RNA and messenger RNA, which is translated into viral proteins (see Fig 4-3). The virus then is released by the host cell. In the process the host cell is often destroyed.[103,104]

Viral Structure

HIV is in the family *Retroviridae*.[105] Included in this family are oncoviruses such as HTLV-I and -II, which primarily induce proliferation of infected cells and formation of tumors. HIV is a lentivirus, a slow-growing type of virus that causes chronic infection. HIV is a 100-nm sphere with an envelope consisting of a lipid membrane through which glycoproteins protrude. The core of the virus contains the genomic RNA and reverse transcriptase. A second strain of HIV called HIV-2 has a different envelope and slightly different core proteins. The host response to this virus is an antibody of a different specificity than that seen with HIV-1 infection. HIV-2 also causes AIDS.[106]

Serologic Response to HIV Infection

Figure 4-4 shows a schematic of the usual serologic findings in an individual who develops HIV infection. There is some controversy as to whether antibody to the envelope (gp41) or to the core proteins (p24) appears first. Shortly after exposure the p24 core protein is detectable in some individuals.[107] Within a few weeks to 6 months, antibodies to both envelope and core proteins are detectable. During the earliest phase of infection the same individuals may have symptoms of a nonspecific acute viral illness.[108] Once antibody appears it seems to increase in titer even though the host is asymptomatic. During this phase of infection, antigen is usually not detectable in the serum; however, viral cultures of patient lymphocytes may demonstrate presence of virus. Immune complexes are present in many patients and on dissociation often reveal the presence of circulating antigen. As infection progresses, changes in the ratio of T4 (helper-inducer) to T8 (suppressor) cells will be observed.[109,110] When this ratio, which is normally 2, begins to fall it is not unusual to find antigen again appearing in the serum. Depending on the host and other unidentified factors, the types of symptoms and the length of time before severe illness occurs is variable. In terminally ill patients antibody to the core proteins may fall in titer and even disappear.[107]

Efforts to protect the safety of the blood supply should be directed to detecting infectious donors as early as possible. It is not known when an exposed individual becomes infectious or how soon infected persons will develop serologically detectable markers of infection. Experience with HBsAg testing demonstrates that no test will detect all potentially infectious donors; therefore, careful donor selection is important to ensure the safety of transfusion. Thus, although the tests to be described later in this chapter will detect most infectious units, it is essential that all prospective donors be given appropriate educational material about activities that increase the risk for HIV infection.[8] Donors must be carefully interviewed using

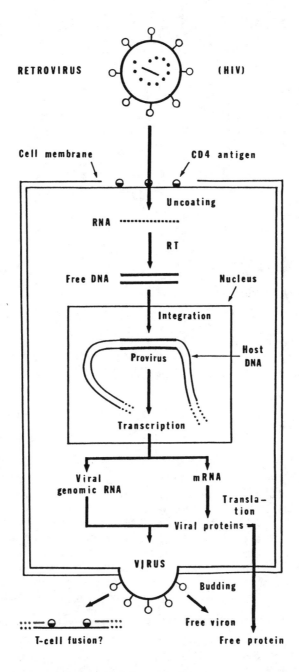

Figure 4-3. The life cycle of a Type C retrovirus (of which HIV is typical). The infection of other cells by cell fusion is postulated, but not proven. RT = reverse transcriptase. (Redrawn after EH Emory by Zuck and Epstein.[104] [(p111)])

STAGES OF HIV INFECTION
ANTIGENS AND ANTIBODIES DETECTABLE

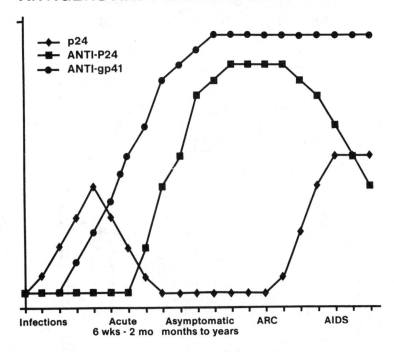

Figure 4-4. The detectability of markers of HIV infection at various stages. The pattern seen will depend on various clinical factors.

direct questions and a self-deferral mechanism.[111] The use of confidential unit exclusion (CUE) is optional (see Chapter 1 for discussion).[112] Testing for HIV markers is only one of the many steps used to protect recipients.[113]

A study by Imagawa et al[114] suggested that in a rare individual in some high risk populations, HIV-1 can be present for up to 36 months before seroconversion is detected.[115] However, additional follow-up of these individuals failed to show they are infected or infectious.[116]

In July of 1992, 26 individuals with a syndrome of immunodeficiency and opportunistic infection who had no evidence of HIV infection [antibody, polymerase chain reaction (PCR) and culture negative] were reported.[117,118] This syndrome has been referred to as idiopathic CD4+ T-lymphocytopenia (ICL). In a few cases reverse transcriptase was found, suggesting infection with a retrovirus.[118] Many of these patients had risk factors similar to those associated with HIV infection. Five had been transfused, including one whose transfusion was in the 1950's. Follow-up of three donors for a patient transfused in 1987 did not reveal any evidence of HIV infection or immunodeficiency in the donors.[117]

Transfusion-Associated AIDS

Recipients have developed AIDS after receiving a single contaminated unit of

WB or any of its components.[119] With the exception of concentrates for treating hemophilia A and B, blood derivatives such as albumin and immune globulins have not been reported to transmit HIV infection. Methods used to purify and/or treat coagulation factor concentrates significantly reduce the risk of HIV infection when these products are made from plasma obtained from anti-HIV negative donors.[6] Several new methods using UV irradiation and/or the addition of photo-activated compounds are being evaluated as means of inactivating viruses in blood components.[120]

As of June 30, 1992 there were 4959 cases of AIDS reported to the CDC in which transfusion or a tissue transplant seemed to be the only identifiable risk.[121] In addition, 2054 cases occurred in patients with hemophilia/coagulation disorders. From July 1990 through June 1992 transfusion-associated AIDS (TAA) represented 1.65% of all AIDS cases (1497/90,516), 4.96% of cases among adult females (561/11,317) and 4.61% of cases in children less than 13 years of age (70/1519). Except for a very few cases[122,123] (21 as of July 1, 1992) the transfusions occurred before routine testing for anti-HIV was available. In 1984 the incubation period between the time of transfusion and diagnosis of AIDS was estimated to be 4.5 years with the 95% confidence interval between 2 and 14 years.[124] This long incubation period and the high mortality rate of transfusion recipients (approximately 50% within 6 months) makes it difficult to determine what the actual risk of TAA was during the period before a specific test for HIV was available. Other factors that must be considered in calculating the risk include the prevalence of the infection in the potential donor population, the efficacy of donor exclusion methods and the sensitivity of any screening test that is used.[122,125] Studies

of recipients who have received tested blood and on pools of donor samples tested by PCR indicate that the risk of HIV-1 infection from screened blood is between 1 in 40,000 to 1 in 225,000 per transfused unit.[126-128]

Recipient and Donor Tracing (Look-Back)

Identification of persons who may have received blood containing HIV is referred to as look-back.[129] With the very long incubation between transfusion and onset of disease, some individuals are unaware of their exposure and may be infectious to others. In order to identify these individuals, blood centers must develop procedures to notify recipients of blood or components when previous donors are found to have been infected with HIV.[8] Look-back should be initiated if anti-HIV is found in a subsequent donation of a donor not previously tested or whose prior test was not reactive. Finding anti-HIV in a donor implicated in a case of TAA is cause to investigate other recipients of the donor's blood. Information that a patient with AIDS has previously been a blood donor is also a reason to initiate look-back.[130]

It is recommended that recipient tracing be done through notification of the patient's physician. Ideally, a mechanism for counseling and testing of the potentially infected individual and, if appropriate, his or her sexual partner will be established. This activity requires counselors with understanding, tact and respect for the confidentiality of the process. If the implicated donor had given on many occasions, look-back can be started with the most recent recipients. If the recipients of units from two successive donations are tested and found negative, it is unlikely that earlier recipients are at risk. Likewise, it is unlikely that a donor was infectious earlier than one year prior to his or her most recent negative screening test. Data from an extensive look-back study in San Francisco show that the recipient's risk for developing AIDS is increased when the time interval between donation and onset of AIDS in the donor is less than 2 years.[119]

The Presidential Commission on the Human Immunodeficiency Virus Epidemic recommended that all recipients of blood between 1977 and the onset of testing in 1985 be contacted and tested.[131] This has not been widely implemented. The look-back procedures described above are more likely to be productive provided that the epidemiologic investigation of AIDS cases and cases of HIV seroconversion includes evaluation of the individual's history of blood donation. If individuals who are prior blood recipients have unusual signs or symptoms or persistent worry about AIDS, testing and counseling by their physicians are indicated.

HIV Testing of Blood Donors

Montagnier's findings that LAV could be propagated in the CEM cell line[101] and Gallo's observation that HTLV-III could be grown in H9 cells[102] led to development of methods for obtaining large quantities of partially purified viral proteins. Using this material, enzyme-linked immunosorbent assays (ELISA or EIA) and Western blot methods for detecting anti-HIV were developed. (See Methods 9.5 and 9.6 and Table 4-4.) On March 2, 1985 licensure in the United States of the first test for use in screening blood donors for anti-HIV was announced and routine testing of all donors was instituted as kits became available.[132]

AABB *Standards* and the *CFR* require that all units of blood and components be nonreactive for anti-HIV-1 and -2 be-fore they are issued for transfusion. Routine screening of all donors is done according to the scheme shown in Fig 4-5. Although there are several methods for detecting anti-HIV (see Table 4-4), screening of donors is usually done with an EIA test.[113,133] Since the consequence of missing a true positive is great, the screening tests are designed to have high sensitivity, ie, [*True Positive*/(TP + *False Negative*)] × 100. In this formula a true positive is an individual who has the disease (in the case of HIV, it is anyone who is infected). In achieving the required sensitivity, specificity, ie, [*True Negative*/(TN + *False Positive*)] × 100, is usually compromised. Specificity is a measure of test accuracy in those tested who do not have the disease (in the case of HIV, it is those not infected). If the prevalence of disease in the test population is low there is a high likelihood that most positives will be false positives. Even with a test that has a sensitivity of 99% and a specificity of 98% the predictive value of a positive test (ratio of true positives to all test positives) is less than 50% until the prevalence of disease in the population is 2% or more.[134]

Confirmation and Reentry

Whenever the EIA screening is repeatedly reactive, a confirmatory test must be done to determine if the donor is positive. Persons who have true positive test results need to be confidentially notified and should be encouraged to obtain counseling and medical follow-up. If the test is not confirmed as a true positive there are both technical problems and biologic causes that can account for the reactivity observed. (See Table 4-5.) Many of the donors initially identified as repeatedly reactive are nonreactive on additional, more specific tests, or are nonreactive on a subsequent donation. Therefore, reentry protocols

Table 4-4. Principles of HIV Test Methods

	EIA				Western Blot	Antigen Capture	IFA
	Enzyme-Labeled Antiglobulin	Sandwich	Competitive Binding	Latex			
Primary reagent	Antigen on solid phase	Recombinant antigens	Antigen on solid phase	Antigen coated latex	Separate viral lysate in SDS-PAGE; transblot to a membrane	Anti-HIV on solid phase	HIV-infected cells on slide
Reaction sample	Diluted unknown	Unknown	Unknown + labeled anti-HIV	Unknown	Unknown	Unknown sample; antibody to specific HIV protein (probe)	Unknown
Probe	Labeled anti-human Ig	Labeled recombinant antigen		Enzyme antibody conjugate	Labeled anti-human Ig	Labeled anti-probe Ig	Fluorescent-labeled anti-human Ig
Detection method	Substrate/chromogen	Substrate/chromogen	Substrate/chromogen	Substrate	Substrate/chromogen	Substrate/chromogen	
Endpoint observed	Measure color (proportional to amount of anti-HIV)	Measure color (proportional to amount of anti-HIV)	Measure color (inversely proportional to amount of anti-HIV)	Observe; color or agglutination	Evaluate bands present	Measure color (proportional to amount of captured antigen)	Read and interpret fluorescent pattern

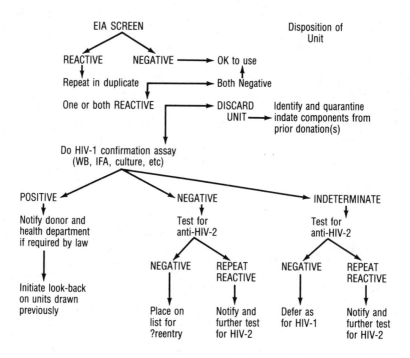

Figure 4-5. Flow diagram for anti-HIV-1/2 testing on donor samples.

were developed by the FDA (see Table 4-6). Critical aspects of the reentry protocol include the 6-month interval between samples to account for possible seronegative donors in the incubation phase, the use of EIA tests based on whole virus lysate and testing with a licensed Western blot to ensure the method has appropriate sensitivity for antibody detection. Licensed immunofluorescence assay (IFA) tests can substitute for the Western blot.[112,136]

Results of Donor Testing

During the first year of donor screening for anti-HIV, repeatedly reactive EIA results ranging from 0.1-0.8% were observed depending on the location of the donor center and the reagents used.[137,138] During this time less than 10% of these samples were confirmed as positive by Western blot. During the second and

Table 4-5. Possible Causes of False-Positive EIA Tests

Initial Reactive (not reproducible)
Technical problems
Improper washing
Improper conjugate/substrate preparation
Edge effect (microtiter plates)
Incorrect reaction temperature

Repeatably Reactive
Decreased reagent specificity
HLA-DR antibodies (seen in anti-HIV tests)
Antibodies cross-reactive with cell culture
contaminants or ?? viral epitope
Patients with increased Ig levels
Passively acquired antibody
Vaccine recipients

Sample Integrity
Lipemia
Hemolysis
Contamination

third years of testing most centers reported repeatedly reactive rates around 0.1-0.2% and found that only 10-20% of these samples were also positive by Western blot.[139] In 1992 detection rates were 5-10 confirmed positives per 100,000 donors.[128] Reports on counseling and interviews with those who are confirmed positive for anti-HIV suggest that most are males who at the time of donation denied existing risk factors or who failed to comprehend the educational material provided but who actually did have risk factors.[140] Self-denial of risk was a major reason for donating.

As the epidemiology of HIV infection evolves, the demographics of confirmed positive donors has also shifted to include more females and fewer males with male-to-male sex as a risk factor.[141]

Anti-HIV Screening

The EIA systems developed to screen blood donors (see Table 4-5) for anti-HIV are based on coating the solid phase material with the appropriate viral epitopes.[133,142] The nonspecific adhesion of protein to polystyrene makes it possible to place the target antigen on

Table 4-6. Reentry of Donors With Repeatedly Reactive (RR) Screening Tests

INITIAL SAMPLE

Test: Anti-HIV-1 or -HIV-1/2[112]	Anti-HIV-2[112]	HBsAg[135]
	NOT ELIGIBLE FOR REENTRY	
Licensed Western blot positive or indeterminate or IFA reactive	Different HIV-2 EIA RR	Confirmed by neutralization or anti-HBc RR
	EVALUATE FOR REENTRY	
Licensed Western blot or IFA nonreactive (NR)	Different HIV-2 EIA NR and licensed Western blot or IFA NR	Not confirmed HBsAg specific and anti-HBc NR

FOLLOW-UP SAMPLE

Test: Anti-HIV-1 or -HIV-1/2	Anti-HIV-2	HBsAg
Sample drawn 6 months later:	Sample drawn 6 months later:	Sample drawn 8 weeks later:
	NOT ELIGIBLE FOR REENTRY	
EIA RR or Western blot positive or indeterminate or IFA reactive	RR HIV-1 or different HIV-2 EIA RR or a licensed Western blot or IFA reactive or indeterminate	HBsAg RR or anti-HBc RR
	ELIGIBLE FOR REENTRY	
Original EIA method nonreactive (NR) and whole virus lysate anti-HIV-1 EIA NR and licensed Western blot or IFA NR	Screening test and a different HIV-2 EIA NR and licensed Western blot or IFA NR	HBsAg NR and anti-HBc NR

microtiter plates or plastic beads. Plastic-coated metal beads have also been used in one system. The antigen is derived from viral cultures by disruption of the infected host cell (H9, CEM). This material is then purified and treated to eliminate the risk of infectivity. Alternate approaches to obtaining antigen are the use of protein prepared by inserting the desired segment of the HIV viral genome into *Escherichia coli* or yeast and harvesting the recombinant material.[143] Synthetic polypeptides containing the desired epitope can also be used.

The other component of most test systems is a set of reagents to detect antibody to HIV bound to the antigen on the solid phase.[133] A polyspecific or monospecific antihuman immunoglobulin (eg, goat, murine monoclonal) labeled with enzyme (eg, horseradish peroxidase, alkaline phosphatase) is used to determine if IgG and/or IgM in the sample has attached to the antigen. (See Table 4-7.) An appropriate chromogenic substrate [eg, tetramethylbenzidine (TMB), O-phenylenediamine·2HCl (OPD), para-nitrophenylphosphate (pNPP)] is used to obtain a colorometric reaction that can be read in a spectrophotometer. In addition to various buffered wash solutions, most

systems also require that a blocking agent be used as part of the sample diluent. Blocking agents include combinations of various animal proteins, powdered milk and proprietary substances that prevent nonspecific binding to the coated solid substrate. Most test systems also use a stop solution (eg, 1N sulfuric acid, sodium hydroxide) to terminate color development after a specified time interval.

Interpretation of the test is based on comparing the absorbance of the sample with a cutoff value calculated from several nonreactive and/or reactive controls (in some systems a correction for a reagent blank is needed). A cutoff value calculated for that run determines which samples are considered reactive. In some systems the cutoff value is determined by adding to the mean of nonreactive controls a value based on a percentage of the mean of reactive controls. In others a fixed value is added to the mean of nonreactive controls. The validity of each run must also be established by evaluating the distribution of values observed on the controls.

Each EIA system and even different reagent lots from the same manufacturer will give varying cutoff values. In order to make comparisons between lots and/or manufacturers it is useful to calculate a ratio or percentage of the sample absorbance to the cutoff.[144]

Table 4-7. Conjugates and Substrates Used in EIA Test Systems

Enzyme*	Chromogen
Horseradish peroxidase (HRPO)	Tetramethylbenzidine (TMB) Ortho phenylenediamine (OPD) 3,3' diaminobenzidine (DAB) 4-chloro-1-napthol (4CN)
Alkaline phosphatase	Paranitrophenylphosphate (pNPP) Nitroblue tetrazolium-5-bromo-4-chloro-3-indolyl phosphate (NBT-BCIP)

*May be enhanced by avidin-biotin sandwich methods.

Competitive Binding EIA

An EIA screening test for anti-HIV based on competitive binding has been widely used for screening blood donors in Great Britain.[145] This test uses microtiter wells coated with chemically inactivated antigen obtained from HIV-1 grown in culture. The antigen is bound to plates that are coated with purified anti-HIV. The unknown sample and reagent anti-HIV labeled with enzyme are added to the plate. After incubation and washing, substrate is added and the amount of color measured. Since the reaction is competitive, the amount of color is inversely proportional to the amount of anti-HIV present in the sample being tested.[133,142]

A competitive format has also been used to detect specific antibodies to envelope and core antigens.[146] These tests use a solid phase coated with recombinant proteins (p24 core or gp41 envelope) and compare competition between the test sample and a labeled polyclonal anti-HIV.

Antigen Capture Assays

HIV polypeptides in serum or in culture supernatant can be detected by coating solid surfaces (microtiter wells, beads) with purified, high-titer anti-HIV and probing with a second antibody after incubation with the test specimen.[107] In one experimental kit the second antibody is a polyclonal enzyme-labeled antibody. Another approach to antigen capture uses a specific antibody to p24 raised in rabbits and enzyme-labeled goat anti-rabbit to detect the presence of antibody bound to the captured antigen. Testing of donor blood for antigen may detect some individuals carrying HIV who have no antibody detectable by current screening assays.[147] A few cases have been reported demonstrating antigen in anti-HIV-1 negative samples from individuals who subsequently seroconverted.[147-149] Studies of large populations of donors in both low and high prevalence areas have failed to demonstrate that routine HIV antigen testing enhances the safety of the blood supply.[150,151]

Validation Assays—Western Blotting

Transblotting was first described by EM Southern[152] (Southern blots) as a method to study DNA. When the technique is applied to study proteins, it is referred to as Western blotting. This technique is useful in detecting the presence of anti-HIV and determining which viral components elicited an antibody response.[133,142] When correctly performed, this test is both sensitive and specific. Unfortunately, its technical complexity and cost preclude its use as a screening test.

The various components of a purified, heat-treated, viral lysate dissolved in sodium dodecyl sulfate (SDS) are separated by polyacrylamide gel electrophoresis (PAGE). Depending on the conditions used, the various viral components will be distributed according to their molecular weights. The proteins are then transferred (transblotted) by use of electrophoresis from the gel to a nitrocellulose membrane. Commercially prepared transblotted membranes are available. In addition to electrophoretically separated viral lysate, it is also possible to prepare membranes using recombinant or synthetic viral proteins.

The membrane is divided into multiple strips. These are incubated with blocking agents prior to addition of the samples. Incubation of the unknown with the strip is followed by washing. To determine if antibodies have reacted with the viral proteins, an indicator system is needed. One method utilizes biotinylated antihuman IgG. After incubation and washing, avidin-labeled alkaline phosphatase is added. This is followed by a nitro blue tetrazolium, 5-bromo-4-chloro-3-indolyl phosphate substrate/stain. Known anti-HIV positive and negative samples must be run with each membrane. It is also useful to run molecular weight standards when doing electrophoresis and transblotting.

Interpretation of Western blot results depends on the bands detected.[133,153-155] (See Fig 4-6.) Most patients with AIDS and donors with anti-HIV show multiple bands representing the various gene

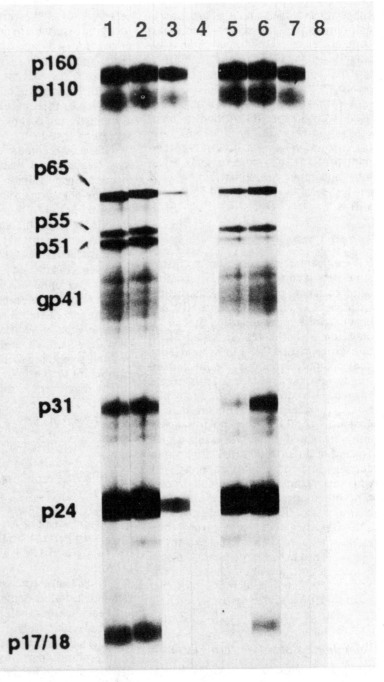

Figure 4-6. A Western blot on several samples included in the CDC Model Performance Evaluation Program. Molecular weights of the viral proteins are indicated on the left and sample numbers are below the individual test strips. Reactive and nonreactive controls are shown on strips 1 and 8, respectively. Strips 2-7 show band patterns that are interpreted as: nonreactive (4), weakly reactive (3, 7) or reactive (2, 5, 6).

products. A positive blot is defined by having bands representing the products of the envelope (env) gene [gp41 (transmembrane env glycoprotein), gp120 (outer env glycoprotein), gp160 (precursor of env glycoprotein)]; the core (gag) gene [p17 and p24 (gag proteins), p55 (precursor of gag proteins)]; and/or the polymerase (pol) gene [p31 (endonuclease component of pol translate), p51 and p66 (reverse transcriptase component of pol translate)]. Criteria for a positive interpretation have been defined for licensed Western blots as well as by the CDC.[154,155] In some cases few bands are seen or the staining intensity of the bands is less than the weak positive control. These blots are called indeterminate and repeat samples should be requested. Individuals with indeterminate blots on the initial test will almost always develop additional bands within 6 months if they are infected with HIV. Several studies on healthy individuals who continue to show indeterminate blots on repeat samples have failed to document HIV infection using additional tests including viral cultures and PCR.[156,157] The significance of the indeterminate blot must be taken in the context of clinical and epidemiologic information.[156,158] If healthy donors who deny HIV risk factors continue to show the same indeterminate pattern for more than 6 months they can be advised that they are not infected with HIV; however, such individuals must be deferred from donating blood. Negative blots have no bands present.

Radioimmunoprecipitation Assay

The radioimmunoprecipitation assay (RIPA) method is similar to the Western blot in that it identifies antibodies to specific viral components and requires an electrophoretic separation step. Disrupted purified virus grown in a culture containing a radioactive amino acid is incubated with the test sample. The immunoglobulin in the sample (including that bound to viral proteins) is separated, washed and subjected to polyacrylamide gel electrophoresis. The presence of antibody attached to various viral proteins is detected by radioautography.[159] This technique is useful in identifying high molecular weight viral proteins, especially labile glycoproteins not easily found by Western blot. The method does require a source of labeled virus and works best when the antibodies have good avidity.

Immunofluorescence Assay

Mixtures of culture cells, some expressing the virus and others without virus, are used as the target for detecting the presence of anti-HIV. An unknown sample can be layered on a slide containing the fixed cell preparation.[160] After incubation and washing a fluorescein-labeled antiglobulin is added. Cells to which anti-HIV has attached will light up when viewed under a fluorescence microscope. Antibodies binding nonspecifically to cell components will attach to both virus-containing and control cells. This test has both good sensitivity and specificity but requires subjective evaluation by individuals trained to read immunofluorescence. The test has been licensed to be used for both screening and confirmation of the presence of anti-HIV-1.[136]

Viral Culture

The growth of virus in a culture system is a definitive way to establish the presence of infection.[159] HIV can be cultured from the plasma or lymphocytes of infected persons. The rate of positive cultures in individuals with antibody to HIV varies, but in some reports is as high as 95%.[104] Virus may be detected in cultures carefully done with repeated supplementation of the medium for up to 4 weeks. The method is slow, tedious and costly.

Detection of Viral DNA

Several methods used in research applications are very sensitive for detection of minute quantities of HIV or other viruses. Polymerase chain reaction, a technique for amplification of specific nucleotide sequences, makes it possible to detect a conserved region of viral genome integrated in the host DNA.[161,162] Though very sensitive and specific, unwanted contamination is a potential problem with this technique. This method is particularly useful in detecting HIV infection in newborns who may have passively transferred maternal anti-HIV.[163]

HIV-2

HIV-2 has been isolated from a number of patients with AIDS. It is found most often in persons from West Africa and has been associated with a case of transfusion-transmitted disease.[164] The first case of HIV-2 infection in the United States was reported in March 1988 in a young West African who had recently immigrated to the US. As of July 1991, approximately 30 cases of HIV-2 infection had been detected in the US. Most patients are from West Africa or have had sexual contact with a person from the endemic area.

HIV-2 is very similar to HIV-1 and some antibodies to HIV-2 crossreact with the viral lysate used in some, but not all, HIV-1 test systems.[106] A licensed test is available for anti-HIV-2 screening. A combination anti-HIV-1/2 screening assay was licensed in September 1991. The FDA required that screening for anti-HIV-2 be implemented by June 1, 1992 using either anti-HIV-2 or the combination test.[112] Donors tested for anti-HIV-2 need not be questioned about their geographic origin. (See Chapter 1.)

HTLV-I

HTLV-I is a retrovirus first isolated in the late 1970's.[165] This virus is primarily associated with a proliferative cell response and is known to cause adult T-cell leukemia/lymphoma (ATL) in some infected individuals. It is associated with cases of tropical spastic paraparesis (TSP) also called HTLV-I associated myelopathy (HAM).[166] Assays to detect anti-HTLV-I may also detect antibodies to a related virus, HTLV-II, which has been isolated from a few patients with hairy-cell leukemia.[167] Although HTLV-I is most frequently found in areas in which the disease is endemic (southern Japan and the Caribbean basin), antibodies have also been found in IV drug abusers. Screening of blood donors and recipients in Kyushu, Japan, has shown that seroconversion does occur in seronegative recipients of seropositive fresh blood.[168] The rate of seroconversion was reduced following the implementation of a passive agglutination screening test for HTLV-I antibody and discarding of reactive donor units.[169] Initial studies in the US identified 2.5/10,000 voluntary donors as reactive by both an EIA screen and confirmation test (Western blot and/or RIPA).[170] It has also been reported that 6/211 multitransfused leukemia patients in New York with no other apparent exposure developed antibodies to HTLV-I.[171]

On November 29, 1988 the FDA licensed tests to screen for antibody to HTLV-I in blood and cellular components donated for transfusions.[171,173] The AABB Board of Directors recommended in February of 1989 that blood centers implement routine testing of donated blood for anti-HTLV-I.[174] (See Table 4-8.)

The screening method is similar to that described for anti-HIV-1 EIA assays.

Table 4-8. Summary of Recommended Actions for HTLV-I Testing[172]

First Donation To Be Tested for HTLV-I Antibodies				Subsequent Donation(s)			
EIA	WB/RIPA	Donation	Donor	EIA	WB/RIPA	Donation	Donor
Repeatedly reactive	Positive	Destroy* all components	Defer and counsel			Not Applicable/Donor Deferred	
Repeatedly reactive	Negative or indeterminate	Destroy* all components	No action	Repeatedly reactive	Negative or indeterminate or positive	Destroy* all components	Defer and counsel
				Non-reactive[†]	Not done	All components acceptable	No action

*Destroyed unless appropriately labeled as positive for HTLV-I antibodies, and labeled for laboratory research use or further manufacture into in-vitro diagnostic reagents.

†Assuming that separate prior donations have been repeatedly reactive for HTLV-I antibody no more than once. If separate prior donations had been repeatedly reactive for HTLV-I antibodies on two or more occasions, the donor should have been either permanently or indefinitely deferred.

It is estimated that 0.1-0.3% of donor units are reactive in screening assays. Supplementary tests with unlicensed reagents including Western blots and RIPAs have been used to confirm the specificity of samples repeatedly reactive for anti-HTLV-I by EIA.

AABB *Standards* requires that all blood for transfusion purposes be tested for anti-HTLV-I/II.[8] It has been recommended that donors who are shown to be positive for anti-HTLV-I using supplementary methods or those who are repeatedly reactive in screening tests on multiple donations be notified and permanently deferred.

Look-back on prior units donated by individuals found to be anti-HTLV-I reactive is recommended.[175] The look-back procedure is similar to that described for anti-HIV-1; however, the time limit for identification and notification of recipient extends back through the five most recent donations from that individual.

Some questions have developed concerning the ability of the current screening tests to detect anti-HTLV-II as well as anti-HTLV-I. Studies show that a large percent of individuals repeatedly reactive in the anti-HTLV-I screening tests actually are infected with HTLV-II, but their antibody crossreacts with HTLV-I protein in the viral lysate.[176] The significance of infection with HTLV-II is unknown at this time since, to date, no disease association has been proven.

Herpes Viruses

Cytomegalovirus

Cytomegalovirus is a DNA virus that characteristically causes intranuclear and intracytoplasmic inclusions in infected cells. Infection with CMV is usually mild and typically results in a period of viral shedding followed by a state of latency.[177] In most populations of blood donors the prevalence of anti-CMV ranges from 40-100%. The number of these seropositive blood donors who are capable of transmitting CMV infection is probably less than 10%.

Transfusion-associated CMV infection was first recognized as a postperfusion mononucleosis syndrome observed following cardiopulmonary bypass surgery. It was thought to be related to use of fresh blood and is rarely observed now since the amount of fresh blood used for cardiac surgery has decreased. CMV infection has also been associated with posttransfusion hepatitis. In a study at the National Institutes of Health, 15% of TAH was associated with CMV infection.[178] Since 1980, new CMV-associated cases have not been identified among patients with TAH. The decrease in this complication is thought to be due to a decrease in the average number of units per patient and elimination of routine use of blood less than 48 hours old.

CMV can cause serious morbidity and mortality in immunosuppressed patients. These patients may present with pneumonitis, hepatitis, retinitis or disseminated disease. The source of infection can be transfusion, particularly in premature infants, bone marrow or organ transplants and severe immunosuppression, as observed in some oncology patients.[179,180] In some of these patients, other sources such as organ transplants from CMV-positive donors or reactivation of latent virus, may be more of a risk than transfusion. In the neonate, transplacental or perinatal exposure to cervical secretions and breast milk are common routes of infection.

Prevention of CMV

AABB *Standards* requires that "where transfusion-associated CMV disease is a problem, cellular components should be selected or processed to reduce that risk to infant recipients weighing less than 1200 grams at birth, when either the infant or the mother is CMV-antibody-negative or that information is unknown"(G6.600).[8(p 27)] The rationale behind this requirement is based on the observation that blood from seronegative donors or blood that has been depleted of leukocytes by freezing-deglycerolization is effective in preventing transfusion-acquired CMV infection.[181] There is also evidence that removal of leukocytes by the use of leukocyte-reduction filters reduces the risk of CMV transmission.[182,183] Administration of CMV immune globulin may also be efficacious in preventing infection in some clinical settings. Current data do not support the use of irradiation or extended storage of blood as methods for preventing transfusion-associated CMV infection. Some studies do not support the need for specialized components in neonates.[180,181] There is also evidence that using only CMV-seronegative blood could increase the susceptibility to infection with CMV in infants whose mothers are seropositive.[179]

Testing for Anti-CMV

Numerous tests are available to detect the presence of CMV antibodies. These include EIA, complement fixation, RIA, IFA, latex agglutination, etc. Donors with recent infection may be more likely to shed virus and hence be more infectious than are chronically infected donors. Thus, detecting IgM anti-CMV that is associated with recent infection should be useful in screening for infectious units.

Epstein-Barr Virus

This ubiquitous herpes virus rarely causes transfusion-associated disease. Infections are usually asymptomatic, but some individuals develop infectious mononucleosis (IM) when exposed to EBV. Cases of IM have been documented in recipients of single units from donors later found to have been incubating IM at the time of donation.[184]

Other Viruses

Parvovirus

Human parvovirus B19 is reported to cause 1) erythema infectiosum (fifth disease), a mild childhood illness, 2) transient aplastic crisis and severe anemia, most often in patients with chronic hemolytic anemia and 3) infection in pregnant women, leading to intrauterine infection and fetal death.[185] Antibody to the virus has been found in from 30-60% of adults. Although transmission is usually by respiratory secretions, it can be transmitted by transfusion of blood and blood derivatives such as coagulation concentrates.[186]

Human Herpesvirus-6

Human herpesvirus-6 (HBLV, HHV-6) has been suspected to be the cause of hepatitis in some organ transplant recipients and possibly after transfusion. HHV-6 is often found in saliva[187] and antibody has been detected by an EIA method in 80-88% of blood donors.[188] A recent prospective study of transfusion recipients (N = 30) failed to show seroconversion or a significant increase in anti-HHV-6 titer.[189]

References

1. Hollinger FB, Kahn NC, Oefinger PE, et al. Posttransfusion hepatitis type A. JAMA 1983; 250:2313-7.
2. Alter HJ. You'll wonder where the yellow went: A 15-year retrospective of posttransfusion hepatitis. In: Moore SB, ed. Transfusion-transmitted viral diseases. Arlington, VA:

American Association of Blood Banks, 1987:53-86.

3. Dienstag JL, Katkov WN, Cody H. Evidence for non-A, non-B hepatitis agents besides hepatitis C virus. In: Hollinger EB, Lemon SM, Margolis H, eds. Viral hepatitis and liver disease. Baltimore, MD: Williams and Wilkins, 1991:349-56.

4. Maynard JE. Epidemic non-A,non-B hepatitis. Semin Liver Dis 1984;4:336-9.

5. Rizzetto M. The delta agent. Hepatology 1983;3:729-37.

6. Centers for Disease Control. Safety of therapeutic products used for hemophilia patients. MMWR 1988;37:441-50.

7. Watson HG, Ludlam CA, Rebus S, et al. Use of several second generation serological assays to determine the true prevalence of hepatitis C virus infection in haemophiliacs treated with non-virus inactivated factor VIII and IX concentrates. Br J Haematol 1992;80:514-8.

8. Widmann FK, ed. Standards for blood banks and transfusion services, 15th ed. Bethesda, MD: American Association of Blood Banks, 1993.

9. Aach RD. Primary hepatic viruses: Hepatitis A, hepatitis B, delta hepatitis and non-A,non-B hepatitis. In: Insalaco SJ, Menitove JE, eds. Transfusion-transmitted viruses: Epidemiology and pathology. Arlington, VA: American Association of Blood Banks, 1987:17-40.

10. Overby L. Comments on hepatitis B markers and update on non-A,non-B. In: Polesky HF, Walker RH, eds. Safety in transfusion practices. Skokie, IL: College of American Pathologists, 1982:28-31.

11. Esteban JI, Gonzales A, Hernandez JM, et al. Evaluation of antibodies to hepatitis C virus in a study of transfusion associated hepatitis. N Engl J Med 1990;323:1107-12.

12. Contreras M, Barbara JAJ, Anderson CC, et al. Low incidence of non-A,non-B post-transfusion hepatitis in London confirmed by hepatitis C virus serology. Lancet 1991;1:753-7.

13. Public Health Service Inter-agency guidelines for screening donors of blood, plasma, organs, tissues and semen for evidence of hepatitis B and hepatitis C. MMWR 1991;40(RR-4):1-17.

14. van der Poel CL, Reesink HW, Lelie PN, et al. Anti-hepatitis C antibodies and non-A,non-B posttransfusion hepatitis in the Netherlands. Lancet 1989;2:297-8.

15. Aach RD, Stevens CE, Hollinger FB, et al. Hepatitis C virus infection in post-transfusion hepatitis: An analysis with first- and second-generation assays. N Engl J Med 1991;325:1325-9.

16. Ebeling F, Naukkarinen R, Leikola J. Recombinant immunoblot assay for hepatitis C virus antibody as predictor of infectivity. Lancet 1990;335:982-3.

17. van der Poel CL, Cuypers HTM, Reesink HW, et al. Confirmation of hepatitis C virus infection by new four-antigen recombinant immunoblot assay. Lancet 1991;337:317-9.

18. Hollinger FB. Specific and surrogate screening tests for hepatitis. In: Insalaco SJ, Menitove JE, eds. Transfusion-transmitted viruses: Epidemiology and pathology. Arlington, VA: American Association of Blood Banks, 1987:69-86.

19. Quinnan GV. FDA recommendations concerning testing for antibody to hepatitis B core antigen (anti-HBc) (memorandum). Bethesda, MD: FDA Center for Biologics Evaluation and Research, September 10, 1991.

20. Dodd RY, Popovsky MA and Members of the Scientific Section Coordinating Committee. Antibodies to hepatitis B core antigen and the infectivity of the blood supply. Transfusion 1991;31:443-9.

21. Werner BG, Grady GF. Accidental hepatitis-B-surface-antigen-positive inoculations: Use of e antigen to estimate infectivity. Ann Intern Med 1982;97:367-9.

22. Stevens CE, Neurath RA, Beasley RP, Szmuness W. HBeAg and anti-HBe detection by radioimmunoassay: Correlation with vertical transmission of hepatitis B virus in Taiwan. J Med Virol 1979;3:237-41.

23. Anti-HCV EIA (Manufacturer's package insert). Raritan, NJ: Ortho Diagnostics, May 1990.

24. Hepatitis C virus encoded antigen (recombinant c100-3,c200 and c22-3) Ortho HCV 2.0 ELISA test system (Manufacturer's product insert). Raritan, NJ: Ortho Diagnostics, March 1992.

25. Valinsky JE, Bianco C. Prevalence of antibodies to hepatitis C virus (HCV) among blood donors. Second International Symposium on HCV (program and abstracts). Secaucus, NJ: Advanced Therapeutics Communications International, 1990:114.

26. Zoon, KC. Revised recommendations for testing whole blood, blood components, source plasma and source leukocytes for antibody to hepatitis C virus encoded antigen (memorandum). Bethesda, MD: FDA Center for Biologics Evaluation and Research, April 23, 1992.

27. Aach RD. Clinical manifestations of viral hepatitis. In: Keating LJ, Silvergleid AJ, eds. Hepatitis. Washington, DC: American Association of Blood Banks, 1981:1-13.

28. Alter HJ, Purcell RH, Feinstone SM, et al. Non-A,non-B hepatitis: A review and interim report of an ongoing prospective study. In: Vyas GN, Cohen SN, Schmid R, eds. Viral hepatitis. Philadelphia: Franklin Institute Press, 1978:359-69.

29. Hepatitis Surveillance Report No. 53. Atlanta: Centers for Disease Control, 1990: 18-31.

30. Yanagi M, Kaneko S, Unoura M, et al. Hepatitis C virus in fulminant hepatic failure. N Engl J Med 1991;324:1895-96.

31. Redeker AG. Chronic hepatitis. Med Clin North Am 1975;59:863-7.

32. Dienstag JL. Non-A,non-B hepatitis: I. Recognition, epidemiology, and clinical features. Gastroenterology 1983;85:439-62.

33. Wands JR, Blum HE. Primary hepatocellular carcinoma. N Engl J Med 1991;325:729-31.

34. Maynard JE, Kane MA, Alter MJ, Hadler SC. Control of hepatitis B by immunization: Global perspectives. In: Zuckerman AJ, ed. Viral hepatitis and liver disease. New York, NY: Alan R. Liss, 1988:967-9.

35. Holland P, Glosova T, Szmuness W, et al. Viral hepatitis markers in Soviet and American blood donors. Transfusion 1980;20:504-10.

36. Starkey JM, MacPherson JL, Bolgiano DC, et al. Markers for transfusion-transmitted disease in different groups of blood donors. JAMA 1989;262:3452-4.

37. Kruskall MS, Popovsky MA, Pacini DG, et al. Autologous versus homologous donors: Evaluation of markers for infectious disease. Transfusion 1988;28:286-8.

38. Sugiura S, Mizokami M, Orito E, et al. DR locus-inclusive HLA in patients with persistent hepatitis B surface antigen. In: Zuckerman AJ, ed. Viral hepatitis and liver disease. New York, NY: Alan R. Liss, 1988:684-7.

39. Kiyosawa K, Sodeyama T, Tanaka E, et al. Interrelationship of blood transfusion, non-A, non-B hepatitis and hepatocellular carcinoma: Analysis by detection of antibody to hepatitis C virus. Hepatology 1990;12:671-75.

40. Polesky HF, Hanson M. Transfusion-associated hepatitis: A dilemma. Lab Med 1983;14: 717-20.

41. Polesky HF, Hanson MR. Transfusion-associated hepatitis C virus (non-A,non-B) infection. Arch Pathol Lab Med 1989;113:232-5.

42. Choo Q-L, Kuo G, Weiner AJ, et al. Isolation of a clone derived from a blood-borne non-A,non-B viral hepatitis genome. Science 1989;244:259-62.

43. Kuo G, Choo Q-L, Alter HJ, et al. An assay for circulating antibodies to a major etiologic virus of human non-A, non-B hepatitis. Science 1989;244:363-4.

44. Esteban JI, Esteban R, Viladomiu L, et al. Hepatitis C virus antibodies among risk groups in Spain. Lancet 1989;2:294-6.

45. Feinman SV, Berris B, Herst R. Anti-HCV in post-transfusion hepatitis: Deductions from a prospective study. J Hepatol 1991;12:377-81.

46. Tremolada F, Casarin C, Tagger A, et al. Antibody to hepatitis C virus in post-transfusion hepatitis. Ann Intern Med 1991;114:277-81.

47. Aach RD, Szmuness W, Mosely JW, et al. Serum alanine aminotransferase of donors in relation to the risk of non-A, non-B hepatitis in recipients: The Transfusion-Transmitted Virus Study. N Engl J Med 1981;304:989-94.

48. Stevens CE, Aach RD, Hollinger FB, et al. Hepatitis B virus antibody in blood donors and the occurrence of non-A,non-B hepatitis in transfusion recipients. Ann Intern Med 1984;101:733-8.

49. Koziol DE, Holland PV, Alling DW, et al. Antibody to hepatitis B core antigen as a paradoxical marker for non-A,non-B hepatitis agents in donated blood. Ann Intern Med 1986;104:488-95.

50. Steane EA. Surrogate testing for non-A,non-B hepatitis (Memo to AABB Institutional Members). Arlington, VA: American Association of Blood Banks, February 11, 1987.

51. Menitove JE. Rationale for surrogate testing to detect non-A,non-B hepatitis. Transfus Med Rev 1988;2:65-75.

52. Chambers LA, Popovsky MA. Decrease in reported posttransfusion hepatitis: Contributions of donor screening for alanine aminotransferase and antibodies to hepatitis B core antigen and changes in the general population. Arch Intern Med 1991;151:2445-8.

53. Donahue JG, Muñoz A, Ness PM, et al. The declining risk of post-transfusion hepatitis C virus infection. N Engl J Med 1992;327:369-73.

54. National household seroprevalence survey feasibility study final report. Research Triangle Park, NC: National Center for Health Statistics, 1990.

55. Stevens CE, Taylor PE, Pindyck J, et al. Epidemiology of hepatitis C virus. A preliminary study in volunteer blood donors. JAMA 1990; 263:49-53.

56. Grady GF, Lee VA, Prince AM, et al. Hepatitis B immune globulin for accidental exposures among medical personnel: Final report of a multicenter controlled trial. J Infect Dis 1978;138:625-38.

57. Abildgaard N, Peterslund NA. Hepatitis C virus transmitted by tattooing needle. Lancet 1991;338:460.

58. Kent GP, Brondum J, Keenlyside RA, et al. A large outbreak of acupuncture associated hepatitis B. Am J Epidemiol 1988;127:591-8.

59. Centers for Disease Control. Viral hepatitis in young women after ear piercing—Washington. MMWR 1973;22:390, 395, 416.

60. Walsh JH, Purcell RH, Morrow AG, et al. Post-transfusion hepatitis after open-heart operations: Incidence after administration of blood from commercial and volunteer donor populations. JAMA 1970;211:261-5.

61. Goldfield M, Bill J, Black H, et al. The consequences of administering blood pretested for HBsAg by third generation techniques: A progress report. Am J Med Sci 1975;270:335-42.

62. Code of federal regulations. Title 21, Part 610, Subpart E. Washington, DC: US Government Printing Office, 1992. (Revised annually.)

63. Peterman T, Jaffe H, Feorino P, et al. Transfusion-associated acquired immunodeficiency syndrome in the United States. JAMA 1985;254:2913-17.

64. Polesky HF, Hanson M. AABB-CAP survey data on hepatitis—incidence, surveillance and prevention. Am J Clin Pathol 1980;74:565-8.

65. Walker RH, Inclan AP. Utilization of the biologic test in posttransfusion hepatitis for the detection of carriers. South Med 1965;58:1131-34.

66. Hanson M, Polesky HF. A method for calculating the risk of donors implicated in transfusion associated hepatitis. In: Hopkins R, Field S. Proceedings of the International Hepatitis Workshop. Edinburgh, Scotland: Nuclear Enterprises, 1982:99-100.

67. Ladd DJ, Hillis A. A new method for evaluating the hepatitis risk of the multiply-implicated donor. Transfusion 1984;24:80-2.

68. Alter HJ. The epidemiology and prevention of post-transfusion hepatitis. In: Polesky HF, Walker RH, eds. Safety in transfusion practices. Skokie, IL: College of American Pathologists, 1982:1-16.

69. Seef LB. The efficacy of and place for HBIG in the prevention of type B hepatitis. In: Szmuness W, Alter HJ, Maynard JE, eds. Viral Hepatitis: 1981 International Symposium. Philadelphia, PA: The Franklin Institute Press, 1982:585-95.

70. Sanchez-Quijano A, Lissen E, Diaz-Torres MA, et al. Prevention of post-transfusion non-A,non-B hepatitis by nonspecific immunoglobulin in heart surgery patients. Lancet 1988;1:1245-9.

71. Conrad ME. Prevention of post-transfusion hepatitis. Lancet 1988;2:217.

72. Hollinger FB, Alter HJ, Holland PV, Aach RD. Non-A,non-B posttransfusion hepatitis in the United States. In: Gerety RJ, ed. Non-A,non-B hepatitis. New York, NY: Academic Press, 1981:49-70.

73. Centers for Disease Control. Immunization Practices Advisory Committee (ACIP). Protection against viral hepatitis. MMWR 1990;39(No. RR-2):1-26.

74. Werzberger A, Mensch B, Kuter B, et al. A controlled trial of a formalin-inactivated hepatitis A vaccine in healthy children. N Engl J Med 1992;327:453-7.

75. Centers for Disease Control. Guidelines for prevention of transmission of human immunodeficiency virus and hepatitis B virus to health-care and public-safety workers. MMWR 1989;38(suppl.6):1-37.

76. Centers for Disease Control. Hepatitis B virus: A comprehensive strategy for eliminating transmission in the United States through universal childhood vaccination. MMWR 1991;40(No. RR-13):1-25.

77. Stevens CE, Taylor PE, Tong MJ, et al. Prevention of perinatal hepatitis B virus infection with hepatitis B immune globulin and hepatitis B vaccine. In: Zuckerman AJ, ed. Viral hepatitis and liver disease. New York, NY: Alan R. Liss, 1988:982-8.

78. Hilleman MR, McAleer WJ, Buynak EB, McLean AA. Quality and safety of human hepatitis B vaccine. Biol Stand 1983;54:3-12.

79. Stevens CE, Taylor PE, Tong MJ, et al. Hepatitis B vaccine: An overview. In: Vyas GN, Dienstag JL, Hoofnagle JH, eds. Viral hepatitis and liver disease. Orlando, FL: Grune and Stratton, 1984:275-91.

80. Davidson M, Krugman S. Immunogenicity of recombinant yeast hepatitis B vaccine. Lancet 1985;1:108-9.

81. Gibas A, Watkins E, Hinkle C, Dienstag JL. Long-term persistence of protective antibody after hepatitis B vaccination of healthy adults. In: Zuckerman AJ, ed. Viral hepatitis and liver disease. New York, NY: Alan R. Liss, 1988:998-1001.

82. Williams WW. Guidelines for infection control in hospital personnel. Infect Control 1983;4(suppl):326-49.

83. Hanson MR, Polesky HF. Hepatitis B surveillance in employees of a community blood center. Transfusion 1985;25:18-20.

84. Page PL. Risk of hepatitis B exposure in regional blood services. Transfusion 1987;27:242-4.

85. Tullis JL, Hinman J, Sproul MT, Nickerson RJ. Incidence of post transfusion hepatitis in previously frozen blood. JAMA 1970;214:719-23.

86. Alter HJ, Tabor E, Meryman H, et al. Transmission of hepatitis B virus infection by transfusion of frozen-deglycerolized red blood cells. N Engl J Med 1978;298:637-42.

87. Haugen RK. Hepatitis after the transfusion of frozen red cells and washed red cells. N Engl J Med 1979;301:393-5.

88. Lim SG, Lee CA, Charman H, et al. Hepatitis C antibody assay in a longitudinal study of haemophiliacs. Br J Haematol 1991;78:398-402.

89. Blanchette VS, Vorstman E, Shore A, et al. Hepatitis C infection in children with hemophilia A and B. Blood 1991;78:285-9.

90. Tabor E, Gerety RJ. Transmission of hepatitis B by immune serum globulin. Lancet 1979;2:1293.

91. Centers for Disease Control. Safety of therapeutic immune globulin preparations with respect to transmission of human T-lymphotropic virus type III/lymphadenopathy-associated virus infection. MMWR 1986;35:231-3.

92. Williams PE, Yap PL, Gillon J, et al. Non-A,non-B hepatitis transmission by intravenous immunoglobulin. Lancet 1988;2:501.

93. Centers for Disease Control. *Pneumocystis* pneumonia—Los Angeles. MMWR 1981;30:250-2.

94. Centers for Disease Control. Kaposi's sarcoma and *Pneumocystis* pneumonia among homosexual men—New York City and California. MMWR 1981;30:305-8.

95. Medley GF, Anderson RM, Cox DR, et al. Incubation period of AIDS in patients infected via blood transfusion. Nature 1987;328:719-21.

96. Brookmeyer R. Reconstruction and future trends of the AIDS epidemic in the United States. Science 1991;253:37-42.

97. Centers for Disease Control. *Pneumocystis carinii* pneumonia among persons with hemophilia A. MMWR 1982;31:365-7.

98. Centers for Disease Control. Possible transfusion-associated acquired immune deficiency syndrome (AIDS)—California. MMWR 1982;31;652-4.

99. Centers for Disease Control. Prevention of acquired immune deficiency syndrome (AIDS): Report of inter-agency recommendations. MMWR 1983;32:101-4.

100. Curran JW. Lawrence DN, Jaffee H, et al. Acquired immunodeficiency syndrome (AIDS) associated with transfusions. N Engl J Med 1984;310:75-9.

101. Montagnier L, Gruest J, Chamaret S. Adaptation of lymphadenopathy associated virus (LAV) to replication in EBV-transformed B lymphoblastoid cell lines. Science 1984;225:63-6.

102. Popvic M, Sarngadharan MG, Read E, Gallo RC. Detection, isolation and continuous production of cytopathic retrovirus (HTLV-III) from patients with AIDS and pre-AIDS. Science 1984;224:497-500.

103. Haseltine WA, Wong-Staal F. The molecular biology of the AIDS virus. Sci Am 1988;259(4):52-72.

104. Zuck TF, Epstein JS. The human immunodeficiency virus: Testing for its presence and strategies for its inactivation. In: Insalaco SJ, Menitove JE, eds. Transfusion-transmitted viruses: Epidemiology and pathology. Arlington, VA: American Association of Blood Banks, 1987:109-25.

105. Smith TF. Structure, classification and replication of viruses. In: Insalaco SJ, Menitove JE, eds. Transfusion-transmitted viruses: Epidemiology and pathology. Arlington, VA: American Association of Blood Banks, 1987:1-16.

106. Denis F, Leonard G, Sangare A, et al. Comparison of 10 enzyme immunoassays for detection of antibody to human immunodeficiency virus type 2 in West African sera. J Clin Microbiol 1988;27:1000-4.

107. Allain JP, Laurian Y, Paul DA, Senn D. Serological markers in early stages of human immunodeficiency virus infection in haemophilacs. Lancet 1986;2:1233-6.

108. Cooper DA, Gold J, Mclean P, et al. Acute AIDS retrovirus infection. Lancet 1985;1:537-40.

109. Melbye M, Goedert JJ, Blattner WA. The natural history of human immunodeficiency virus infection. In: Gottlieb MS, Jeffries DJ, Mildvan D, et al, eds. Current topics in AIDS: Vol 1. Chichester, UK: John Wiley and Sons, 1987:57-93.

110. McDougal JS, Nicholson JKA, Mawle A. Effects of HIV infection on the immune system. In: Madhok R, Forbes CD, Evatt BL, eds. Blood, blood products, and AIDS. Baltimore, MD: The Johns Hopkins University Press, 1987:51-88.

111. Chiavetta JA, Nusbacher J, Wall A. Donor self-exclusion patterns and human immunodeficiency virus antibody test results over a twelve-month period. Transfusion 1989;29:81-3.

112. Zoon KC. Revised recommendations for the prevention of human immunodeficiency virus (HIV) transmission by blood and blood products (memorandum). Bethesda, MD: FDA Center for Biologics Evaluation and Research, April 23, 1992.

113. Dodd RY. Donor screening for HIV in the United States. In: Madhok R, Forbes CD, Evatt BL, eds. Blood, blood products, and

AIDS. Baltimore, MD: The Johns Hopkins University Press, 1987:143-60.

114. Imagawa DT, Lee MH, Wolinsky SM, et al. Human immunodeficiency virus type 1 in homosexual men who remain seronegative for prolonged periods. N Engl J Med 1989; 320:1458-62.

115. Haseltine WA. Silent HIV infection. N Engl J Med 1989;320:1487-9.

116. Imagawa D, Detels R. HIV-1 in seronegative homosexual men. N Engl J Med 1991;325: 1250-1.

117. Centers for Disease Control. Unexplained CD4+ T-lymphocyte depletion in persons without evident HIV infection—United States. MMWR 1992;41:541-5.

118. Laurence J, Siegal FP, Schattner E, et al. Acquired immunodeficiency without evidence of infection with human immunodeficiency virus types 1 and 2. Lancet 1992;340: 273-4.

119. Perkins HA, Samson S, Garner J, et al. Risk of AIDS for recipients of blood components from donors who subsequently developed AIDS. Blood 1987;70:1604-10.

120. Prodouz KN, Fratantoni JC. Inactivation of virus in blood products. Transfusion 1988; 28:2-3.

121. HIV/AIDS surveillance report. Atlanta, GA: Centers for Disease Control, July 1992.

122. Ward JW, Holmberg SD, Allen JR, et al. Transmission of human immunodeficiency virus (HIV) by blood transfusions screened as negative for HIV antibody. N Engl J Med 1988;318:473-8.

123. Conley LJ, Holmberg SD. Transmission of AIDS from blood screened negative for antibody to the human immunodeficiency virus. N Engl J Med 1992;326:1499-1500.

124. Lui KJ, Lawrence DN, Morgan WM, et al. A model-based approach for estimating the mean incubation period of transfusion-associated acquired immunodeficiency syndrome. Proc Natl Acad Sci USA 1987;83: 3051-5.

125. Kleinman S, Secord K. Risk of human immunodeficiency virus (HIV) transmission by anti-HIV negative blood: estimates using the lookback methodology. Transfusion 1988;28: 499-501.

126. Busch MP, Eble BE, Khayam-Bashi H, et al. Evaluation of screened blood donations for human immunodeficiency virus type 1 infection by culture and DNA amplification of pooled cells. N Engl J Med 1991;325:1-5.

127. Nelson K, Donahue J, Muñoz A, et al. Transmission of HIV by transfusion of screened blood. N Engl J Med 1990;323:1709.

128. Dodd RY. The risk of transfusion-transmitted infection. N Engl Med 1992;327:419-20.

129. Bove JR, Rigney R, Kehoe PM, Campbell J. Look-back: Preliminary experience of AABB members. Transfusion 1987;27:201-2.

130. Busch MP, Samson SM, Perkins HA. Is lookback doing the job? Transfusion 1987;27: 503-4.

131. Watkins JD. Report of the Presidential Commission on the Human Immunodeficiency Virus Epidemic. Washington, DC: US Government Printing Office, 1988:78-80.

132. Petricciani JC. Licensed tests for antibody to human T-lymphotropic virus type III. Ann Intern Med 1985;103:726-9.

133. Polesky HF. Anti-HIV (human immunodeficiency virus) testing: Methods and results. In: Insalaco SJ, Menitove JE, eds. Transfusion-transmitted viruses: Epidemiology and pathology. Arlington, VA: American Association of Blood Banks, 1987:87-107.

134. Galen RS, Gambino SR. Beyond normality: The predictive value and efficiency of medical diagnosis. New York, NY: John Wiley and Sons, 1975.

135. Esber EC. Recommendations for the management of donors and units that are initially reactive for hepatitis B surface antigen (HBsAg) (memorandum). Bethesda, MD: Food and Drug Administration, December 2, 1987.

136. Zoon KC. Use of Fluorognost HIV-1 immunofluorescent assay (IFA)(memorandum). Bethesda, MD: FDA Center for Biologics Evaluation and Research, April 23, 1992.

137. Schorr JB, Berkowitz A, Cummings PD, et al. Prevalence of HTLV-III antibody in American blood donors. N Engl J Med 1985;313:384-5.

138. Kuritsky JN, Rastogi SC, Faich GA, et al. Results of nationwide screening of blood and plasma for antibodies to human T-cell lymphotrophic III virus, type III. Transfusion 1986;26:205-7.

139. AABB/CAP viral markers survey: Set W-B. Skokie, IL: College of American Pathologists 1988:9-10.

140. Ward JW, Grindon AJ, Feorini PM, et al. Laboratory and epidemiologic evaluation of an enzyme immunoassay for antibodies to HTLV-III. JAMA 1987;256:357-61.

141. Haley NR, Williamson PB. Trends of HIV-1 positivity among blood donors in a large southeastern blood region 1985-1991. In: Program and abstracts of the Fifth National Forum on AIDS, Hepatitis, and Other Blood-Borne Diseases, Atlanta, March 29-April 1, 1992. Princeton, NJ: Symedco, 1992:69.

142. Mortimer PP, Clewley JP. Serological tests for human immunodeficiency virus. In: Gottlieb MS, Jeffries DJ, Mildvan D, et al, eds. Current topics in AIDS: Vol 1. Chichester, UK: John Wiley and Sons, 1987:133-54.

143. Thorn RM, Beltz GA, Hung C-H, et al. Enzyme immunoassay using a novel recombinant polypeptide to detect human immunodeficiency virus env antibody. J Clin Microbiol 1987;25:1207-12.

144. Polesky HF, Hanson MR. Human immunodeficiency virus type 1 proficiency testing. Arch Pathol Lab Med 1990;114:268-71.

145. McClelland DBL. Blood donor screening for HIV infection: Introduction in the United Kingdom and Europe and its impact on transfusion medicine. In: Madhok R, Forbes CD, Evatt BL, eds. Blood, blood products, and AIDS. Baltimore, MD: The Johns Hopkins University Press, 1987:161-81.

146. Frosner GG, Erfle V, Mellert W, Hehlmann R. Diagnostic significance of quantitative determination of HIV antibody specific for envelope and core proteins. Lancet 1987;1:159-60.

147. Stramer SL, Heller JS, Coombs RW, et al. Markers of HIV infection prior to IgG antibody seropositivity. JAMA 1989;262:64-9.

148. Gilcher RO, Smith J, Thompson S, et al. Transfusion-associated HIV from anti-HIV non-reactive, HIV antigen reactive donor blood (abstract). In: Book of Abstracts from the ISBT/AABB Joint Congress. Arlington, VA: American Association of Blood Banks, 1990:60.

149. Irani MS, Dudley AW, Lucco LJ. Case of HIV-1 transmission by antigen-positive, antibody-negative blood. N Engl J Med 1991;325:1174-5.

150. Alter HJ, Epstein JS, Swenson SG, et al. Prevalence of human immunodeficiency virus type 1 p24 antigen in US blood donors—an assessment of the efficacy of testing in donor screening. N Engl J Med 1990;323:1312-17.

151. Bäcker U, Weinauer F, Gathof G, Eberle J. HIV antigen screening in blood donors. Lancet 1987;2:1213.

152. Southern EM. Detection of specific sequences among DNA fragments separated by gel electrophoresis. J Mol Biol 1975;98:503-17.

153. The Consortium for Retrovirus Serology Standardization. Serological diagnosis of human immunodeficiency virus infection by Western blot testing. JAMA 1988;260:674-9.

154. Centers for Disease Control. Interpretation and use of the Western blot assay for serodiagnosis of human immunodeficiency virus type 1 infections. MMWR 1989;38(no. S-7):1-7.

155. Centers for Disease Control. Interpretive criteria used to report Western blot results for HIV-1-antibody testing—United States. MMWR 1991;40:692-5.

156. Dock NL, Lamberson HV, O'Brien TA, et al. Evaluation of atypical human immunodeficiency virus immunoblot reactivity in blood donors. Transfusion 1988;28:412-8.

157. Jackson JB, MacDonald KL, Cadwell J, et al. Absence of HIV infection in blood donors with indeterminate Western blot tests for antibody to HIV-1. N Engl J Med 1990;322:217-22.

158. Dock NL, Kleinman SH, Rayfield MA, et al. Human immunodeficiency virus infection and indeterminate western blot patterns: Prospective studies in a low prevalence population. Arch Intern Med 1991;151;525-30.

159. Levinson SS, Denys GA. Strengths and weaknesses in methods for identifying the causative agent(s) of acquired immunodeficiency syndrome. CRC Crit Rev Clin Lab Sci 1988;26:277-302.

160. Sandstrom EG, Schooley RT, Ho DD, et al. Detection of human anti-HTLV-III antibody by indirect immunofluorescence using fixed cells. Transfusion 1985;25:308-12.

161. Kwok S, Mack DH, Mullis KB, et al. Identification of human immunodeficiency virus sequences by using in vitro enzymatic amplification and oligomer cleavage detection. J Virol 1987;61:1690-4.

162. Jackson JB. The polymerase chain reaction in transfusion medicine. Transfusion 1990;30:51-7.

163. Rogers MF, Ou C, Rayfield M, et al. Use of the polymerase chain reaction for early detection of the proviral sequences of human immunodeficiency virus in infants born to seropositive mothers. N Engl J Med 1989;320:1649-54.

164. Horsburgh CR, Holmberg SD. The global distribution of human immunodeficiency virus type 2 (HIV-2) infection. Transfusion 1988;28:192-5.

165. Poiesz BJ, Ruscetti FW, Gazdar AF, et al. Detection and isolation of type C retrovirus particles from fresh and cultured lymphocytes of a patient with cutaneous T-cell lymphoma. Proc Natl Acad Sci USA 1980;77:7415.

166. Sandler SG, Fang C. HTLV-I and other retroviruses. In: Moore SB, ed. Transfusion-transmitted viral diseases. Arlington, VA: American Association of Blood Banks, 1987:19-35.

167. Rosenblatt JD, Golde DW, Wachsman W, et al. A second isolate of HTLV-II associated with atypical hairy-cell leukemia. N Engl J Med 1986;315:32-5.

168. Okochi K, Sato H, Hinuma YA. A retrospective study on transmission of adult T cell leukemia virus by blood transfusion: Seroconversion in recipients. Vox Sang 1984;46:245-53.

169. Inaba S, Sato H, Okochi K, et al. Prevention of transmission of human T-lymphotropic virus type 1 (HTLV-1) through transfusion by donor screening with antibody to the virus: One-year experience. Transfusion 1989;29:7-11.

170. Williams AE, Fang CT, Slamon DJ, et al. Seroprevalence and epidemiological correlates of HTLV-I infection in US blood donors. Science 1988;240:643-6.

171. Minamoto GY, Gold JWM, Scheinberg DA, et al. Infection with human T-cell leukemia virus type I in patients with leukemia. N Engl J Med 1988;318:219-22.

172. Parkman PD. HTLV-I antibody testing (memorandum). Bethesda, MD: FDA Center for Biologics Evaulation and Research, November 29, 1988.

173. Centers for Disease Control. Licensure of screening tests for antibody to human T-lymphotropic virus type I. MMWR 1988;37:736-47.

174. Menitove JE. Blood donor HTLV-I antibody testing. Transfusion 1989;29:1-2.

175. Sherman LA. Guidelines for notification and counseling of recipients of HTLV-I/II positive blood (Memo to AABB institutional members). Arlington, VA: American Association of Blood Banks, May 26, 1989.

176. Lee HH, Swanson P, Rosenblatt JD, et al. Relative prevalence and risk factors of HTLV-I and HTLV-II infection in US blood donors. Lancet 1991;337:1435-39.

177. Tegtmeier GE. Blood transfusion and the transmission of cytomegalovirus. In: Moore SB, ed. Transfusion-transmitted viral diseases. Arlington, VA: American Association of Blood Banks, 1987:87-118.

178. Alter HJ, Purcell RH, Feinstone SM, Tegtmeier GE. Non-B hepatitis: Its relationship to cytomegalovirus, to chronic hepatitis, and to direct and indirect test methods. In: Szmuness W, Alter HJ, Maynard JE, eds. Viral Hepatitis: 1981 International Symposium. Philadelphia, PA: Franklin Institute Press, 1982:279-94.

179. Tegtmeier GE. The use of cytomegalovirus-screened blood in neonates. Transfusion 1988;28:201-3.

180. Hillyer CD, Snydman DR, Berkman EM. The risk of cytomegalovirus infection in solid organ and bone marrow transplant recipients: transfusion of blood products. Transfusion 1990;30:659-66.

181. Preiksaitis JK, Brown L, McKenzie M. Transfusion-acquired cytomegalovirus infection in neonates: Prospective study. Transfusion 1988;28:205-9.

182. Gilbert GL, Hayes H, Hudson IL, James J. Prevention of transfusion acquired cytomegalovirus infection in infants by blood filtration to remove leucocytes. Neonatal Cytomegalovirus Infection Study Group. Lancet 1989;1:1228-31.

183. Eisenfeld L, Silver H, McLaughlin J, et al. Prevention of transfusion-associated cytomegalovirus infection in neonatal patients by removal of white cells from blood. Transfusion 1992;32:205-9.

184. McMonigal K, Horowitz CA, Henle W, et al. Post-perfusion syndrome due to Epstein-Barr virus: Report of two cases and review of the literature. Transfusion 1983;23:331-5.

185. Centers for Disease Control. Risks associated with human parvovirus B19 infection. MMWR 1989;38:81-97.

186. Mortimer PP, Luban NLC, Kelleher JF, Cohen BJ. Transmission of serum parvovirus-like virus by clotting-factor concentrates. Lancet 1983;2:482-4.

187. Fox JD, Briggs M, Ward PA, Tedder RS. Human herpesvirus 6 in salivary glands. Lancet 1990;2:590-3.

188. Saxinger C, Polesky H, Eby N, et al. Antibody reactivity with HBLV (HHV-6) in US populations. J Virol Methods 1988;21:199-208.

189. Lunel F, Agut H, Robert C, et al. Is human herpes virus 6 (HHV-6) infection associated with posttransfusion hepatitis? Transfusion 1991;31:872.

5

Cryopreservation of Blood

Cryobiology is the study of the effects of subfreezing temperatures on biological systems. The application of this scientific discipline to cellular preservation began in 1949 with the freezing and recovery of live fowl sperm, using glycerol as a cryoprotectant.[1] In 1950, glycerol techniques were applied to the freezing of red blood cells.[2]

Cold Injury and Cryoprotective Agents

Meryman has suggested[3] that cell injury occurring during the freeze-thaw process results from: 1) cellular dehydration and/or 2) mechanical trauma caused by the formation and growth of intracellular ice crystals as shown in Fig 5-1. At relatively slow rates of freezing (less than 10 C/min) extracellular water freezes earlier than intracellular water, causing an osmotic gradient such that water diffuses from inside the cell to outside the cell. Consequently, the cell loses water volume and becomes dehydrated. Such moderate to severe dehydration and intracellular hypertonicity cause significant cell injury.

At more rapid rates of freezing the osmotic gradient has almost no time to develop and dehydration and volume reduction are minimal. The problem with rapid freezing, however, is the spontaneous formation of intracellular ice crystals and accompanying cell damage.

The ideal would be to find a cooling rate just less than that which causes intracellular freezing. At such an ideal cooling rate, enough water would leave the cell to produce mild intracellular hypertonicity and retard intracellular ice formation, but not so much as to cause significant dehydration. Cryoprotective agents that penetrate the cell combine with intracellular solutions and lower the temperature at which ice crystals form. Cells thus treated can be stored at below freezing temperatures without excessive ice crystal formation, thereby avoiding damage due to intracellular ice crystal formation and excessive cellular dehydration. Only two cryoprotective agents are in current clinical use—glycerol and dimethyl sulfoxide (DMSO).[4]

Glycerol, a trihydric alcohol, is a clear, colorless, syrup-like fluid with a sweet taste. It is miscible with water. Pharmacologically, glycerol is relatively inert, and systemic effects from infusion are negligible except for the shifts in intracellular fluid that occur if improperly deglycerolized cells are exposed to circulating plasma.

DMSO is a colorless liquid with a sulfur-like smell and has several medical uses. For instance, it is used for symptomatic treatment in patients with interstitial cystitis. It is highly polar and dis-

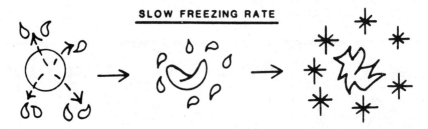

SLOW FREEZING RATE

Large amounts of water leave cell, causing dehydration injury.

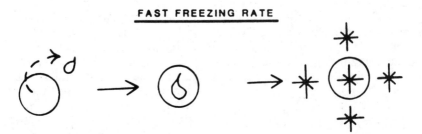

FAST FREEZING RATE

Little water leaves cell allowing for intracellular ice formation.

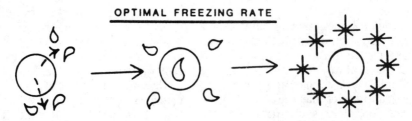

OPTIMAL FREEZING RATE

Only part of water leaves cell resulting in minimal dehydration injury and retarded intracellular ice formation.

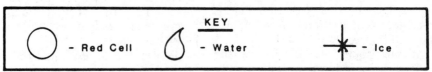

Figure 5-1. Illustration of effects of varied freezing rates. (Modified from Meryman.[3])

solves many water- and lipid-soluble substances. DMSO given intravenously may cause nausea, vomiting, local vasospasm and an objectionable garlic-like odor and taste.

Freezing Red Cells

Previously frozen deglycerolized red cells (D-RBCs) were first successfully transfused in 1951.[5] D-RBCs did not become clinically useful until the 1960's, after the development of effective techniques for removing glycerol. Several mechanical devices for deglycerolization are now available.[6] Preparation of frozen cells fits easily into component preparation programs.

It is possible to obtain both platelets and fresh frozen plasma (FFP) from a donor unit, and then freeze the red cells. Frozen preservation of red cells is particularly advantageous for storing units with rare blood types and for autologous transfusion. Frozen cells can be effectively stockpiled for military mobilization or civilian disasters. They are less useful in routine inventory management due to the high cost and due to the fact that D-RBCs are licensed only for a 24-hour shelf life. Recently, a specially designed plastic bag system that allows removal of glycerol in a closed system has been described.[7] With the new method, D-RBCs can be stored for 35 days.[7]

Processing Methods

There are three basic methods that have been used to cryopreserve red cells,[8-11] as shown in Table 5-1 (also refer to Methods 10.6 and 10.7). This chapter will discuss in detail only the high-concentration glycerol technique, which is used by most blood banks that freeze red cells.

A recent modification of the high-concentration glycerol method using an 800 mL primary collection container for freezing has been adopted by the Department of Defense.[12] See Method 10.7. Since both the addition of cryoprotective agent and freezing are in the original collection container, there is less chance of contamination and/or identification error. In addition, the amount of extracellular glycerol is smaller and it is more efficient to store and ship units prepared by this method.[12]

Many different instruments are available to process frozen blood. The manufacturer of each instrument provides detailed instructions for using that instrument. Many different techniques exist for glycerolizing, freezing, storing, thawing and deglycerolizing blood.[13,14]

Blood for subsequent freezing can be collected in CPD or CPDA-1 and stored as WB or RBCs (including RBCs in AS-1 or AS-3). Ordinarily, blood should be glycerolized and frozen within 6 days of collection.[15,16] RBCs preserved in AS-1 and AS-3 can be frozen after up to 42 days of liquid storage.[17,18] These products can be licensed if the red cells were collected in CPD or CPDA-1.

Prior to glycerolization, some procedures require removal of most of the plasma or additive from the RBCs, while others do not.[19,20]

Glycerol is used for freezing in concentrations hypertonic to blood, and its rapid introduction can cause damage to red cells. This damage becomes manifest as hemolysis only after thawing. Therefore, glycerol and red cells should be well mixed as they are transferred into the storage container.

Practical methods for cryopreservation of red cells using glycerol are available[8-12] as described in Methods 10.6 and

Table 5-1. Comparison of the Three Basic Methods of Red Blood Cell Cryopreservation

Consideration	High-Concentration Glycerol	Agglomeration[8]	Low-Concentration Glycerol[9-11]
Final glycerol concentration (w/v)	Approx. 40%	Approx. 40%	Approx. 20%
Initial freezing temperature	−80 C	−80 C	−196 C
Freezing rate	Slow	Slow	Rapid
Freezing rate control	No	No	Yes
Type of freezer	Mechanical	Mechanical	Liquid nitrogen
Storage temperature (maximum)	−65 C	−65 C	−120 C
Change in storage temperature	Can be thawed and refrozen	Cannot be refrozen	Critical
Type of storage	Polyvinyl chloride; polyolefin	Polyvinyl chloride	Polyolefin
Shipping	Dry ice	Dry ice	Liquid nitrogen
Special deglycerolizing equipment required	Yes	No	No
Deglycerolizing time (minutes)	20–40	35	30
Hematocrit	0.55–0.70	0.85	0.50–0.70
WBC removed (%)	94–99	80–90	95

10.7. Red cells can be rejuvenated and frozen up to 3 days after expiration.

Freezing and Storage

Storage Containers

There is some evidence that the composition of the storage container may be important in minimizing hemolysis.[16] For reasons not clearly understood, less hemolysis occurs with freezing in polyolefin than in polyvinyl chloride (PVC) containers.[10] Red cells in contact with the container surface seem to sustain some injury that does not affect cells in the central portions. These differences in hemolysis are not large. Although PVC containers have given satisfactory results for freezing RBCs in a high concentration of glycerol, polyolefin bags are currently more popular for the high-concentration glycerol method, since they are less brittle at −80 C and can be handled and shipped with less likelihood of breakage. Valeri et al, however, have demonstrated that breakage rates with the 800-mL PVC bag may be as low as 1% with in-facility storage and 3% even when shipped.[21]

Freezing Conditions

Red cells with a final glycerol concentration of 40% may be stored at temperatures of –65 C or lower, in containers made of either PVC or polyolefin. Either kind of container may crack if bumped or handled roughly when frozen. Glycerolized red cells are usually placed in cardboard or metal canisters for protection during freezing, storage and thawing. Up to 18 hours at room temprature can elapse between glycerolizing and freezing without increased postthaw hemolysis; however, freezing should be accomplished as soon as practical.[10] With the currently used high-concentration glycerol methods, freezing is accomplished by placing the RBC container into a –80 C freezer. Control of the freezing rate is unnecessary. However, it is recommended that no more than 4 hours elapse between the time the glycerol is added and the unit is placed in the freezer.

No controlled studies exist that establish a maximum storage time for red cells kept at –65 C or colder. Many units stored 10-21 years have been transfused successfully.[6,21] The FDA licenses Red Blood Cells Frozen for storage up to 10 years. AABB *Standards for Blood Banks and Transfusion Services* allows frozen storage of blood for routine transfusion up to 10 years. For blood of rare phenotypes, a facility's medical director may wish to extend the storage period. The medical director should document and record the unusual nature of such units and the reason for retaining them past the 10-year storage period. Since new donor screening tests are being continuously introduced, it is prudent to freeze samples of serum from units to be frozen to allow additional testing in the future. Frozen rare RBCs not tested for the new markers should be distributed only if suitable alternative units are not available. The label should indicate that the unit has not been tested or that the donor was subsequently negative for a given marker.

Thawing and Deglycerolizing

Frozen red cells, in their protective canister, may be placed in either a 37 C waterbath or 37 C dry warmer. Units frozen in the primary collection bag system should be thawed at 42 C.[12] Prolonged immersion in a waterbath is not recommended. Gentle agitation in the waterbath may be used to speed thawing. The thawing process takes at least 20-25 minutes and should not exceed 40 minutes. Glycerol must be properly removed from thawed cells to avoid in vivo and/or in vitro hemolysis. The intracellular environment of glycerolized cells is hypertonic relative to plasma and the first solution used for deglycerolization must also be somewhat hypertonic. This allows the glycerol to begin diffusing out of the red cell while the intracellular environment remains hypertonic.

The three basic deglycerolization procedures—high-concentration glycerol, low-concentration glycerol and agglomeration—use different hypertonic solutions and wash protocols, but the principle is the same: equilibration of the thawed red cells with a hypertonic solution, followed by washing with solutions progressively less hypertonic and final suspension of red cells in an isotonic electrolyte solution containing glucose.

Any of the commercially available instruments for batch or continuous flow washing can be used to deglycerolize cells frozen in a high concentration of glycerol.[11,17] A procedure for deglycerolization is described in Method 10.6. With longer postthaw storage (past 24 hours) there may be an increase in the amount of hemolysis observed.

When the final component is prepared for issue, the integrally connected tubing must be filled with an aliquot of rbcs and sealed in such a manner that it will be available for subsequent compatibility testing.[15] The label must identify the collecting facility as well as the facility preparing the D-RBCs.[15]

Since there are so many small but potentially important variations in deglycerolization protocols for each instrument, the reader should follow the individual manufacturer's specific recommendations.

Red Cells With Hemoglobin S

Red blood cells from persons with sickle trait tolerate glycerolizing, freezing and thawing normally but form a jelly-like mass and hemolyze during deglycerolization. In many cryopreservation programs, cells are screened for the presence of hemoglobin S before freezing is undertaken, but there may be occasions when cells from sickle trait donors must be frozen, especially for autologous transfusions. Such units may not be suitable for neonatal exchange transfusions.[15] The hypertonic deglycerolizing solutions appear to cause sedimentation of the abnormal red cells, such that glycerol is not adequately removed from the red cells, which then hemolyze when suspended in normal saline. Satisfactory deglycerolization can be achieved if the thawed red cells are massively diluted with 0.2% dextrose in 0.9% sodium chloride after equilibration with 12% sodium chloride and the hypertonic washing solution is omitted.[22] Deglycerolizing a unit of frozen sickle trait cells requires intensive technical attention and the manual operation of the cell washer, with more washes than are necessary for normal cells.

Storing Red Blood Cells Deglycerolized

When glycerolizing or deglycerolizing requires entering the container, it is considered an "open" system. Therefore, D-RBCs so prepared can be stored for only 24 hours at 1-6 C. A longer postthaw shelf life would make frozen RBCs more useful for inventory management. A sterile connection device or a specially designed plastic container configuration can be used to prepare frozen red cells and to glycerolize them in a closed system. Even with presently used open systems, bacterial growth in D-RBCs is very rare.[23] The deglycerolizing process reduces the number of organisms present, and those remaining grow very slowly during refrigerated storage. In experimental studies, when D-RBCs are stored up to 7 days, the most important change that occurs is increased concentration of potassium and hemoglobin in the supernatant fluid,[24] which can easily be removed just before transfusion. AS-1 has been used to decrease postthaw hemolysis and to allow 14 days of storage at 4 C after thawing.[24]

Refreezing Red Blood Cells Deglycerolized

It may occasionally be desirable to refreeze thawed units of red cells, either after unintentional thawing or after deglycerolization of units that are not used. One study of cells frozen with the high-concentration glycerol method showed there was no loss of ATP, 2,3-DPG or in-vivo survival in units that were deglycerolized, stored 20 hours at refrigerator temperature and then reglycerolized and refrozen.[25] In a different study,[26] units of red cells subjected three times to glycerolizing, freezing and thawing exhibited 27% loss of total hemoglobin. AABB *Standards* does not address refreezing thawed units, since this should not be considered routinely as a desirable practice. To avoid losing units of high-priority blood, a responsible physician in a blood bank who decides to refreeze thawed units should document the valuable nature of such units and the reasons for refreezing them.

Transportability

Red cells that are cryopreserved with high concentrations of glycerol tolerate fluctuations in temperature from –85 to –20 C without any significant effects on in-vitro recovery or 24-hour posttransfusion survival.[6,7] These RBCs can be transported on dry ice or in a container that will guarantee maintaining the temperature at –65 C or lower. AABB *Standard*s requires that components ordinarily stored frozen should be transported in a manner designed to maintain them frozen.[15]

Quality Assurance

See Chapter 22.

Clinical Considerations

Deglycerolized red cells are comparable in volume, hematocrit and efficacy to a unit of RBCs. Since virtually all the plasma and anticoagulant and most of the leukocytes and platelets have been removed, the deglycerolized unit consists essentially of red cells in an electrolyte solution. Red cells filtered using the new filters to remove leukocytes are preferred over deglycerolized RBCs when leukocyte-reduced RBCs are needed. The absence of potassium in the supernatant may be advantageous for selected patients with hyperkalemia. In-vivo survival and function are comparable to *freshly* drawn, liquid-stored red cells because ATP levels, 2,3-DPG content and oxygen dissociation curves are unchanged from pre-freeze values.

Immunologic Activity

The long storage life of frozen red cells is, in some circumstances, a significant advantage over liquid-stored red cells; their unique composition makes them potentially advantageous in certain clinical situations. Deglycerolized red blood cells have very little plasma protein and can be used for IgA-deficient patients with anti-IgA antibodies, or others with severe immune reactions to transfused plasma proteins. Most hematologists use D-RBCs for patients with paroxysmal nocturnal hemoglobinuria because plasma, leukocyte and platelet content are all low. Since red cells are usually frozen within 6 days of collection or after appropriate rejuvenation, 2,3-DPG levels are nearly normal in D-RBCs. This may be advantageous when transfusing newborns. Glycerolizing and deglycerolizing red cells remove granulocytes and platelets, but some lymphocytes survive. Transfusing D-RBCs prevents reactions in patients with granulocyte or platelet antibodies, but other less costly blood components may be equally effective. Since some viable lymphocytes are present,[27] D-RBCs could theoretically cause graft-vs-host disease (GVHD) in immunodeficient patients. For patients at risk for GVHD from transfusion, irradiation of the D-RBCs is recommended.

Disease Transmission

Alter et al[28] demonstrated in 1978 that human blood in which the plasma was seeded with hepatitis B virus before freezing could transmit the virus to chimpanzees after processing, freezing and deglycerolization. D-RBCs have also been shown[29] to transmit hepatitis B to human recipients. It is also likely that retroviruses such as HIV could be present in a unit of D-RBCs.

Hepatitis B virus exists in plasma. Cytomegalovirus (CMV) is usually found in white cells. The use of D-RBCs to reduce transmission is an acceptable alternative to CMV-negative RCBs. In low birth weight premature infants, selected transplant recipients and other severely immunosuppressed individuals, CMV-seronegative units are used to reduce CMV infection. The freeze-thaw process is an effective alternative way to reduce the likelihood of CMV transmission in selected recipients.[30]

Immunization to HLA Antigens

D-RBCs contain reduced numbers of elements that express HLA antigens—granulocytes, lymphocytes and platelets. Transfusing deglycerolized cells instead of WB reduces immunization to HLA antigens.[31] D-RBCs were initially indicated to reduce the risk of HLA immunization in dialysis patients awaiting a cadaveric kidney transplant, but transfusion of blood components containing HLA-active material was shown to improve survival of transplanted kidneys.[32] In patients treated with cyclosporin this transfusion effect may not be significant. Until recently, most recipients of kidney transplants have been given RBCs as the transfusion component of choice.[33] Since lymphocytes responsive to phytohemagglutinin stimulation have been found in D-RBCs,[27] irradiation should be considered for patients at risk for GVHD.

Freezing Other Cells

Platelets

Frozen storage of autologous platelets is highly desirable for patients with non-hematologic diseases whose therapy will cause bone marrow ablation, for alloimmunized patients in remission and for patients with expected episodic needs for platelets.

Several cryoprotectants have been used to freeze platelets,[34] but DMSO is the agent that is preferred.[35] Use of DMSO no longer requires filing for investigational new drug approval, and several medical centers have developed protocols for collecting, storing and transfusing cryopreserved autologous platelets. Platelets preserved in the frozen state have been used clinically.[35-38] Platelet recovery is significantly lower than for the recovery of cryopreserved RBCs (approximately 30-50%), so the use of cryopreserved platelets is not widespread. Procedures for freezing platelets are described in Methods 10.16 and 10.17.

Granulocytes

Treating the severely granulocytopenic, septic patient with granulocytes is difficult for two reasons. Granulocytes rapidly lose function upon storage at room temperature and, once infused, granulocytes have only an 8-hour half-life. Granulocytes are much more sensitive to freezing, thawing and hyperosmotic stress than are red cells, lymphocytes or platelets.[39]

Human granulocyte cryopreservation was first reported in 1963.[40] Since then, a variety of cryoprotectants, freezing rates, storage temperatures and isolation procedures have been tried, with questionable success.[41,42] It is difficult to monitor the safety and therapeutic effectiveness of transfused cryopreserved granulocytes in part because infusion of freshly drawn granulocytes causes little measurable increase in peripheral count and efficacy can only be inferred by clinical response. Labeling granulocytes with indium-111 may prove helpful in studying both freshly drawn and cryopreserved granulocytes. In-vivo migration of these tagged cells to sites of infection can be observed directly, allowing more immediate inferences about function than is obtained by counting circulating white cells or observing changes in body temperature.[43]

Lymphocytes

Frozen with a final concentration of 10% DMSO and kept in the vapor phase of liquid nitrogen, lymphocytes maintain their cellular immune reactivity when thawed.[44,45] Lymphocyte freezing is used primarily for preserving cells used in laboratory tests. The HLA reactivity of a patient's cells can be tested against previously frozen cells of known antigenic composition. Homozygous typing cells with a double dose of HLA-D antigens can be stored frozen. Reagent cells or patient's cells can be frozen to maintain viability during shipping. Lymphocytes in 10% DMSO are more sensitive to the cooling rate than RBCs in high concentrations of glycerol. The cooling rate should be about 1 C/min, and not exceed 10 C/min. Controlled addition of cryopreservative and dilution protocols for its removal after thawing yield high recoveries.

References

1. Polge C, Smith AU. Revival of spermatozoa after vitrification and dehydration at low temperature. Nature 1949;164:666.
2. Smith AU. Prevention of hemolysis during freezing and thawing of red blood cells. Lancet 1950;2:910.
3. Meryman HT. Cryopreservation of blood and marrow cells: Basic biological and biophysical considerations. In: Petz LD, Swisher SN, eds. Clinical practice of blood transfusions. New York: Churchill Livingstone, 1981:313-31.
4. Meryman HT. Cryoprotective agents. Cryobiology 1971;8:173-83.
5. Mollison PL, Sloviter HA. Successful transfusion of previously frozen human red cells. Lancet 1951;2:862.
6. Meryman HT. The cryopreservation of blood cells for clinical use. Prog Hematol 1979;11:193-227.
7. Lovric VA, Klarkowski DB. Donor blood frozen and stored between –20 C and –25 C with 35-day post-thaw shelf life. Lancet 1989;1:71-3.
8. Huggins CE. Practical preservation of blood by freezing. In: Red cell freezing. Washington, DC: American Association of Blood Banks, 1973:31-53.
9. Rowe AW, Eyster E, Kellner A. Liquid nitrogen preservation of RBCs for transfusion. A low glycerol-rapid freeze procedure. Cryobiology 1968;5:119-28.
10. Hornblower M, Meryman HT. Influence of the container material on the hemolysis of glycerolized red cells after freezing and thawing. Cryobiology 1974;11:317-23.
11. Rowe AW. Preservation of blood by the low glycerol-rapid freeze process. In: Red cell freezing. Washington, DC: American Association of Blood Banks, 1973:55-71.
12. Valeri CR, Valeri DA, Anastasi J, et al. Freezing in the primary polyvinylchloride plastic collection bag: A new system for preparing and freezing nonrejuvenated and rejuvenated red blood cells. Transfusion 1981;21:138-41.
13. Red cell freezing. Washington, DC: American Association of Blood Banks, 1973.
14. Dawson RB, ed. Clinical and practical aspects of the use of frozen blood. Washington DC: American Association of Blood Banks, 1977.
15. Widmann FK, ed. Standards for blood banks and transfusion services. 15th ed. Bethesda, MD: American Association of Blood Banks, 1993.
16. Valeri CR. Factors influencing the 24-hour posttransfusion survival and the oxygen transport function of previously frozen red cells preserved with 40% w/v glycerol and frozen at –80 C. Transfusion 1974;14:1-15.
17. Rathbun EJ, Nelson EJ, Davey RJ. Posttransfusion survival of red cells frozen for 8 weeks after 42-day liquid storage in AS-3. Transfusion 1989;29:213-7.
18. Brecher ME, Zylstra-Halling VW, Pineda AA. Rejuvenation of erythrocytes preserved with AS-1 and AS-3. Am J Clin Pathol 1991;96:767-9.
19. Meryman HT, Hornblower M. A method for freezing and washing RBCs using a high glycerol concentration. Transfusion 1972;12:145-56.
20. Valeri CR. Simplification of the methods for adding and removing glycerol during freeze-preservation of human red blood cells with high or low glycerol methods: Biochemical modification prior to freezing. Transfusion 1975;15:195-218.
21. Valeri CR, Pivacek LE, Gray AD, et al. The safety and therapeutic effectiveness of human red cells stored at –80 C for as long as 21 years. Transfusion 1989;29:429-37.

22. Meryman HT, Hornblower M. Freezing and deglycerolizing sickle-trait red blood cells. Transfusion 1976;16:627-32.

23. Simpson MB, Radcliffe JH. Bacteriological safety of cryopreserved erythrocytes. In: Dawson RB, Barnes A Jr, eds. Clinical and practical aspects of the use of frozen blood. Washington, DC: American Association of Blood Banks, 1977:37-59.

24. Ross DG, Heaton WAL, Holme S. Additive solution for the suspension and storage of deglycerolized red blood cells. Vox Sang 1989; 56:75-9.

25. Kahn RA, Auster M, Miller WV. The effect of refreezing previously frozen deglycerolized red blood cells. Transfusion 1978;18:204-5.

26. Myhre BA, Nakasako YUY, Schott R. Studies on 4 C stored frozen reconstituted red blood cells. III. Changes occurring in units which have been repeatedly frozen and thawed. Transfusion 1978;18:199-203.

27. Kurtz SR, Van Deinse WH, Valeri CR. The immunocompetence of residual leukocytes at various stages of red cell cryopreservation with 40% w/v glycerol in an ionic medium at −80 C. Transfusion 1978;18:441-7.

28. Alter HJ, Tabor E, Meryman HT, et al. Transmission of hepatitis B virus infection by transfusion of frozen-deglycerolized RBCs. N Engl J Med 1978;298:637-42.

29. Haugen RK. Hepatitis after the transfusion of frozen red cells and washed red cells. N Engl J Med 1979;301:393-5.

30. Brady MT, Milam JD, Anderson DC, et al. Use of deglycerolized red cells to prevent post-transfusion infection with cytomegalovirus in neonates. J Infect Dis 1984;150:334-9.

31. Polesky HF. Frozen deglycerolized versus washed red blood cells in transplantation and HLA-sensitization. In: Dawson RB, Barnes A Jr, eds. Clinical and practical aspects of the use of frozen blood. Washington, DC: American Association of Blood Banks, 1977:113-23.

32. Opelz G, Terasaki PI. Improvement of kidney-graft survival with increased numbers of blood transfusions. N Engl J Med 1978;299:799-803.

33. Walker RH. Transfusion support of clinical transplantation. Laboratory Medicine 1987;18: 834-8.

34. Taylor MA. Cryopreservation of platelets: An in-vitro comparison of four methods. J Clin Pathol 1981;34:71-5.

35. Schiffer CA, Aisner J, Dutcher JP. Platelet cryopreservation using dimethyl sulfoxide. Ann NY Acad Sci 1983;411:161-9.

36. Daly PA, Schiffer CA, Aisner J, Wiernik PH. Successful transfusion of platelets cryopreserved for more than 3 years. Blood 1979; 54:1023-7.

37. Schiffer CA, Aisner J, Wiernik PH. Frozen autologous platelet transfusion for patients with leukemia. N Engl J Med 1978;299:7-12.

38. Valeri CR. SOP freeze preservation of pooled human platelets or apheresis platelets with 6% DMSO. Available from: Naval Blood Research Laboratory, Boston University School of Medicine, Boston, MA. (No date available.)

39. Meryman HT. Cryopreservation of blood cells for clinical use. In: Brown EB, ed. Progress in hematology, volume XI. New York: Grune and Stratton, Inc., 1979:193-228.

40. Rowe AW, Kaczmarek CS, Cohen E. Low temperature preservation of leukocytes in dimethylsulfoxide. Fed Proc 1963;22:170.

41. Bank H. Granulocyte preservation circa 1980. Cryobiology 1980;17:187-97.

42. Valeri CR. Current state of platelet and granulocyte cryopreservation. CRC Crit Rev Clin Lab Sci 1981;14:21-74.

43. McCullough J, Weiblen BJ, Clay ME, Forstrom L. Effect of leukocyte antibodies on the fate in vivo of indium-111-labeled granulocytes. Blood 1981;58:164-70.

44. Strong DM, Sell KW. Frozen cell banking in immunology. In: Simatos D, Strong DM, Turc JM, eds. Cryobiology. Paris: INSERM, 1977: 101-5.

45. Glassman AB, Bennett CE. Cryopreservation of human lymphocytes: A brief review and evaluation of an automated liquid nitrogen freezer. Transfusion 1979;19:178-81.

6

Tissue Banking and Organ Transplantation

Introduction

A hospital transfusion service or a blood center may have a tissue bank and/or be involved in the support of an organ recovery/transplantation program. A transfusion service or a blood center could be active in one or more of the following activities: donor selection; procurement; testing for infectious disease markers; processing, storage and distribution of tissues; and provision of blood components for organ transplantation. The field of tissue banking and organ transplantation, although not new, is rapidly evolving. A number of different acceptable procedures exist now that will change as new information becomes available. If the blood bank assumes responsibility for this activity, all phases of tissue/organ (T/O) recovery should be under the control of the blood bank medical director.

Consent and Donor Suitability

Written consent for specific tissue or organ donation must be obtained from the living donor or next of kin of the deceased donor for T/O recovery. Generally, tissue banks obtain this documentation even though the deceased may carry a signed and witnessed organ donor card, in order to ensure that next of kin have no objections and that the deceased had not decided to revoke the card. The tissues and organs to be recovered should be specific-ally documented in the consent form. Most, if not all, states have "required request" statutes, requiring that the next of kin or responsible party be asked for tissue or organ donations whenever a suitable donor dies. There are exceptions and these laws are not very effective. To avoid conflict of interest, the person declaring death should not be the requestor. Living donors and families of deceased donors should not be responsible for expenses involved in recovery and processing of T/O. They should not receive compensation for the donation.

Each potential donor should be evaluated for each specific T/O because some donors cannot donate certain tissue (eg, deceased newborns are not suitable for bone donation because of their cartilaginous skeletal structure, but they are candidates for heart donation). Although exceptions may be made in specific cases, ideally, there should be:

1. No evidence of infection by history, physical examination, laboratory tests or autopsy (if performed).
2. An afebrile hospital course.
3. A short duration of ventilator-dependent respiratory assistance.
4. Absence of clinical sepsis and a lack of pathogens in blood and urine cultures, if taken.
5. No history of intravenous drug use or other high risk behaviors for HIV infection.

6. No history of prolonged high dose steroid therapy.
7. No history of malignancy other than carcinoma of the skin or cancer in situ of the uterine cervix.
8. No history of hepatitis, syphilis, HIV or slow virus (Creutzfeldt-Jakob) infection.
9. No history of currently active autoimmune disease.

Bone donors should preferably be under the age of 50-60 years (especially women) to ensure strength when bone grafts are used for weight-bearing purposes. However, frozen femoral heads removed from elderly patients undergoing total hip arthroplasty are widely used even in weight-bearing applications. The age of the donor may preclude donation of other T/O depending upon the clinical application. Generally, a medical history similar to that used for a blood donation can be applied to determine tissue donor suitability.

Tissue Recovery

Candidate donors for organs (kidneys, livers, pancreata, hearts, heart/lungs) must be declared brain dead but cardiopulmonary function can be maintained artificially with life support techniques to ensure adequate perfusion to the organs to be recovered. These organs must be recovered in the surgical suite using sterile technique. Tissues, such as skin, bone or fascia do not require a heart-beating donor and are recovered by orthopedic surgeons or specially trained technicians. Eyes are usually removed by eye bank technicians who should be certified by the Eye Bank Association of America (EBAA) or other accrediting agencies. Skin, bone and fascia should be recovered within 24 hours of death, while eyes should be recovered within 6 hours of death.

Sterile Technique

Tissues are recovered in a similar manner to organs in an aseptic environment. Frequently, the operating room is used at night so as not to interfere with the surgical schedule.

Clean, But Nonsterile Technique

In this approach, tissues are recovered in the funeral home or autopsy room without aseptic technique but using instruments and methods that minimize microbial contamination of the tissues. Tissues collected and processed under clean conditions are then secondarily sterilized either by exposure to ethylene oxide (ETO) gas or gamma radiation using cobalt-60. Specific techniques for the recovery of tissues are given in the *Technical Manual for Tissue Banking* (*TMTB*) of the American Association of Tissue Banks (AATB).[1] Removal of corneas is described in the *Eye Bank Tissue Procedure Manual* of the EBAA.[2]

Sterility

Tissue specimens collected by sterile technique should be cultured for aerobic and anaerobic microorganisms. Representative final tissue products, or 10% of all specimens that have undergone secondary sterilization, should also be cultured. Fragments of tissue and swabs of the surface, or both, may be used. Details of the culture techniques are given in the *TMTB* of the AATB.[1] Preservation times vary according to the T/O to be preserved. Approximate storage times[1,2] are listed in Table 6-1.

Serologic Testing

The donor of tissues and organs must be tested for HBsAg, anti-HIV-1/2, anti-HCV and other tests for infectious disease markers required by such agencies as the AATB and the United Network for

Table 6-1. Approximate Preservation Times for Various Tissues and Organs

Tissue/Organ	Storage Time	Storage Temperature
Kidney	48–72 hours	4–10 C
Liver	4–24 hours	4–10 C
Heart	3–5 hours	4–10 C
Heart-lung	3–5 hours	4–10 C
Pancreas	12–24 hours	4–10 C
Corneas	7–10 days	4–10 C
Skin	5 years or longer	−65 C or colder
Bone, freeze dried	5 years or longer	Room
Bone, frozen	5 years	−65 C or colder
Bone marrow	Up to 5 years	−196 C

Organ Sharing (UNOS). The anti-HIV-1 and anti-HCV tests must be repeated after 6 months on donors of semen and surgical bone before these tissues can be released for use. A serologic test for syphilis (STS) and Rh typing should be performed on donor blood for fresh and surgical bone allografts. ABO grouping is required in organ grafts. HLA typing is essential for bone marrow and kidney grafts (see Chapter 13). Other tests, such as anti-CMV, may be performed on organ donors. Ideally, serologic tests should be performed on pretransfusion/infusion blood samples to avoid false-negative results due to hemodilution.

Bone Banking

Processing

Fresh Frozen

Cadaveric bone is obtained under sterile technique and extraneous tissues are excised. Antibiotic solutions may be used topically after cultures of a piece of tissue or surface swabs are obtained for microbiologic study. The cortical bone may be cut into "matchsticks" or "cubes" etc, prior to freezing. The bone units are double- or triple-wrapped in sterile moisture-proof material. Airtight packaging is preferred. Bone removed during surgery is widely used and is described in greater detail in Methods 10.20-10.24.

Freeze-Drying

Freeze-drying (lyophilization) has several advantages over the freeze-preservation of bone. Freeze-dried (FD) tissue can be stored at room temperature and has a shelf life of 5 years. It is ideal for shipping. Bone to be processed should first be cleared of unwanted tissue, and defatted. If the bone has been obtained under sterile conditions, it can be freeze-dried directly. Bone obtained using an unsterile technique must be sterilized either before or after freeze-drying.

Several different freeze-driers are available. The procedure used should either follow the manufacturer's instructions or, if modified, should yield a product documented to be equivalent to that obtained by the unmodified technique. The processing of each batch of FD material should be documented including the instrument used, method, length of cycle (if applicable), FD items, and length, temperature and vacuum pressure of each step of the cycle.

Demineralization

Weak transplantation antigens (hydrophobic glycopeptide) in allogeneic bone may cause an immune response in the recipient.[3] Immunogenicity can be reduced by treating the bone with a mixture of chloroform and ethanol followed by extraction and demineralization with weak hydrochloric acid. Following treatment with buffer, the bone is frozen. Bone treated in this manner is referred to as autolyzed antigen-extracted bone.[4]

Storage

Packaging

Freeze-dried bone is commonly stored in glass containers. Frozen bone is generally stored in heat-sealed plastic containers. Heat-sealing under vacuum is often used. Fresh frozen or cryopreserved massive bone allografts or bone-tendon-bone allografts are stored in several layers of impermeable wrapping material. Frozen femoral heads obtained from living donors are stored in single or double plastic bags or glass jars.

Frozen Storage

Frozen bone should be stored at –65 C or colder. This can be accomplished in either a mechanical freezer or in the vapor or liquid phase of liquid nitrogen. Bone has an indefinite storage life if maintained under these conditions. The freezers should be monitored continuously and alarm systems should be in place. Long-term (longer than 6 months) bone storage at temperatures warmer than –20 C is not recommended.[1]

Shelf Life

Bone should be stored according to directions supplied by the tissue bank providing the tissue. Bone specimens that are lyophilized (less than 5% residual mois-

ture) and stored in a vacuum have an indefinite shelf life as long as the vacuum is maintained. Bone that is not fully dehydrated and/or not packed under vacuum has a finite shelf life as determined by the medical director. ETO-sterilized bone specimens may be reprocessed at or before the expiration date in order to increase the shelf life. Such reprocessing should be done only according to established protocol. Shelf life of frozen bone stored at –65 C or colder is usually 5 years.

Skin Banking

General

Allogeneic or autologous skin may be recovered. Allogeneic donors are generally between the ages of 14 and 75 years of age. Cultures for aerobic and anaerobic bacteria are obtained to ensure safety. The techniques used and criteria for rejection are detailed in the *TMTB* of the AATB.[1] Skin should be recovered using a sterile dermatome and strict aseptic technique.

Storage

Skin may be preserved and stored in tissue culture nutrient media and antibiotics at 4 C for several days or cryopreserved in a mechanical freezer at –65 C or in the vapor phase or submerged in liquid nitrogen at –100 C to –196 C. Various preservative and cryoprotective solutions are described in the *TMTB* of the AATB.[1]

Distribution

Skin should be transported to the operating room on ice if stored at 4 C or on dry ice if cryopreserved. Labeling, thawing and application of the skin graft are described in the *TMTB* of the AATB.[1]

Semen Banking

Donor semen can be cryopreserved for future artificial insemination. Several medical indications exist for such a procedure. In addition, depositors may elect to preserve their own sperm because of planned surgical or therapeutic procedures that might render them sterile. Semen from donors who are not married to the intended recipient should be cryopreserved and these donors should be retested after 6 months for infectious disease markers.

Donor Screening

Potential sperm donors, other than the husband, are screened by interview for demographic, medical and family histories. The donor's blood is tested using an STS and for the presence of HBsAg, anti-HIV, anti-HCV and other disease markers. For sperm donors other than the husband, the anti-HIV and anti-HCV tests are repeated on a new sample from the donor 6 months or more after the sperm collection date. Frozen semen should be used only if the original and repeat tests at 6 months are both negative. Chromosome, red cell and biochemical studies may be indicated in special situations. Allogeneic donors are usually between the ages of 18 and 40.

Semen Analysis

The ejaculate is examined for sperm concentration, motility, spermatozoal abnormalities and for the presence of *N. gonorrhoeae.*

Freezing

The seminal fluid is prepared for freezing by mixing with 5-10% glycerol or glycerol plus an extender. Details are given in the *TMTB* of the AATB.[1] Seminal fluid is stored in liquid nitrogen at –196 C.

Heart Valves and Blood Vessels

Hearts from cadaveric donors that are not used for various reasons as whole organs for cardiac transplants can be dissected using aseptic technique to obtain pulmonary and aortic valves, which can be used for valve replacement. The isolated valves are treated with antibiotics and cryopreserved using liquid nutrient medium and a cryoprotective agent, such as dimethyl sulfoxide (DMSO). They are subsequently stored in vapor phase of liquid nitrogen (–100 C).

Blood vessels, especially saphenous veins, are processed in a similar manner. The vessel is dissected free of surrounding tissue, treated with antibiotics and stored in liquid nitrogen with DMSO and liquid nutrient medium. Saphenous vein allografts are used for revascularization of the lower limbs, for coronary artery bypass and for arteriovenous fistula for chronic hemodialysis when autologous veins are not available and when the use of prosthetic material is not desirable.

Tracking of Tissues

Facilities that process, store, ship, receive or issue tissues must have a system in place to identify and track the tissue from the donor (or supplier source) to the recipient. Records must be retained indefinitely to show the source facility, the original numeric or alphanumeric donor or lot identification and all recipients or other final disposition of each tissue. Records to be retained for a minimum of 5 years (or as required by applicable state and federal laws) include storage temperatures, control testing and all superseded procedures and manuals.[4]

Transfusion Service Support for Organ Transplantation

The blood bank is a vital part of the support team for a clinical transplantation program. Close communication with the transplant surgeon and other professionals involved in the program is essential. Morbidity, mortality and graft survival rates can be measurably influenced by the transfusion of blood components in the peritransplant period.

Candidates for bone marrow and solid organ transplants are generally available for study well before the transplant, so there is ample time to obtain historical information and perform pretransplant laboratory tests. Information of special importance to the blood bank includes:

1. History of prior pregnancy, transfusion or transplantation.
2. Laboratory tests should include at least: ABO and Rh type, DAT, IAT and anti-CMV. CMV-negative recipients may require CMV-negative blood components. HLA typing and HLA antibody studies are routine for organ and bone marrow recipients (see Chapter 13).

Additional tests might include subgrouping of those patients who are group A or AB and an antibody detection test in the recipient using enzyme-treated rbcs. Phenotyping rbcs of the donor and the patient may be performed in order to follow engraftment of transplanted bone marrow.

ABO Grouping

The ABO antigens are of major importance in transplantation because they constitute very strong histocompatibility antigens. Since they are expressed on vascular endothelium, major ABO mismatching can cause rapid graft rejection due to endothelial damage by ABO antibodies with subsequent widespread thrombosis within the graft. Therefore, ABO matching is crucial to the success of vascularized grafts, ie, kidney, heart, liver and pancreas. ABO matching is not important in tissue grafts, ie, fascia, bone and cornea.

The definition of an ABO-compatible graft is the same as that for a red cell transfusion. The group O donor tissue or organ is a universal donor and can be transplanted into recipients of all blood groups. Case reports document rare successful organ transplants with major ABO incompatibility in organs but these are biological curiosities.[5] It is recognized that A_2 donor kidneys can be successfully transplanted into group O recipients and that their survival may be comparable to that of O donor kidneys.[6]

Kidney Transplants

The Role of Pretransplant Transfusions

Historically, blood transfusions were avoided in patients awaiting kidney transplants because of the belief that they would immunize the recipient to transplantation antigens found on the transfused leukocytes. However, transfusions were often unavoidable since the early hemodialysis units required priming with blood. In addition, the patients were anemic as a result of their kidney disease. Erythropoietin is now routinely given to these patients and has reduced the transfusion requirements considerably. Kissmeyer-Nielsen et al[7] demonstrated that hyperacute rejection of renal allografts was associated with preformed humoral cytotoxic antibodies directed against white blood cells. In 1973, Opelz et al[8] noted that kidney allograft survival was gradually decreasing in the late 1960's and early 1970's. This was a period when hemodialysis units avoided the blood prime and intentionally limited the pretransplant blood transfusions. They suggested that these two phenomena may have a cause-and-effect relationship (ie, limiting the blood transfusions may interfere with renal allograft survival). As a result of this startling apparent association, transplant centers began using intentional pretransplant blood transfusion protocols in the mid 1970's. Data accumulated from transplant centers all over the world supported the thesis of Opelz et al that pretransplant blood transfusions enhanced renal allograft survival.[9,10]

Although numerous protocols exist, until recently many transplant centers have transfused at least five units of blood to all new dialysis patients awaiting renal transplants.[11] These are usually given in the form of WB, although RBCs, deglycerolized RBCs and buffy coat transfusions are effective alternatives to WB.

Timing of pretransplant transfusions seems to be important. Perioperative blood transfusions are usually not as effective as those given prior to surgery. Three to 6 months prior to transplantation appears to be the optimal time for the transfusion.[12]

The minimum number of pretransplant transfusions that will achieve maximal benefit for graft survival is controversial. Horimi et al[13] found that the more transfusions given, the better the result. However, Persijn[14] found the same benefit with a single transfusion.

In 1980, Salvatierra et al[15] reported that transplant recipients could be specifically primed for enhancement of renal allografts by transfusing the intended recipient with blood from the intended living donor. Such transfusions are termed donor-specific transfusions (DST). The original protocol involved transfusing the intended recipient with 200 mL of fresh WB from the donor at 2-week intervals. Numerous modifications have evolved. Salvatierra et al[15] used DSTs for haploidentical donor-recipient pairs with high mixed lymphocyte culture (MLC) reactivity. An unexpected 94% 1-year graft survival was observed.

However, DSTs also resulted in a 30% sensitization rate, which precluded transplantation in those donor-recipient pairs. In addition, the rapid onset of rejection episodes (DST-type rejection) occurred within 10 days following transplantation in about one third of the patients who were successfully transplanted.[15]

Anderson et al[16] found that the use of azathioprine (AZA) together with DSTs reduced the incidence of humoral immunization without compromising the beneficial effect of the DSTs. AZA + DST also caused a reduction in the DST-type rejections.

Explanations for the Beneficial Effect

Numerous theories exist to explain the beneficial effect of pretransplant blood transfusions on renal graft survival.

Selection

It is well known that blood transfusions frequently elicit the production of HLA antibodies in transfused patients. However, detectable HLA antibody is not a consistent outcome and some recipients fail to respond. Thus, blood transfusions can serve to define responders and nonresponders in terms of HLA antibody production. Nonresponders (those who do not develop antibodies to HLA following transfusion) are expected to have a negative pretransplant crossmatch and are also expected to tolerate the transplantation antigens of the kidney allograft, resulting in good graft survival. Responders (those who develop antibodies to HLA following transfusion), on the other hand, are difficult to crossmatch and therefore are either not transplanted or require a better HLA-matched graft.

Suppressor T-Cell Activation

Lymphocytes from some transfused humans are less responsive to a variety of soluble antigens, mitogens and allogeneic cells in the MLC in comparison to lymphocytes before transfusion.[17] Kaplan, Sarniak and Levy have shown diminished helper/suppressor ratios and natural killer cell activity in peripheral blood lymphocytes obtained from transfused patients as compared to nontransfused control patients.[18] Although there does not appear to be a specific subset of T-suppressor cells generated following transfusion, there is evidence for a nonspecific suppression which may be mediated by macrophages, monocytes and T cells.[12]

Clonal Deletion

Terasaki proposed that the blood transfusions prime alloreactive T cells, which marks them for selective elimination when they respond to the secondary stimulation of the graft and are then destroyed by the initiation of immunosuppressive therapy in the first few days posttransplant.[19]

Idiotype Network

This theory suggests that blood transfusions cause the clonal expansion of donor-reactive T cells, which in turn stimulate B cells to produce anti-idiotype antibodies. The anti-idiotype antibodies block the antigen-specific T-cell receptors so that the allograft antigens are not recognized. Thus, the anti-idiotype antibodies serve as blocking antibodies to the nonself antigens. Such antibodies have been detected by their ability to inhibit the primary MLC response to a donor in patients following DST + AZA treatment immediately prior to kidney transplantation.[20]

Prostaglandin Activity

Prostaglandins such as PGE_2 have been demonstrated to prolong allograft survival in animal models.[21,22] Increased production of PGE_2 by splenic macrophages in mice

has been reported following injection of sheep erythrocytes.[21,22] High levels of PGE_2 have been shown to suppress cell-mediated immune (CMI) responses, although low levels enhance CMI responses.

Current Status

The "transfusion effect" has greatly diminished since the advent of cyclosporine A (CSA) and many centers are now finding that pretransplant blood transfusions offer little benefit in CSA-treated renal allograft patients.[23,24] However, the large multicenter UCLA Transplant Registry continues to document benefit from blood transfusions in CSA-treated patients.[10,25] There is also some evidence that pretransplant blood transfusions are of value in reducing the frequency of rejection episodes and prolonging patient survival in heart allograft recipients.[26,27] Nonetheless, use of pharmacologic agents, such as cyclosporin and erythropoietin, and the increased appreciation of risks of transfusion-transmitted infections have resulted in a marked decrease in pretransplant blood transfusions.

Excess of Group O Patients

There is an excess of group O patients with end-stage renal disease awaiting renal allografts. This is a serious nationwide problem in that group O patients must wait a disproportionate time for a transplant since they can only receive group O (or in some instances A_2) kidneys. The excess of group O patients awaiting kidney transplants is due primarily to an imbalance in the number of cadaver kidneys obtained from O donors.[28]

Liver Transplants

A clinical liver transplant program presents one of the greatest challenges to the donor center and hospital transfusion service. The demands of a liver transplant program require that the support be maximal in terms of preparedness, supply and responsiveness. Institutions that begin a liver transplant program must make a major commitment to this support. Cooperation and communication are required between the hospital administration, staff of the operating room, intensive care unit, respiratory therapy, radiology, gastroenterology, anesthesiology, coagulation laboratory, transfusion service and the regional donor center. The institutional commitment must extend 24 hours a day and on weekends and holidays. Advance notice of a liver transplant is not more than a few hours. Additional staff for the hospital blood bank must be available on a regular on-call basis in order to meet the transfusion requirements. The surgical procedure frequently takes place at night or on weekends because of the availability of the donor organ and in order not to disrupt the operating room schedule. The transplant procedure may take 6-24 hours and involve several surgical teams.

As soon as the donor organ becomes available and the decision for transplant is made, the blood bank is notified and the preparations begin. The blood bank alerts its staff, including on-call personnel, and obtains a generous blood sample from the recipient(s) for crossmatching. The institution may have more than one patient waiting for the liver transplant and the surgeons may be undecided as to the specific recipient when the liver is recovered. Therefore, the blood bank may have to crossmatch more than one patient. This could involve patients with different ABO and Rh types. One pretransplant protocol[29] involves type and screen and crossmatching the patient with 20 units of RBCs. All additional units are released after an immediate-spin crossmatch if the antibody detection test is negative.

The protocol[29] also involves the provision of the first 10 units of RBCs as Rh– if the patient is Rh–. Subsequent units issued may be Rh+ until near the end of the procedure. Then, the last 10-15 units are provided as Rh–. An attempt is made to provide all Rh– blood for younger female adults and children. The same policy has been used for patients with specific clinically significant alloantibodies; the first 10 units are antigen negative. Next, additional units are antigen untested and the last 10-15 are antigen negative. Additionally, 10-20 units of FFP are thawed for initial transplant availability. Some centers also pool multiple units of CRYO for the surgery. Additional units of RBCs, FFP and CRYO are supplied upon demand.

The transfusion service must make special arrangements to staff the laboratory with personnel who will be dedicated to the constant supply of blood and components throughout the surgical and postsurgical time period. This includes serologic testing, thawing of frozen units of FFP and CRYO, tagging blood units, paperwork and billing.

The orders can be initiated by telephone, dedicated operating room communication system or runner. Completion of request forms and transfusion records can be facilitated if the blood bank has its own copy of the plastic patient identification card for imprinting the forms. Consideration should be given to the placement of a monitored blood bank refrigerator in the operating room for easy access of the prepared blood components to the operating room personnel. Alternatively, a cooler system can be used for transport and temporary storage. The surgical suite should provide an aide to expedite delivery of blood components and blood samples to and from the operating room/recovery room and the blood bank. Adults use approximately 20 units of RBCs, 24 units of FFP, 25 units of PCs and 8 units of CRYO. Children

Table 6-2. Examples of Units of Blood Components Transfused in Adult Liver Transplant Patients[29, 30]

Component	Number of Units, Median (Range in Parentheses)		
	Intraoperative	Postoperative	Total
Red Blood Cells	12 (1-202)	4 (0-75)	19 (3-211)
Fresh Frozen Plasma	12 (0-189)	14 (0-123)	24 (0-201)
Platelets	15 (0-70)	15 (0-420)	25 (0-449)
Cryoprecipitated AHF	8 (0-119)	1 (0-180)	8 (0-290)

may use up to one-half of these amounts. Median and ranges of blood and component use for a liver transplant are shown in Table 6-2.

Heart Transplants

Blood bank support for cardiac transplantation is very similar to that routinely used for other types of open-heart surgery in which cardiopulmonary bypass is employed. See Table 6-3. The blood bank can also provide ABO testing and assist in release of ABO-compatible organs to prevent ABO-mismatched organ transplantation.

Pancreas Transplants

Pancreatic transplants have fewer transfusion requirements. However, either a type and screen or the complete crossmatching of a few RBC units should be established as a routine.

Bone Marrow Transplantation

The term "bone marrow transplantation" (BMT) should be modified by a word denoting the source of the marrow: autologous or allogeneic. Furthermore, clinical differences make it important to know if the source of allogeneic marrow is an HLA-identical sibling, a phenotypically matched relative, a partially mis-

Table 6-3. Examples of Routine Preoperative Surgical Blood Orders for Organ Transplantation*

Component	Number of Units					
	Living Donor Nephrectomy	Kidney	Heart	Pancreas	Bone Marrow	Liver
Red Blood Cells	0[†]–2	0[†]–2	5–10	0[†]–4	0	20
Platelets	0	0	8	0	0	20
Fresh Frozen Plasma	0	0	2	0	0	20

*Postoperative needs vary according to individual clinical circumstances, but for the typical organ recipient, postoperative blood components are not needed. Exceptions for the bone marrow and liver transplant recipient are explained in text.

† = Type and Screen or no blood orders.

matched relative or a donor unrelated to the recipient.

Autologous Bone Marrow Transplantation

Autologous BMT is used to "rescue" a patient from an otherwise lethal dose of radiation and/or chemotherapy given to treat malignancies of the marrow and metastatic or recurrent solid tumors. For acute leukemias, marrow is obtained during remission, often treated to remove any potentially remaining leukemic cells, cryopreserved, and reinfused during relapse or a subsequent remission after massive antileukemic therapy. For solid tumors, the collected marrow is also often treated to remove any contaminating malignant cells before being cryopreserved for later reinfusion. Reliable in-vitro assays to determine the efficacy of these techniques for removing or killing malignant or leukemic cells are not yet available. Furthermore, it is not certain if they are needed; malignant and leukemic cells may not survive frozen storage.

Another way to avoid the reinfusion of potentially viable malignant or leukemic cells is to obtain progenitor cells from the peripheral blood using apheresis techniques. Timing the collections after certain types of chemotherapy (eg, cytoxan) and administering growth factors to the autologous donor allow the number of peripheral blood progenitor cells (PBPCs), also known as stem cells (PBSCs), collected to be greatly enhanced. Optimal methods to collect and use PBPCs for autologous reconstitution are still under investigation.

Collection

Bone marrow is usually aspirated from multiple sites in the iliac crest under general or spinal anesthesia at 10-30 mL per kg of patient body weight. It is desirable to remove at least $1\text{-}2 \times 10^8$ mononuclear cells per kg body weight to ensure engraftment and reconstitution. Pluripotent stem cells constitute less than 1% of the mononuclear cells present.[31] Since 1-2 liters of marrow are removed in heparinized syringes, autologous RBC transfusions are sometimes given to replace the loss of rbc mass. The rbcs can be obtained from a prior donation or recovered from the processed marrow. Allogeneic cellular components transfused just prior to and following the collection of bone marrow must be irradiated to prevent transfusion-associated graft-vs-host disease (GVHD). The autologous bone marrow *must not* be irradiated.

The use of autologous transplantation with peripheral blood progenitor cells is increasing. PBPCs are collected in the mononuclear cell fraction using blood cell separators (apheresis machines). Each procedure takes at least 4 hours and multiple procedures are usually needed to collect sufficient numbers of mononuclear cells to provide satisfactory reconstitution.

Processing

The aspirated marrow diluted with peripheral blood is filtered through a sterile stainless steel sieve to separate bone spicules and fat globules. The marrow may then be centrifuged to remove red cells or the marrow may be subjected to sedimentation with polymers or density gradient centrifugation. The RBCs may be transfused back to the patient. The goal is to concentrate the mononuclear cell fraction, which contains the progenitor cells, and minimize contamination with other cellular elements. The mononuclear cells are sometimes subjected to further purification to remove malignant cells by the use of monoclonal antibodies or other purging techniques. Unfortunately, specific in-vitro assays for the quantitation and viability of human pluripotent hematopoietic stem cells are unavailable. Two recent publications on bone marrow processing are valuable resources for additional information.[32,33]

Storage

Liquid

Studies using in-vitro assays for colony-forming units suggest that unseparated marrow can be stored at 4 C for up to 3 days.[34] It is not certain how reliable such in-vitro assays are in predicting in-vivo marrow repopulation. Also, most chemotherapeutic preparative regimens take longer than 3 days. Thus, most transplant physicians prefer to store the autologous marrow (or PBPCs) frozen.

Frozen

The processed marrow can be frozen for long-term storage in plastic vials or bags in liquid nitrogen at −196 C using a cryoprotective agent such as glycerol, DMSO or polyvinylpyrrolidone (PVP). DMSO at a concentration of about 10-20% is a very popular cryoprotective agent. It rapidly penetrates the cells and does not have to be removed upon thawing since intravenous infusion is relatively safe and without toxicity. Addition of autologous serum or plasma to DMSO in order to achieve a final concentration of about 20% improves recovery of viable cells following thawing.[35]

The rate of cooling during freezing must be controlled at 1-2 C/minute. More rapid freezing may promote intracellular ice formation, while slower rates may cause protein damage from osmotic forces subsequent to increased solute concentration during ice crystal formation. Equipment especially designed for controlled freezing rates is commercially available.

Thawing

The frozen marrow is thawed rapidly in a 37-40 C waterbath and can then be transfused intravenously without washing or further processing.

Allogeneic Bone Marrow Transplantation

Transfusions prior to allogeneic BMT for aplastic anemia adversely affect the chances for long-term disease-free survival. BMT should be considered and performed, if possible, promptly after the diagnosis of severe aplastic anemia is made. Prior to BMT for any indication, family members should not be used as donors for blood or blood component because one of them might be a marrow donor and sensitization to their antigens should be avoided. Unfortunately, most BMT candidates have diseases such as aplastic anemia or leukemia in which transfusions are often necessary. Transfusions from other than family members are less likely to diminish chances for long-term disease-free survival after BMT for leukemia.[36]

Following BMT, the recipient must receive transfusion support until engraftment occurs and blood cell production is adequate. RBCs are usually given to maintain the hemoglobin at 90-100 g/L (9-10 g/dL). This usually requires 6-20 units in the 10-week period posttransplant.[36] All cellular blood components (except those from the marrow donor) must be irradiated (25-50 Gy) to prevent GVHD from viable donor lymphocytes being superimposed on the effects of the marrow transplant itself. Steps must be taken to prevent the transmission of CMV infection to the transplant recipient, especially if both the recipient and the marrow donor are CMV antibody-negative. This can be accomplished by using CMV antibody-negative blood component donors or by using high performance filters for the removal of leu-

Table 6-4. Potential Problems in ABO- and Rh-Incompatible Bone Marrow Transplantation

Incompatibility	Example		Potential Problems
	Donor	Patient	
ABO*			
Major incompatibility	A	O	Hemolysis of rbcs in donor marrow; failure of engraftment
Minor incompatibility	O	A	Hemolysis of patient's rbcs by antibody in marrow or produced after engraftment; GVHD due to anti-A
Rh	Positive	Negative	GVHD due to anti-Rh (unlikely)
	Negative	Positive	Hemolysis of patient's rbcs by (donor) antibody produced after engraftment
	Positive	Negative anti-D	Hemolysis of rbcs from newly engrafted bone marrow stem cells

(Reproduced with permission from McCullough.[37])
*Major incompatibility = recipient serum contains antibodies that react with ABO antigens on donor's rbcs.
Minor incompatibility = donor serum contains antibodies that react with ABO antigens on recipient's rbcs.

kocytes from components not tested for CMV.

Platelet support may also be needed for BMT recipients. HLA-identical or haploidentical family members are the ideal donors for the preparation of apheresis platelets, but this is not always possible and random-donor platelets are often used. These platelet transfusions may be continued every 2-4 days to maintain the platelet count in the recipient above 10-20 × 10^9/L (10-20,000/μL). If patients become refractory to platelet transfusions, therapy with HLA-matched platelets becomes more important but is not always beneficial. Prophylactic granulocyte transfusions during marrow hypoplasia are not indicated. In fact, even therapeutic granulocyte transfusions are rarely used.

Since an HLA-identical donor is usually required for bone marrow transplantation, the donor (usually a sibling) may not have the same ABO and/or Rh types as the patient. ABO and Rh identity or compatibility between the donor and the recipient are not required for success of the BMT, but incompatibilities may pose special problems for the blood bank (Table 6-4).[37] A detailed description and review of this topic have been given by Petz.[38]

Major ABO Incompatibility

If the donor and recipient have a major ABO incompatibility (ie, donor is group A, recipient is group O), then the group A rbcs in the aspirated bone marrow may be rapidly hemolyzed when the marrow is transfused into the recipient. This could cause a significant problem as a result of immune hemolysis from the large amount of the rbc mass in the aspirated material. The problem can be resolved by processing the aspirated marrow to deplete it of contaminating rbcs.[38] Fortunately, stem cells do not express A and B antigens.

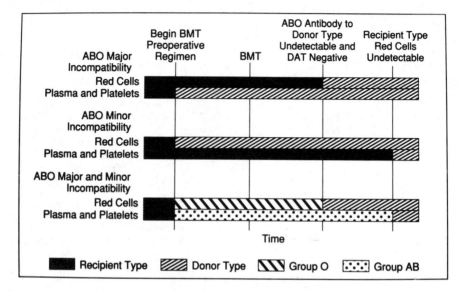

Figure 6-1. Recommended ABO group of blood components for use in patients receiving ABO-incompatible bone marrow. BMT indicates bone marrow transplant; DAT, direct antiglobulin test. (Reproduced with permission from McCullough et al.[37])

The group O recipient transplanted with group A marrow may continue to produce anti-A and anti-B for 3-4 months or, in rare instances, for 10-20 months posttransplant. The grafted marrow will begin to produce a new population of blood cells. Group A red cells will appear in the circulation when the recipient's anti-A disappears.

Hemolysis of the newly produced group A rbcs may be noted about 2 months posttransplant. This may last for approximately 3 weeks and result in a temporary drop in the patient's hemoglobin. If transfusions are necessary, washed group O RBCs can be given (Fig 6-1).[37] These components should be CMV– if the patient has been determined to be CMV–. In addition, all blood components transfused to BMT recipients should be irradiated to prevent GVHD.

Circulating donor white blood cells are usually found about 2-½ weeks posttransplant and platelets follow at about 4 weeks posttransplant.

Minor Side ABO Incompatibility

When marrow from a group O donor is to be transfused into a non-group O recipient, the plasma should be removed to decrease the amount of incompatible antibody given to the recipient. The marrow transfusion then is analogous to a unit of group O RBCs used as a universal donor unit. However, in approximately 10-15% of such BMTs, there is the rather abrupt onset of immune hemolysis, which begins about 7-10 days posttransplant and may last for 2 weeks. The DAT is positive and anti-A and/or anti-B can be recovered in the eluate. The hemolysis may result in hemoglobinemia and hemoglobinuria. An additional 30% of such BMT recipients may develop a positive DAT but not manifest gross hemolysis. This phenomenon is due to passenger B lymphocytes in the bone marrow that are producing alloantibody. This hemolysis is transient but may persist for up to 2 weeks and may require transfusion.

Irradiated group O RBCs may be used (Fig 6-1).[37] This same phenomenon may develop following solid organ transplants of kidney, liver, lung, pancreas and spleen. Typically there is an abrupt onset during the first 2-3 weeks posttransplant. Although usually transient, the hemolysis may continue for up to 6 months. Swanson et al[39] have reported a transient hemolytic anemia in a kidney transplant recipient due to anti-D.

Chimerism

In spite of the intensive pretransplant chemotherapy and irradiation, some of the host's hematopoietic cells may survive and subsequently co-exist with the transplanted donor's cells. This results in what has been termed hematopoietic chimerism and thus the recipient may have a dual cell population.[40]

National Bone Marrow Donor Registry

This registry was established for those patients who do not have a suitably matched family member to serve as a donor but who need a bone marrow transplant. All potential volunteer donors for unrelated patients in the registry are now HLA typed for A and B antigens; some are also typed for DR.

A preliminary search can be initiated by an individual hematologist or oncologist by calling the National Bone Marrow Donor Program (NBMDP) at 1-800-654-1247. The following information should be avail-able at the time of the call:

- Patient's name (last, first, middle initial).
- Patient's date of birth.
- Patient's sex and race.
- Referring physician's name, address, phone number.
- Patient's diagnosis.
- Patient's disease status.
- Patient's previous history of blood transfusion (for patients with aplastic anemia).
- Patient's HLA antigens (performed by accredited lab)—A, B and DR.
- Date of primary diagnosis.
- Current activity status.
- Blood counts.
- Insurance coverage.

The results of the preliminary search will be mailed to the physician in a few days. If matches are found, a formal search can then be initiated. For more details call the NBMDP at the phone number given above.

After preliminary HLA-A and -B matching, -DR typing and MLC tests are performed as needed. The relative importance of matching for Class I or Class II histocompatibility antigens is not well understood. The serologic detection of Class II antigens is less satisfactory than it is for Class I; newer techniques involving the polymerase chain reaction and the identification of specific molecular differences between HLA-DR subtypes are rapidly being applied to marrow transplantation and may lead to better matching and better results from unrelated-donor marrow transplantation. The MLC reaction or DNA typing methods are currently being used in matching donor and recipient.

When a match is found and the volunteer donor wishes to proceed, the marrow may be aspirated at a marrow collection center convenient to that donor. The aspirated marrow is then carried by a trained courier, traveling by the most expeditious method available, to the transplant center of the recipient.

It is clear that BMTs from unrelated donors (when matched, related donors are not available) are feasible for the treatment of many diseases for which a marrow transplant is appropriate. However, transplant recipients of marrow from unrelated donors generally have a more difficult course and much more severe

GVHD than those who are transplanted from matched siblings. Access to the registry for a preliminary computerized search can be made by a patient's private hematologist-oncologist or through a participating transplant center; activating the search to evaluate thoroughly potential donors must be done through a participating transplant center.

References

1. Technical manual for tissue banking. McLean, VA: American Association of Tissue Banks, 1992.

2. Eye bank tissue procurement manual. Washington, DC: Eye Bank Association of America, 1987.

3. Urist MR. Bone transplants and implants. In: Urist MR, ed. Fundamental and clinical bone physiology. Philadelphia: JB Lippincott, 1980: 331-68.

4. Widmann FK, ed. Standards for blood banks and transfusion services. 15th ed. Bethesda, MD: American Association of Blood Banks, 1993:47.

5. Alexandre GPJ, Squifflet JP, DeBruyere M, et al. ABO-incompatible related and unrelated living donor renal allografts. Transplant Proc 1986;18:1090-2.

6. Breimer ME, Brynger H, Rydberg L, et al. Transplantation of blood group A2 kidneys to O recipients. Biochemical and immunological studies of group A antigens in human kidneys. Transplant Proc 1985;17:2640-3.

7. Kissmeyer-Nielsen F, Olsen S, Petersen VP, et al. Hyperacute rejection of kidney allografts, associated with preexisting humoral antibodies against donor cells. Lancet 1966;2:662.

8. Opelz G, Sengar DPS, Mickey MR, Terasaki P. Effect of blood transfusion on subsequent kidney transplants. Transplant Proc 1973;5:253-9.

9. Terasaki PI, Toyotome A, Mickey MR, et al. Patient, graft, and functional survival rates: An overview. In: Terasaki PI, ed. Clinical kidney transplants, 1985. Los Angeles: UCLA Tissue Typing Laboratory, 1985:11.

10. Tokunaga K, Terasaki PI. The transfusion effect. In: Terasaki PI, ed. Clinical kidney transplants, 1986. Los Angeles: UCLA Tissue Typing Laboratory, 1986:175.

11. Norman DJ, Opelz G. Blood transfusions in transplantation. In: Garovoy MR, Guttmann RD, eds. Renal transplantation. New York: Churchill Livingstone, 1986:355-82.

12. Rodey GE. Blood transfusions and their influence on renal allograft survival. In: Brown EB, ed. Progress in hematology, Volume XIV. New York: Grune and Stratton, Inc, 1986:99-122.

13. Horimi T, Terasaki PI, Chia D, et al. Factors influencing the paradoxical effect of transfusions on kidney transplants. Transplantation 1983;35:320-3.

14. Persijn GG, Cohen B, Lansbergen Q, et al. Retrospective and prospective studies on the effect of blood transfusions in renal transplantation in the Netherlands. Transplantation 1979;28:396-401.

15. Salvatierra O, Vincenti F, Amend W, et al. Deliberate donor-specific transfusions prior to living related transplantation: A new approach. Ann Surg 1980;192:543-52.

16. Anderson CB, Sicard GA, Etheredge EE. Pretreatment of renal allograft recipients with azathioprine and donor-specific blood products. Surgery 1982;92:315-21.

17. Shelby J, Wakely E, Corry RJ. Suppressor cell induction in donor specific transfused mouse heart recipients. Surgery 1984;96:296-301.

18. Kaplan J, Sarnaik S, Levy J. Transfusion-induced immunologic abnormalities not related to the AIDS virus. N Engl J Med 1985;313:1227.

19. Terasaki PI. The beneficial transfusion effect on kidney graft survival attributed to clonal deletion. Transplantation 1984;37:119-25.

20. Burlingham WJ, Sparks-Mackety EMF, Wendel T, et al. Beneficial effect of pretransplant donor-specific transfusions: Evidence for an idiotype network mechanism. Transplant Proc 1985; 17:2376-9.

21. Keown DA, Descamps B. Improved renal allograft survival after blood transfusions: A non-specific, erythrocyte-mediated immuno-regulatory process. Lancet 1979;1:20-2.

22. Webb DR, Osheroff PL. Antigen stimulation of prostaglandin synthesis and control of immune responses. Proc Natl Acad Sci USA 1976; 73:1300.

23. Kahan BD, Mickey R, Flechner SM, et al. Multivariate analysis of risk factors impacting on immediate and eventual cadaver allograft survival in cyclosporine-treated recipients. Transplantation 1987;43:65-70.

24. Time to abandon pretransplant blood transfusion? (editorial) Lancet 1988;1:567-8.

25. Cats S, Terasaki P, Perdue S, Mickey MR. Effect of HLA typing and transfusions on cyclosporine-treated renal-allograft recipients. N Engl J Med 1984;311:675.

26. Keogh A, Baron DW, Spratt P, et al. The effect of blood pretransfusion on orthotopic cardiac transplantation. Transplant Proc 1987;19:2845-6.

27. Katz MR, Barnhart GR, Goldman MH, et al. Pretransplant transfusions in cardiac allograft recipients. Transplantation 1987;43:499-501.

28. Callender CO. Organ donation in the black population: Where do we go from here? Transplant Proc 1987;19:36-40.

29. Jenkins DE, Israel LB. Adaptation of a large blood bank to an active liver transplant service. In: Winter PM, Yang YG, eds. Hepatic transplantation—anesthetic and perioperative management. New York: Praeger Scientific, 1986:229-40.

30. Marengo-Rowe AJ, Leveson J, Larsen N, et al. Blood and blood component transfusion experience in an established liver transplantation program (abstract). SCABB Journal 1987;28: 13.

31. Gorgone BC. Tissue banking of bone marrow: Collection, processing and storage. In: Fawcett KJ, Barr AR, eds. Tissue banking. Arlington, VA: American Association of Blood Banks, 1987: 125.

32. Areman EM, Deeg HJ, Sacher RA eds. Bone marrow processing: A manual of current techniques. Philadelphia, PA: FA Davis, 1992.

33. Gee AP, ed. Bone marrow processing and purging: A practical guide. Boca Raton, FL: CRC Press, 1991.

34. Lasky LC, McCullough J, Zanjani ED. Liquid storage of unseparated human bone marrow. Transfusion 1986;26:331-4.

35. Schaefer VW. Preservation of bone marrow for transplantation. In: van Bekkum DW, Lomenberg B, eds. Bone marrow transplantation. New York: Marcel Dekker, Inc, 1985:526.

36. Petz LD, Scott EP. Supportive care. In: Blume KG, Petz LD, eds. Clinical bone marrow transplantation. New York: Churchill Livingstone, 1983:177-205.

37. McCullough J. The role of the blood bank in transplantation. Arch Pathol Lab Med 1991; 115:1195-1200.

38. Petz LD. Immunohematologic problems associated with bone marrow transplantation. Transfus Med Rev 1987;1:85-100.

39. Swanson J, Sebring E, Sastamoinen R, et al. Gm allotyping to determine the origin of the anti-D causing hemolytic anemia in a kidney transplant recipient. Vox Sang 1987;52:228-30.

40. Branch DR, Gallagher MT, Forman SJ, et al. Endogenous stem cell repopulation resulting in mixed hemapoietic chimerism following total body irradiation and marrow transplantation for acute leukemia. Transplantation 1982; 34:226-8.

7

Immunohematology

Introduction

The ability to mount an immune response resides in a system of interrelated cells, tissues and organs that collectively constitute the immune system. There are two categories of immunity: innate and adaptive. Innate immunity is more primitive and is probably the first line of defense against invading pathogenic organisms. Adaptive immunity evolved to combat the divergent nature of pathogenic viruses, bacteria and other microorganisms. Adaptive immunity has the properties of specificity, recall and memory, as well as the ability to discriminate between "self" and "nonself." This unique feature of the adaptive immune response is established early in embryogenesis, but how this discrimination is achieved is not fully understood, although it undoubtedly involves specific selection processes within the thymus. Thus, the human fetus acquires the ability to distinguish between normal constituents of its own body and those that are foreign or nonself. Whatever is present before this mechanism is established will be regarded as self. Substances or molecules encountered after that time are regarded as foreign.[1,2]

The response to foreign substances can be either the production of antibodies, called the *humoral response*; or a *cell-mediated response*, which reflects actions of T-lymphocyte subsets. *Immu-*nohematology is concerned primarily with the causes and effects of humoral immunity, but should be understood in the broader context of the whole (or complete) immune response.

Lymphohematopoiesis

The mature blood cells that carry oxygen (erythrocytes), effect host defenses against infection and tissue rejection (lymphocytes, granulocytes and macrophages) and maintain hemostasis (macrophages and platelets) derive from only a very few specialized cells found in the bone marrow. These so-called pluripotent stem cells comprise approximately 0.001% to 0.003% of all nucleated bone marrow cells and are capable of both 1) self-renewal, ie, they have the capacity to replicate into identical daughter progeny, and 2) differentiation into committed hematopoietic progenitor cells, which then give rise to all lymphohematopoietic cells of the body.[1,3]

The regulation of hematopoiesis may include both stochastic events (those events involving chance or probability) as well as environmental influences, termed deterministic events.[4,5] The pluripotent stem cell gives rise to a series of early, high-proliferative potential stem cell types, collectively termed colony-forming unit, spleen (CFU-S). These cells then give rise to myeloid or lymphoid stem cells, which also have replicative ability. Maturation at this very immature cell stage proceeds with continued loss of potential, in terms of both the numbers and types of cells that individual progenitor cells can produce. Eventually, progenitor cells restricted to producing a single blood-cell type arise, marking the origin of specific differentiation lineages. These unipotent progenitor cells continue to mature, giving rise to the morphologically identifiable hematopoietic cells and finally to nongrowing, functional blood cells (see Fig 7-1).

Proliferation, differentiation and function are regulated at multiple levels. Soluble humoral factors, termed cytokines, influence the direction of lymphohematopoietic development.[6-8] Cytokines comprise a group of regulatory proteins and glycoproteins termed colony-stimulating factors (CSFs) and the interleukins (IL-1 through IL-13). These cytokines, along with additional growth-relevant polypeptides, including the tumor necrosis factors, interferons and transforming growth factors, serve as stimulators or inhibitors of lymphohematopoiesis, and can also be inducing agents for functional differentiation (see Table 7-1).

The development of culture techniques using semisolid medium was the major breakthrough that allowed for the in-vitro study of the growth of hematopoietic cells.[9,10] The initial culture methods allowed for the identification and study of colonies of mature macrophages and granulocytes when hematopoietic cells of bone marrow origin were immobilized in a soft gel, such as agar, and provided with "growth factors" contained in various crude extracts. These colony-forming assays resulted in the identification and subsequent study of CSFs for macrophage (CSF-1), granulocyte (G-CSF), granulocyte-macrophage (GM-CSF), and erythroid [IL-3, erythropoietin (Epo)] production. Further advances in cell culture

techniques and molecular cloning have allowed for the identification of numerous other cytokines and cytokine receptors involved in lymphohematopoietic cell development. It is now clear that specific low- and/or high-affinity receptors, unique for each type of hematopoietic cytokine, are found on several cell lines, on normal hematopoietic tissues and also on primary myeloid leukemic cells. The cellular distribution of the receptors matches the known biological specificities of each cytokine, and these receptors are generally low in number on normal cells.[7]

The number of cytokines able to influence lymphohematopoietic cell survival, growth and differentiation stands at more than 40 and continues to grow. Table 7-1 lists some of the more important hematopoietic cytokines. Understanding the complex network of interaction of these cytokines, which orchestrate the development and function of mature blood cells, will undoubtedly require many more years of investigation.

Cytokines

Myeloid Growth Factors

Epo was the first humoral agent shown to regulate hematopoietic cell differentiation. Unlike the other blood cell growth factors, it has an absolute requirement for glycosylation for its in vivo biologic activity. Epo is a lineage-restricted myeloid growth factor, or unipoietin, that acts at the intermediate stem cell level [ie, burst-forming unit, erythroid (BFU-E) and colony-forming unit, erythroid (CFU-E)] to induce both proliferation and differentiation of erythroid cells. Recent evidence suggests Epo may also stimulate megakaryocyte development. It is produced largely by the kidney although 5-10% appears to be extrarenal in origin and may be produced by cells of the mononuclear phagocyte

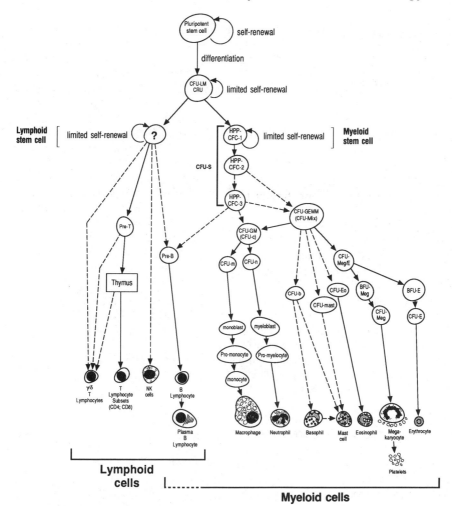

Figure 7-1. Hierarchy of lymphohematopoiesis. Solid lines indicate probable pathways. Broken lines indicate speculated pathways. CFU-LM, colony-forming unit, lymphoid, myeloid; CRU, competitive repopulating unit; HPP-CFC, high proliferative potential colony-forming cell; CFU-S, colony-forming unit, spleen; CFU-GM, colony-forming unit, granulocyte/macrophage; CFU-c, colony-forming unit, culture; CFU-m, colony-forming unit, macrophage; CFU-n, colony-forming unit, neutrophil; CFU-GEMM, colony-forming unit, granulocyte/erythroid/macrophage/megakaryocyte; CFU-Mix, colony-forming unit, mixed cellular; CFU-Meg/E, colony-forming unit, megakaryocyte/erythroid; BFU-Meg, burst-forming unit, megakaryocyte; CFU-Meg, colony-forming unit, megakaryocyte; CFU-mast, colony-forming unit, mast cell (postulated); CFU-b, colony-forming unit, basophil (postulated); CFU-Eo, colony-forming unit, eosinophil; BFU-E, burst-forming unit, erythroid; CFU-E, colony-forming unit, erythroid. Other cell types may precede the CFU-S compartment; these include pre-CFC$_{multi}$, pre-colony-forming cell, multilineage; and CFU-Bl, colony-forming unit, blast cell. There is good evidence for the myeloid stem cell; however, the lymphoid stem cell is postulated. B lymphocytes share features of both lymphocytes and myeloid cells, particularly, properties of macrophages [from Branch DR. Cytokine regulation of mouse macrophage proliferation (thesis). Edmonton, Canada: University of Alberta, 1992].

Table 7-1. Partial List of Growth-Relevant Cytokines

Name	Descriptive Name	Effect on Cell Growth or Function	Human Gene Location
Epo	Erythropoietin	Stimulation; differentiation	7q
G-CSF	Granulocyte colony-stimulating factor	Stimulation; inhibition; differentiation	17q
GM-CSF	Granulocyte-macrophage colony-stimulating factor	Stimulation; inhibition	5q
CSF-1	Macrophage colony-stimulating factor (M-CSF)	Stimulation; inhibition; differentiation	5q
IL-1α	Endogenous pyrogen hemopoietin 1	Stimulation; inhibition	2q
IL-1β	Lymphocyte-activating factor	Stimulation; inhibition	2q
IL-2	T-cell growth factor	Stimulation; differentiation	4q
IL-3	Multipotent colony-stimulating factor (multi-CSF)	Stimulation	5q
IL-4	B-cell stimulatory factor I	Stimulation; inhibition; differentiation	5q
IL-5	B-cell growth factor II T-cell-replacing factor; eosinophil differentiation factor	Stimulation; differentiation	5q
IL-6	Interferon beta2; hybridoma growth factor; B-cell-stimulating factor-2; hepatocyte growth factor	Stimulation; inhibition; differentiation	7p
IL-7	Lymphopoietin 1; pre-B cell growth factor	Stimulation; inhibition	
IL-8	Monocyte-derived neutrophil chemotactic factor; neutrophil-activating protein 1 (NAP-1)	Chemotaxis	
IL-9	T-cell growth factor P40; erythroid enhancing factor	Stimulation	5q
IL-10	Cytokine synthesis-inhibitory factor	Inhibition; stimulation	
IL-11	Stromal cell-derived cytokine	Stimulation	
TNFα	Tumor necrosis factor; cachectin	Stimulation; inhibition	6p
TNFβ	Lymphotoxin	Stimulation; inhibition	6p
LIF	Leukemia inhibitory factor	Stimulation; inhibition	
MIPα	Macrophage inflammatory protein-alpha	Inhibition	
MIPβ	Macrophage inflammatory protein-beta	Inhibition	
SLF	Steel factor; mast cell growth factor; stem cell factor (SCF); *c-kit* ligand (KL)	Stimulation	12
IFNγ	Interferon-gamma; immune interferon	"Activation;" inhibition; differentiation	12
TGFα	Transforming growth factor-alpha	Stimulation; inhibition	
TGFβ	Transforming growth factor-beta	Stimulation; inhibition; IgA switch factor	

lineage. Epo is a classical endocrine hormone. Serum levels correlate with the degree of hypoxia and nothing else can replace it in stimulating the later stages of erythrocyte production.[11]

G-CSF, like Epo, is a lineage-restricted myeloid growth factor. The main target cell for G-CSF is a progenitor cell, which proliferates and differentiates into colonies consisting primarily of neutrophils. Under appropriate stimuli, G-CSF can be produced by a variety of normal cell types including macrophages, fibroblasts, endothelial cells and brain astrocytes. Stimulation of G-CSF production from monocyte-macrophages usually requires endotoxin or inflammatory molecules such as IL-1, or tumor necrosis factor-α (TNFα), suggesting that G-CSF production may play some role in inflammatory reactions. G-CSF also can induce differentiation of certain malignant cells in vitro and, thus, may be a major differentiation agent.

GM-CSF is a pluripoietin, which is a growth-promoting agent for many different cell types including granulocyte, macrophage, mast cell, megakaryocyte and erythroid. Many cell types produce GM-CSF under appropriate conditions, including T lymphocytes, macrophages, fibroblasts, endothelial cells, mesangial cells, keratinocytes, placental cells and brain astrocytes. There are indications that GM-CSF may be important as a cellular regulatory molecule in the bone marrow stroma or play an important physiologic role in the inflammatory response. Since GM-CSF becomes detectable in serum only during infection, a possible physiologic role for GM-CSF may also involve bacterial and parasitic infections.

CSF-1, also known as macrophage colony-stimulating factor (M-CSF), was the first CSF to be identified and purified to homogeneity. It is a homodimeric sialoglycoprotein, which stimulates the survival, proliferation and differentiation of mononuclear phagocytes and may also play a role in placental development as well as in the control of immune function in the glomerulus of the kidney. CSF-1 may also be an important cytokine for early CFU-S proliferation. CSF-1 is produced by a variety of cells including monocyte-macrophages, fibroblasts, placental cells, mesangial cells, keratinocytes, and activated T and B lymphocytes. Human CSF-1 has a normal range in blood of between 350-700 U/mL (about 100-200 pM). Serum CSF-1 levels become high only transiently following aggressive cytotoxic treatment or injection of bacterial endotoxin. However, very high serum levels (10 to 100 times normal levels) may be detectable throughout pregnancy.

IL-3, also known as multi-CSF, was first identified in splenic lymphocytes from nude mice. Subsequent to its purification, IL-3 was also found to be a growth-promoting agent for many different cell types including granulocyte, macrophage, eosinophil, mast cell, megakaryocyte, natural killer (NK), erythroid and even early T and B lineage cells. Thus, IL-3 may be a true pluripoietin. The major, and possibly only, source of IL-3 is from activated T lymphocytes. Although no clear physiologic role for IL-3 has been firmly established, it may function as a short-range paracrine survival and differentiation factor, primarily for very early hematopoietic cells and cells of the erythroid lineage.

Lymphocyte and Other Growth-Relevant Cytokines

Many additional cytokines having effects on lymphohematopoietic development have been identified (See Table 7-1). Many of these cytokines (IL-1, IL-2, IL-4 through IL-7, IL-10) were originally described for their single effect on immune cells, ie, T or B lymphocytes (see below). With the availability of these cytokines in a pure recombinant form, further study has shown these proteins to be pleotropic. That is, a given cytokine can act on a variety of cell types and has the potential to induce different functional activity (not only mitogenic stimulation) depending upon the cellular target. Thus, many of these molecules have now been assigned an interleukin designation. However, at present, a uniform nomenclature does not exist for cytokines, such as the clusters of differentiation (CD) terminology developed for leukocyte cell-surface proteins. Perhaps a definitive nomenclature at this time is premature, but mRNA and protein amino acid sequences, membrane receptor cross-binding studies, receptor sequences and homologies, and genomic DNA structures, in progress, may ultimately allow a rational grouping and acceptable nomenclature for these important proteins.

Cells of the Immune System

Lymphocytes

Lymphocytes are heterogeneous in size and function. They are capable of very precise recognition of foreign molecules and cells and of responding to successive contacts with previously encountered foreign materials.

B Lymphocytes (B Cells)

The B cells have the capacity to synthesize heavy and light immunoglobulin chains and assemble them into an immunoglobulin molecule. The combining site of the immunoglobulin molecule (V_L and V_H domains) are proteins encoded for by five genes, three for the heavy chain (V_H, D and J_H) and two for the light chain (both κ and λ), V_L and J_L.[1,2,12,13] There are 500-1000 different V_H genes, 10 D genes

and 4 J_H genes to encode for the protein sequences of the V_H chain, and at least 200 V_L genes and 6 J_L genes to encode for the protein sequence of the V_L chain. The result is an enormous variation in the structure of the variable region of the immunoglobulin. During differentiation of the B cell, a complex series of "gene rearrangements" within the germline genome results in a particular V_HDJ_H/V_LJ_L code. This, coupled with imprecise joining of these gene segments, point mutations and allelic exclusion (whereby only one chromosomal haplotype will be expressed, either the maternal or paternal chromosome, for a particular heavy or light chain, respectively), means that a unique immunoglobulin is expressed for each B cell. At least 10^7-10^8 unique immunoglobulin molecules can be expressed on 10^7-10^8 individual B cells (one unique immunoglobulin for each B cell). This series of gene translocations has been described as the "one cell-one antibody" theory and is independent of antigen. Although each B cell, and all progeny of that B cell, will synthesize the same immunoglobulin, the reproducing B cell, after contact with an antigen, may mutate to produce an immunoglobulin of higher affinity for the particular antigen. Point mutations, a one-nucleotide substitution, have a 100,000 times greater chance of happening in dividing B cells than in other dividing cells. This somatic mutation "tailors" an antibody, establishing a better fit, or affinity, for a foreign antigen. It is this ability to adapt to the foreign antigen that allows the immune response to perform with such specificity.

B cells are produced in the bone marrow. The circulating, unstimulated, resting B lymphocytes have immunoglobulin molecules, usually monomeric IgD and IgM, on their surface. This feature makes them easy to identify in tissue or in mixed cell populations. They also have surface receptors for complement and express HLA-DR antigens.[1,2]

T Lymphocytes (T Cells)

Immature T cells (having the phenotype CD4– CD8–) are "educated" in the thymus where T-cell clones having T-cell receptors (TCRs), which recognize self antigen in the context of self major histocompatibility complex (MHC), are deleted. The mature T cells that emerge from the thymus have one of two phenotypes (CD4+8– or CD4–8+). CD4+8– (or CD4) T cells are termed helper/inducer T cells. These T cells are required for normal humoral and cell-mediated immunity, and recognize processed foreign antigen in the context of self-MHC Class II molecules when expressed on the surface of antigen-presenting cells (APCs; see below). CD4–8+ (or CD8) T cells are also called cytotoxic T cells. These T cells are responsible for cell-mediated immunity (particularly in response to viruses) and recognize processed antigen in the context of self-MHC Class I molecules.

T cells do not have surface-bound immunoglobulin. However, they have distinct receptors (TCRs) that recognize specific protein antigenic sequences when these are associated with self-MHC molecules. These TCRs are heterodimers composed of α and β polypeptides in about 90% of T cells, and γ and δ polypeptides in about 10% of T cells.[14-17] These chains have variable region domains and, as with B cells, are encoded by V, D and J genes. A series of rearrangements, similar to those that occur in the B cells, ensure that a unique and specific receptor is synthesized for each T cell. This diversification process is independent of antigen stimulation both for T and B cells, and is called *lymphoneogenesis*. The TCR is also called Ti for idiotypic T cell. The TCR is located on the T-cell surface in close association with CD3,[18-20] an antigen marker on mature T lymphocytes. The association between CD3 and TCR is essential for antigen recognition; the entire association is called the TCR complex.[1,2]

Antigen-Presenting Cells (APCs)

APCs can be phagocytic cells (ie, macrophages, dendritic cells) or other cells (ie, B cells) that have the ability to endocytose protein antigens, degrade these proteins into small peptide fragments (termed "antigen processing") and then present these "processed" antigens on their surface. The cell surface-associated processed antigen can then be recognized by the TCR of a single antigen-specific T cell. This specific recognition, however, requires that the processed antigen be associated with another APC molecule. This molecule is an integral membrane protein that serves as a self-restriction element, which, as stated above, must be associated with the processed antigenic peptide before the entire complex can be recognized by the TCR complex. These restriction elements are glycoproteins and are encoded for by genes within the MHC.

There are two classes of MHC molecules and these are recognized by the two major classes of T cells. The T cells with receptors for molecules encoded by the Class I MHC genes, the HLA-A, -B and -C antigens, are known as CD8 cytotoxic T lymphocytes. These cells were previously termed cytotoxic/suppressor T cells. However, the existence of a distinct suppressor T-cell subset is now uncertain. The T cells with receptors for restriction molecules encoded by the Class II MHC genes, first described as Ia molecules in mice and later as HLA-D and HLA-DR antigens in humans, are known as CD4 helper/inducer T lymphocytes. Most mature functional T cells will be positive for either CD4 or CD8, never both. It has been shown that the presence or absence of a particular MHC antigen will determine the ability or inability of an antigen to induce an immune response.[1,2]

To summarize, APCs have the ability to take up antigens, process them into small peptide fragments, associate these peptides with Class II MHC (a process known as determinant selection) and then display this processed antigen (in the context of self MHC) on the cell surface. Endogenous peptides associated with self Class I MHC molecules can be presented to CD8 T cells (recognition is through the TCR complex), while peptides associated with self Class II MHC are recognized by CD4 T cells.

Clonal Selection

The clonal selection theory is the central dogma of modern immunology.[2] The underlying assumption is that the B and T cells (which secrete antibody and help B cell antibody production, respectively) are preprogrammed to respond to antigen. Thus, an antigen does not instruct the immune system in what specificity to generate; rather, it selects those B and T cells displaying a receptor of the appropriate specificity (ie, TCR on T cells, immunoglobulin on B cells), inducing them to proliferate and differentiate, resulting in expansion of specific clones having one unique specificity. It has been calculated that a given individual has 10^7-10^8 preprogrammed immunoglobulin specificities, thus allowing for the recognition of the "universe" of possible antigens.

Antigens

An *antigen* is a substance that is capable of eliciting an immune response when introduced into the tissues of an immunocompetent individual, often referred to as the *host*, and of being recognized by an antibody and/or sensitized cells produced as the result of an immune response. A single antigen may possess many different epitopes (antigenic determinants) each capable of eliciting an antibody response and each the target of the antibody so produced. An epitope may contain 5-6 amino acids in a precise spatial arrangement. The ability of the antigen to react with the products of a specific immune response is its *antigenicity*.[21] The antigenicity of materials is usually affected by its size, shape, rigidity, location of determinants and tertiary structure. Antigens must normally be foreign to the host, and are usually greater than 40,000 daltons in molecular weight, although rarely they can be as small as 4000 daltons.[22] Some antigens are proteins or polysaccharide, while others, such as penicillin or methyldopa, are small chemical structures. Smaller molecular structures weighing less than 4000 daltons can elicit an antibody response if they are coupled to a "carrier" protein. The smaller molecule is called a "hapten." The "hapten-carrier" complex is capable of eliciting an immune response; the hapten will combine with the resulting antibody.

The ability of a material (antigen, drug, etc) to elicit an immune response is its *immunogenicity*, and the material eliciting that response is an *immunogen*. A *complete antigen* is a material that can elicit an immune response and react with the product of that immune response. Thus a complete antigen is both an antigen and an immunogen. A *hapten* is a chemically active material that is usually of low molecular weight, that cannot induce an immune response by itself, but must combine with a larger molecule (hapten-carrier) to become immunogenic.[21]

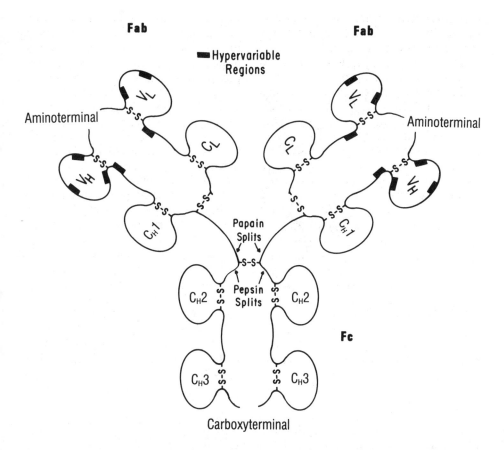

Figure 7-2. The basic four-chain immunoglobulin unit. Specificity of antibody activity derives from amino acid sequence in the hypervariable regions of the variable domains of heavy and light chains (V_H and V_L). Class-specific characteristics derive from amino acid sequences in the constant domains of the heavy chains (C_H1, C_H2, C_H3).

Antibodies

Polypeptide Chains

Immunoglobulins are proteins that possess antibody activity. Approximately 82-96% of the immunoglobulin molecule is polypeptide and approximately 4-18% is carbohydrate. The basic immunoglobulin unit consists of two identical light (L) chains, each containing about 220 amino acids, and two identical heavy (H) chains, each containing about 440 amino acids (Fig 7-2). The four chains are held together by disulfide bonds and noncovalent bonds.

Heavy and light chains have regions called *domains*, each consisting of about 110 amino acids. Serological and biological actions of antibodies result from the amino acid sequence within these domains. Amino acid sequences in amino-terminal ends of heavy and light chains vary from one antibody to another. This sequence is called the *variable (V) domain*; the variability of amino acids provides the ability to combine with specific antigens. Within the variable domain are regions that are exceptionally variable and are called the *hypervariable* or the *complementarity-determining regions*. These appear to contain amino acids that constitute the antibody's combining site. The H chains have four hypervariable regions and the L chains have three hypervariable regions. The regions on either side of the hypervariable regions are less variable and are called *framework regions*. Light chains consist of the variable domain and a single *constant (C) domain*, located at the carboxyterminal end of the chain, in which the amino acid sequence is essentially identical for all chains of a given isotype. Heavy chains consist of one variable domain and three constant domains, numbered C_H1, starting from the aminoterminal end, to C_H3. IgM and IgE have an extra C domain, C_H4, at the carboxyterminal end.[23,24]

Cleavage by Enzymes

Antibody molecules can be cleaved into different characteristic fragments by proteolytic enzymes (Fig 7-3). Papain cleaves heavy chains at the aminoterminal end just above the disulfide bonds that link them. The light chain remains attached to half of the heavy chain, leaving intact the antigen-binding site on each of the two identical fragments. These two identical fragments are called *Fab (fragment antigen binding)* fragments. The linked portions of the heavy chains, containing the constant-region domains that confer biological activity, such as macrophage binding of IgG1 and IgG3 and binding of IgE to tissue cells, are called the *Fc (fragment crystallizable)* fragment. Pepsin cleaves the heavy chain at the carboxyterminal end at a site below the disulfide bonds linking the heavy chains, producing a single fragment containing both antigen-binding sites, the *F(ab')₂* fragment; the rest of the Fc region is degraded. Individual Fab fragments can combine with separate antigen molecules. Neither Fab nor F(ab')₂ fragments have the biological properties of intact antibody molecules because they lack the Fc portion (Fig 7-3).

Idiotypes

Antibody molecules of any individual specificity have a unique amino acid sequence in the variable domains that form the antigen-binding (Fab) portion of the molecule. The amino acid sequence confers the three-dimensional configuration that allows the antibody to interact with its specific antigen. The amino acid sequence characteristic of the antibody's specificity can, itself, serve as an antigen and elicit an antibody response if suitably introduced into a susceptible host. The unique antigenic feature of an antibody molecule's Fab domain is called its *idiotype* (see Table 7-2); antibodies that react with the combining site of an antibody molecule of any given specificity are called anti-idiotypes. For example, IgG antibodies from one person, directed against different antigens, would have the same isotype (antigen differences that characterize the class and subclass of the H chains and the type and subclass of the L chains) and allotype (polymorphic form of H and L chains) but different idiotypes.

In 1973, Jerne proposed a theory based on idiotypes to explain how the immune system regulates itself.[2] The *network theory* allows the immune system to regulate itself using only self.[2] The theory is based on the ability of the immune system not only to produce antibody, but also to respond to the resultant antibody by producing an anti-antibody directed to the Fab idiotype of the first antibody (Ab1). The second antibody (Ab2), the anti-idiotype to Ab1, can then regulate the production of the initial antibody. The concept central to the network the-

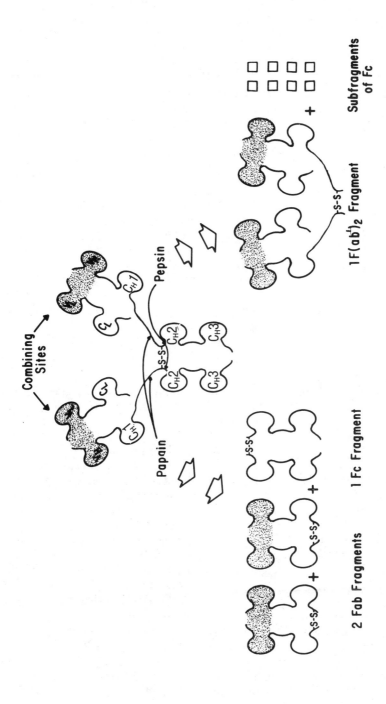

Figure 7-3. The different sites at which papain and pepsin cleave the immunoglobulin heavy chains.

Table 7-2. Classification of Immunoglobulins

Type of Variation	Refers to	Examples
Isotypic	Ig classes and subclasses present in *all* members of the species.	IgG, IgA, IgM, etc; IgG1, IgG2, etc
Allotypic	Variations in the amino acid structure of heavy and light chains unrelated to antibody specificity. Present in some but *not all* members of the species.	Gm and Km allotypes
Idiotypic	Idiotypes that are the antigen binding sites on the antibody molecule. Present in some but not all antibody molecules within an individual member of the species.	Fab regions of antibody molecules

ory is that all possible antigens (idiotypes) are reflected in the production of anti-idiotypes. Thus, the immune system has the capability of modulating any immune response through the network. Rarely, an Ab2 anti-idiotype is produced where its idiotype looks exactly like the antigen to which the Ab1 was originally produced. This "internal image" Ab2 can, in fact, mimic antigen; it can even cause disease, such as thyrotoxicosis, in which the Ab2 antibody mimics thyroid stimulating hormone.

Immunoglobulin Classes

An assembled immunoglobulin molecule consists of two identical H and two identical L chains. Distinctive amino acid sequences of the heavy chains characterize individual immunoglobulin classes that are called *isotypes* (Table 7-2). The iso-type of the heavy chain determines the immunoglobulin class of the molecule; IgA, IgD, IgE, IgG and IgM molecules have respectively, alpha(α), delta(δ), epsilon(ϵ), gamma(γ) and mu(μ) heavy chains. The amino acid sequence in the constant domains are comparable to or identical within each isotype.

Many H chains have a region between the first and second C domain (C_H1 and C_H2), the *hinge region*, which is flexible and allows the two combining sites of the molecule to move in relationship to each other. This disulfide bond region holds the two H chains together. IgM molecules have the hinge region located between the C_H2 and C_H3 domains.

Within immunoglobulin classes, the light chains may be either kappa (κ) or lambda (λ). About 60% of immunoglobulin molecules have κ chains and 40% have λ chains. In any one mole-

Table 7-3. Human Immunoglobulins[22, 23, 25]

Class	IgG	IgA	IgM	IgD	IgE
Structure					
H-chain isotype	γ	α	μ	δ	ε
Number of subclasses	4	2	1	?	?
L-chain, types	k,λ	k,λ	k,λ	k,λ	k,λ
Molecular weight (daltons)	150,000	180,000-500,000	900,000	180,000	200,000
Exists as polymer	no	yes	yes	no	no
Electrophoretic mobility	γ	γ	between γ and β	between γ and β	fast γ
Sedimentation constant (in Svedberg units)	6-7S	7-15S	19S	7S	8S
Gm allotypes (H chain)	+	0	0	0	0
Km allotypes (Kappa L chain; formerly Inv)	+	+	+	?	?
Am allotypes	0	+	0	0	0
Serum concentration (mg/dL)	1000-1500	200-350	85-205	3	0.01-0.07
Total immunoglobulin (%)	80	16	4	<0.1	<0.1
Synthetic rate (mg/kg/day)	33	24	6–7	<0.4	<0.02
Serum half-life (days)	23	6	5	2-8	1-5
Distribution (% of total in intravascular space)	45	42	76	75	51
Present in epithelial secretions	no	yes	no	no	no
Antibody activity	yes	yes	yes	probably no	yes
Serologic characteristics	Usually nonagglu-tinating	Usually nonagglu-tinating	Usually agglu-tinating	?	?
Fixes complement	yes	no	yes	no	no
Crosses placenta	yes	no	no	no	no

cule, the light chains are always of the same isotype. Different isotypes, for both heavy and light chains, characterize different species, ie, the μ chains of human IgM molecules are all very similar, and differ somewhat from the μ chains of rabbit IgM. Table 7-3 shows some characteristics of human immunoglobulin molecules.

IgG

IgG constitutes approximately 80% of the total serum immunoglobulins and is also found in extravascular fluid. It exists only as the single basic immunoglobulin unit of 2H chains and 2L chains. Four subclasses of IgG molecules (*IgG1, IgG2, IgG3* and *IgG4*) exist. Respectively, they represent approximately 60-70%, 14-20%, 4-8% and 2-6% of the IgG molecules. The subclasses differ in the amino acid sequence of the H chain and the arrangement of interchain disulfide bonds. The L chain can be either κ or λ and either or both can be found in each immunoglobulin subclass. IgG is the only immunoglobulin that crosses the placenta from the mother to the fetus with IgG2 being the most inefficient.

IgG is capable of binding complement.[25] The order of efficiency is IgG3>IgG1>>IgG2. IgG4 is incapable of fixing complement by the classical pathway, but may participate in the alternative pathway.

IgM

IgM constitutes approximately 4% of the total serum immunoglobulin and characteristically exists as a pentamer consisting of five basic immunoglobulin units and a short additional polypeptide chain called the J (for joining) *chain*. Although the pentameric molecule has 10 antigen-combining sites, all 10 sites on any one molecule can react simultaneously only with small antigens such as haptens. The valency (availability of combining sites) falls to 5 when larger antigens react simultaneously, probably because of a limited flexibility within each μ chain of this molecule, resulting in a steric restriction of the number of antigen-binding sites available for attachment of the antigen. Although the antigenic sites of IgM usually have low binding affinity, this is balanced by the presence of multiple antibody-binding sites, which increases the avidity of binding.

IgM is the first class of immunoglobulin produced as the fetal immune system matures and is the predominant class produced in the early stages of a primary antibody response. Plasma is the only body fluid that contains signif-

icant amounts of IgM. IgM and IgD are the major immunoglobulins expressed on the surface of unstimulated, resting B lymphocytes.

IgM antibodies are highly effective agglutinins that activate complement very efficiently. A single molecule bound to the surface of an rbc can initiate complement-mediated lysis of that cell. Gentle reduction of IgM with 2-mercaptoethanol or dithiothreitol (see Method 4.4) separates the five subunits and also releases the J chain. Both hemolyzing and direct agglutinating activity are destroyed by this treatment.

IgA

IgA is the predominant immunoglobulin in body secretions. It exists both as a monomer and as polymers. Most serum IgA exists as IgA1, is produced in the bone marrow and is in the monomeric form, although a small proportion has the J chain and exists as multimers of the basic unit. In saliva, tears, bronchial secretions, nasal mucosa, prostatic fluid, vaginal secretions and mucus secretions of the small intestines, IgA exists as predominately IgA2, principally as a dimer, including not only the J chain but also a polypeptide chain of epithelial origin called the *secretory component*. Thus the secretory and serum IgA molecules have different biochemical and immunochemical properties. The large concentration of IgA in secretions has led to speculation that the primary function of this immunoglobulin is to prevent access of foreign agents to the general immune system. The predominant role of serum IgA has been suggested to be the removal of antigenic substances without the generation of an inflammatory response. However, aggregated IgA can activate complement via the alternative pathway and IgA can trigger cell-mediated events.[26,27] In humans two antigenically distinct subclasses have been described, designated IgA1 and IgA2 with IgA2 existing as two allotypic (AM) variants IgA2m(1) and IgA2m(2). (See Fig 7-4 and Table 7-3.)

IgD

IgD is found in trace amounts in the plasma. It exists as a monomer slightly larger than IgG. Most IgD is present as a membrane immunoglobulin on unstimulated, resting B lymphocytes, where it may serve as a receptor for antigen, along with monomeric IgM. No blood group antibodies have been reported to belong to this class.

IgE

IgE exists as a monomer at extremely low concentrations in plasma. Virtually all the body's IgE molecules are bound to circulating basophils or their tissue equivalent, mast cells. Binding results from interactions between a receptor on the basophil's membrane and a portion of the heavy chain. The combining sites of the antibody remain free to bind to antigen. Combination of the IgE molecule with its specific antigen triggers the basophil to release histamine and other vasoactive substances from its granules. The clinical effects of these substances may include anaphylactic shock and death, edema from increased vascular permeability, skin rashes, respiratory tract constriction and increased secretions from epithelial surfaces, depending upon the site involved (see Hypersensitivity, p 169).

Allotypes

The amino acid sequence in certain segments of the constant regions of human γ and α H chains, and κ L chains, varies to produce heritable traits called *allotypes*, determined by allelic genes. At least 28 different allotypic sequences have been described in human γ chains (the Gm allotypes), two different sequences for the α chain, (the Am allotypes), and three different sequences for the κ chains (the Km allotypes, formerly called Inv). In any one person all the γ or α chains will have the same Gm or Am allotype and all κ chains will have the same Km allotype, because the immunoglobulin chain structure reflects the allelic genes present in that person. Allotypes are used as markers in paternity testing, population genetics and more recently to determine the source of immunoglobulin produced in transplanted patients.[28]

Fc Receptors

The effector portion of immunoglobulin molecules is the Fc region. Specific receptors existing on specialized cell types recognize this region (Table 7-4). Attachment results in phagocytosis, release of inflammatory or allergic mediators, or both.

Complement

General Concepts

The two major functions of complement are to promote the inflammatory response and to alter biological membranes to cause direct cell lysis or enhanced susceptibility to phagocytosis. Cell lysis occurs when antibody-mediated complement activation leads to sequential interaction of the entire complement cascade. Intermediary products in the complement sequence attract white cells (chemotaxis), promote the efficiency of phagocytic activity and alter vascular permeability and stability of cell membranes, notably those of platelets and granulocytes.

Complement consists of at least 25 different glycoproteins with varying electrophoretic mobilities. Most circulate in an inactive precursor form and develop proteolytic activity upon activation. Together they constitute approximately 4-5% of the total serum protein. Many complement proteins are designated by C, followed by identifying numbers and letters. Many components are present in small or trace quantities although C4, C3, factor B and C1 inhibitor are each present in concentrations greater than 0.1 g/L (10 mg/dL). Complement proteins undergo activation either by attaching to or associating with other proteins or, more often, by undergoing proteolytic cleavage, such that removal of part of the molecule leaves the residual portion enzymatically or biologically active. The sequence whereby each component undergoes activation and then activates the next component is often described as a cascade reaction.[29]

Sequential Interactions

Cleavage of many components generates a small fragment, which enters the surrounding milieu, and a larger residual molecule, which attaches to the cell surface and continues the reaction sequence. The complement cascade, like the coagulation cascade, requires the presence of cations; both calcium and magnesium are necessary for the classical pathway initiated by antibody activity, but only magnesium ions are needed for the alternative pathway (see later). The major controls on the system are: 1) inhibitory proteins acting at the critical C1 and C3 activation steps, 2) spontaneous decay of the enzymatically active proteins produced during the cascade sequence and 3) rapid clearance of active fragments.

Complement may be activated through the *classical* or the *alternative* pathways (see Fig 7-4). The classical pathway is activated following specific antigen-antibody reactions. It is the primary amplifier of the biologic effects of humoral immunity. The alternative pathway amplifies nonantibody defense against microbial infection and other biologic alterations. By convention, individual complement components are designated C1, C4, C2, etc; cleavage fragments of complements are designated C4a, C3d, etc; the activated components are designated by placing a bar over the numbered component; capital letters are used for components of the alternative pathway, eg, Factors B and D.

Classical Pathway

Attachment

The first component of complement, C1, interacts directly with the Fc portion of

Table 7-4. Receptors for the Fc Region of Immunoglobulin

Receptor (CD Designation)	Ligand	Receptor-Positive Cells
FcγRI (CD64)	IgG1, IgG3	Mononuclear phagocytes
FcγRII (CDw32)	IgG complexes	Mononuclear phagocytes, granulocytes, B cells
FcγRIII (CD16)	IgG complexes	Macrophages, neutrophils, K and NK cells, some T cells, platelets
FcεRI	IgE	Mast cells, basophils
FCεRII (CD23)	IgE	B and T cells, platelets, eosinophils, Langerhans cells, follicular dendritic cells

CD = clusters of differentiation

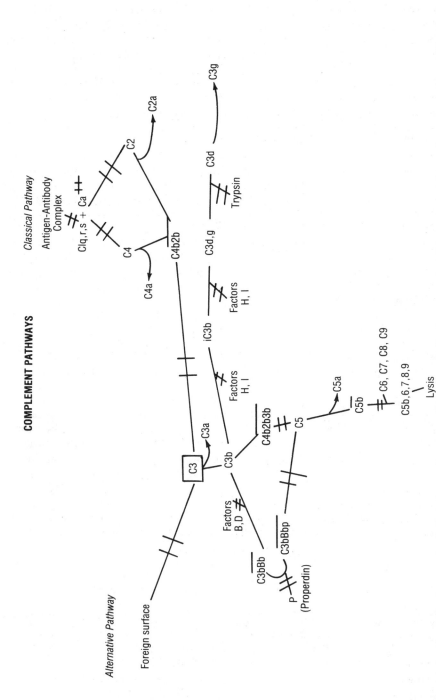

Figure 7-4. A schematic representation of complement pathways. || indicates enzyme action on a complement component, resulting in the cleavage of that component. → points to the product cleaved from the complement component and released into the fluid phase.

those immunoglobulin molecules that have the appropriate binding site in the C_H2 domain of the heavy chain. All μ chains have this site, and most γ chains. C1 is composed of three subunits, C1q, C1r and C1s, which are held in close association by calcium ions. C1q consists of 18 polypeptide chains wound together into six subunits; each subunit can bind to the Fc region of one immunoglobulin. C1q attaches only to those antibody molecules that have bound their corresponding antigen. The reaction of antibody with antigen may cause some conformational change in the antibody molecule, exposing or altering the site where C1q attaches, or it may simply bring the binding sites of several Fc segments close together so that a C1q molecule can interact with them. At least two of the six C1q subunits must bind to the Fc region of an immunoglobulin. A single IgM pentamer attached to a cell surface antigen can provide sufficient binding sites, but for IgG two separate molecules (a doublet) are required, and these must be close enough together on the cell surface that one C1q molecule can bind to them simultaneously. Individual IgG molecules attached to antigen sites widely separated on a cell surface are ineffective in activating complement regardless of the number of IgG molecules actually present. F(ab')₂ fragments are unable to activate complement, even though they may crosslink nearby antigen sites because the binding site resides in the C_H2 region of the Fc fragment.

Activation

Bound C1q undergoes a conformational change that activates C1r. This in turn activates C1s, the part of the molecule that propagates the complement sequence by cleaving C4 into C4a and C4b, and cleaving C2 to uncover a labile binding site. C4b contains a binding site through which

it attaches to the cell membrane. C4a is released into the body fluid where it has a number of biologic actions collectively described as *anaphylatoxic* activity. *Anaphylatoxins* stimulate mast cell degranulation and histamine release, thereby increasing vascular permeability. They also induce contraction of smooth muscle and release of lysosomal enzymes from neutrophils.

Once C4b is bound to the cell membrane, C2 can attach to it or closely adjacent to the C4b. The larger fragment, C2b (C2a in some texts), combines with C4b to produce C4b2b (C4b2a), also called *C3 convertase*, which has enzymatic activity. Each site of C1q attachment to an Fc chain can generate 100-200 C4b2b complexes attached to the cell membrane.

Amplification

C4b2b is called *C3 convertase* because it cleaves the inactive C3 molecule into C3a and C3b. One C4b2b molecule can cleave hundreds of C3 molecules. The smaller fragment, C3a, is released into the plasma, where it acts as an anaphylatoxin. The larger fragment, C3b, either binds promptly to the cell membrane or decays in solution. C3b fragments by themselves are not active catalytically and do not promote cell lysis, but the presence of C3b on a cell membrane greatly increases the susceptibility of that cell to phagocytosis because macrophages and neutrophils have receptors for C3b. A substance whose presence on the cell surface enhances susceptibility to phagocytosis is called an opsonin. C3b and the Fc portion of IgG molecules are powerful opsonins.

Some C3b fragments join C4b2b to form the next catalytic unit, C4b2b3b, which is called C5 convertase and has proteolytic activity against C5. C4b2b3b splits C5 into C5a and C5b. As with C4a and C3a, C5a is released into the plasma

Table 7-5. Receptors for C3-Derived Complement Fragments[29]

Receptor (CD Designation)	Ligand	Receptor-Positive Cells
C3aR	C3a	Mast cells, mononuclear phagocytes, neutrophils, basophils
CR1 (CD35)	C3b	Rbcs, mononuclear phagocytes, T and B cells, neutrophils, eosinophils
CR2 (CD21)	C3d, C3dg	B cells, thymocytes, follicular dendritic cells
CR3 (CD11b/CD18)	iC3b	Mononuclear phagocytes, neutrophils, eosinophils, K and NK cells
CR4 (CD11c/CD18)	iC3b	Monocytes, macrophages, neutrophils, K and NK cells
CR5	C3dg, C3d	Neutrophils, platelets

CD = clusters of differentiation

where it is a potent anaphylatoxin. It also acts as an attractant for polymorphonuclear leukocytes and as a stimulant to intracellular processes involved in inflammation.

Attack

In the presence of C5b, molecules of C6, C7, C8 and a variable number of C9 molecules assemble themselves into aggregates called the *membrane attack unit*. This molecular complex causes a change in membrane permeability, allowing water to enter the cell such that it swells and bursts. It is not clear whether the membrane attack unit produces a pore in the rbc membrane or whether its presence causes a rearrangement of the phospholipid bilayer that alters permeability, or both. The membrane attack unit remains active for only a very short time, after which it loses its affinity for the cell membrane.

Complement Receptors

Immunohematology is mostly concerned with the C3-derived components of complement as deposition of C3 on rbcs or platelets can lead to lysis of these cells. Specific cell surface receptors exist for a number of complement components.[30] Those for C3-derived fragments are shown in Table 7-5.

Alternative Pathway

In the alternative pathway, cleavage of C3 and activation of the remainder of the complement cascade occur independently of complement-fixing antibodies. Triggers for the alternative pathway include particulate polysaccharide and lipopolysaccharides such as those on the surfaces of some microorganisms; endotoxin; trypsin-like enzymes; and antigen/antibody complexes involving antibodies, such as IgA and IgG4, that do not activate C1.

Molecules of C3 in normal plasma and other body fluids undergo cleavage at a continuous low level, apparently due to interaction with factor B in the fluid phase. Normally, the resulting C3b, which is in fluid phase and not bound to any surface, is rapidly degraded by control proteins in plasma. If, however, the C3b comes in contact with particulate activators of the alternative pathway, the surface of these activators provides protection from the control proteins in fluid and acts as a sheltered environment in which C3b and factor B can associate. The bound C3b-factor B complex interacts with an active serum protease, *factor D*, which cleaves factor B to produce C3bBb. C3bBb is an effective C3 convertase, generating additional C3b, which attaches to the complex and amplifies its activities. The association (on the surface of a microorganism or an aggregate of protein) of numerous C3b units, factor Bb and a stabilizing protein called *properdin* (P) has potent activity as a C5 convertase. With cleavage of C5, the remainder of the complement cascade continues as in the classical pathway. The action of C3bBb or C3bBbP on C3 generates C3a as well as C3b, and the C5 convertase activity of C3bBbP generates C5a as well as C5b, so the alternative pathway produces both the anaphylatoxic effects and the lytic effects of complement activation.

Inactivation of C3b

In both the classical and the alternative pathway, C3b binds to the surfaces of cells through a thioester bond. Several serum proteins may act on the C3b molecule to abolish its enzymatic effects. *Factor H* (formerly called C3 binding protein or β_{1H}) attaches to C3b and renders it susceptible to the proteolytic effects of *factor I* (formerly called C3b inactivator). Factor I cleaves C3b into iC3b and subsequent cleavage by factor I produces fragments of C3dg and C3c. The C3c escapes into the fluid phase and the C3dg fragment remains permanently bound to the membrane. Factors H and I often exert this inhibitory effect on the bound C3b when there is in-vivo complement activation; coating of cells with

C3dg is frequently seen as the residual effect of antibodies acting in vivo against blood cells.

What was once thought to be C3d on the red cell membrane in vivo is now known to be C3dg. However, in vitro, C3dg can be cleaved by serine proteases such as trypsin to form C3d, which remains bound to the cell membrane, and C3g, which escapes into the fluid phase.[31,32] This fact forms the basis for the standardization of anti-C3d antiserum used in blood banks. (See Chapter 8.)

In vivo, the C3dg complex has no activating effect on the complement sequence but may interact with receptors on certain cells (see Table 7-5).

Factor I may also cleave cell-bound C4b, to leave enzymatically inert C4d attached to the cells. C4d is the antigenic determinant recognized by anti-Chido/Rogers (see Chapter 12). A number of membrane and plasma proteins also exist to regulate complement deposited on cell surfaces. The largest group of *regulator proteins* is directed at C3 convertases and includes *CR1* (C3b/C4b receptor), *decay-accelerating factor* (DAF) and *membrane cofactor protein*.[33] These plasma and membrane proteins will break down the C3 convertase or will serve as a cofactor for the proteolytic inactivation of C3b or C4b by plasma factor I. DAF is of special clinical interest because it is deficient in patients with paroxysmal nocturnal hemoglobinuria whose rbcs have increased sensitivity to complement-mediated lysis. DAF may also be involved in the down regulation of complement activation.

The Immune Response

The cells principally involved in the adaptive immune response are macrophages, B lymphocytes (B cells) and T lymphocytes (T cells).[1,2,21,22] Since the 1960's it has been apparent that the T cell is the major cell responsible for cell-mediated immunity, while the B cell is the major effector cell for humoral immunity, ie, production of antibody. However, the actions of T cells affect, in most cases, the activity of B cells. The macrophage plays an important role in many aspects of the immune response (see Fig 7-5).

Humoral Immunity

When a foreign antigen is introduced into a living system (in higher species), before it can initiate an immune response, that antigen is usually processed by being broken down into small peptide fragments, then presented to helper T lymphocytes in the context of self MHC. The cells responsible for the processing and presentation of foreign antigens are the APCs. They can be B cells, monocytes, macrophages, fixed tissue histocytes, dendritic cells, Langerhans cells, etc. See Fig 7-6. The APCs are found in highest concentration in lymphoid organs (ie, lymph nodes and the spleen), but are present in all tissue.

The APCs first capture and internalize the foreign antigen, subjecting it to various enzymes, thereby breaking the antigen into its smaller protein fragments. A process known as "determinate selection" results in certain protein fragments associating with the MHC Class II molecules of the APC. These small protein fragments, or epitopes, are distributed upon the surface of the effector cells in the context of self MHC, where they may be recognized by the T-cell receptor of lymphocytes as they migrate past these cells.

Primary Immunization

The usual mechanism to initiate the production of antibody is a series of interactions of specific cells. First, as foreign antigen is introduced into the body, it comes into contact with an APC. The antigen interacts with the APC, it is ingested, processed and presented on the outer surface of that cell along with the self MHC Class II antigens (see Fig 7-6). The APCs may circulate until they interact with a CD4, helper/inducer T cell that recognizes the foreign antigen, in combination with the MHC complex, through its TCR. Conversely, an antigen-specific T cell may circulate until it recognizes, through its TCR, an APC expressing on its surface the corresponding ligand (peptide plus MHC). When the CD4 cell reacts with the presented foreign antigen along with the MHC antigens, a series of changes begins to occur. The APCs secrete cytokines such as IL-1, which stimulates CD4 cells to enlarge. Simultaneously, signaling through the TCR causes CD4 cell surface antigen recognition sites to decrease and *transferrin* and *IL-2* receptors to increase. These activated CD4 cells begin to secrete cytokines (IL-2, which autostimulates the T cell to proliferate) and *interferon* (IFNγ, which further stimulates the APC to produce more IL-1). These changes allow the CD4 cell to undergo clonal expansion. After clonal expansion of the CD4 T cells, large numbers of these cells can circulate and find the single B cell expessing the same processed antigen (in the context of self MHC) that these clonally expanded T cells recognize. At this point, B cells are "helped" through stimulation by the CD4 cell-derived cytokines *IL-2* and *IL-4*, and the B cell will begin to divide. The B cells are further stimulated by *IL-4* and undergo clonal expansion to produce daughter cells that are genetically identical.[2,34] (See Fig 7-6.) Under the influence of additional cytokines (IL-6 and IL-7) the daughter cells develop into either *plasma cells*, the cells that actually secrete antibody, or *memory B cells*, which enter the circulating lymphocyte pool and persist for months or years.

Antibody produced in the primary response is predominantly IgM. In a *primary immune response*, when the host

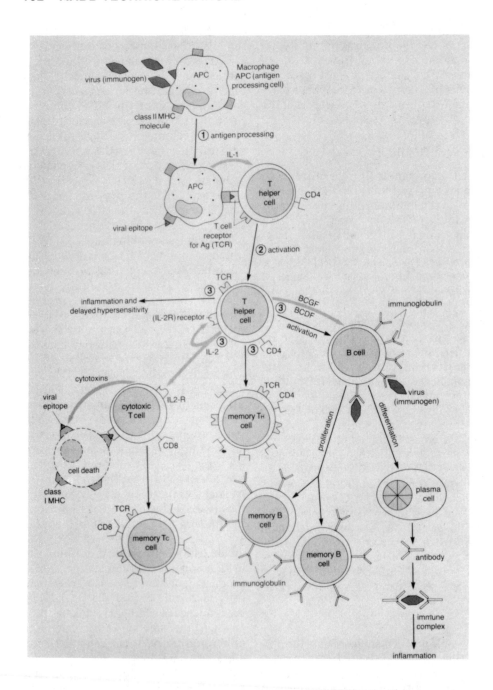

Figure 7-5. Grand scheme of adaptive immune system. 1) Antigen processing, 2) T-helper cell activation and 3) T-helper cell responses to activation. (Used with permission from Stites DP, Terr Al. Basic human immunology. Norwalk: Appleton & Lange, 1991.)

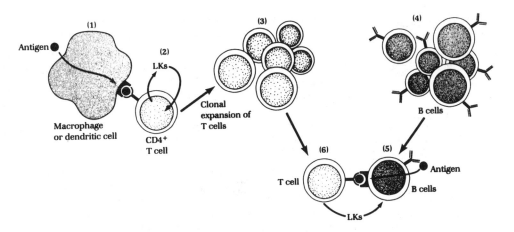

Figure 7-6. A model for the roles of antigen presentation by macrophages versus B cells during a primary antibody response (1). Antigen enters the system and is processed and presented by macrophages or dendritic cells. (2) Antigen-specific CD4+T cells respond to the presented antigen plus Class II MHC by producing cytokines, also known as lymphokines (LKs), that stimulate the T cell to proliferate. The cells in the expanded clone of T cells (3) are now more likely to contact a relatively rare antigen-specific B cell (4), which has taken up and processed the antigen after specific binding to cell-surface Igs (5). The specific T cell finds the B cell (relatively easily because the T cell now has many copies) and responds to the processed antigen (plus Class II MHC) presented by the B cell by releasing LKs (6), which stimulate clonal expansion and differentiation of the specific B cell. Note that this model requires that the carrier and hapten be linked in order for the expanded T cell to contact the appropriate B cell, and that the LKs act only at short range. (Used with permission from Golub and Green.[2])

first encounters a particular antigen, several days to several weeks elapse before detectable antibody is found; this is called the *lag period*. During the lag period the B cell undergoes reorganization of genetic material, assembly of ribosomes, initiation of DNA synthesis and, ultimately, mitosis. This is a key aspect of the immune response because, if DNA synthesis and mitosis are disturbed, the amount of antibody produced is drastically reduced.

By a series of signals from the T cells, and sometimes mutations of the B cells, the immunoglobulin production can be switched from IgM to IgG, IgA, IgD or IgE or to the same immunoglobulin but of a higher affinity than initially produced.

Not all B cells are stimulated to produce antibody by the above mechanism.

Some large molecules, especially those with multiple repeating polysaccharide antigenic determinants, can induce antibody production without intervention from T cells and are called *T-cell-independent* antigens.

Secondary Immunization

It is the memory B cell that responds to subsequent contact with antigens to produce the secondary immune response. The *secondary*, or *anamnestic, response* occurs very rapidly and results in production of more antibody than the primary response because the memory B cells have already been exposed to antigen and have produced daughter cells that will recognize that antigen. On a subsequent encounter with the same antigen, more cells are able to respond. IgG is the major class of antibody produced in a secondary response. IgM production occurs in the same cells that originally produced IgM, through an imperfectly understood switching mechanism that permits synthesis of IgG antibody with specificity for the same antigen.

The antibody molecules produced by the B cells cannot by themselves destroy foreign substances. However, they mark these substances for destruction via the activation of complement (see p 156), or by interacting with macrophages, which have receptors for the Fc region of immunoglobulins. The macrophages phagocytose and digest the antibody-coated foreign cells.

Regulation of the Immune Response

Once an adaptive immune response has been initiated, it is important that mechanisms to regulate its magnitude or terminate it exist. The following mechanisms may be involved in limiting antibody production: 1) individual plasma cells survive only a few days and, unless new plasma cells evolve, antibody production ceases; 2) antibody produced in the immune response coats macrophage-bound antigen so that it no longer stimulates clonal expansion; 3) active suppression causes inhibition of lymphocyte function; 4) the antigen that initially elicited the response is often degraded or eliminated from the body; and 5) anti-idiotypic antibodies are produced, which modulate B-cell antibody production.

Cytotoxic Immune Reaction

Viral infection and foreign transplanted antigens can generate T cells that are cytotoxic for the virus-infected cells or for the allograft. When virus-infected cells or foreign allografts are recognized by the CD4 T cells, these T cells are activated and IL-2 is released. The proliferating CD4 T cells and the release of IL-2 stimulate the proliferation of cytotoxic effec-

tor cells among the CD8 T cells (see Fig 7-5). These cytotoxic cells bind effectively to the target cell (virus-infected cell or allograft). Lesions appear at the site of attachment and the membrane permeability of the target cell increases, eventually resulting in membrane disruption and cell death.

In-Vitro Detection of Antigen-Antibody Reactions

Once antibody has been formed in vivo there are various ways in which it can be detected in vitro. These include, but are not limited to, the following processes.

Agglutination

Agglutination is the clumping of particles that have antigen on their surface by antibody molecules forming bridges between antigenic determinants on adjacent cells. Agglutination, the endpoint for most tests involving red cells and blood group antibodies, can be observed either through direct techniques such as ABO testing, or indirect techniques such as the antiglobulin test. Agglutination is discussed in more detail in a later section.

Precipitation

Precipitation is the formation of a visible, insoluble complex when soluble antibody reacts with soluble antigen. Such complexes are detected in test tubes as a sediment and in agar gels as a white line appearing where the antigen and antibody interact. Precipitation is the basis of procedures such as immunodiffusion and immunoelectrophoresis.

Precipitation does not always occur, even though soluble antigen and its specific antibody are present. It depends on the formation of a lattice structure that requires the presence of equivalent amounts of antigen and antibody. If antibody is present in excess, there are too few antigen sites with which the molecules can crosslink, and the lattice structure is not formed. This is called a *prozone phenomenon*. The prozone phenomenon can occur in agglutination tests when: 1) antibody is in very high concentration and there are few antigen-bearing particles or 2) the antigen concentration on the surface of cells is very low.

Hemolysis

Hemolysis is the rupture of rbcs with release of intracellular hemoglobin. Cells of other types may undergo lysis, due to disruption of the membrane from a variety of causes. Antibody-mediated hemolysis requires activation of complement and does not occur if the antigen and antibody interact in the absence of complement or in plasma when an agent that chelates calcium and magnesium ions is present. Hemolysis is interpreted as a positive result in tests for red cell antibodies because it indicates the presence of a complement-activating antibody. Pink or red supernatant fluid after incubation of antibody with rbc is an important observation because antibodies that are lytic in vitro are likely to cause intravascular hemolysis in vivo.

Inhibition of Agglutination

In agglutination inhibition tests the presence of antigen or antibody is detected by inhibition of previously documented agglutination. For example, the saliva of persons who are secretors normally contains soluble blood group antigens. Their presence can be detected by incubating boiled saliva with a standardized dilution of anti-A or anti-B and then adding A and B red cells. If the saliva contains blood group substance it will complex with the antibody and neutralize its agglutinating properties so that subsequently added red cells will not be agglutinated. Inhibition of agglutination indicates that the corresponding antigen is present in the test material. Conversely, agglutination of the indicator cells denotes the absence of the corresponding antigen.

Another important example of inhibition of agglutination is unwanted inactivation of antihuman globulin serum. Unbound globulin combines with antiglobulin molecules before they can react with rbc-bound globulins. If rbcs used in either direct or indirect antiglobulin testing are not thoroughly washed and free of serum, residual globulin can inhibit the antihuman globulin reagent and cause a false-negative result (see p 180).

Immunofluorescence

Immunofluorescence allows identification and localization of antigens on cell surfaces and in cells. A fluorochrome such as fluorescein or phycoerythrin can be attached to an antibody molecule, rendering it intensely fluorescent without destroying its specificity or ability to bind antigen. After a fluorescent-labeled antibody reacts with cellular antigens, the antibody-coated cell appears sharply visible and yellow-green or red (depending on the fluorochrome) when examined with a fluorescence microscope. The amount of fluorescence can also be determined by flow cytometry.

Immunofluorescence can be used as either a direct or an indirect procedure, analogous to direct and indirect antiglobulin testing. In a direct test a specific antibody is fluorescent-labeled and reacted with tissues or cells. In an indirect test a fluorescent-labeled antiglobulin serum is added to cells that have been incubated with unlabeled antibody (eg, anti-D). Immunofluorescence is commonly used to detect surface antigens of T cells and to identify the immunoglobulins present on and in B cells. More recently, flow cytofluorometry has been used to measure the amount of IgG on rbcs, quantitate fetal-maternal hemorrhage, follow transfused rbcs for rbc survival studies and differentiate homozygotes from heterozygotes.[35,36]

Radioimmunoassay

Radioimmunoassay procedures use a suitable radionuclide as a marker for either antigen or antibody and are suitable for either direct or indirect tests. In a direct test, antibody is radiolabeled without destroying its specificity. Following exposure to the antigen, the quantity of antibody bound can be very accurately measured. The indirect technique is based on localization of the antigen upon fixed, unlabeled antibody. Tests for HBsAg have used this method. Unlabeled anti-HBs is coupled to a solid material and test material added. If HBsAg is present it combines with the fixed antibody and remains capable of reacting with subsequently added radiolabeled anti-HBs. A gamma counter quantifies very precisely the amount of radiolabeled anti-HBs that has attached to the previously bound antigen.

Radiolabeling is also used in competitive binding procedures. Here the principle that labeled and unlabeled antibody of the same specificity have the same reactivity with the corresponding antigen is employed. Calculating the proportion of a known dose of labeled material bound in a test system permits calculation of the amount of unlabeled material that must have been present.

Enzyme-Linked Immunosorbent Assay

Enzyme-linked immunosorbent assays (ELISAs) are used to measure either antigen or antibody. Enzymes such as alkaline phosphatase can be linked to antibody without destroying either the antibody specificity or the enzyme activity. The enzyme acts as a quantifiable label, similar to radiolabeling. Enzyme labels are far more stable than radioactive labels; are safer, cheaper and simpler to measure; and in many cases, provide results that are comparably sensitive. A number of tests for HAV, HBV and HIV markers use this principle. ELISA has been used for detecting rbc-bound IgG and detecting fetal-maternal hemorrhage. When rbcs are used the test is often called an enzyme-linked antiglobulin test.

Solid-Phase Red Cell Adherence Tests Using Indicator RBCs

Solid-phase microplate techniques, used in immunologic assays for many years (eg, for HBsAg tests), are now being used to identify rbc antigens or antibodies.[37,38] In a direct test, antibody is coated to the sides of a microplate well and rbcs are added to the wells. If the appropriate antigen is on the rbcs, they will adhere to the sides of the well (eg, if the wells are coated with anti-A, group A rbcs will adhere to the wells). If there is no antigen-antibody reaction, the rbcs will settle to the bottom of the well. In an indirect test, rbcs are adhered to the sides of the wells by pretreating the well with compounds such as glutaraldehyde, poly L-lysine, or a monoclonal or potent serum antibody. The patient's serum is added to these rbc-coated wells and allowed to react with the rbcs. The plates are then washed free of serum. Anti-IgG coated rbcs (indicator rbcs) are added and the plate is centrifuged. A reaction is positive if the indicator rbcs adhere to the sides of the well. If the indicator rbcs settle to the bottom of the wells, no antigen-antibody reaction has occurred.

Factors Affecting Agglutination

Rbc agglutination is thought to occur in two stages: 1) physical attachment of antibody to rbcs, called sensitization, and 2) formation of bridges between the sensitized red cells to form the lattice that constitutes agglutination. A number of variables affect each stage.

The First Stage

The association of antigen with antibody is reversible. The amount of antibody attached to antigen at equilibrium is affected by the equilibrium constant, or affinity constant, of the antibody. In general, the larger the equilibrium constant, the greater the rate of association and the slower the rate of dissociation. The association of antigen with antibody is affected by the concentration of antigen and antibody and by various physical conditions such as pH, ionic strength and temperature. Altering the physical conditions of agglutination tests can increase or decrease their sensitivity.

Temperature

Most blood group antibodies show reactivity over a restricted temperature range; some, such as anti-P_1, react optimally at 18 C and some, such as anti-Fy^a, react optimally at 37 C. Generally, IgM antibodies are more reactive at lower temperatures (4-27 C),[39] whereas IgG antibodies are detected better at 37 C.[40,41] Methods for antibody detection often cover a range of temperatures (eg, 22-37 C or 30-37 C). Antibodies that react in vitro only at temperatures below 37 C usually are considered to have no clinical significance; they rarely cause destruction of transfused rbcs.[39,40] A notable exception is the anti-P found in the serum of some patients with paroxysmal cold hemoglobinuria. Some cold-reactive IgM antibodies may activate complement at temperatures above 30 C but cause only minimally shortened survival of transfused incompatible rbcs. Identification of these antibodies is discussed in Chapter 15. Clinically significant antibodies are those that cause rbc destruction in vivo. This is usually reflected by reactivity in vitro at 37 C.[41]

pH

The optimal pH for antibodies of most blood group systems has not been determined. Some antibodies, such as anti-M, react best at low pH. Hughes-Jones et al[42] reported an optimum of between 6.5 and 7.0 for anti-D. Practically, a pH of around 7.0 should be used for routine work. Since the pH of stored saline may be 5.0-6.0, some workers use buffered saline in serologic testing.

Incubation Time

The time needed to reach equilibrium differs for different blood group antibodies. Significant variables include the class of immunoglobulin involved and how well it combines with its specific antigen. Studies with serum and saline-suspended red cells have shown that, of the total amount of Rh antibody ultimately bound, approximately 25% will be taken up in the first 15 minutes and 75% within the first hour.[42] The addition of various enhancing agents (eg, to produce a lower ionic strength) can increase the amount of antibody taken up in the first 15 minutes and, therefore, decrease the incubation time needed to reach equilibrium.

Ionic Strength

In normal saline, Na^+ and Cl^- ions cluster around and partially neutralize opposite charges on antigen and antibody molecules. This shielding effect, which hinders the association of antibody with antigen, is reduced by lowering the ionic strength of the reaction medium. In general, the speed of antibody uptake is enhanced by lowering the salt concentration of the reaction medium.[43]

Antigen-Antibody Ratio

The speed with which antigen and antibody bind is affected by the number of antibody molecules in the medium and the number of antigen sites per cell. Increasing the quantity of antibody present can increase the sensitivity of the test. By raising the serum-to-cell ratio, more molecules of antibody are available relative to the number of antigen sites. If a low ionic strength saline (LISS) system is used, the proportion of LISS must be adjusted appropriately to achieve the desired final ionic strength.

The Second Stage

Distance Between Cells

There are several theories about the mechanism whereby sensitized rbcs are linked into a lattice. The size of the IgG molecule is too small to span the distance between rbcs, which are separated from one another by repulsion of like charges.[44] Red cells have a net negative charge at their surface; interaction with ions in the suspending medium alters this surface charge, resulting in a reduction in the strength of this charge, which, when measured at the surface of shear, is called the *zeta potential*. The distance between rbcs is proportional to the zeta potential. Reducing the effective charge separating rbcs allows them to come closer together and may permit agglutination by IgG molecules.

Steane and Greenwalt[45] favor the water hydration theory. Water tightly bound at the surface of the rbcs keeps them separated in solution by maintaining a hydration shell around them, much like bubbles of water insulating the surface. They suggest that antibody binding to an antigen on the surface decreases the hydration layer and increases the tendency to agglutinate.

Effects of Enzymes

Proteolytic enzymes (eg, papain, ficin) used in serologic tests reduce the surface charge of the rbc by cleaving sialoglycoproteins from the cell surface. Neuraminidase reduces the charge on the cell surface by cleaving N-acetylneuraminic acid (NeuNAc, a sialic acid) molecules from polysaccharide chains. If the net charge keeps cells apart, any mechanism that reduces the net charge on the cell surface should therefore enhance agglutination. Cells pretreated with proteolytic enzymes often show enhanced agglutination by IgG molecules, but cells pretreated with neuraminidase demonstrate no comparable increase in agglutinability. Steane and Greenwalt[45] postulate that each type of enzyme removes a different amount of water, or insulation, from the polypeptides that are cleaved by these enzymes and that this accounts for the difference in the results.

The proteolytic enzymes used most often in immunohematology laboratories are bromelin, ficin and papain. The actions of these enzymes on the rbc surface, in addition to enhancing agglutination of rbcs coated with some antibodies, also eliminate the antigen-binding sites for other antibodies such as anti-M, -N, -S, -Fy^a and -Fy^b.

Effect of Positively Charged Molecules

The behavior of NeuNAc-deficient rbcs (eg, T or Tn polyagglutinable rbcs and protease-treated rbcs) with macromolecules such as Polybrene® gives additional information about the physical aspects of agglutination. Polybrene® (a positively charged polymer) causes normal rbcs to aggregate spontaneously, an effect many workers believe results from neutralizing the negative surface charge contributed by sialic acid. NeuNAc-deficient rbcs do not aggregate in Polybrene®. Steane and Greenwalt[45] postulated that hydration is the important factor, that water is extruded from the rbc surface as the macromolecules bind to oppositely charged groups and the insulating shell of water molecules is removed.

Other Considerations

Stratton et al[46] suggested that proteolytic enzymes affect the first stage of agglutination. They postulated that polypeptides protruding from the rbc surface cause steric interference in antibody binding, and that enzyme-mediated removal of these polypeptide chains facilitates antibody attachment. Van Oss and colleagues [47,48] emphasized that erythrocyte shape is important in the agglutination reaction. They postulated that rbcs of abnormal shape come into closer contact than normal rbcs and thus overcome the electrostatic repulsion normally present.

It is also possible that antigen mobility, antigen clustering and membrane flexibility play a role in the agglutination reaction. The exact mechanisms have yet to be determined.

Immunologically Mediated Diseases

The actions of the immune system are essential for good health but in many circumstances immune responses cause unpleasant, dangerous or even fatal effects in the host. The harmful effects of immunity are often collectively described as *hypersensitivity*; allergy and anaphylaxis are terms applied to certain restricted immune-mediated disorders. Hypersensitivity reactions may cause illness or tissue damage through a variety of mechanisms.

Hypersensitivity

Gell, Coombs and Lachman[32] have proposed four mechanisms of hypersensitivity (see Table 7-6). Types I, II and III depend on interaction between antigen and humoral antibody, with or without complement or other mediators. Type IV involves a cell-mediated immune response (CD4 T cells) and has a protracted course. The systemic anaphylactic reactions to IgA that occur in IgA-deficient persons and the allergic-IgE-mast cell reactions responsible for the atopic diseases, anaphylaxis and urticaria are examples of Type I. Transfusion reactions due to blood group antibodies, autoimmune hemolytic anemia and hemolytic disease of the newborn are considered Type II. Hemolytic conditions resulting from drug/antidrug immune complexes can be considered Type III reactions. Contact dermatitis and, probably, some aspects of graft-vs-host disease, such as that seen in some bone marrow recipients, are examples of Type IV.

Delayed Type Hypersensitivity

Cell-mediated delayed type hypersensitivity (DTH; also called Type IV hypersensitivity) is one of the body's defenses against viruses, fungi, mycobacteria and other organisms that replicate intracellularly, and may be involved in antitumor effects. The mode of primary immunization differs from that described for humoral immunity. Once the CD4 T cell has been activated by the APC, there is a delay period, allowing for the synthesis of cytokines and the effects of these cytokines to occur.[34] Table 7-1 lists the major T cell-derived cytokines, which include IL-2, IL-3, IFNγ and TNFβ. Other cytokines, GM-CSF and IL-8, attract and

Table 7-6. Classification of Immune-Mediated Tissue Damage*

Type	Descriptive Terms	Ig Class	Effectors	Time Course at Onset	Examples of Pathologic Conditions
I	Reaginic Atopic Anaphylactic	E, ?IgG4	Histamine and other substances from basophil granules	Minutes	Anaphylaxis Some asthma Urticaria Hay fever
II	Membrane-reactive	G, M	Complement Phagocytic cells Proteolytic enzymes	Minutes to hours	Transfusion reactions Autoimmune hemolysis Hemolytic disease of the newborn Some types of glomerulonephritis Myasthenia gravis
III	Immune complex Serum sickness	G, M	Complement Neutrophils	Minutes to hours	Some drug-induced hemolysis Post-streptococcal glomerulonephritis Many manifestations of lupus erythematosus Some pulmonary allergies Arthus reaction
IV	Cell-mediated	None	T lymphocytes Macrophages Lymphokines	Days to weeks	Allograft rejection Graft-vs-host disease Lung changes in tuberculosis Some chronic hepatitis

*Modified from Gell, Coombs and Lachman.[32]

keep the mononuclear phagocytes and polymorphonuclear granulocytes in the area of cytokine release. *IFNγ*, a cytokine previously called macrophage-activating factor, and, most likely, TNFβ enhance the cytolytic activity of the accumulated macrophages. Failure to eliminate the antigen could cause an accumulation of macrophages and the formation of a granuloma. This T-cell-dependent immune reaction is usually manifested by an inflammatory reaction at the site of antigen accumulation, usually the skin (ie, contact dermatitis such as occurs with poison ivy). This reaction reaches its peak in 24-48 hours. Other actions of IFN and TNF secreted by DTH cells may stop the growth of tumor cells.

Transfer of Immunoglobulin From Mother to Fetus

The transfer of immunoglobulin and other proteins from the mother to fetus is independent of molecular size; IgG (150,000 daltons) is transferred much more readily than albumin (64,000 daltons). Selective distribution must occur because IgG primarily enters the fetal blood while albumin primarily enters the amniotic fluid.[49] In humans, IgM does not reach the fetus and IgA is not readily transferred, although low levels have been found in the newborn infant.

All four subclasses of IgG are transported across the placenta, but the rate varies between individual mother-fetus pairs. Early in pregnancy IgG probably passes from mother to fetus by diffusion and concentration in fetal serum is low for all subgroups. Between 20 and 33 weeks of gestation, fetal IgG levels rise markedly, apparently due to maturation of a selective transport system. IgG1, the predominant subclass in maternal blood, is transported in greatest quantity. Part of the placental transport system seems to involve specific protein receptors on the membrane of placental cells[50] but other mechanisms are also involved.

Monoclonal Antibodies

Hybridomas

In 1975 Köhler and Milstein[51] showed that antibody-secreting cells from immunized animals could be fused with cultured myeloma cells capable of indefinite reproduction. The resulting hybrid cells grow continuously in culture and secrete the antibody characteristic of the parent cell. This technique is called somatic cell hybridization and the multiplying hybrid cell culture a hybridoma.

The standard technique for selecting successful hybrid cells uses a myeloma cell that has lost the ability to secrete hypoxanthine-guanine-phosphoribosyltransferase (HGPRT). This enzyme is needed to synthesize nucleotides, the coding elements of nucleic acids essential for preservation and transfer of genetic information. Absence of HGPRT is not a problem for the myeloma cell in standard culture medium because it has an alternative metabolic pathway for producing nucleotides. Growing the cell fusion mixture in a medium that blocks the other pathway makes the cells dependent on HGPRT. Normal lymphocytes possess HGPRT. In hybrid cells, the lymphocyte provides HGPRT and the ability to produce antibody; the myeloma cell provides the ability to reproduce indefinitely. In the selective medium, unfused myeloma cells die out because they lack HGPRT and normal lymphocytes die out because they cannot reproduce themselves through many generations. Only successful hybrid cells will remain viable.

The supernatant fluid from a successful culture of hybrid cells must be tested to determine the presence and the specificity of antibody. With appropriate selection and culture conditions, large numbers of antibody-producing cells can be isolated. Antibody can be harvested from the supernatant culture. Higher concentrations are obtained if the cells are injected into the peritoneal cavity of mice where they multiply and secrete antibody into the resulting ascitic fluid. A practical approach is to inject some of the cultured cells into mice, and store the remaining cells frozen until more ascitic fluid is required. This also ensures that the original antibody specificity can be maintained for long periods of time, because hybrid cells become unstable if maintained in tissue culture conditions indefinitely.

Epstein-Barr Virus Infected Human B Cells

Another method of producing monoclonal antibodies is to use human B cells infected with Epstein-Barr virus (EBV).[52,53] In this process, B cells are harvested from a recently stimulated donor (eg, a D– person recently stimulated to make anti-D). EBV will transform some B cells, immortalizing and activating them to produce antibody. EBV-infected cells will begin to synthesize DNA in approximately 48 hours, turn into blast cells and divide into antibody-producing plasma cells. This technique was used to produce anti-D, but cell lines usually ceased antibody production after a few weeks or months. Thompson et al[54] modified this procedure by collecting B cells, infecting them with EBV and then fusing the EBV-infected cells with mouse myeloma cells. These heterohybridomas produced IgM and IgG antibodies over a 14-month period, allowing large quantities of anti-D to be collected. Another technique, involving fusion of a human lymphoblastoid cell line with the B cells from an immunized donor, has also resulted in a stable culture of monoclonal anti-D.[55]

Applications

Monoclonal antibodies have many applications in the field of immunohematology, eg, typing the subsets of T and B cells and as HLA typing sera. Numerous monoclonal reagents that recognize red cell antigens have been identified. Those recognizing ABO and Rh antigens, as well as hybridoma-derived monoclonal antiglobulin reagents, are of particular interest to blood bank workers.

The selection of reagents for the blood bank serology laboratory requires that they be able to react with antigen-positive rbcs, including some examples of rbcs showing a weaker-than-expected expression of the antigen subgroups.[56]

Monoclonal reagents, by definition, are directed against a single epitope (antigen-binding site) on an antigen used to immunize the host. They contain only one immunoglobulin type (having only one type of light chain and heavy chain) produced by the host after exposure to what may be a complex antigen. Since the monoclonal antibody reacts with only one epitope on an antigen molecule, it may not react with all subgroups within a blood group. For this reason many commercial monoclonal reagents are a blend of two or more monoclonal antibodies; this broadens the specificity of the reagent to a blood group determinant.

Monoclonal sera are now harvested using large culture systems. This is easier and less time-consuming than reinoculating mice and collecting and standardizing ascitic fluid. Monoclonal reagents can be produced in large batches. This reduces the dependence of the manufacturers on collecting, processing and testing large numbers of human sera.

The ABH monoclonal sera are usually powerful IgM agglutinins. Some blends of anti-A will give strong reactions when tested with various subgroups of A. Monoclonal sera will not react with T-activated rbcs nor will the anti-B sera react with the acquired B antigen. In addition to the ABH sera, monoclonal reagents are commercially available as antiglobulin sera (see p 177). These sera offer the same advantages of the ABH sera, with less lot-to-lot variability and fewer false-positive reactions. They have also been used extensively in research and have been helpful in identifying the differences in immunoglobulin molecules[57] (see p 171).

Monoclonal anti-D sera are also available commercially. These reagents, derived from tissue cultures of EBV-transformed cell lines or human-human monoclonal reagents, must meet the same standards as described for the ABH sera (eg, the anti-D must detect the D antigen and weak examples of the D antigen and react with examples of $D_{variant}$ or weak D rbcs). Once again, due to the nature of monoclonal sera, a blended reagent is necessary to meet these demands (see Chapter 11).

References

1. Paul WE, ed. Fundamental immunology, 2nd ed. New York, NY: Raven Press Ltd., 1989.
2. Golub ES, Green DR. Immunology: A synthesis, 2nd ed. Sunderland, MA: Sineau Associates, 1991.
3. Clark SC, Kamen R. The human hematopoietic colony-stimulating factors. Science 1987;236:1229-37.
4. Till JE, McCulloch EA. A direct measurement of the radiation sensitivity of normal mouse bone marrow cells. Radiat Res 1961;14:213.
5. Curry JL, Trentin JJ. Hemopoietic spleen colony studies. I. Growth and differentiation. Dev Biol 1967;15:395.
6. Golde DW, Gasson JC. Hormones that stimulate the growth of blood cells. Sci Am 1988;259:62-70.
7. Nicola NA. Hemopoietic cell growth factors and their receptors. Annu Rev Biochem 1989;58:45.
8. Herrmann F, Mertelsmann R. Polypeptides controlling hematopoietic cell development and activation. Blut 1989;58:117-28.
9. Pluznik DH, Sachs L. The cloning of normal "mast" cells in tissue culture. J Cell Comp Physiol 1965;66:319.
10. Bradley TR, Metcalf D. The growth of mouse bone marrow cells in vitro. Aust J Exp Med Sci 1966;44:287.
11. Eaves AC, Eaves CJ. Erythropoiesis in culture. In: McCulloch EA, ed. Clinics in hematology. Toronto: WB Saunders, 1985:371.
12. Nossal GJV. Current concepts: Immunology. The basic concepts of the immune system. N Engl J Med 1987;316:1320-5.
13. Levitt D, Cooper MD. Lymphocytes II. B Cell. In: Stites DP, Stobo JD, Wells JV, eds. Basic and clinical immunology. 6th ed. Los Altos, CA: Appleton & Lang, 1987:72-81.
14. Alberts B, Bray D, Lewis J, et al. Molecular biology of the cell. New York: Garland, 1983.
15. Williams AF. The T-lymphocyte antigen receptor—elusive no more. Nature 1984;308:108-9.
16. Blann AD. T lymphocyte surface molecules: Structure and function. Med Lab Sci 1987;44:220-36.
17. Stobo JD. Lymphocytes I. T cells. In: Stites DP, Stobo JD, Wells JV, eds. Basic and clinical immunology. 6th ed. Los Altos, CA: Appleton & Lang, 1987:65-72.
18. Bernard A, Bernstein I, Baumsell L, et al. Nomenclature for clusters of differentiation (CD) of antigens on human leukocyte populations. Bull WHO 1984;62:809-11.
19. Knapp W, Dörken B, Rieber P, et al. CD antigens 1989. Blood 1989;74:1441-50.
20. Knapp W, Rieber P, Dörken B, et al. Toward a better definition of human leucocyte surface molecules. Immunol Today 1989;10:253-8.
21. Sell S. Immunology immunopathology and immunity. 4th ed. New York: Elsevier, 1987.
22. Roitt I. Essential immunology. 6th ed. Oxford: Blackwell Scientific Publications, 1988.
23. Goodman JW. Immunoglobulins I: Structure and function. In: Stites DP, Stobo JD, Wells JV, eds. Basic and clinical immunology. 6th ed. Los Altos, CA: Appleton & Lang, 1987:27-36.
24. Burton DR. The conformation of antibodies. In: Metzger H, ed. Fc receptors and the action of antibodies. Washington, DC: American Society for Microbiology, 1990:31-54.
25. Myrvik QN, Weiser RS. Fundamentals of immunology. 2nd ed. Philadelphia: Lea and Febiger, 1984:62.
26. Kerr MA. The structure and function of human IgA. Biochem J 1990;271:285-96.
27. Schumaker VN, Poon PH. Activation of the classical and alternative pathways of complement by immune complexes. In: Metzger H, ed. Fc receptors and the action of antibodies. Washington, DC: American Society for Microbiology, 1990:181-206.
28. Steinberg AG. Immunoglobulin allotypes. In: Atassi MZ, van Oss CJ, Absolom DR, eds. Molecular immunology. A textbook. New York: Marcel Dekker Inc, 1984:231-53.
29. Garratty G. The significance of complement in immunohematology. CRC Crit Rev Clin Lab Sci 1984;20:25-56.
30. Erdei A, Fust G, Gergely J. The role of C3 in the immune response. Immunol Today 1991;12:332-7.
31. Freedman J. The significance of complement on the red cell surface. Transfus Med Rev 1987;1:58-70.
32. Gell PGH, Coombs RRA, Lachman PJ, eds. Clinical aspects of immunology. 3rd ed. Oxford: Blackwell Scientific, 1975.
33. Lublin DM, Atkinson JP. Decay-accelerating factor: Biochemistry, molecular biology, and function. In: Paul WE, Fathman CG, Metzger H, eds. Annual review of immunology. Palo Alto: Annual Reviews Inc, 1989;7:35-58.
34. Smith KA. Lymphokine regulation of T cell and B cell function In: Paul WE, ed. Funda-

mental immunology. New York: Raven Press, 1984:559-76.

35. Nance ST. Applications of flow cytometry in blood transfusion science. In: Moore SB, ed. Progress in immunohematology. Arlington, VA: American Association of Blood Banks, 1988:1-30.

36. Garratty G. Flow cytometry: Its applications to immunohaematology. Baillière's Clin Haematol 1990;3:267-87.

37. Rosenfield RE, Kochwa S, Kaczera Z. Solid phase serology for the study of human erythrocytic antigen-antibody reactions. Paper presented at the 15th Congress of the International Society of Blood Transfusion, Paris. July 1978.

38. Plapp FV, Rachel JM, Beck ML, et al. Blood antigens and antibodies: Solid phase adherence assays. Laboratory Management 1984; 22:39-46.

39. Issitt PD. Antibodies reactive at 30 centigrade, room temperature, and below. In: Butch SH, Beck M, eds. Clinically significant and insignificant antibodies. Washington, DC: American Association of Blood Banks, 1979:13-28.

40. Garratty G. Clinical significance of antibodies reacting optimally at 37 C. In: Butch SH, Beck M, eds. Clinically significant and insignificant antibodies. Washington, DC: American Association of Blood Banks, 1979:29-49.

41. Arndt P, Garratty G. Evaluation of the optimal incubation temperature for detecting certain IgG antibodies with potential clinical significance. Transfusion 1988;28:210-3.

42. Hughes-Jones NC, Gardner B, Telford R. Studies on the reaction between the blood-group antibody anti-D and erythrocytes. Biochem J 1963;88:435-40.

43. Elliot M, Bossom E, Dupuy ME, Masouredis SP. Effect of ionic strength on the serologic behavior of red cell isoantibodies. Vox Sang 1964;9:396-414.

44. Pollack W, Hager HJ, Reckel R, et al. A study of the forces involved in the second stage of hemagglutination. Transfusion 1965;5:158-83.

45. Steane EA, Greenwalt TJ. Erythrocyte agglutination. In: Sandler SG, Nusbacher J, Schanfield MS, eds. Immunobiology of the erythrocyte. Progress in clinical and biological research. Vol 43. New York: Alan R. Liss, 1979:171-88.

46. Stratton F, Rawlinson VI, Gunson HH, Phillips PK. The role of zeta potential in Rh agglutination. Vox Sang 1973;24:273-9.

47. Van Oss CT, Mohn JF, Cunningham RK. Influence of various physicochemical factors on hemagglutination. Vox Sang 1978;34:351-61.

48. Van Oss CJ, Mohn JF, Cunningham RK. Physicochemical aspects of hemagglutination. In: Mohn JF, Plunkett RW, Cunningham RK, Lambert RM, eds. Human blood groups. Basel: S Karger, 1977:56-64.

49. Wild AE. Transport of immunoglobulins and other proteins from mother to young. In: Dingle JT, ed. Lysosomes in biology and pathology. Vol 3. New York: American Elsevier, 1973.

50. Gitlin JD, Gitlin D. Protein binding by specific receptors on human placenta, murine placenta, and suckling murine intestine in relation to protein transport across these tissues. J Clin Invest 1974;54:1155-66.

51. Köhler G, Milstein C. Derivation of specific antibody-producing tissue culture and tumor lines by cell fusion. Eur J Immunol 1976;6:511-19.

52. Boylston AW, Gardner B, Anderson RL, Hughes-Jones NC. Production of human IgM anti-D in tissue culture by EB virus transformed lymphocytes. Scand J Immunol 1980;12:355-8.

53. Koskimies S. Human lymphoblastoid cell line producing specific antibody against Rh-antigen D. Scand J Immunol 1980;11:73-7.

54. Thompson KM, Melamed MD, Eagle K, et al. Production of human monoclonal IgG and IgM antibodies with anti-D (rhesus) specificity using heterohybridomas. Immunology 1986;58:157-60.

55. Lowe AD, Green SM, Voak D, et al. A human-human monoclonal anti-D by direct fusion with a lymphoblastoid line. Vox Sang 1986; 51:212-6.

56. Edelman L, Back JF, Reviron J. Monoclonal antibodies against blood group antigens. International Symposium on Monoclonal Antibodies. Standardization of their characterization and use. Paris, France, 1983. Dev Biol Stand 1984;57:43-7.

57. Issitt PD. The impact of monoclonal antibodies in blood group serology. Transfusion 1989; 29:58-64.

The Antiglobulin Test

In 1945, Coombs, Mourant and Race[1] described a test for detecting nonagglutinating (coating) antibodies in serum. Later, the same test was used to demonstrate in-vivo coating of rbcs with antibody[2] and with complement components.[3] This test is now known as the antiglobulin test.

Two forms of antiglobulin testing are used in immunohematology, the direct antiglobulin test (DAT) and the indirect antiglobulin test (IAT). The DAT is a diagnostic procedure used to demonstrate in-vivo coating of rbcs with antibody and/or complement. It is used in investigating autoimmune hemolytic anemia (AIHA), drug-induced hemolysis, hemolytic disease of the newborn and alloimmune reactions to recently transfused rbcs. The IAT is used to demonstrate in-vitro reactions between rbcs and coating antibodies, as in antibody detection, antibody identification, blood grouping and compatibility testing.

Principles of the Antiglobulin Test

The antiglobulin test is based on the following simple principles:
1. Antibody molecules and complement components are globulins.
2. Injecting an animal with human globulin stimulates the animal to produce antibody to the foreign protein, ie, antihuman globulin (AHG). The animal serum, after adsorption to remove unwanted agglutinins, will react specifically with human globulins. Hybridoma technology (see Chapter 7) is also used to prepare AHG reagents. Serologic tests employ a variety of AHG reagents reactive with various human globulins including anti-IgG, antibody to the C3d component of human complement; and polyspecific reagents that contain both anti-IgG and anti-C3d activity.
3. AHG will react with human globulin molecules either bound to rbcs or free in serum. Unbound globulins may react with and neutralize AHG added to a system containing both coated rbcs and free globulin molecules. Unless rbcs are washed free of unbound globulin before testing with AHG, the unbound globulins may neutralize AHG and cause a false-negative result.
4. Washed rbcs coated with human globulin are agglutinated by AHG, as shown in Fig 8-1. The Fab portion of the AHG molecule reacts with the Fc portion of the human antibody molecules attached to each of two separate rbcs. Uncoated rbcs are not agglutinated. The strength of the observed agglutination reaction is proportional to the amount of globulin coating the rbcs.

175

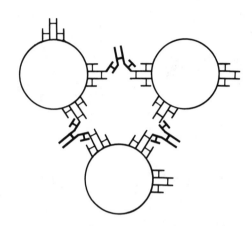

Figure 8-1. The antiglobulin reaction. Rabbit IgG molecules with antihuman globulin specificity are shown reacting with the Fc portion of human IgG molecules coating adjacent red cells (eg, anti-D coating D+ red cells).

Antihuman Globulin Reagents

The FDA Center for Biologics Evaluation and Research has established definitions for a variety of AHG reagents, as shown in Table 8-1. The properties and applications of these reagents are discussed below.

Polyspecific AHG

Polyspecific AHG reagents are used for routine compatibility tests, alloantibody detection and the DAT. They contain antibody to human IgG and to the C3d component of human complement. Other anticomplement antibodies may be present, including anti-C3b, anti-C4b and anti-C4d. Commercially prepared polyspecific AHG contains little, if any, activity against IgA and IgM heavy chains; it may react with IgA or IgM molecules, however, since it may contain antibodies to κ and λ light chains common to all immunoglobulin classes.

Since most clinically significant antibodies are IgG, the most important function of polyspecific AHG is to detect the presence of IgG. These reagents are prepared and standardized to detect a wide variety of IgG antibodies. In addition, the FDA requires that reagents marketed as polyspecific AHG contain anti-C3d activity at a level that equals or exceeds the FDA's anti-C3d reference serum.

The importance of anticomplement activity in reagents used for antibody detection and compatibility tests is debatable, since antibodies detectable only by their ability to bind complement are quite rare.[4-9] Anti-C3d activity is, however, important for the DAT in the investigation of AIHA,[5,7,10-11] because C3dg may be the only globulin detectable on rbcs in AIHA (see Chapter 16).

Antihuman globulin (rabbit and murine monoclonal) consists of a blend of rabbit antihuman IgG and mouse monoclonal anti-C3b and -C3d. The reagent is prepared by pooling optimum proportions of the immune rabbit sera (anti-

Table 8-1. Antihuman Globulin Reagents

Reagent	Definition*
Polyspecific (rabbit polyclonal; rabbit/murine monoclonal blend; and murine monoclonal)	Rabbit polyclonal contains anti-IgG and anti-C3d (may contain other anticomplement and other anti-immunoglobulin antibodies); rabbit/murine monoclonal blend contains a blend of rabbit polyclonal anti-human IgG and murine monoclonal anti-C3b and -C3d; murine monoclonal contains murine monoclonal anti-IgG, -C3b and -C3d.
Anti-IgG (rabbit polyclonal; IgG heavy chains; monoclonal IgG)	Rabbit polyclonal contains anti-IgG with no anticomplement activity (not necessarily gamma chain specific); IgG heavy chains contain only antibodies reactive against human gamma chains; monoclonal IgG contains murine monoclonal anti-IgG.
Anti-C3d and anti-C3b, (rabbit polyclonal) and anti-C3d, -C4b, -C4d (rabbit polyclonal)	Contain only antibodies reactive against the designated complement component(s), with no anti-immunoglobulin activity.
Anti-C3d (murine monoclonal) and anti-C3b, -C3d (murine monoclonal)	Contains only antibodies reactive against the designated complement component, with no anti-immunoglobulin activity.

*As defined by the FDA: *Code of Federal Regulations 21 CFR 660 55(d)*.

IgG) and the ascitic fluid of two sets of mice, one injected with anti-C3b secreting hybridoma and one injected with anti-C3d secreting hybridoma. Alternatively, tissue culture supernatant fluid can be used instead of ascitic fluid. The resulting polyspecific AHG does not contain anti-C4.

Polyspecific antihuman globulin (murine monoclonal) consists of a blend of antibodies secreted by three cell lines of the following specificities: anti-IgG, -C3b and -C3d. By definition this reagent does not contain anti-C4 or anti-light-chain immunoglobulins.

Anti-IgG

Reagents labeled "anti-IgG" contain no anticomplement activity. Their major component is antibody to human γ chains, but unless labeled as "heavy chain specific," they may react with light chains com-

mon to all immunoglobulin classes. Anti-IgG is largely used as an alternative to polyspecific AHG in antibody detection and compatibility tests. Some workers prefer anti-IgG over polyspecific AHG, because it does not react with complement bound to cells by clinically insignificant cold-reactive autoantibodies such as anti-I (see Chapter 15).

Anti-IgG not designated "heavy chain specific" must be considered capable of reacting with light chains of IgA or IgM. A positive DAT with anti-IgG not specific for γ chains does not prove IgG is present, but it is rare for cells to be coated, in vivo, with IgA or IgM, without IgG. In a 10-year study of 347 patients with immune hemolytic anemia, Petz and Garratty[11] detected no patients with rbcs coated exclusively with IgM, and only two of 104 patients with rbcs coated exclusively with IgA.

Monospecific AHG Reagents

Monospecific antibodies to human globulins are prepared by injecting animals with immunogens such as IgG, IgA, IgM, C3 or C4. These sera generally require adsorption of unwanted antibodies in order to ensure the purity of the monospecific reagent.

Monospecific antisera licensed by the FDA are 1) anti-IgG and 2) anti-C3b,C3d. The FDA has established labeling requirements for other anticomplement reagents, including anti-C3b, anti-C4b and anti-C4d, but these products are not generally available.

Monospecific AHG reagents are used to determine the proteins responsible for a DAT positive with polyspecific AHG. (See Chapter 16.) Anti-IgG (heavy chains) and anti-C3d are also used in the IAT to distinguish patterns of reactivity produced when a single serum contains both complement-binding and non-complement-binding antibodies, for example, anti-Le^a and anti-E.

Anti-C3b,C3d

Anti-C3b,C3d reagents prepared by animal immunization contain no activity against human immunoglobulins, and are used in the situations described for anti-C3d. This type of anti-C3d characteristically reacts with C3b and possibly other epitopes present on C3-coated cells.

Murine monoclonal anti-C3b,C3d is a blend of ascitic fluids collected from mice injected with either anti-C3b or anti-C3d secreting hybridomas or antibodies obtained by cell culture. Murine monoclonal anti-IgG is a blend of a few monoclonal antibodies secreted by single murine hybridoma cell lines. Tissue culture supernatant fluid could be used instead of ascitic fluid. Monoclonal anti-C3d, in contrast to that obtained by animal immunization, might be less likely to react with C3b.

Antiglobulin Techniques

Direct Antiglobulin Test

The DAT is used to demonstrate in-vivo coating of rbcs with globulins, in particular IgG and C3dg. Washed rbcs from a patient or donor are tested directly with AHG reagents (see Method 3.6).

Indirect Antiglobulin Testing

The IAT is used to demonstrate in-vitro coating of rbcs with antibody or complement, achieved by incubating serum with rbcs, then washing the rbcs to remove unbound globulins. Agglutination after the addition of AHG indicates that the serum contains antibody reactive with antigens present on the rbcs. The antibody specificity may be known, as in blood grouping tests with coating antibodies such as anti-Fy^a, or the antigenic composition of the rbcs may be known, as in antibody detection and identification tests. In the antiglobulin crossmatch, neither is known; the test is used to determine whether an antigen-antibody interaction occurs. Individual uses of the IAT are detailed in other chapters, where specific procedures are described.

Reagents used for blood group testing using the IAT can be processed in the following ways to eliminate the need to wash the serum/cell suspension before the addition of AHG. The first technique involves adsorption of specific antibody to antigen-positive rbcs and disassociation of the antibody (usually by preparing an eluate of the rbcs) from the rbcs.[12] Since the processed sera are not contaminated with unwanted human globulin capable of neutralizing the AHG reagents, there is no need to wash the rbc suspension before the addition of the AHG reagents. The second technique uses a microtube filled with mixtures of gel or beads, buffer and sometimes reagents.[13] An antiglobulin test can be performed by adding a suspension of rbcs (a DAT) or a serum and rbc mixture that has been incubated for the appropriate amount of time at 37 C (an IAT) to a microtube containing gel/beads to which the antiglobulin sera has been added. The tube is centrifuged, and agglutinates will be "fixed" in the top gel/bead layer, while unagglutinated rbcs will form a pellet at the bottom of the tube. Again, no washing phase is required for the antiglobulin test.

Factors Affecting the Sensitivity of Indirect Antiglobulin Tests

The following variables affect the in-vitro attachment of antibody molecules to rbcs, and are not relevant to the DAT.

Temperature

Red cells and serum are normally incubated at 37 C, since most clinically significant coating antibodies react optimally at this temperature.[14] Incubation at lower temperatures usually decreases the rate of association between antigen and antibody, while incubation above 37 C may damage rbcs or antibody molecules.

Ionic Strength

Rbcs may be suspended in various media, including isotonic saline, albumin solutions, low ionic strength saline (LISS) reagents, or additive reagents such as polyethylene glycol (PEG)[15] or hexadimethrine bromide (Polybrene®)[16,17] can be added to the test system. In isotonic saline, Na^+ and Cl^- ions cluster around and partially neutralize oppositely charged sites on antigen and antibody molecules. This shielding effect, which hinders the association of antibody with antigen, is reduced by lowering the ionic strength of the reaction medium.[18] Consequently, lowering the salt concentration of the reaction medium enhances antibody uptake and with some antibodies may enhance the quantity of antibody bound.[19-21] The use of LISS solutions has occasionally been associated with weaker-than-expected reactions with some examples of antibodies in the Kell blood group system. Albumin solutions, unless used under low ionic conditions, do little to promote antibody uptake.[22] Rather, albumin influences the second stage of hemagglutination (see Chapter 7).

A Polybrene® additive solution works in a different way. In a manual antibody detection or crossmatch test, Polybrene® is added to rbcs that have been incubated at low ionic strength and low pH. Polybrene® is added, causing the rbcs to aggregate very closely. The aggregation is disassociated by the addition of a salt solution (ie, sodium citrate). If the rbcs were coated with antibody at the time Polybrene® was added, the rbcs would stay agglutinated and not disperse in the presence of salt solutions, thereby giving a positive reaction.

PEG reacts differently also. PEG makes water unavailable, which effectively concentrates antibody (if too high a concentration of PEG is added to the test mixture, it could cause proteins to precipitate). This concentration of antibody enhances antibody uptake and in many cases results in stronger reactions.[23,24] Since anti-IgG is the antiglobulin reagent of choice in PEG tests, one would expect to see diminished reactivity or nonreactivity with test serum containing IgM antibodies, including Le[a], Vel and ABO antibodies.

Proportion of Serum to Cells

Increasing the ratio of serum to rbcs increases the degree of antibody coating. A commonly used ratio is 2 drops of serum to 1 drop of a 2-5% rbc suspension. Alternatively, reducing the rbc suspension from 5% to 2-3% could double the serum-to-rbc ratio. By increasing the ratio of serum to rbcs, Mollison[25] detected weakly reactive antibodies that were not demonstrable under standard test conditions. It is sometimes useful to increase the volume of serum to 10 or even 20 drops, particularly when investigating a hemolytic transfusion reaction in which routine testing reveals no antibody.

In techniques using LISS as the suspending medium, one volume of serum is used with one volume of LISS-suspended rbcs.[22,26-30] Increasing the serum volume without increasing the volume of LISS increases the ionic strength of the reaction medium. When LISS is used as an additive reagent, the manufacturer's direction circular must always be followed. It is important to use the specified volumes when performing LISS tests, especially when incubation time is 15 minutes or less.

Incubation Time

For saline or albumin techniques, 30 minutes of incubation at 37 C is adequate to detect most clinically significant coating antibodies. With some weakly reactive antibodies, however, antigen-antibody association may not reach equilibrium at 30 minutes, and extended incubation is necessary to demonstrate their presence. Extending incubation times beyond 30 minutes has few disadvantages, except for the extra time involved. In LISS and PEG tests, equilibrium for most antigen-antibody reactions is attained within 10-15 minutes,[15,27-30] due to the increased rate of association that occurs under low-ionic test conditions.[19-21]

Sources of Error

False-Negative Results

Direct and Indirect Tests

The following considerations apply to tests using either direct or indirect antiglobulin techniques.

1. Failure to wash rbcs adequately is a major cause of false-negative antiglobulin tests, since globulins not bound to rbcs will neutralize AHG. One volume of human serum diluted as much as 1:4000 in saline will neutralize an equal volume of AHG. The washing process must ensure adequate removal of unbound globulins. Correctly functioning automated cell washers achieve this objective,[31] as do three or four manual washes, providing the test tubes are filled at least three-quarters full with saline and the rbc button is thoroughly resuspended each time saline is added. Washing removes unbound globulins by dilution, so it is important to decant supernatant saline thoroughly at each wash phase. Rbcs must be resuspended completely with each new addition of saline; the rbc button should be shaken briskly, and saline added in a forceful stream. The tube should not be inverted against finger or palm, partly because this endangers the worker's health and partly because it can introduce globulins into the wash solution if the hands are contaminated with blood or reagent.

2. False-negative reactions can occur if testing is interrupted or delayed. The entire washing process must be undertaken as quickly as possible, to minimize loss of bound antibody by elution from the rbcs. AHG must be added immediately after washing is completed; otherwise, bound globulins may elute, leaving too little IgG on the cells to react when AHG is added. Once AHG has been added, tests should be centrifuged and read immediately, since reactions due to IgG coating may become perceptibly weaker after incubation. (See Note below.)

3. AHG reagents can lose activity following improper storage, bacterial contamination or contamination with hu-

man serum. AHG reagents are usually stored between 2 C and 8 C. They should never be frozen, since this may impair antibody reactivity. AHG reagents, like all blood bank reagents, should be inspected visually with each use and should not be used if they appear turbid or discolored. The entire contents of a vial of AHG will be neutralized if contaminated with whole human serum or with another reagent such as anti-D grouping serum. This may not be apparent visually, and will only be detected when globulin-coated rbcs are not agglutinated.

4. AHG may not be present in the test. Addition of AHG to the test is sometimes inadvertently omitted when multiple tests are performed simultaneously. The use of a colored AHG reagent provides an indication the AHG is present, but provides no indication as to its activity.

5. Improper centrifugation influences the sensitivity of antiglobulin tests. Undercentrifugation provides suboptimal conditions for agglutination, while overcentrifugation packs rbcs so tightly that the agitation required to resuspend them may break up fragile agglutinates.

6. The number of rbcs present in an individual test influences reactivity. Weak reactions occur if too many rbcs are present, while too few rbcs make it difficult to read agglutination reactions accurately.

7. Prozone reactions are sometimes cited as a possible cause of nonreactive antiglobulin tests (see Chapter 7). Prozones are rarely a problem with licensed AHG reagents that are standardized by the manufacturer. The manufacturer's directions must, however, be followed.

8. The presence of an IgG cryoprecipitable paraprotein in a patient's serum may inhibit anti-IgG, even after six washes using conventional automated or manual washing techniques.[32] The paraprotein inhibition can be averted if 1) the patient's blood samples are maintained at 37 C, and the serum or plasma is separated and tested at 37 C (including washing the patient's rbcs at 37 C) or 2) the serum is incubated overnight at 4 C, centrifugation is performed in the cold and the supernatant plasma or serum is removed from the cryoprecipitated paraprotein before testing.

9. Saline solutions, particularly those of low pH or those autoclaved and stored in plastic containers, can result in decreased sensitivity or false-negative results if they are used in the wash phase of the antiglobulin test.[33] The optimal saline solution suggested for this test is a phosphate-buffered saline, pH 7.0 to 7.2. However, if a commerical saline is used, the laboratory should ensure that the pH of the saline is above 6.0, and that saline autoclaved and stored in plastic bottles is not used for the wash phase of the antiglobulin test.

Note: A negative DAT does not necessarily mean absence of coating globulins. Polyspecific and anti-IgG reagents will only detect approximately 200 molecules of IgG per rbc.[11] Adding IgG-coated rbcs to nonreactive tests will demonstrate impaired AHG activity for reasons cited in items 1 through 4, but will not detect other causes of false-negative antiglobulin tests. AABB *Standards for Blood Banks and Transfusion Services*[34] requires use of IgG-coated rbcs to check negative results on antiglobulin tests performed in antibody detection and crossmatching procedures. These, however, are commonly performed with rbcs coated too heavily with IgG to provide an effective test. Heavily coated Coombs control cells may react with partially neutralized anti-IgG, thereby giving a false sense of security.

Direct Antiglobulin Tests

The following additional consideration applies only to direct tests:

Complement coating may not be apparent as agglutination upon immediate reading. All manufacturers recommend that the test be incubated at room temperature for approximately 5 minutes and examined after centrifugation when maximal sensitivity for complement detection is desired. This incubation can convert a negative DAT into a positive DAT when rbcs are coated with complement or IgA.[35] IgG-coated rbcs may give weaker reactions after incubation than at immediate reading, so incubation before reading should never *replace* an immediate reading. Although tests may be centrifuged and read immediately and then incubated and read again, optimal sensitivity is achieved by setting the test up in duplicate and reading one tube after immediate centrifugation, the other after incubation.

Indirect Antiglobulin Tests

The following additional considerations apply only to indirect tests:

1. Rbcs and serum lose reactivity if improperly stored. Exposure to excessive heat or repeated freezing and thawing impairs antibody reactivity. Rbcs may be damaged at temperatures above 37 C, but some antigens undergo more subtle changes above 6 C.
2. Occasional examples of anti-Jk[a] and anti-Jk[b] may be detected only in the presence of active complement (eg, polyspecific AHG).[9] Most anticoagulants chelate calcium and magnesium ions that are essential for complement binding; the use of plasma instead of serum can lead to failure to detect these antibodies. Old or improperly stored serum also has impaired complement activity.

3. Temperature and incubation time affect attachment of antibody or complement to rbcs. For most clinically significant coating antibodies, the optimal temperature is 37 C.[14] Incubation for 30 minutes is satisfactory for saline or albumin tests, but 10-15 minutes is adequate for LISS or PEG techniques.
4. An optimal proportion of serum to rbcs should be achieved. If the usual 2 or 3 drops of serum are used, one drop of a 2-5% rbc suspension is adequate for routine tests (the lower the rbc concentration the greater the sensitivity). Too heavy an rbc suspension will result in inadequate coating, and too weak a suspension will provide insufficient rbcs to read agglutination reactions accurately. Specified volumes of serum and rbcs are required when using LISS techniques (see Methods 3.1.2 and 3.1.3).

False-Positive Results

Direct and Indirect Tests

The following considerations apply to both direct and indirect tests:

1. Rbcs may be agglutinated before they are washed. If this is not noted, agglutination observed after adding AHG may be incorrectly interpreted as the result of IgG or complement coating. Rbcs from patients with potent cold-reactive autoantibodies agglutinate in whole blood samples kept at or below room temperature. This can be recognized by observing the appearance of washed rbcs suspended in 6% bovine albumin, inert serum or AHG reagent diluent. In indirect procedures, some antibodies cause direct agglutination of rbcs prior to the addition of AHG. This constitutes an antigen-antibody reaction, but the seemingly positive AHG result should not be inter-

preted as indicating coating with IgG or complement components.

2. Saline stored in glass bottles may contain colloidal silica particles, leached from the container, that can cause false-positive antiglobulin tests.[25] Saline stored in metal containers, or used in equipment with metal parts, may contain metallic ions that mediate nonspecific attachment of proteins to rbcs.[25] The problems are both defined and solved by demonstrating nonreactive tests using saline from a different container (eg, plastic or glass).

3. Improperly cleansed glassware may be contaminated with dust, detergent or other material that causes rbcs to aggregate. It is worthwhile to use test tubes from another source when all tests on different blood samples are weakly reactive.

4. Overcentrifugation packs rbcs so tightly that they cannot be dispersed completely. This leads to rbc aggregation, which can be mistaken for agglutination.

5. Improperly prepared AHG reagent may contain trace amounts of antihuman species antibodies, and agglutinate uncoated rbcs. Enzyme-treated rbcs have enhanced reactivity with antispecies antibodies and may react directly with those AHG reagents containing this contaminating activity. Although this was a problem in the past,[36] all manufacturers now test their AHG reagents with enzyme-treated rbcs.

Direct Antiglobulin Tests

The following additional considerations apply only to the DAT:

1. Complement components, primarily C4, may bind to rbcs from clotted blood samples and donor segments in CPDA-1 kept at 4 C, and occasionally when these samples are kept at room temperature.[5,37] This results from the activity of naturally occurring cold-reactive autoagglutinins often present in human serum[18] and accounts for false-positive antiglobulin tests observed with potent anticomplement reagents.[5,10] Red cells from blood anticoagulated with EDTA, ACD or CPD should be used for the DAT. These anticoagulants chelate calcium and magnesium ions that are essential for in-vitro complement activation, but do not affect complement components already bound to rbcs following an immune reaction in vivo.

2. False-positive DAT results may occur with blood samples collected into tubes containing silicone gel. Geisland and Milam[38] found eight of 60 (13%) blood samples collected into such tubes had a spuriously positive DAT. Complement coating alone was demonstrable in all eight cases.

3. Blood samples collected from intravenous fluid lines used to administer solutions, such as 5% or 10% dextrose in distilled water, may have complement present on the rbcs.[39] The gauge of the needle used in the intravenous line and the volume of blood obtained influence the strength of the DAT; strongest reactions are observed when large-bore needles are used or when the sample volume obtained is less than 0.5 mL.

4. Septicemia in a patient or bacterial contamination of stored specimens may cause a positive DAT. Microbial agents can cause rbcs to become T-activated, resulting in agglutination by the person's own anti-T that is present in the serum for some time before it disappears.[36]

Indirect Antiglobulin Tests

The following additional consideration applies only to IATs. Rbcs with a positive DAT will give positive IATs with all sera. Rbcs coated with IgG cannot be tested with blood grouping reagents that react only by IAT, such as anti-Fy^a.

Procedures for removing IgG from in-vivo coated rbcs such as heat treating, chloroquine or ZZAP are given in the Methods section. When these procedures are used, sufficient IgG can often be removed from rbcs to render them suitable for typing with antisera that react solely by IAT.[40,41] The use of ZZAP reagent destroys all rbc antigens normally denatured by enzymes—ie, LW^a, Fy^a, Fy^b, S, s, Yt^a, Ch, Rg, Pr and Tn, as well as all Kell blood group system antigens.[42] This reagent should only be used to remove IgG from rbcs when other techniques, such as gentle heat treatment or chloroquine, have failed and when testing for antigens not affected by ZZAP. Any of the above techniques may alter rbc antigens, and tests with blood grouping reagent may give discrepant results, particularly with the Kell blood group system. Therefore, it is essential that control and test rbcs be treated in the same manner and tests be performed in parallel. (See Methods section.)

Role of Complement in the Antiglobulin Reactions

Complement components may coat rbcs, either in vivo or in vitro, through either of two mechanisms:

1. Complement-binding antibodies attach complement to the rbc surface when they react with rbc antigens.
2. Immune complexes present in plasma activate complement components that may be adsorbed to rbcs in a nonspecific manner. The antigen-antibody reaction does not involve specific rbc antigens and the rbcs to which complement is adsorbed are often described as innocent bystanders.

Whichever mechanism is involved, rbcs become coated with elements of the complement cascade, which may or may not proceed to hemolysis. If the rbcs do not undergo hemolysis, the presence of bound complement can be detected by AHG reagents containing anticomplement activity. C3 is the complement component most readily detected, since activity of only a few antibody molecules can bind several hundred C3 molecules to the rbc. C4 coating can also be detected, but C3 coating has more clinical significance.

Anticomplement Activity of AHG

C3b is bound to rbcs following the action of C4b2b (see Chapter 7). If the complement cascade does not proceed to hemolysis, factor I (formerly called C3b inactivator), in the presence of factor H, cleaves most of the C3b into C3c and C3dg. Only C3dg remains firmly attached to rbcs. To detect in-vivo complement coating, AHG reagents must contain adequate anti-C3d.

Human C3b molecules have epitopes that interact with antibodies to C3d. Some reagent anti-C3d react not only with residual C3d but also with C3b that has not been cleaved by factor I. The FDA designates such reagents anti-C3b,-C3d (see Table 8-1). In contrast, some monoclonal anti-C3d reagents react weakly, if at all, with intact C3b on rbcs coated with C3b by a low-ionic-strength method.[43] This may be due to the fact that the epitopes for monoclonal anti-C3d are not fully expressed on intact C3b molecules.

Antibody-Mediated Complement Binding

Some blood group antibodies bind complement to rbc membranes.[3-10,31,37] Most examples of anti-A,-B and -Tj^a (PP$_1$ P^k) and some examples of anti-Vel, -Jk^a and -Le^a do this very effectively, and may cause lysis of rbcs both in vivo and in vitro. Other examples of anti-Le^a and some examples of anti-Le^b, -Jk^b and -P$_1$, coat rbcs with complement components either in vivo or in vitro, but do not hemolyze normal rbcs in vitro unless they have been pretreated with a proteolytic enzyme. Yet other examples of these antibodies, and some examples of anti-K, -Fy^a, -Fy^b, -S, -s, -I, -i and -HI, cause in-vitro coating with complement components but do not cause in-vitro hemolysis. The clinical significance of these complement-binding antibodies is also variable. It is not understood why some blood group antibodies coat rbcs with sufficient C3 to give strongly reactive antiglobulin tests without causing hemolysis.

Most complement-binding antibodies coat rbcs. Some, including anti-A, -B, -I, -i, -HI and -Le^a, are IgM, and cause agglutination as well as complement coating. Other rare IgM antibodies do not cause agglutination under normal conditions, but coat rbcs with sufficient complement that their presence is demonstrable using the antiglobulin test. Still others, including most examples of anti-Jk^a and anti-Jk^b, are IgG antibodies that also bind complement. With these antibodies, the antiglobulin test detects both IgG and complement coating. In a few instances the IgG coating is weak and the complement coating is strong.[4,6-10,25,31,37] This has been noted especially with anti-Jk^a and anti-Jk^b, both in vivo and in vitro.[6-8,25,31]

Complement as the Only Coating Globulin

Complement alone, without immunoglobulin, may be present on washed rbcs in certain situations.
1. IgM antibodies reacting with the rbcs in vitro occasionally coat the rbcs without causing direct agglutination. IgM coating is difficult to demonstrate in antiglobulin tests because IgM molecules tend to dissociate during the washing process and polyspecific AHG contains little, if any, anti-IgM activity.

Since IgM antibodies often bind complement, the reaction of antibody with antigen can best be recognized by reactivity with the anticomplement components of AHG, since each IgM molecule binds several hundred C3 molecules to rbcs.
2. About 10%-20% of patients with warm autoimmune hemolytic anemia have rbcs with a positive DAT due to C3 coating alone. No IgG, IgA or IgM coating is demonstrable using routine procedures. Some of these patients have low levels of IgG on their rbcs, but in amounts below the threshold of sensitivity for the standard DAT.[11,37]
3. In cold hemagglutinin disease the cold-reactive autoantibody reacts at temperatures up to 32 C. Skin temperature is at this level, so rbcs become coated with autoantibody. The autoantibody then binds complement to rbcs, which may not proceed to hemolysis. If rbcs escape hemolysis, they return to the central circulation where the temperature is 37 C. Autoantibody dissociates from the rbcs, but complement components remain firmly bound and their presence can be detected with anticomplement reagents. The complement component detectable by antiglobulin reagents currently in use is C3dg.
4. Rbcs may become coated with complement components that have been activated by immune complexes that form in the plasma and bind weakly and nonspecifically to rbcs. The activated complement remains firmly bound to the rbc surface but the immune complex dissociates from the cells. C3 remains as the only surface globulin and can be detected by the antiglobulin test. An example of this mechanism is the positive DAT that sometimes occurs in patients with antibodies to phenacetin or quinidine.[11,44]

References

1. Coombs RRA, Mourant AE, Race RR. A new test for the detection of weak and "incomplete" Rh agglutinins. Br J Exp Pathol 1945;26:255-66.
2. Coombs RRA, Mourant AE, Race RR. In-vivo isosensitisation of red cells in babies with haemolytic disease. Lancet 1946;1:264-6.
3. Dacie JV, Crookston JH, Christenson WN. "Incomplete" cold antibodies: Role of complement in sensitization to antiglobulin serum by potentially haemolytic antibodies. Br J Haematol 1957;3:77-87.
4. Garratty G, Petz LD. An evaluation of commercial antiglobulin sera with particular reference to their anticomplement properties. Transfusion 1971;11:79-88.
5. Garratty G, Petz LD. The significance of red cell bound complement components in development of standards and quality assurance for the anti-complement components of antiglobulin sera. Transfusion 1976;16:297-306.
6. Issitt PD, Issitt CH, Wilkinson SL. Evaluation of commercial antiglobulin sera over a two-year period. Transfusion 1974;14:93-102.
7. Petz LD, Garratty G. Antiglobulin sera—past, present and future. Transfusion 1978;18:257-68.
8. Wright MS, Issitt PD. Anticomplement and the indirect antiglobulin test. Transfusion 1979;19:688-94.
9. Howard JE, Winn LC, Gottlieb CE, et al. Clinical significance of the anti-complement component of antiglobulin antisera. Transfusion 1982;22:269-72.
10. Chaplin H. Clinical usefulness of specific antiglobulin reagents in autoimmune hemolytic anemias. Prog Hematol 1973;8:25-49.
11. Petz LD, Garratty G. Acquired immune hemolytic anemias. New York: Churchill-Livingstone, 1980.
12. Gale SM. Red cell antigen typing using eluted antibodies in a modified antiglobulin test. Med Lab Sci 1987;44:160-4.
13. Lapierre Y, Rigal D, Adam J, et al. The gel test: A new way to detect red cell antigen-antibody reactions. Transfusion 1990;30:109-13.
14. Arndt P, Garratty G. Evaluation of the optimal incubation temperature for detecting certain IgG antibodies with potential clinical significance. Transfusion 1988;28:210-3.
15. Nance SJ, Garratty G. Polyethylene glycol: A new potentiator of red blood cell antigen-antibody reactions. Am J Clin Pathol 1987;87:633-5.
16. Lalezari P, Jiang AF. The manual Polybrene® test: A simple and rapid procedure for detection of red cell antibodies. Transfusion 1980;20:206-11.
17. Lalezari P. The manual hexadimethrine bromide (Polybrene®) test: Effects of serum proteins and practical applications. Transfusion 1987;27:295-301.
18. Moore BPL. Antibody uptake: The first stage of the hemagglutination reaction. In: Bell CA, ed. Seminar on antigen-antibody reactions revisited. Arlington, VA: American Association of Blood Banks, 1982:47-66.
19. Hughes-Jones NC, Gardner B, Telford R. The effect of pH and ionic strength on the reaction between anti-D and erythrocytes. Immunology 1964;7:72-81.
20. Hughes-Jones NC, Polley MJ, Telford R, et al. Optimal conditions for detecting blood group antibodies by the antiglobulin test. Vox Sang 1964;9:385-95.
21. Elliot M, Bossom E, Dupuy ME, Masouredis SP. Effect of ionic strength on the serologic behavior of red cell isoantibodies. Vox Sang 1964;9:396-414.
22. Case J. Potentiators of agglutination. In: Bell CA, ed. Seminar on antigen-antibody reactions revisited. Arlington, VA: American Association of Blood Banks, 1982:99-132.
23. Wenz B, Apuzzo J, Shah DP. Evaluation of the polyethylene glycol-potentiated indirect antiglobulin test. Transfusion 1990;30:318-21.
24. deMan AJM, Overbeeke MAM. Evaluation of the polyethylene glycol antiglobulin test for detection of red blood cell antibodies. Vox Sang 1990;58:207-10.
25. Mollison PL, Engelfriet CP, Contreras M. Blood transfusion in clinical medicine. 9th ed. Oxford: Blackwell Scientific Publications, 1993.
26. Löw B, Messeter L. Antiglobulin test in low-ionic strength salt solution for rapid antibody screening and cross-matching. Vox Sang 1974;26:53-61.
27. Moore HC, Mollison PL. Use of a low-ionic-strength medium in manual tests for antibody detection. Transfusion 1976;16:291-6.
28. Wicker B, Wallas CH. A comparison of low ionic strength saline medium with routine methods for antibody detection. Transfusion 1976;16:469-72.
29. Rock G, Baxter A, Charron M, Jhaveri J. LISS—an effective way to increase blood utilization. Transfusion 1978;18:228-32.
30. Fitzsimmons JM, Morel PA. The effects of red blood cell suspending media on hemagglutination and the antiglobulin test. Transfusion 1979:19:81-5.
31. Issitt PD. Applied blood group serology, 3rd ed. Miami: Montgomery Scientific Publications, 1985.
32. Ylagen ES, Curtis BR, Wildgen ME, et al. Invalidation of antiglobulin tests by a high thermal amplitude cryoglobulin. Transfusion 1990;30:154-7.

33. Bruce M, Watt AH, Hare W, et al. A serious source of error in antiglobulin testing. Transfusion 1986;26:177-81.
34. Widmann FK, ed. Standards for blood banks and transfusion services. 15th ed. Bethesda, MD: American Association of Blood Banks, 1993.
35. Sturgeon P, Smith LE, Chun HMT, et al. Autoimmune hemolytic anemia associated exclusively with IgA of Rh specificity. Transfusion 1979;19:324-8.
36. Beck ML, Hicklin B, Pierce SR. Unexpected limitations in the use of commercial antiglobulin reagents. Transfusion 1976;16:71-5.
37. Gilliland BC, Leddy JP, Vaughan JH. The detection of cell-bound antibody on complement-coated human red cells. J Clin Invest 1970; 49:898-906.
38. Geisland JR, Milam JD. Spuriously positive direct antiglobulin tests caused by silicone gel. Transfusion 1980;20:711-3.
39. Grindon AJ, Wilson MJ. False-positive DAT caused by variables in sample procurement. Transfusion 1981;21:313-4.
40. Edwards JM, Moulds JJ, Judd WJ. Chloroquine dissociation of antigen-antibody complexes: A new technique for typing red blood cells with a positive direct antiglobulin test. Transfusion 1982;22:59-61.
41. Branch DR, Petz LD. A new reagent (ZZAP) having multiple applications in immunohematology. Am J Clin Pathol 1982;78:161-7.
42. Wilkinson SL. Serological approaches to transfusion of patients with allo- or autoantibodies. In: Nance SJ, ed. Immune destruction of red blood cells. Arlington, VA: American Association of Blood Banks, 1989:227-61.
43. Fruitstone MJ. C3b-sensitized erythrocytes (correspondence). Transfusion 1978;18:125.
44. Garratty G, Petz LD. Drug-induced immune hemolytic anemia. Am J Med 1975;58:398-407.

9

Genetics

The information necessary to determine specific biologic structures and processes resides in specific genes, which are present on chromosomes. In normal humans, there are 46 chromosomes in each nucleated cell, 22 homologous *autosomal* pairs and one pair of sex chromosomes. The Y chromosome carries the genes for male sex determination and is paired with an X chromosome. The sex chromosome pairs are XX in females and XY in males.

Terminology

Genes occupy specific positions or *loci* on chromosomes. Alternative forms of genes that occupy a single locus on homologous chromosomes are called *alleles*; for example, the Kell blood group system includes two alleles, *K* and *k*. An individual who inherits identical alleles at the *KEL* locus on both chromosomes (eg, *KK* or *kk*) is *homozygous* for either *K* or *k*, respectively. In the *heterozygous* condition, *Kk*, the alleles present at the *KEL* locus on each chromosome are nonidentical. Loci present on the same chromosome are *syntenic* with one another, regardless of the distance between loci. When two alleles occupy syntenic loci, they are in *cis* position; when they are on opposite chromosomes, they are in *trans* position. Figure 9-1(A) serves as an example: the alleles N and S (or M and s)

are in *cis* position, whereas N and s (or M and S) are in *trans* position.

In some blood group systems, persons who have inherited identical genes have more antigen on their rbcs than persons with different allelic genes. For example, rbcs from a person whose genotype is *KK* have a "double dose" of K antigen, while those from a *Kk* person have a "single dose." The difference in amount of antigen on rbcs between a homozygote and a heterozygote may be detected serologically. For example, some anti-K may give the following pattern of reactivity:

Antibody	Genotype of rbc donor	
	KK	*Kk*
Anti-K	3+	2+

This variation in strength of antigen reactivity is called *dosage* effect. Dosage effects are not seen with all blood group antigens or all antibodies of a given specificity.

Gene Transmission

The genes on an individual chromosome may not be transmitted as an intact unit in a gamete, either sperm or egg. During metaphase of the reductive (second) division of meiosis there is exchange of material between paired chromosomes. This process is called *crossing over*, resulting in a *recombination* of genetic information on these chromosomes. Re-

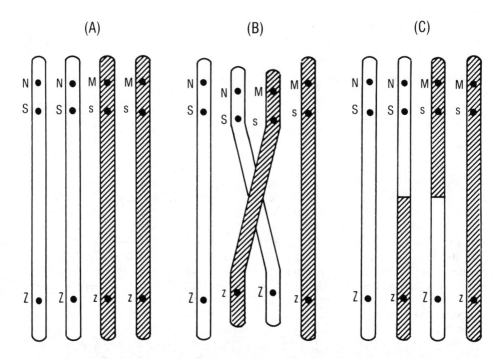

Figure 9-1. Crossing over is one kind of recombination. It occurs between chromatids during meiosis, resulting in segregation of alleles on the same chromosome. Very closely linked loci are rarely affected by crossing over so that alleles of those loci are inherited together (N and S, M and s in the example shown). Loci on the same chromosome that are not closely linked (the *Ss* locus and the *Zz* locus shown) demonstrate crossing over.

combination involves an exchange of a portion of DNA strands of homologous chromosomes. For example, a parent who is heterozygous at two loci on the same chromosome (*MN* at one locus and *Zz* at the second locus) may transmit any one of four different gametes to a child, *MZ, Mz, NZ, Nz.* See Fig 9-1(C). The chance of inheriting *any of the four combinations of two alleles* is influenced by the genetic distance between the loci. The genetic distance between loci (which is not the same as physical distance) is measured in *centi-Morgans* (cM), *map units* or *recombination units.* Alleles at loci far apart on the same chromosome (as shown in Fig 9-1) or alleles at loci on different chromosomes *segregate* randomly (Mendel's First

Law is followed). In the example shown (Fig 9-1) one fourth of the children would inherit *MZ*, one fourth *Mz*, etc, because the map distance is great and there is a high probability of recombination between locus *MN* and locus *Zz*. In the general population, however, the frequencies of the combinations *MZ, Mz, NZ* and *Nz* are dependent on the frequency in the population of each allele *M* and *N, Z* and *z*. Over many generations, recombination events cause independence of genes on separate loci that are syntenic. When there is "linkage equilibrium" the alleles at two loci associate in frequencies that depend on their individual allele frequencies. For example, if the alleles are in the population with frequencies:

M	0.53	Z	0.30
N	0.47	z	0.70
	1.00		1.00

then the frequencies of the combination should be the product of the frequency of each allele:

MZ 0.53 × 0.3 = 0.16
Mz 0.53 × 0.7 = 0.37
NZ 0.47 × 0.3 = 0.14
Nz 0.47 × 0.7 = 0.33
               1.00

In such a case the alleles are in *equilibrium* since they are inherited independently.

Linkage

An important exception to the rule of independent segregation of alleles is *linkage*. The alleles of linked loci do not segregate independently and are transmitted to the gametes in a nonrandom fashion. The closer the linkage (ie, the less genetic distance between the loci) the less likely it is that a crossover will occur between them and the more likely that the alleles occupying those loci will be inherited together. The MN blood group system provides a good example. As shown in Fig 9-1, S and s are alleles at a locus situated very close to the locus for M and N and the alleles on the same chromosome occupying these loci are characteristically transmitted together. These two linked loci are not linked to the hypothetical Zz locus. Thus, alleles of the Zz locus segregate independently of alleles at the MN locus or of the Ss locus. Notably, over many generations, the alleles of even closely linked loci reach equilibrium and associate according to their individual frequencies in the population.

Linkage Disequilibrium

When two loci are closely linked, recombination is decreased and alleles that occupy those loci on the same chromosome tend to be inherited *en bloc*. They are said to constitute a *haplotype*. For example, in the MN blood group system the locus controlling expression of M and N determinants is closely linked to the locus controlling expression of S and s. The approximate frequencies of the alleles are:

M	= 0.53	S	=	0.33
N	= 0.47	s	=	0.67

If the alleles segregated independently, the observed frequencies of each haplotype would be the product of the frequencies of the individual alleles. (Over many generations, alleles would freely associate.) However, the observed frequencies are not those expected:

	Expected frequency			Observed frequency
MS =	0.53 × 0.33	=	0.17	0.24
Ms =	0.53 × 0.67	=	0.36	0.28
NS =	0.47 × 0.33	=	0.16	0.08
Ns =	0.47 × 0.67	=	0.31	0.40
			1.00	1.00

This is an example of *linkage disequilibrium*: alleles of linked loci are associated more or less frequently than is expected from allele frequencies and recombination over many generations.

Another commonly cited example of linkage disequilibrium occurs in the HLA system. (See Chapter 13.) The *HLA-A1,B8* haplotype occurs approximately five times more frequently ("positive" linkage disequilibrium) than would be expected on the basis of frequencies of the individual alleles.[1] (Linkage disequilibrium may be positive or negative and it may indicate a selective advantage of one haplotype over another, insufficient time for a mutation to reach equilibrium, inhibition of recombination of some DNA sequences, etc.)

Gene Action

The genetic message is carried on chromosomes as a sequence of nucleotides in deoxyribonucleic acid (DNA). The sequence of DNA is transcribed into messenger ribonucleic acid (mRNA), which is processed and results in a manufactured sequence of amino acids (a peptide). The direct product of an allele (DNA) is a transcribed sequence of RNA; peptides are the translated cellular products of gene action. Processed peptides form the named proteins and variants known to immunohematologists (eg, the various Rh phenotypes).

Blood group antigens are inherited characteristics, but they are not all protein structures. Carbohydrates constitute the ABO blood group antigens. (See Chapter 10.) Since the end products of gene action are proteins, one could predict that ABO alleles encode for proteins that are enzyme variants. Thus, genetically determined carbohydrate antigens are the result of an enzymatic transfer of carbohydrate to a protein chain.

Enzyme Effects

A and B determinants consist of a lipid (in red cell membranes) or a protein (in secretions) structure to which sugars are sequentially added. The attachment of a sugar occurs only when an enzyme specific for that sugar is present and active. The enzymes, *glycosyltransferases*, which catalyze the addition of sugars to precursor molecules, are the protein products of gene action. The *A* allele encodes an *N*-acetyl-*D*-galactosamine transferase; the *B* allele encodes a *D*-galactose transferase. The transferases must have available a specific acceptor for their respective sug-

ars. For A and B activity, the acceptor is H substance, which, itself, arises from the action of the transferase encoded by an *H* allele at the *H/h* locus. The H immunodominant sugar, *L*-fucose (Fuc), is added to its oligosaccharide acceptor by the action of the fucosyltransferase determined by the *H* allele. If the *H* gene is absent, there will be no fucosyltransferase, no H substance produced and no acceptor for the A and B immunodominant sugars. Persons whose genotype is *hh* (rather than *HH* or *Hh*) have no H, A or B antigens on the rbc membrane, a condition called the Bombay (O_h) phenotype.

From the serologic standpoint, the product of the *O* allele is not directly observable. It is "silent" (an "amorph" or "null" allele) because of mutation in the DNA encoding for transferase. There is an expressed protein that lacks transferase activity.[2] Therefore in group O persons, neither N-acetyl-D-galactosamine (GalNAc) nor D-galactose (Gal) is attached to the H acceptor.

The specificities of certain other blood group antigens also reside on carbohydrate molecules (eg, those of the Lewis,[3] and P[4] blood group systems). In other carbohydrate-rich blood groups (eg, the MN system), differences in antigen specificity result directly from differences in amino acid sequence of a sialoglycoprotein (glycophorin A for M and N and glycophorin B for S and s antigens).[5]

Dominant and Recessive Traits

Traits are the observed expressions of genes. A trait that is observable when the determining allele is present in a heterozygote is called *dominant*. A *recessive trait* is observable only when the allele is present in the homozygous state. It is important to note that these terms are properly used to describe traits (observable characteristics, phenotypes); they should not be applied to loci. The observable traits that are determined by testing A_1 and A_2 rbcs with anti-A_1 are called phenotypes. In an A^1A^2 person, the presence of the A^2 allele cannot be inferred by phenotyping the rbcs; and the product of the A^1 allele is said to be dominant to the product of the A^2 allele. In the A^2O person, however, the product of the A^2 allele is dominant to expression of the product of the O allele. In these examples the genetic formulas A^1A^2 and A^2O represent the *genotypes* of the individuals.

Describing traits as dominant and recessive depends on the method used to detect gene products. Consider again the A_1 and A_2 phenotypes. Based on rbc testing, the product of the A^1 allele is dominant to that of the A^2 allele in an A^1A^2 heterozygote. Techniques that identify the specific gene products, the transferases, reveal that an A^1A^2 heterozygote generates the products of both alleles, ie, both A_1 transferase and A_2 transferase.[6] Similarly, an immunologically determined transferase-like protein, the product of O-allele translation), can be demonstrated in the serum of an A^2O heterozygote.[2] In terms of protein production, A^1, A^2 and O genes are *codominant*.

Blood group antigens, as a rule, are expressed as codominant traits; heterozygotes express the products of both alleles. For example, the rbcs of an Fy^aFy^b individual express Fy^a and Fy^b antigens, and the rbc phenotype is Fy(a+b+).

Patterns of Inheritance

The genetic loci of most blood groups have been mapped to the 22 pairs of autosomes. The Rh and Duffy loci are on chromosome 1, and the ABO genes are on chromosome 9. No blood group genes have been discovered on the Y chromosome; the *Xg* and *XK* loci are the only

blood group systems mapped to the X chromosome. The known chromosome assignments of the blood group loci are given in Table 9-1.[7-10]

Autosomal Dominant or Codominant Inheritance

An autosomal dominant trait shows a characteristic pattern of inheritance. The trait appears whenever the allele has been inherited by either males or females. (See the discussion on dominant and recessive traits in this chapter for a more detailed explanation.) Most blood group and histocompatibility antigens fit into this category. Figure 9-2(A) presents a pedigree showing the pattern of autosomal dominant inheritance. Characteristically, each generation contains one or more persons with the trait if it is present within a family.

Table 9-1. Blood Group Locus Assignments to Chromosomes[7-10]

Chromosome	Locus*
1	RH
	SC
	FY
	CROMER
4	MNS
6	CH/RG
7	CO
	YT
	KEL
9	ABO
18	JK
19	LE
	LW
	LU
	H
22	P1
X	XG
	XK

*ISBT designation

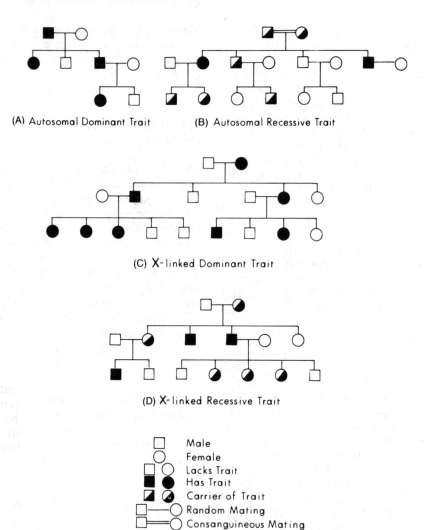

(A) Autosomal Dominant Trait

(B) Autosomal Recessive Trait

(C) X-linked Dominant Trait

(D) X-linked Recessive Trait

□	Male
○	Female
□ ○	Lacks Trait
■ ●	Has Trait
◪ ◑	Carrier of Trait
□——○	Random Mating
□══○	Consanguineous Mating

Figure 9-2. Four pedigrees showing different patterns of inheritance.

Autosomal Recessive Trait

Traits inherited in either autosomal dominant or autosomal recessive fashion occur with equal frequency in males and females. People who exhibit a recessive trait are homozygous for the encoding allele. Their parents may either have or lack the trait. Parents who lack the trait, however, must necessarily be *carriers*, ie, heterozygotes for an allele whose presence is not phenotypically apparent.

If a recessive trait is rare, because the population frequency of the variant encoding allele is low, the trait occurs only in members of one generation and not in preceding or successive generations. Related persons are more likely to carry the same rare gene than unrelated persons from a random population. When offspring are homozygous for a rare allele (frequency: <1:10,000) and display the trait, the parents are often blood relatives (a consanguineous mating). See Fig 9-2(B). Autosomal recessive traits tend to skip generations in families carrying the alleles encoding for the trait.

Sex-Linked Dominant or Codominant Inheritance

A male always receives his single X chromosome from his mother. Therefore, the predominant feature of X-linked inheritance of a given trait, both dominant and recessive, is absence of male-to-male (father-to-son) transmission of the trait. A male passes his single X chromosome to all of his daughters. Therefore, all daughters of a man possessing a *dominant* X-linked trait also express the trait. If a woman expresses a dominant trait but is heterozygous (expresses the trait on only one X chromosome), each child, male or female, has a 50% chance of inheriting that trait. If the mother expresses the dominant trait on both X chromosomes, all her children will express the trait. A sex-linked dominant trait of interest in blood group genetics is the Xg^a blood group. See Fig 9-2(C). An X-linked dominant trait tends to appear in each generation, but without male-to-male transmission.

Sex-Linked Recessive Trait

Hemophilia A provides a classic example of X-linked recessive inheritance. See Fig 9-2(D). Among the children of an affected male and a female who lacks the disease allele, all sons are normal and all daughters are carriers. Males inherit the trait from carrier mothers or, very rarely, from an affected mother homozygous for the allele. In the mating of a normal male and a carrier female, one-half of the male offspring are affected and one-half of the females are carriers.

If the recessive allele carried on the X chromosome is rare, males exhibit the trait almost exclusively. If the X-linked allele is not infrequent in the population, affected females will be seen, since the chances of an affected male mating with a carrier female increase and 50% of daughters of these couples will be homozygous for the trait.

Gene Interaction

Quite often, a trait is modified from interaction among alleles or the products of different loci. Among the blood groups, one major example involves competition between the *H* and *Le* transferases and effects of the *Se* gene. This interaction gives rise to the three rbc phenotypes: Le(a+b–), Le(a–b+) and Le(a–b–). (See Chapter 10.)

Terms such as *suppressor* and *modifier* are used to describe genes that affect the expression of other genes, but the mechanisms of these postulated gene interactions are unknown. Some phenomena in blood group serology that have been explained by gene interaction are weakening of the D antigen when the C-determining gene is in *trans* position, and suppression of Lutheran antigenic expression by the dominant modifier gene, *In(Lu)*. The reader is referred to *Blood Groups in Man*[11] for a discussion of other examples of gene interaction.

Gene interaction of the kind exemplified by the failure to express A or B traits because of an absence of H substance is referred to as *epistasis*; two different loci are sequentially important in the development of a biochemical end product.

Blood Group Nomenclature

There have been concerted attempts to establish rational, uniform criteria on which to designate rbc phenotypic, genotypic and locus notations used in blood group genetics. Nomenclature for the hemoglobins, immunoglobulin allotypes, histocompatibility antigens and some other serum protein and red cell enzyme systems follow generally accepted principles established by international committees. Attempts to standardize blood group notations by the International Society of Blood Transfusion (ISBT) Working Party on Terminology for Red Cell Surface Antigens have met with some success.[7,8] Some examples of past difficulties are:

1. An allele that determines a dominant trait is signified by a capital letter, and an allele determining a recessive trait by a lowercase letter. In rbc immunogenetics the *A* and *B* genes of the ABO system are signified by a capital letter. The traits of both of these are considered dominant to the *O* trait, which is also capitalized. Without prior knowledge, it would be impossible to recognize that these characters represent allelic products in a blood group system.

2. In rbc genetics, unlike classical Mendelian genetics, some codominant traits have been designated with capital letters and lowercase letters, for example, K and k of the Kell blood group system and C and c of the Rh system.

3. Some codominant traits have different superscript symbols but identical base symbols such as Fy^a and Fy^b (Duffy system) and Lu^a and Lu^b (Lutheran system).

4. Sometimes authors have denoted absence of a serologic specificity with a symbol devoid of superscripts or other modifications. Thus, in the Lutheran system, the assumed amorphic gene is not called *lu* but rather *Lu*.

In 1984, Issitt and Crookston presented guidelines for the nomenclature and terminology of blood groups.[12] Genes encoding for the expression of blood group antigens are written in italics, or if italics are not available, they are underlined. If antigens are designated by a superscript or a number (ie, Fy^a, Fy1), their names are written in normal (Roman) script with numeric designations written on the same line as the letters. The superscripts usually are presented as lowercase letters (eg, Fy^a). Various methods are used to write the phenotype results obtained using specific blood grouping reagents or antibodies. These results usually are written as + or –, when antigen phenotypes are expressed using letter designations. The + and – symbols appear on the same line as the letter(s) of the antigen, and if the antigen is designated with a superscript letter, that letter is placed in parentheses on the same line as the letter defining the antigen—eg, K+, K–, Fy(a+), Fy(a–). If the phenotype is expressed with numbers, the letters defining the antigen are notated in capital letters followed by a colon followed by the number representing the antigen tested. Plus signs do not appear when test results are positive, but a minus sign is placed before negative test results; eg, K:1, K:–1. If several antigens within one blood group have been typed, the phenotype would be designated by the letter(s) of the locus or blood group system followed by a colon, followed by the different antigen numbers separated by commas (eg, K:–1,2,–3,4). Only specifically tested antigens are listed; if an antibody for a specific antigen was not used, then the number of the antigen is not listed (eg, K:–1,–3,4). Antibodies are notated by the prefix "anti-" plus the antigen they define (eg, anti-K, anti-Fy^a, etc). These rules apply to antigens and genes of the Kell, Lutheran, Duffy and Kidd blood group systems.

The ISBT Working Party on Terminology for Red Cell Surface Antigens has devised a numerical nomenclature suitable for computerization.[8] The committee used a six-digit numerical system to denote each blood group specificity. The first three numbers identify the blood group system and the last three numbers identify one unique specificity. A sampling appears in Table 9-2.

Parentage Testing

Since many of the blood group antigens are expressed as codominant traits with simple Mendelian modes of inheritance, they are useful in parentage analyses. If one assumes maternity and that test results are accurate, then exclusion of paternity may be demonstrated in two ways:

1. *Direct* exclusion of paternity is established when a genetic marker is present in the child, but is absent from the mother and the alleged father. Example:

Child	Mother	Alleged Father
B	O	O

Provided that neither the mother nor the biologic father is of the rare O_h phenotype, the child has inherited a *B* allele, which could not be inherited from either the mother or the alleged father. The *B* gene, based on the phenotypes of mother and child, must have been inherited from the biologic father and is therefore called a paternal *obligatory* allele.

2. Evidence of exclusion is *indirect* when a child lacks a genetic marker that it necessarily should have inherited from the alleged father, given his observed phenotype. Example:

Child	Mother	Alleged Father
Jk(a+b−)	Jk(a+b−)	Jk(a−b+)

Table 9-2. Nomenclature* for Red Cell Specificities and Genes[7-10]

System	Specificity			Allele	
	Letter	Number	ISBT Number	Letter	ISBT Designation
ABO	A	—†	001001	A	ABO*1
	B	—	001002	B	ABO*2
MN	M	—	002001	M	MNS*1
	N	—	002002	N	MNS*2
	S	—	002003	S	MNS*3
	s	—	002004	s	MNS*4
Kell	K	K1	006001	K	KEL*1
	k	K2	006002	k	KEL*2
	Kp^a	K3	006003	Kp^a	KEL*3
Lutheran	Lu^a	Lu1	005001	Lu^a	LU*1
	Lu^b	Lu2	005002	Lu^b	LU*2
Duffy	Fy^a	Fy1	008001	Fy^a	FY*1
	Fy^b	Fy2	008002	Fy^b	FY*2
	—	Fy3	008003	—	FY*3
	—	Fy4	008004	—	FY*4
	—	Fy5	008005	—	FY*5

*This list is not complete, but is presented in part to give examples of the nomenclatures.
†— No term in that system.

In this case, the alleged father is presumably homozygous for Jk^b and should have transmitted Jk^b to the child.

Direct exclusionary evidence is more convincing than indirect evidence that the alleged father is not the biologic father. Rarely can the test results be explained by known genetic mechanisms (eg, gene interaction). Apparent indirect exclusionary findings, however, can sometimes result from the presence of a silent allele. In the example above, the alleged father could be genotype Jk^bJk and could have transmitted the silent allele (Jk) to the child. Thus, the child's genotype could be Jk^aJk. The interpretation of phenotypic data must include all known biologic and analytic factors that influence results.

Parentage testing laboratories determine a probability of paternity that is calculated when the alleged father cannot be excluded from paternity. The probability that the alleged father transmitted the paternal obligatory alleles is compared with the probability that some other man (selected at random from the same racial population as the alleged father) transmitted the obligatory alleles. The result is expressed as a likelihood ratio (paternity index) or as a percentage (posterior probability of paternity given some prior probability). The reader is referred to other references on parentage analysis for additional information.[13,14] Standards for laboratories that carry out parentage studies have been developed by AABB.[15] Methods include study of many genetic systems other than blood groups, including restriction fragment length polymorphisms of DNA.[16]

Population Genetics

Some understanding of population genetics is important in both parentage testing and in clinical situations (eg, pre-

dicting the likelihood of finding blood compatible with a serum that contains multiple antibodies). Calculations depend on observations of phenotype frequencies.

Phenotype Frequencies

Phenotype frequencies of rbc antigens are determined by testing a large number of randomly selected people of the same race, and calculating the proportion of positive or negative reactions with a given antibody. The sum of phenotype frequencies in a given blood group system should equal 100% or 1.00. For example, if rbcs from a large number of randomly selected Caucasians are tested with anti-Jk^a, the frequency of persons who are Jk(a+) is expected to be 77%. The frequency of Jk(a–) individuals is expected to be 23%. If blood is needed for a patient with anti-Jk^a, 23% or approximately one in four ABO-compatible units of blood should be compatible.

Calculations for Combined Phenotypes

If a patient has multiple blood group antibodies, it may be useful to estimate the number of units that will have to be screened with the patient's serum (or blood grouping reagent) to find units of blood negative for the appropriate antigens. The estimate is a measure of the difficulty of finding compatible donors. For example, if a patient has anti-c, anti-K and anti-Jk^a, how many ABO-compatible units of blood will have to be tested to find four units of the appropriate phenotype?

	Phenotype Frequency %
c–	20
K–	91
Jk(a–)	23

To calculate the frequency of the combined phenotype, the individual frequencies are multiplied because the phenotypes are independent of one another. Thus, the proportion of persons that are c– is 20%. Of that 20%, 91% are K– (18%). Of persons both c– and K–, 23% are also Jk(a–) (4%):

$$0.2 \times 0.91 \times 0.23 = 0.04$$

Approximately 100 units would have to be tested to find four compatible ones. If there are only 25 ABO-compatible units available, one is expected to be compatible and it is most unlikely that sufficient units of compatible blood will be found for the patient without the assistance of the local blood supplier or reference laboratory.

Allele (Gene) Frequencies

An allele's frequency, which is calculated from phenotype frequencies, is its proportion of the total allelic pool. The sum of allele frequencies at a given locus must equal 1.00. For a two-allele system and with some assumptions about the Caucasian population, one can determine the frequencies of Jk^a and Jk^b from the observation that 77% of blood samples are Jk(a+), using the Hardy Weinberg equation for a two-allele system:

$$p^2 + 2pq + q^2 = 1$$

In the equation:

p = frequency of Jk^a
q = frequency of Jk^b
p^2 = frequency of Jk^aJk^a
$2pq$ = frequency of $Jk^aJk^b \times 2$
$q2$ = frequency of Jk^bJk^b

Then

$p^2 + 2pq$ = frequency of persons who are Jk(a+) and carry the allele Jk^a
= 0.77

$q^2 = 1 - (p^2 + 2pq)$ = frequency of persons who are Jk(a–) Jk^bJk^b (homozygous for Jk^b)
$q^2 = 1 - 0.77$ = 0.23
q = $\sqrt{0.23}$
q = 0.48 (allele frequency of Jk^b)

Since the sum of frequencies of both alleles must equal 1.00,

$p+q$ = 1
p = 1 – q
p = 1 – 0.48
p = 0.52 (allele frequency of Jk^a)

Once the allele frequencies have been calculated, the number of Jk(b+) individuals (both homoyzgous and heterozygous) can be calculated as:

$2pq + q^2$ = frequency of Jk(b+)
= 2 (0.52 × 0.48) + (0.48)^2
q = 0.73

If both anti-Jk^a and anti-Jk^b are available, allele frequencies can be determined more easily by direct counting. As shown in Table 9-3, the random sample of 100 people tested for Jk^a and Jk^b antigens possess 200 total alleles in the Kidd blood group system; each person inherits two alleles (one from each parent), (2 × 100). The frequency of Jk^a is 105 ÷ 200 = 0.52 and the frequency of Jk^b is 95 ÷ 200 = 0.48.

More information on population genetics as applied to blood groups is available in Walker[14] or Steane.[17]

Molecular Genetics

Molecular genetics has growing application to transfusion medicine. It is already important in understanding disease etiology, in diagnosis, in parentage analysis, in recombinant DNA therapeutics and in HLA typing. Erythropoietin (Epo), granulocyte colony-stimulating factor, Factor VIII and many other products can be manufactured by recombinant DNA technology. Recombinant products can be given to patients as substitutes for blood or component transfusion (eg, Factor VIII), or to stimulate endogenous production of cells (eg, Epo) or proteins.

Each chromosome contains one double strand of DNA. DNA is composed of the sugar deoxyribose, a phosphate group, the purine bases adenine (A) and guanine (G), and the pyrimidine bases thymine (T) and cytosine (C). A double strand of DNA consists of two complementary (nonidentical) single strands that are bound together by hydrogen bonds between specific base pairings of A-T and G-C. The two strands form a double helix configuration with the sugar-phosphate backbone on the outside and paired bases on the inside. Phosphate groups serve to bridge the sugar groups between the fifth carbon atom of one sugar and the third carbon atom of the adjacent sugar.[18]

Along the DNA strands are linear base sequences called *genes*. Most genes tend to occupy constant locations in the DNA of specific chromosomes (eg, a gene can be mapped to a specific locus). These regions consist of sequences of bases that code for a particular amino acid sequence (peptide). The base pairs are arranged in groups of three called *codons*; 64 codons have been identified. Most codons encode for 21 amino acids but others are signal codons (eg, terminator codons). Several "triplet codes" may encode for the same amino acid. The degeneracy of the genetic code provides code flexibility, message stability and protection against adverse point mutations. Within a given locus, a base sequence may vary, giving rise to DNA polymorphism. Some base sequences within a locus do not code for peptide manufacture and are not expressed. Variation in expressed DNA sequences of bases produces allelism (eg, protein polymorphisms).

Transcription

The information contained in base sequences of DNA, located in the nucleus of the cell, is initially transferred to a molecule of messenger RNA (mRNA). The structure of RNA is similar to that of a single strand of DNA, with ribose replacing deoxyribose and uracil (U) replacing the pyrimidine base thymine. The transfer of genetic information is accomplished by RNA polymerase, which separates the DNA double strand, and uses one strand (anticoding) as a template on which to build the mRNA (coding). This process starts at the 3' end of the DNA template, and the ribonucleotides are added by pair-

Table 9-3. Gene Frequencies in the Kidd Blood Group System Calculated Using Direct Counting Method

Phenotype	Individuals	Kidd Genes	Jk^a	Jk^b
Jk(a+b−)	28	56	56	0
Jk(a+b+)	49	98	49	49
Jk(a−b+)	23	46	0	46
Totals	100	200	105	95

ing of their pyrimidine-purine bases (A-U and G-C). The mRNA is then made functional by "capping" its 5' end with a 7-methylguanosine linked to a triphosphate. The 3' end is completed when a polymerase enzyme adds several adenine (A) residues to form a polyadenylated tail (poly A).[19] Nucleated cells contain genes with both coding and noncoding sequences. Along the DNA chain the sequences that encode for amino acids are called *exons*, and the intervening sequences (interrupting the exonic sequence) that do not code for amino acids, are called *introns*. In order for the mRNA to carry only the coded information from DNA, first a copy is made of both intronic and exonic sequences of the DNA chain. Then the intervening sequences are removed (*splicing*).

When the above three processes (capping, the addition of the poly A tail and the RNA splicing) are completed, the mRNA moves from the nucleus. When the mRNA transcription is completed, the DNA template hybridizes with its complementary strand and returns to its double-stranded configuration.

Translation

The single-stranded mRNA moves to the cytoplasm where it binds to ribosomal RNA (rRNA), which is a large globular structure. The rRNA supports the building of polypeptides from amino acids, each of which is carried by its own small transfer RNA (tRNA) molecule. The tRNA is a small (75-90 nucleotide) molecule arranged in a series of base-paired stems and unpaired loops, creating a "cloverleaf" (four arms). One arm of this structure carries an anticodon loop, and the acceptor arm opposite this loop carries a specific amino acid that binds to tRNA. As the rRNA moves down the mRNA sequence of bases, it binds specific tRNA molecules to the complementary codons

of mRNA. The binding end of each tRNA consists of three base pairs, which code for a specific amino acid. The bases on the tRNA are called *anticodons*, because they are complementary to (and pair with the bases of) the codon sequence on mRNA. As a subsequent tRNA combines with the next codon of mRNA, the amino acid deposited by the first tRNA forms a peptide bond with the amino acid carried by the next tRNA to form the primary structure of a peptide beginning with the N-terminus. Each tRNA is removed as the subsequent tRNA is added. This process continues until a termination triplet is encountered, and releases the entire polypeptide chain.

The process of transcription and translation can be artificially interrupted and changed.[19] Artificial interventions have allowed workers to synthesize and clone DNA and mRNA. The cloned code sequences can then be inserted into various cells of various species to produce specific human protein in large quantities.

References

1. Miller WV. The HLA system. In: Petz LD, Swisher SN, eds. Clinical practice of blood transfusion. New York: Churchill Livingstone, 1981:149-68.
2. Yamamoto F, Marken J, Tsuji T, et al. Cloning and characterization of DNA complementary to human UDP-GalNAc:Fuc1→2Galα1→3GalNAc transferase (histo-blood group A transferase) mRNA. J Biol Chem 1990;265:146-51.
3. Marcus DM, Cass LE. Glycosphingolipids with Lewis blood group activity: Uptake by human erythrocytes. Science 1969;164:553-4.
4. Naiki M, Marous DM. An immunochemical study of the human blood group P^1, P and P^k glycosphingolipid antigens. Biochemistry 1975; 14:4837-41.
5. Dahr W, Uhlenbruck G, Janssen E, Schmalisch R. Different N terminal amino acids in the MN-glycoprotein from *MM* and *NN* erythrocytes. Hum Genet 1977;35:335-43.
6. Schacter H, Michaels MA, Tilley CA, et al. Qualitative differences in the N-acetyl-D-galactosaminyltransferases produced by A^1 and A^2 genes. Proc Natl Acad Sci USA 1973;70:220-4.

7. Lewis M, Anstee DJ, Bird GWG, et al. Blood group terminology 1990. Vox Sang 1990;58:152-69.

8. Lewis M, Anstee DJ, Bird GWG, et al. ISBT Working Party for Red Cell Surface Antigens: Los Angeles Report. Vox Sang 1991;61:158-60.

9. Zelinski T, Coghlan C, Myal Y, et al. Genetic linkage between the Kell blood group system and prolactin-inducible protein loci: Provisional assignment of KEL to chromosome 7. Ann Hum Genet 1991;11:137-40.

10. Zelinski T, White L, Coghlan G, et al. Assignment of the YT blood group locus to chromosome 7q. Genomics 1991;11:165-7.

11. Race RR, Sanger R. Blood groups in man. 6th ed. Oxford: Blackwell Scientific Publications, 1975.

12. Issitt PD, Crookston MC. Blood group terminology: Current conventions. Transfusion 1984;24:2-7.

13. Silver H, ed. Probability of inclusion in paternity testing. Arlington, VA: American Association of Blood Banks, 1982.

14. Walker R. Mathematical genetics. In: Wilson JK, ed. Genetics for blood bankers. Washington, DC: American Association of Blood Banks, 1980:55-100.

15. Standards for parentage testing laboratories. 1st ed. Arlington, VA: American Association of Blood Banks, 1990.

16. Dykes DD. Parentage testing using restriction fragment length polymorphisms (RFLPs). In: Lasky C, Edwards-Moulds JM, eds. Clinical applications of genetic engineering. Arlington, VA: American Association of Blood Banks, 1987:59-85.

17. Steane EA. Basic genetics. In: Pittiglio DH, ed. Modern blood banking and transfusion practices. Philadelphia: FA Davis Co, 1983:23-53.

18. Klug WS, Cummings MR. Concept of genetics. Columbus, Ohio: Charles E. Merrill Publishing Co, 1983.

19. Pogo AO, Miller KS, Chaudhuri A, et al. The cloning of blood group genes. In: Edwards-Moulds J, Tregellas WM, eds. Introductory molecular genetics. Arlington, VA: American Association of Blood Banks, 1986:53-76.

10

ABO, H and P Blood Groups and Structurally Related Antigens

Introduction

ABO, H, P, I and Lewis blood group antigens are constructed on structurally related carbohydrate molecules through the activity of gene-encoded glycosyltransferase enzymes. Since it is possible for the carbohydrate molecules to carry the determinants of more than one of these blood groups, the activities of the genes of one of these blood groups may affect the expression of the antigens of another. The antigens appear when transferases add specific sugars to the ends of carbohydrate chains called oligosaccharides. The sugars are referred to as immunodominant sugars since the sugars confer specific antigenic activity to the terminal portions of the converted precursor oligosaccharide chains.[1]

Oligosaccharides consist of chains of sugars that can be attached to either glycoprotein or glycosphingolipid carrier molecules. In glycoproteins, oligosaccharides are linked via galactosamine (GalNAc) to polypeptide backbones. Structurally similar oligosaccharides are attached via glucose (Glc) to ceramide residues in glycosphingolipids. Glycosphingolipids form part of rbc membranes and also the membranes of most endothelial cells. Soluble forms are present in plasma, but are not secreted in body fluids. Soluble glycoproteins with blood group antigen activity exist in the body's serous and mucous secretions. Membrane-associated glycoproteins are present on rbcs and other body cells.[2]

The ABO System

A series of tests performed by Karl Landsteiner in 1900 led to the discovery of the ABO blood groups and to the development of routine blood grouping procedures. Landsteiner tested blood samples from his colleagues by mixing each person's serum with suspensions of rbcs from the others. Noting agglutination in some mixtures but not in others, he was able to classify the blood samples into one of three groups, now named A, B and O. (The fourth group, AB, was discovered in 1902 by Landsteiner's pupils von Decastello and Sturli.) Landsteiner recognized that the presence or absence of only two antigens, A and B, was sufficient to explain the three blood groups he saw. He also demonstrated that the serum of each person contained an antibody directed against the antigen absent from that person's rbcs. The first blood group system to be discovered, ABO, remains the most significant for transfusion practice. It is the only system in which the reciprocal antibodies are consistently and predictably present in the sera of normal people whose rbcs lack the corresponding antigen(s)—"Landsteiner's Rule" (see Table 10-1). Testing to detect ABO incompatibility between a recipient and

203

Table 10-1. Routine ABO Grouping

Reaction of Cells Tested With		Reaction of Serum Tested Against			Interpre- tation	Frequency (%) in US Population			
Anti-A	Anti-B	A Cells	B Cells	O Cells	ABO Group	Whites	Blacks	American Indians*	Orientals*
0	0	+	+	0	O	45	49	79	40
+	0	0	+	0	A	40	27	16	28
0	+	+	0	0	B	11	20	4	27
+	+	0	0	0	AB	4	4	<1	5

+ = agglutination; 0 = no agglutination.
*Composite figures, calculated from Mourant et al.[3]

the donor is the foundation on which all other pretransfusion testing rests.[4]

Antigens of the ABO System

Biochemical and Genetic Considerations

Glycosphingolipids carrying A or B oligosaccharides are integral parts of the membranes of rbcs, epithelial and endothelial cells (Fig 10-1); they are also present in soluble form in plasma. Glycoproteins that carry identical oligosaccharides are responsible for the A and B activity of secreted body fluids such as saliva. A and B oligosaccharides that lack carrier protein or lipid molecules are found in milk and urine.

Genes at three separate loci (ABO, Hh and Sese) control the occurrence and the location of the A and B antigens. Three common alleles—A, B and O—are located at the ABO locus on chromosome 9. The A and B genes encode glycosyltransferases that produce the A and B antigens, respectively.[5] The O gene is considered to be nonfunctional since no detectable blood group antigen results from the action of its protein product. The rbcs of group O persons lack A and B, but carry an abundant amount of H antigen. H antigen is the precursor material on which A and B antigens are built.

Family studies have shown that the genes at the remaining two loci, Hh and Sese (secretor), are closely linked on chromosome 19.[6] It is suggested that one of these loci may have arisen through gene duplication of the other.[7] Two recognized alleles reside at each locus. Of the two alleles at the H locus, one of these, H, produces an enzyme that acts at the cellular level to construct the antigen on which A or B are built. The other allele at this locus, h, is very rare. No antigenic product has been linked to h, so this gene is also considered an amorph. The possibility exists that other alleles occur at the Hh locus that differ from H in that they cause the production of only very small amounts of H antigen.[8]

The Se gene is directly responsible for the expression of H (and indirectly responsible for the expression of A and B) on the glycoproteins in epithelial secretions such as saliva. Eighty percent of the population are secretors; they have inherited the Se gene and produce H in their secretions that can be converted to A and/or B (depending on the genetic background of the secretor). The se gene, having no demonstrable product, is an amorph.

Oligosaccharide chains on which the A and B antigens are built can exist as simple structures of a few sugar mole-

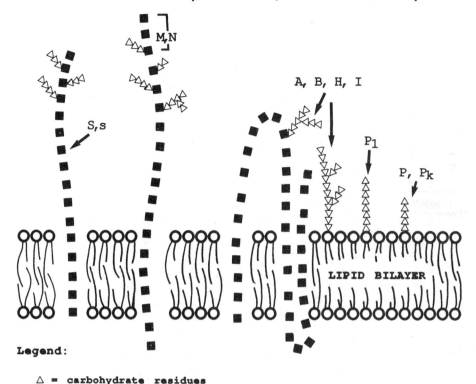

Figure 10-1. Diagrammatic representation of some membrane glycoproteins and glycosphingolipids that carry blood group antigens.

cules linked together in linear fashion. They can also exist as more complex structures that are composed of many sugar residues connected together in branching chains. It has been proposed that the differences in cellular A, B and H activity seen between specimens from infants and adults may be related to the number of branched structures carried on the cellular membranes of each group.[9] The rbcs of infants are thought to carry A, B and H antigens built predominantly on linear oligosaccharides. Linear oligosaccharides have only one terminus to which the H, then A and B, sugars can be added. In contrast, the rbcs of adults appear to carry a high proportion of branched oligosaccharides. Branching creates additional portions on the oligosaccharide

that can be converted to H and then to A and B antigens.

A and *B* genes do not produce antigens directly but, instead, produce enzymes called glycosyltransferases that add specific sugars to oligosaccharide chains that have been converted to H by the action of the product of the *H* gene. H antigens are constructed on precursor (core) oligosaccharide chains ending in Type 1 and Type 2 linkages between the sugars β-D-galactose (Gal) and N-acetylglucosamine (GlcNAc) (see Fig 10-2).[1,5] The number 1 carbon of the terminal 6-carbon sugar Gal is linked to the number 3 carbon of subterminal GlcNAc in Type 1 chains and to the number 4 carbon of GlcNAc in Type 2 chains. In both chain types, the subterminal GlcNAc is attached via a β(1→3) linkage to Gal residue. Type 1 A, B and H antigens are carried on free oligosaccharides in milk and urine and on glycolipids in plasma.[10] Type 1 A, B and H are also found on endodermally derived tissues such as the epithelial lining of the gut. Type 1 chains are also the main carriers of A, B and H in body fluids and secretions. In saliva, A, B and H are carried on glycoproteins with Type 1 and Type 2 chains.[9-11]

Glycolipid A, B and H antigens produced by the rbcs have been thought to be formed exclusively on Type 2 chains. About 75% are part of highly branched oligosaccharide chains attached to glycoproteins known as bands 3 and 4.5. The remaining antigens are bound to glycolipids. Recent studies have indicated that more complex core molecules called Type 3 and Type 4 chains may be involved also. It is estimated that the number of potential A, B and H sites on rbcs is in excess of 2 million.[12,13]

At the cellular level, the *H* gene produces a fucosyltransferase that adds fucose (Fuc) in α(1→2) linkage to the terminal Gal of Type 2 chains (see Fig 10-3). The *A* and *B* gene transferases can only attach their immunodominant sugars when the Type 2 (or Type 1) chains have been substituted with Fuc (ie, changed to H); thus, the A and B antigens are constructed at the expense of H. The *A* gene-specified *N*-acetylgalactosaminyltransferase and the *B* gene-specified galactosyltransferase add GalNAc and Gal, respectively, in α(1→3) linkages to the same Gal acted on by the *H* gene transferase.

Until recently, it was believed that addition of A and B sugars to core molecules terminated chain growth. No glycosyltransferase was thought to utilize A or B as acceptor substrates. The discovery of glycolipids in which two A structures appeared linked in tandem altered this view[10,11,14,15] (see Fig 10-4).

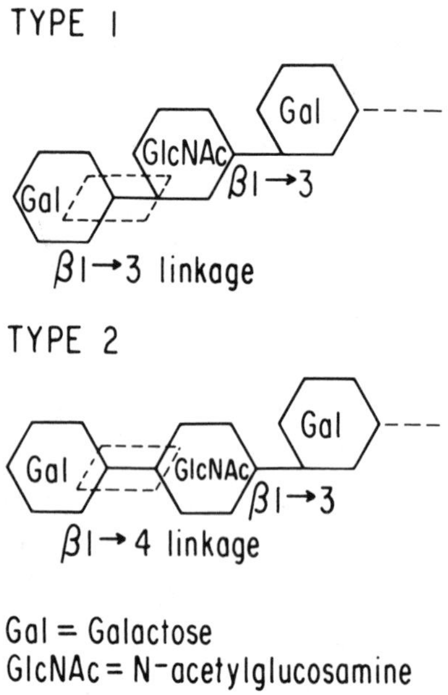

Figure 10-2. Type 1 and Type 2 oligosaccharide chains differ only in the linkage between the GlcNAc and the terminal Gal.

ABO Genes at the Molecular Level

Yamamoto and Hakomori have shown that *A* and *B* genes differ from one another by seven single base substitutions.[16,17] This results in four possible amino acid substitutions (at positions 176, 235, 266 and 268) in the protein chains of the A and B transferases. Substitutions at positions 266 and 268 were found to be most critical in determining sugar-nucleotide specificity, although the amino acid substitution that occurred at position 235 also had some effect. It has been proposed that alleles of *A* and *B* that result in subgroups (phenotypes of A and B that differ from each other with respect to the amount of antigen carried on the rbcs) produce transferases exhibiting additional amino acid substitutions resulting in enzymes of slightly different abilities to convert H.

The base sequence of the *O* gene appears to be similar to that of *A* except for a single base deletion (nucleotide position 258) in the coding region close to the N-terminus of the resulting protein. The deletion shifts the reading frame, resulting in the translation of a protein, unrelated to A and B transferases, that does not produce a blood group antigen.[16] Thus, there are three primary genes in the ABO system; two are functional and one is nonfunctional.

The secretions of *sese* persons contain Type 1 and Type 2 chains with no H, A or B activity. It has been suggested that the *H* and *Se* genes each encode a different fucosyltransferase.[7,18] The enzyme produced by *H* acts primarily on Type 2 chains and in rbc membranes. The enzyme produced by *Se* prefers (but does not limit its action to) Type 1 chains and acts primarily in the secretory glands. Studies performed on the secretions of persons with the rare O_h phenotype support the concept that two types of H antigen exist.[8] Persons of this phenotype, who are genetically *hh* and *sese*, have no H and, therefore, no A or B antigens on their rbcs or in their secretions. However, H, A and B antigens are found in the secretions of some genetically *hh* persons, who, through family studies, appear to possess at least one *Se* gene.

A and B antigens are detected in direct agglutination tests with anti-A and

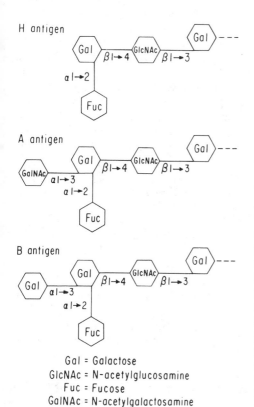

Gal = Galactose
GlcNAc = N-acetylglucosamine
Fuc = Fucose
GalNAc = N-acetylgalactosamine

Figure 10-3. Gal added to the subterminal Gal confers B activity; GalNAc added to the subterminal Gal confers A activity to the sugar. Unless the fucose moiety that determines H activity is attached to the number 2 carbon, galactose does not accept either sugar on the 3 carbon.

GalNAcα(1→3)Galβ(1→4) GalNAcα(1→3)Galβ(1→4)GlcNAcβ (1→3)--

| α(1→2) | α(1→2)
Fuc   Fuc

└──────────────────┘└──────────────────────┘
Repetitive A structure   Type 2 A antigen

Figure 10-4. Type 3 A antigen structure.[10]

anti-B reagents. ABO reagents frequently produce weaker reactions with the rbcs of newborns than with rbcs from adults. Weaker reactions are encountered because A and B antigens are not fully developed at birth, even though they can be detected on the rbcs of embryos 5-6 weeks old.[4,18,19] By the time a person is 2-4 years old, rbc A and/or B antigen expression is fully developed. Antigenic expression remains fairly constant throughout life.

Subgroups of A

Subgroups of A are phenotypes that differ from others of the same ABO group with respect to the amount of A antigen carried on rbcs and, in secretors, present in the saliva. (See Table 10-2.) The two principal subgroups of A are A_1 and A_2. It is known that the glycosyltransferases produced by the A_1 and A_2 genes differ and that there are both quantitative and qualitative differences between the A_1

and A_2 antigens produced. Rbcs of both A_1 and A_2 persons react strongly with anti-A reagents in direct agglutination tests. The serologic distinction between A_1 and A_2 is based on results obtained in tests with reagent anti-A_1 prepared from group B human serum or the lectin of *Dolichos biflorus* seeds. Under prescribed testing conditions, anti-A_1 reagents agglutinate A_1 but not A_2 rbcs. The rbcs of approximately 80% of group A or group AB persons are agglutinated by anti-A_1 and, thus, are classified as A_1 or A_1B. The remaining 20%, whose rbcs are agglutinated by anti-A, but not by anti-A_1, are called A_2 or A_2B.[19,20]

Anti-A_1 occurs as an alloantibody in the serum of 1-8% of A_2 persons and 22-35% of A_2B persons.[19,21] Anti-A_1 can cause discrepancies in ABO testing and incompatibilities in crossmatches with A_1 or A_1B rbcs. It is considered to be clinically insignificant unless it reacts at 37 C. It is not necessary to test group A rbcs routinely with anti-A_1 to determine

Table 10-2. Serologic Reactions Observed in Persons With A and B Phenotypes*

Red Blood Cell Phenotype	Reaction of Cells With Known Antiserum to					Reaction of Serum Against Reagent Red Blood Cells				Saliva of Secretors Contains
	A	B	A,B	H	A_1	A_1	A_2	B	O	
A_1	+ + + +	0	+ + + +	0	+ + + +	0	0	+ + + +	0	A & H
A_{int}	+ + + +	0	+ + + +	+ + +	+ +	0	0	+ + + +	0	A & H
A_2	+ + + +	0	+ + + +	+ +	0	†	0	+ + + +	0	A & H
A_3	+ + ^{mf}	0	+ + ^{mf}	+ + +	0	†	0	+ + + +	0	A & H
A_m	0/±	0	0/±	+ + + +	0	0	0	+ + + +	0	A & H
A_x	0/±	0	+/+ +	+ + + +	0	+ +/0	0/+	+ + + +	0	H
A_{el}	0	0	0	+ + + +	0	+ +/0	0	+ + + +	0	H
B	0	+ + + + + + + +	0			+ + + + + + + +		0	0	B & H
B_3	0	+ ^{mf}	+ + ^{mf}	+ + + +		+ + + + + + + +		0	0	B & H
B_m	0	0	0/±	+ + + +		+ + + + + + + +		0	0	B & H
B_x	0	0/±	0/+ +	+ + + +		+ + + + + + + +		0	0	H

+ to + + + +, agglutination of increasing strength; ±, weak agglutination; mf, mixed-field pattern of agglutination; 0, no agglutination.
*Modified from Beattie[19]
†The occurrence of anti-A_1 is variable in these phenotypes. A_2 persons frequently have anti-A_1; A_3 persons usually do not, but a few A_3 individuals with anti-A_1 in the serum have been found.

their subgroup status. This information is useful only when working with samples from people whose sera contain anti-A_1.

Subgroups weaker than A_2 occur infrequently and, in general, are characterized by decreasing numbers of A antigen sites on the red cells and a reciprocal increase in H antigen activity. The genes responsible constitute less than 1% of the total pool of *A* genes. Classification of weak subgroups is generally based on the[18]:

1. Degree of rbc agglutination by anti-A and anti-A_1.
2. Degree of rbc agglutination by anti-A,B.
3. Degree of H reactivity of the rbcs.
4. Presence or absence of anti-A_1 in the serum.
5. Presence of A and H substances in the saliva of secretors.

See Table 10-2 for the serologic characteristics of A phenotypes.

Rbcs of the A_x, A_{el}, A_{int} or A_3 subgroups are seen only infrequently in transfusion practice. A_x rbcs are, in general, agglutinated by human anti-A,B but not by human anti-A. A_x rbcs may react with some murine monoclonal anti-A reagents, a characteristic dependent on the type of monoclonal antibody selected for the reagent.[22] A_{el} rbcs are not agglutinated by anti-A or anti-A,B of any origin. Adsorption and elution studies are necessary to show that these rbcs carry the A antigen. Rbcs of the A_{int} phenotype can be identified only if tests with anti-A_1 are performed. A_{int} rbcs react more weakly than A_1 rbcs with anti-A_1, yet more strongly with anti-H than do A_2 rbcs. A_3 rbcs produce a characteristic mixed-field pattern of small agglutinates among many free rbcs in tests with anti-A and anti-A,B. Weak subgroups of A such as A_x, A_m and A_{el} cannot be identified on the basis of blood grouping tests alone. Saliva studies and adsorption/elution studies must be performed.

Subgroups of B are even less common than subgroups of A. Criteria for their differentiation resemble those for subgroups of A (see Table 10-2).

Antibodies to A and B

Ordinarily, individuals possess antibodies directed toward the A or B antigen absent from their own rbcs. (See Table 10-1.) This predictable complementary relationship permits serum grouping in addition to rbc ABO grouping tests (see Methods 2.2 and 2.3). One hypothesis for the appearance of these antibodies is based on the fact that the immunoreactive configurations that confer A and B specificities to molecules of the rbc membrane also exist in other biologic entities, notably bacterial cell walls. Bacteria are widespread in the environment and it appears that their presence in intestinal flora, dust, food and other widely distributed agents ensures a constant exposure of all persons to A-like and B-like antigens. Immunocompetent persons react to the environmental antigens by producing antibodies to those that are absent from their own systems. Thus, anti-A occurs in the sera of group O and group B persons and anti-B occurs in the sera of group O and group A persons. Group AB people, having both antigens, make neither antibody. As mentioned previously, the emergence of anti-A and anti-B due to environmental stimulants is only a hypothesis and may not be found correct as more knowledge is gained regarding the immune response.

Time of Appearance

Anti-A and anti-B production generally begins after the first few months of life. Occasionally, infants can be found already producing these antibodies at the time of birth,[4] although most antibodies in cord sera are of maternal origin. Antibody production is reported to peak at

5-10 years of age and decline with advancing years. In elderly people, anti-A and anti-B levels may be lower than those seen in young adults.[4,23] Since antibody production normally begins after birth, results obtained with the sera of newborns or infants younger than about 4-6 months cannot be considered valid because the antibodies may have been acquired through the placental transfer of maternal IgG anti-A and anti-B.

Reactivity of Anti-A and Anti-B

Anti-A produced by group B persons and anti-B produced by A persons are composed predominantly of IgM molecules.[4] Small quantities of IgG molecules are also present in the sera of these two groups. IgG is the dominant form of anti-A and anti-B of group O serum. The IgG forms readily cross the placenta and can cause ABO HDN. Because of the predominance of IgM antibodies in the sera of group A or B persons, ABO hemolytic disease is rarely seen in ABO-incompatible infants born of group A or B mothers.[4,19]

The distinguishing features of IgM and IgG anti-A and anti-B are given in Table 10-3. Both immunoglobulin types preferentially agglutinate red cells at room temperature (20-24 C) or below. Both are efficient activators of complement at 37 C. The complement-mediated lytic capabilities of these antibodies are most apparent when an incubation phase at 37 C is added to serum grouping tests. Occasionally, patients or donors can be found whose sera cause the hemolysis of ABO-incompatible rbcs at temperatures below 37 C. Hemolysis by ABO antibodies in serum grouping tests should be suspected when a pink to red discoloration appears in the supernatant fluid or when the buttons of reagent ABO grouping rbcs are reduced in size or are missing. Hemolysis must be interpreted as a pos-

itive result. Hemolysis of rbcs will not occur if reagent rbcs are suspended in solutions that contain EDTA or other anticoagulants that prevent complement activation.

Anti-A,B (Group O Serum)

Serum from group O persons contains an antibody designated as anti-A,B because it reacts with A and B rbcs. Specificities for both rbc groups cannot be separated by differential adsorption. Eluates prepared from group A rbcs that have been used to adsorb group O serum contain anti-A and an antibody that reacts with both A and B rbcs. Similar findings are obtained when B rbcs are used for adsorption. Saliva from A or B secretors inhibits the activity of this antibody with either A or B rbcs.

Group O sera have been used to prepare potent typing reagents capable of agglutinating A and B cells. Similar reagents, called anti-A,B, can be manufactured by blending monoclonal antibodies with apparent A and B specificities. Human polyclonal or monoclonal reagent anti-A,B will not agglutinate group O red cells. Depending on the antibodies selected to prepare this reagent, monoclonal anti-A,B may react as well as, or better

Table 10-3. Distinguishing Characteristics of IgM and IgG Anti-A and Anti-B

	IgM	IgG
Reactions enhanced		
—with enzyme-treated rbcs	yes	yes
—by lowering temperatures	yes	no
Readily inhibited by soluble A or B antigens	yes	no
Inactivated by 2-ME or DTT	yes	no
Predominant in non-immunized group A and B donors	yes	no

than, natural human anti-A,B with rbcs of weak A phenotypes.

Anti-A$_1$

The anti-A of group B serum appears, from simple studies, to contain separable anti-A and anti-A$_1$. In direct tests, group B serum agglutinates A$_1$ and A$_2$ rbcs, yet following adsorption with A$_2$ rbcs, group B serum reacts only with A$_1$ rbcs. If further tests are performed, the differences between A antigen expression on A$_1$ and A$_2$ rbcs appears to be quantitative more than qualitative. Further adsorption of group B serum with A$_2$ rbcs will remove all serum activity for A$_1$ rbcs. The apparent anti-A$_1$ made by adsorption of group B serum can be thought of as a weakened form of anti-A. It reacts with A$_1$ rbcs because they have more A antigen than do A$_2$ rbcs. The sera of persons of certain weak subgroups of A may contain anti-A$_1$ that is serologically similar to the anti-A$_1$ of group B adsorbed serum.

Adsorbed group B serum can be used at the practical level to differentiate between A$_1$ and A$_2$ subgroups. More frequently, however, anti-A$_1$ reagents are employed that are manufactured from the lectin of *Dolichos biflorus*. (See Method 2.12.) The lectin will react with A$_1$ and A$_2$ rbcs unless it has been diluted appropriately. Reagent anti-A$_1$ lectins have been diluted by the manufacturer to react with A$_1$, but not A$_2$, rbcs.

Routine Testing for ABO

Rbc grouping tests, using anti-A and anti-B to determine the presence or absence of the antigens, are often referred to as direct or forward grouping tests. Serum grouping tests, using reagent A$_1$ and B rbcs to detect serum anti-A and anti-B, are sometimes called reverse grouping tests. Routine grouping of donors and patients must include both rbc and serum

tests, each serving as a check on the other.[24,25] It is permissible to test only rbcs when ABO grouping is performed to confirm the group of donor blood that has already been labeled with a blood group designation or when testing is performed on samples from infants less than 4 months of age. Routine procedures for ABO grouping by slide, tube or microplate tests are described in Methods 2.1, 2.2 and 2.3.

Some ABO rbc grouping reagents are prepared from pools of sera from persons who have been stimulated with A or B blood group substances to produce antibodies of high titer. Other ABO grouping reagents are manufactured from monoclonal antibodies derived from cultured cell lines. Both types of reagents are potent and agglutinate most antigen-positive rbcs on direct contact without centrifugation. Serum testing is most reliably performed by tube or microplate methods. Anti-A and anti-B occurring in the sera of patients and donors are frequently too weak to agglutinate rbcs without centrifugation. Therefore, it is not recommended that serum grouping tests be performed on slides.

B(A) Phenotype

In 1984, Yates et al[26] reported that a 10,000-fold concentrate of purified *B* gene-specified galactosyltransferase, isolated from the sera of group B individuals, has the capacity, in vitro, to attach small amounts of A sugar to human milk fucosyllactose, a blood group H-like structure. That high levels of *B* gene-associated glycosyltransferases have the capacity to synthesize blood group A-active structures in vivo has been demonstrated by Beck et al.[27] They found that the rbcs of some group B individuals reacted with an FDA-licensed anti-A blood grouping reagent that was formulated, in part, with a murine monoclonal antibody, MHO4. Subsequently, sera from these group B donors were shown to contain excessively high levels of *B* gene-specified galactosyltransferase. The designation B(A) has been used to describe this blood group phenotype.

Reports on the incidence of B(A) among group B individuals are conflicting, and range from a high of 1% (Beck et al[27]) to below 0.1%. Recognition of the B(A) phenotype is usually made with the discriminating monoclonal anti-A grouping reagent. The reaction of B(A) rbcs with this monoclonal anti-A is variable. The majority of examples react weakly, and the agglutinates are fragile and easily dispersed. Some examples have been reported as strong as 2+. Except for newborns and immunocompromised patients, serum grouping should distinguish an $A_{sub}B$ sample with anti-A_1 from a B(A) sample containing anti-A that reacts with both A_1 and A_2 rbcs. Transferase studies should provide conclusive data; *A* gene-specified *N*-acetylgalactosaminyltransferase should be present in the $A_{sub}B$ sample and absent in the B(A) sample.

Nonroutine ABO Testing

On occasion, other reagents are incorporated into ABO grouping procedures. These include anti-A,B (rbc grouping) and reagent A_2 and O rbcs (serum grouping). Some workers elect to use anti-A,B routinely in grouping tests to avoid mistakenly classifying weakly reactive A or B rbcs as group O. Unfortunately, there exists a misconception that anti-A,B of human origin is more potent than either anti-A or anti-B and, thus, will detect most weak subgroups of A or B. With the exception of A_x, human anti-A,B does not agglutinate the rbcs of less common subgroups that fail to react with anti-A or anti-B.[19] Human-source anti-A,B does not react well with A_x rbcs in immediate-spin tests. The reagent and rbcs must be incu-

bated together for 10-60 minutes at room temperature for reactions to occur. In contrast, A_x cells, or red cells of other weak ABO subgroups, may react well with monoclonal anti-A,B in immediate-spin tests. If the manufacturer's directions recommend using anti-A,B for the detection of weak subgroups, it means that its reactivity against A_x rbcs has been demonstrated.[24] AABB *Standards for Blood Banks and Transfusion Services*[25] does not require the use of anti-A,B to detect weak A or B subgroups since such blood samples often distinguish themselves from group O by failing to produce the expected serum grouping results (see Table 10-2). Moreover, the adverse consequences associated with the transfusion of weak subgroups of A and B to group O recipients are minimal.[4,28]

Some commercially prepared reverse grouping reagents contain A_2 and O rbcs in addition to A_1 and B rbcs. The sole purpose of A_2 rbcs in these reagents is to facilitate the recognition of anti-A_1 in the sera of persons who are subgroups of A.[28] Since the majority of A blood does not contain anti-A_1, many workers employ this reagent only when discrepancies between rbc and serum tests are encountered. Group O rbcs of reverse grouping sets can be used to identify those sera that contain cold-reactive agglutinins that may interfere with serum grouping tests. Generally, such rbcs cannot be used for the detection or identification of unexpected antibodies since they have not been manufactured to meet the requirements of the FDA for these purposes.

Manufacturers of ABO reagents provide, with each reagent package, detailed instructions for the use of the reagent. Instructions may vary from one manufacturer to another in testing requirements. Therefore, it is important to follow the directions supplied with the specific reagent in use.

Discrepancies Between Red Blood Cell and Serum Tests

Table 10-1 shows the results and interpretations of routine ABO rbc and serum testing. A discrepancy exists when the interpretation of rbc typing tests is at odds with that of serum tests. When a discrepancy is encountered, the discrepant results should be recorded. ABO interpretation must be delayed until the discrepancy is resolved. If the blood under test is from a donor unit, the unit may not be released for transfusion until the discrepancy is resolved. When the blood is from a potential recipient, the clinical condition of the patient may make it necessary to administer group O RBCs of the appropriate Rh type before the investigation is completed. It is important to obtain sufficient amounts of a patient's pretransfusion blood to permit any additional studies that may be required to resolve the discrepancy.

Discrepancies between rbc and serum tests occur because of technical errors, intrinsic rbc or serum factors, or extrinsic test factors. Technical problems can lead to ABO testing discrepancies either because negative results are obtained in place of positive results, or positive results are found when tests should have been negative.

Technical and clerical problems leading to falsely negative ABO rbc or serum test results include the failure to:
1. Add serum or blood grouping reagent to a test.
2. Identify hemolysis as a positive reaction.
3. Use the appropriate ratio of serum (or blood grouping reagent) to rbcs.
4. Centrifuge tests correctly (undercentrifugation).
5. Incubate tests at temperatures of 20-24 C or below.
6. Use active reagents.
7. Interpret or record test results correctly.

Technical and clerical problems that produce falsely positive tests include:
1. Overcentrifugation of tests.
2. Use of contaminated blood grouping reagent, rbcs or saline.
3. Use of dirty glassware.
4. Incorrect interpretation or recording of test results.

Some discrepancies are caused by problems in rbc grouping tests.
1. Samples obtained from patients who have received transfusions recently or who have received a bone marrow transplant may produce unexpected reactions if the samples contain a mixture of rbcs that differ from each other in their ABO group (transfusion or transplantation chimera).
2. Rbcs from persons who have inherited variant *A* or *B* genes may carry poorly expressed antigens. Weak antigens may also be found on the rbcs of some people with diseases such as leukemia.[4] Samples from these people may fail to produce the expected reactions in direct agglutination tests with anti-A and anti-B.
3. Abnormalities of an inherited or acquired nature, leading to what is referred to as polyagglutinable states, can result in rbcs with modified membranes. The modified rbcs can be unexpectedly agglutinated by reagent anti-A, anti-B or both.[29-31]
4. Abnormal concentrations of serum proteins and the presence of macromolecules (or in cord blood samples, the presence of Wharton's jelly) may cause nonspecific aggregation that simulates agglutination if rbcs are suspended in their own serum.
5. High concentrations of A or B blood group substances in the serum have been found, on rare occasions, to inhibit the activities of reagent antibodies to such an extent that unexpected negative reactions are

obtained when serum- or plasma-suspended rbcs are used.[19,32]

6. The sera of some persons contain antibodies to the dyes used to color anti-A and anti-B reagents. These antibodies can cause falsely positive agglutination reactions if serum- or plasma-suspended rbcs are used in testing.[19]

7. Rbcs of persons producing potent cold-reactive autoagglutinins may be coated with antibody to the extent that the rbcs agglutinate spontaneously in the diluent used to prepare the reagent, thus producing unexpected positive results.

Discrepancies also occur that are caused by problems in serum grouping tests.

1. Frequently, small fibrin clots occur in ABO grouping tests employing plasma or incompletely clotted serum. The fibrin clots may be mistaken for true agglutination.

2. The sera of patients who have abnormally high concentrations of abnormal proteins in their serum, who have altered serum protein ratios or who have received plasma expanders of high molecular weight or intravenous contrast materials can produce nonspecific rbc aggregation in serum grouping tests that is difficult to distinguish from true agglutination.

3. Antibodies other than anti-A and anti-B in a test sample can cause the unexpected agglutination of reagent A_1 and B rbcs if those rbcs carry the corresponding antigen.

4. False-positive results can be obtained if the test sample contains antibodies to chemical constituents of the diluents used to preserve reagent A_1 and B rbcs. The lattice formed by the interaction between the antibodies and the chemicals traps the rbcs nonspecifically to produce the unexpected agglutination reactions.[19,33]

5. Unexpected weak or negative serum test results may be encountered if the sample under test is from a person who is immunodeficient due to disease or therapy and who has depressed immunoglobulin levels. Weak serum ABO tests can also be seen with samples from elderly patients whose antibody levels have declined with age and with samples from patients whose antibodies have been greatly diluted by plasma exchange procedures.

6. Negative or weak results are seen if serum tests are performed on specimens from infants under 4-6 months of age. Serum tests are not routinely done on samples from newborns since antibodies that are found are generally derived in utero from the mother.[4]

7. The patient's serum may contain unusually potent anti-A and anti-B that bind the complement component C1 to the extent that C1 interferes with antibody binding and agglutination in serum grouping tests. This phenomenon has been reported in serum grouping tests using red cells suspended in diluents that lack EDTA.[34]

8. If the patient has received a bone marrow transplant of a compatible, but dissimilar, ABO group, the rbc type may not match that of the serum type. For example, a group A person transplanted with group O marrow (minor mismatch) will produce O rbcs, and yet produce only anti-B.

9. Unexpected reactions may be obtained if the recipient has recently received sufficient volumes of blood components containing plasma of an ABO group other than that of the patient.

Resolving ABO Discrepancies

Since many discrepancies occur as the result of technical errors, the first step that should be taken to resolve the problem is, simply, to repeat the tests on the same sample. If initial tests were performed with serum- or plasma-suspended rbcs, repeat testing should incorporate rbcs that have been washed and resuspended in saline. If the discrepancy persists, the following procedures can be incorporated into the investigation.

1. Obtain a new blood specimen from the donor unit or patient and repeat tests with the new sample. This action will assist with the identification of discrepancies due to mislabeled or contaminated specimens.
2. Wash the test and reagent rbcs several times to remove serum or chemical constituents that may be causing unexpected positive reactions.
3. Test the rbcs with anti-A,B, anti-A_1 or anti-H as appropriate for the individual problem.
4. Test the serum against group A_2 rbcs if interfering reactions due to anti-A_1 are suspected.
5. Test group O rbcs of adults and autologous rbcs to detect interfering activity of cold-reactive auto- or alloagglutinins other than anti-A or anti-B.
6. Incubate rbc and serum tests at room temperature for 30 minutes to facilitate the detection of weak antigens or antibodies. Tests can also be incubated at 4 C providing the appropriate controls are tested in parallel. Results obtained at 4 C with group O and autologous controls should be evaluated before reactions with A_1 or B rbcs are considered valid. Autoagglutinins capable of reacting with the rbcs of all adults (such as anti-I and anti-IH) are more likely to be detected at 4 C.

Resolving discrepancies due to absence of expected antigens. Rbcs of most A or B people are strongly agglutinated (3–4+) by their respective reagent antibody. The corresponding sera of these samples usually agglutinate A_1 or B reagent rbcs strongly (3–4+). The reaction strengths that are obtained in rbc or serum grouping tests often indicate what is causing the discrepancy. For example, serum that fails to agglutinate A_1 rbcs, but strongly agglutinates group B rbcs, suggests that the test specimen is group A, even though the corresponding rbcs fail to react with anti-A and anti-B. As mentioned previously, discrepancies due to weakened forms of A or B antigens occur in persons who have inherited variant alleles, or in patients in whom disease has decreased antigen activity. In such cases, the antigens can be depressed to the extent that they will not be detected in routine direct agglutination tests. The following procedures can be used to facilitate detection of weakly expressed antigens.

1. Test washed rbcs with anti-A and anti-A,B for 30 minutes at room temperature or at 4 C. Extended incubation at room temperature or 4 C can facilitate the detection of weak A or B antigens by reagent antibodies. If tests are performed at 4 C, group O and autologous control rbcs *must* be tested in parallel to ensure that reactions observed are due to anti-A and anti-B and not to other cold-reactive agglutinins.
2. Treat the patient's rbcs with proteolytic enzymes (such as ficin, papain or bromelain). Enzyme-treated group A and B rbcs react more strongly with their respective antibodies. In some instances, reactions between reagent anti-A and rbcs expressing weak A antigens will become detectable at room temperature within 30 minutes if enzyme-treated rbcs are employed. Group O rbcs that have been treated with enzyme must be tested in a similar manner to serve as controls in ABO grouping tests employing enzyme-treated rbcs.
3. Incubate an aliquot of rbcs at room temperature or at 4 C with anti-A or anti-B (depending on the discrepancy) to adsorb antibody to the rbc antigens.

(Do not use anti-A_1 lectin.) Group O rbcs should be handled in a similar manner to serve as a control of the procedure. Following incubation, wash the rbcs thoroughly, then prepare an eluate. Test the eluate against group A_1, B and O cells. If the rbcs carried the A antigen, the eluate will agglutinate A_1, but not B or O rbcs. Eluates prepared from group B rbcs will agglutinate only other B rbcs. (See Method 2.4.) The eluates prepared from group O control rbcs should be nonreactive. Activity in the group O control eluate invalidates results obtained with patient rbc and can mean either the anti-A or anti-B sera contained other antibodies, or that the adsorption/elution procedure was not performed correctly.

4. Test the saliva for the presence of A or B and H substances. (See Method 2.5 for hemagglutination-inhibition tests for salivary antigens.) Saliva tests are helpful only if the person is a secretor.

Resolving discrepancies due to unexpected reactions with anti-A and anti-B. In some instances, unexpected positive reactions are obtained in rbc grouping tests. For example, the rbcs of a sample are agglutinated weakly in tests with anti-A even though the corresponding serum produced reactions expected of a normal group B or O. Situations such as this can arise through the inheritance of a variant allele at the *ABO* locus, or from other problems unrelated to the actions of *ABO* genes. The following paragraphs describe those events that can lead to the appearance of unexpected reactions in ABO grouping tests and the steps that can be taken to identify their causes.

Acquired B Phenotype

The acquired B state should be considered when the serum of a patient contains anti-B and the patient's rbcs appear to be group AB with a weak B antigen. The acquired B phenotype arises through the modification of the A antigen by microbial enzymes called deacetylases. The enzymes modify cellular A immunodominant sugars (GalNAc) so they become more like the B sugar (Gal). A_1 rbcs are the only group that exhibits acquired B activity in vivo.[29] The acquired B antigen is made at the expense of A; therefore, a concomitant decrease in the strength of A may be seen in the acquired B state. When present in sufficient numbers, acquired B antigens react with human anti-B in direct agglutination tests. While many examples of rbcs with acquired B antigens react weakly with anti-B, some examples can be found that are agglutinated quite strongly. These same rbcs may fail to react with some monoclonal anti-B reagents but react strongly with others. An increased incidence in the detection of acquired B antigens has been observed through the use of some FDA-licensed monoclonal anti-B blood grouping reagents.[35] To confirm that group A_1 rbcs carry the acquired B structure:

1. Check the patient's diagnosis. Acquired B antigens tend to be associated with carcinoma of the colon or rectum, infection with gram-negative organisms and intestinal obstructions. Nevertheless, acquired B antigens have been found on the rbcs of normal blood donors.[35]

2. Test the patient's serum against his or her own rbcs. The anti-B in the patient's serum will not agglutinate his or her own rbcs when they carry the acquired B determinant.

3. Test the rbcs with monoclonal anti-B. Some monoclonal reagents, unlike human-source antibodies, do not react with the acquired B phenotype. Such information may be carried in the instructions that accompany the monoclonal reagent.

4. Test the rbcs with human anti-B serum acidified to pH 6.0. Acidified human anti-B reagents do not react with the acquired B receptor.[36]
5. If the patient is a secretor, test saliva for the presence of A and B substances. Patients whose rbcs carry acquired B structures will have A, but not B, substance in their saliva.
6. Treat the rbcs with acetic anhydride. A marked reduction in the reactivity of acquired B rbcs is seen after reacetylation of the B-like antigen by this reagent. Normal group B rbcs remain reactive following treatment while acquired B rbcs become nonreactive.[36(p167)]

Acquired A-Like Antigens

ABO discrepancies are sometimes associated with Tn polyagglutination.[19] Tn-activated rbcs have glycoproteins that carry abnormally formed oligosaccharides. Such structures appear when there is a genetic dysfunction in a hematopoietic stem cell resulting in a deficiency of a particular glycosyltransferase. When group O, Tn or group B, Tn rbcs are tested, they may behave as if they have acquired an A-like antigen reacting with human or monoclonal anti-A reagents. The A-like antigen of Tn rbcs can be differentiated from A arising through the action of an *A* gene transferase if rbcs are treated with proteolytic enzymes before testing. A-like antigens of Tn rbcs are destroyed by enzymes.

Other forms of polyagglutination may interfere in ABO grouping tests. These phenomena are described by Beck.[30] See Method 2.12 to classify polyagglutinable red cells using lectins.

Mixed-Field Agglutination

In some cases, samples are encountered that contain two distinct, separable populations of rbcs. Usually a mixture occurs because group O rbcs were transfused to a group A (or group B) patient. Rbc mixtures also occur in a condition called chimerism, resulting either from the intrauterine exchange of erythropoietic tissue by fraternal twins or from mosaicism arising through dispermy. Less frequently, it occurs when a patient has received a transplant of bone marrow that is of an ABO group different from the patient's own. In all such circumstances, rbc grouping tests may give a mixed-field pattern of agglutination. The mixed-field reactions due to transfusion last only for the life of the transfused rbcs. Mixed-field reactions that arise through chimerism persist throughout the life of the donor. In the case of bone marrow transplantation, the mixed-field reaction will usually disappear when the patient's own rbcs are no longer produced. However, many instances of persistent mixed cell populations have been reported following bone marrow transplantation. A description of procedures used to separate two dissimilar rbc populations due to chimerism or transfusion can be found in Beattie.[19]

Mixed-field agglutination is characteristically seen when A₃ rbcs are tested with anti-A. If the agglutinated rbcs are removed and the remaining rbcs again tested with anti-A, mixed-field agglutination occurs in the residual population as well. Mixed-field agglutination may also be seen with rbcs carrying A antigens weakened by diseases such as leukemia or with Tn rbcs.[30]

Antibody-Coated Red Blood Cells

Rbcs from infants with HDN, or from adults suffering from AIHA or HTRs may be heavily coated with IgG antibody molecules. Such rbcs often agglutinate spontaneously in the presence of high-protein diluents (18-22%) of some types of anti-D. In some cases, sensitization is such that the rbcs also agglutinate in low-protein (6-12%) ABO reagents. Gentle elution at 45 C (see Method 2.14 and Chapter 16) can be used to remove much of this antibody from the rbcs so they can then be tested reliably with anti-A and anti-B.

Rbcs coated heavily with IgM cold-reactive autoagglutinins will agglutinate spontaneously in saline tests. If the rbc suspension is incubated briefly at 37 C, then washed several times with saline warmed to 37 C, the antibodies can be eluted from the rbc membranes. If the IgM-related agglutination is not dispersed by this technique, the rbcs can be treated with the sulfhydryl compound dithiothreitol (DTT).[37] (See Method 2.13.)

Resolving discrepancies due to unexpected serum reactions. The following paragraphs describe those events that can lead to unexpected or erroneous serum grouping results and the steps that can be taken to resolve them.

1. Patients with immunodeficiency diseases such as agammaglobulinemia or hypogammaglobulinemia may not produce detectable levels of anti-A and anti-B. These antibodies are also absent from the sera of newborns and from many elderly patients.

2. Prozone reactions leading to false-negative results in serum tests have been associated with abnormally high concentrations of anti-A and anti-B. (See Judd et al.[34]) In these instances, the ABO group can be inferred by rbc tests, dilution of the serum or by the use of EDTA-treated serum.[36]

3. Anti-A_1 in the serum of persons of the A_2, A_2B or other subgroups may agglutinate A_1 reagent rbcs in serum grouping tests. To identify anti-A_1 as the cause of the discrepancy:

   a. Test the serum against several examples of group A_1, A_2 and O rbcs (preferably three of each). The antibody is anti-A_1 only if it agglutinates all A_1 rbcs but none of the A_2 or O rbc samples.

   b. Test the rbcs of the antibody producer with anti-A_1. Rbcs of the A_2 subgroup can be differentiated from A_1 rbcs by this lectin.

   Anti-A_1 can cause crossmatches with A_1 units to be incompatible. Most often, examples of this antibody react only at temperatures below 30 C, and are considered to be clinically insignificant. Some examples can be found, however, that react at 37 C. Antibodies active at this temperature should be considered clinically significant and only A_2 or O rbcs should be used for transfusion.

4. When cold-reactive autoagglutinins, such as autoanti-I, are of sufficient strength, they can agglutinate rbcs of all adults, including those used to prepare reagent rbcs. With few exceptions, agglutination caused by the cold-reactive agglutinin is weaker than that caused by anti-A and anti-B. The following can be done when the reactivity of the autoagglutinin interferes to the point that interpretation of serum grouping tests is difficult.

   a. Warm serum and reagent red cells to 37 C before mixing and testing. Read serum tests at 37 C and convert them to the antiglobulin phase. Note: Weakly reactive examples of anti-A or anti-B may not be detected by this method because 37 C is above the reactive optimum for these antibodies. Further, in patients other than those who are group O, ABO antibodies are predominantly of the IgM class. IgM antibodies will not be detected in routine antiglobulin tests since they employ anti-IgG reagents; thus, examples of anti-A and anti-B that contain little or no IgG can go undetected.

b. Adsorb the cold-reactive autoagglutinin from the serum using a cold autoadsorption method as described in Method 6.1. The adsorbed serum can then be tested against A_1 and B reagent rbcs.

c. Treat the serum with DTT and test the treated serum against A_1 and B reagent rbcs. Since DTT destroys the agglutinating activity of IgM antibodies, serum grouping tests that use DTT-treated serum must be converted to the AHG test where the presence of IgG forms of the antibodies might be detected. (See Method 4.4.) Since many group A or B persons do not produce more than minute quantities of IgG anti-A or anti-B, negative tests should be interpreted with caution.

5. Unexpected alloantibodies, such as anti-P_1 or anti-M, react at room temperature and may agglutinate the reagent rbcs used in serum grouping if they carry the corresponding antigen. In general, reagent rbcs used for antibody detection will also be agglutinated at room temperature. (Rarely, the serum may react with an antigen on the rbcs other than A and B that is not present on the antibody detection rbcs.) To determine the correct ABO group of sera containing other cold-reactive alloantibodies:

a. Identify the alloantibody, as described in Chapter 15.

b. Test the reagent A_1 and B rbcs to determine which reagent, if either, carries the corresponding antigen.

c. Test the serum against examples of A_1 and B rbcs that lack the corresponding antigen. For instance, if anti-M is identified, test the serum against A_1,M– and B,M– rbcs to resolve the discrepancy.

If the antibody detection test is negative, repeat serum ABO tests with several examples of A_1 and B rbcs. Since the antibody is directed against an antigen of low incidence, most randomly selected A_1 and B rbcs will lack the corresponding antigen.

6. Serum from patients with abnormally high concentrations of serum proteins, who have altered serum protein ratios or who have received plasma expanders of high molecular weight can cause reagent rbcs to appear agglutinated. Some of these samples cause rouleaux to occur. Rouleaux formation can be easily recognized microscopically if the rbcs aggregate in what has been described as a "stack of coins" formation. More often, such sera cause aggregates that appear as irregularly shaped clumps that closely resemble antibody-mediated agglutinates. The results of serum grouping tests can often be corrected if the following procedures are employed:

a. Dilute the serum to abolish the aggregating properties of the serum. Make a 1 in 4 dilution of the serum and test the dilution against autologous rbcs. If no aggregation is seen, then test the diluted serum against reagent rbcs. In most cases, but not all, anti-A and anti-B alloantibodies will react at this dilution.

b. Respin the serum-cell mixture when rouleaux formation is suspected. Remove the serum with a pipet and replace it with an equal volume of saline. Spin the serum-saline mixture, then resuspend the button. Rouleaux will disperse but true agglutination will remain.

The H System

As mentioned previously, the genes of the H system are *H* and *h*. *H* leads to the production of the H antigen that serves as the precursor molecule on which A and B antigens are built. The amount of H antigen is, in order of diminishing quantity, $O>A_2>B>A_2B>A_1>A_1B$.[18] H-like antigens are found in nature. Persons of the rare O_h phenotype, whose rbcs lack H, have (in addition to anti-A and anti-B) potent anti-H in their serum that is considered to be clinically significant.[38] Occasionally, group A_1, A_1B or (less commonly) B persons have so little unconverted H antigen on their rbcs that they may produce anti-H. In such situations the antibody is relatively weak and virtually always reacts at room temperature or below.

O_h Phenotype

The term "Bombay" has been used for the O_h phenotype because examples of such rbcs were first discovered in Bombay, India. The symbol O_h has been selected to denote the phenotype because results obtained in routine ABO grouping tests mimic those of group O persons. O_h rbcs are not agglutinated by anti-A, anti-B or anti-A,B. That a sample is O_h (and not group O) is generally not recognized until serum from the O_h person is tested against group O rbcs. Group O rbcs are agglutinated by O_h sera as strongly as A and B rbcs. The anti-H of O_h persons reacts well over a wide thermal range (from 4-37 C) with all rbcs except those of other O_h people. O_h patients must be transfused with only O_h blood because their anti-H rapidly destroys the H+ rbcs of the other ABO groups.[39] The O_h phenotype can be proven if the rbcs are tested with the anti-H lectin of *Ulex europeaus*. Anti-H lectin fails to agglutinate O_h rbcs, although it agglutinates group O rbcs quite strongly. Further confirmation testing can be performed if other examples of O_h rbcs are available. The serum of a suspected O_h person will be compatible only with the rbcs of other O_h persons.

Para-Bombay Phenotypes, A_h and B_h

A_h and B_h rbcs lack serologically detectable H antigen but carry small amounts of A or B, depending on the genotype of the individual. Weak reactions are obtained in grouping tests with anti-A or anti-B.[18,19] The rbcs are nonreactive with anti-H lectin or with the anti-H sera of O_h persons. The para-Bombay phenotype is thought to result from the inheritance of variant *H* genes that produce only minute amounts of H antigen. At the rbc level, all of the H is converted to A or B by the products of the *A* and *B* genes, respectively. The sera of A_h and B_h people contain anti-H in addition to the expected anti-A or anti-B.

The Lewis Antigens

The common Lewis antigens, Le^a and Le^b, are not intrinsic to rbcs, but are carried on plasma glycosphingolipids that are adsorbed from plasma to the rbc membranes. Their presence or absence in plasma and on rbcs is dependent, in part, on whether a person has inherited one *Le* or two *le* genes. The *Le* gene encodes a fucosyltransferase that adds Fuc in $\alpha(1\to4)$ linkage to the subterminal GlcNAc of Type 1 oligosaccharides.[18] (See Fig 10-2.) The resulting structure has Le^a activity. Persons who have inherited the dominant *Se* gene in addition to *Le* produce an antigen called Le^b. When Le^b is produced, it is adsorbed preferentially over Le^a to rbc membranes. Le^b is made when Type 1 chains are first modified into H by the *Se* gene transferase. The *Le* gene transferase then adds Fuc to this structure to form Le^b. The *le* gene is an amorph. Persons who have the genotype *lele* produce no Le^a and no Le^b antigens.

Table 10-4. Phenotypes and Frequencies in the Lewis System

Reactions With Anti-			Adult Phenotype Frequency %	
Le^a	Le^b	Phenotype	Whites	Blacks
+	0	Le(a+b−)	22	23
0	+	Le(a−b+)	72	55
0	0	Le(a−b−)	6	22
+	+	Le(a+b+)	rare	rare

Table 10-4 shows the Lewis phenotypes and their frequencies in the population. Rbcs that type as Le(a+b+) are only rarely found when human antisera are used in blood grouping. Such rbcs are seen more frequently when more potent monoclonal anti-Le^a and anti-Le^b reagents are used.[40,41]

Lewis Antibodies

Lewis antibodies occur almost exclusively in the sera of Le(a–b–) persons, and usually without known rbc stimulus. Persons whose rbc phenotype is Le(a–b+) do not make anti-Le^a because small amounts of unconverted Le^a are present in their saliva and plasma. It is unusual to find anti-Le^b in the serum of a Le(a+b−) person. Anti-Le^a and anti-Le^b may occur together in sera. They are composed mostly of IgM molecules and do not cross the placenta. Because of this, and because Lewis antigens are poorly developed at birth, the antibodies have not been implicated in HDN. Lewis antibodies may bind complement. Fresh sera that contain anti-Le^a (or infrequently anti-Le^b) may cause the in-vitro hemolysis of incompatible rbcs. In-vitro hemolysis is more often seen with enzyme-treated rbcs than with untreated rbcs.

Most Lewis antibodies agglutinate saline-suspended rbcs of the appropriate phenotype. The resulting agglutinates are often fragile and are easily dispersed if rbc buttons are not resuspended gently after centrifugation. Agglutination sometimes is seen after incubation at 37 C, but rarely of the strength seen in tests incubated at room temperature. Some examples of anti-Le^a, and less commonly anti-Le^b, can be detected in the antiglobulin phase of the IAT. In some cases this is due to complement bound by the antibody. Complement can be detected if polyspecific antiglobulin is used. In other cases, antiglobulin reactivity is due to an IgG component of the antibody.[4]

Sera with anti-Le^b activity can be divided into two categories. The most common examples react best with rbcs of group O and A$_2$ rbcs. These antibodies have been designated as anti-Le^{bH}. Those that react equally well with the Le^b antigen on rbcs of all ABO phenotypes are called anti-Le^{bL}. Anti-Le^{bH}, but not anti-Le^{bL}, is neutralized by saliva from group O, Le(a–b–) persons

Table 10-5. Serologic Behavior of the Principal Antibodies of the Lewis and P Blood Groups

Antibody	In-Vitro Hemolysis	Saline		Albumin		Enzyme		Associated With	
		4 C	22 C	37 C	AGT	37 C	AGT	HDN	HTR
anti-Le^a	some	most	most	some	many	most	most	no	few
anti-Le^b	rare	most	most	few	some	some	some	no	no
anti-P$_1$	occ.	most	some	occ.	rare	some	few	no	rare
anti-P	some	most	some	some	some	some	some	no	?
anti-P$_1$ + P + P^k	some	most	some	some	some	some	some	rare	?

who are secretors of H substance. Table 10-5 lists the serologic behavior of the common Lewis system antibodies.

Two other antibodies (anti-Le^c and -Le^d) have been given Lewis designations although in the case of two of these (anti-Le^c and -Le^d) the determinants with which they react are not the products of Lewis gene transferases. Anti-Le^c has been reported in one human subject as a cold-reactive agglutinin.[42] This antibody agglutinates the rbcs of Le(a–b–) persons who have the genotype *sese* and are therefore nonsecretors of H substance. The antibody called anti-Le^d agglutinates the rbcs of Le(a–b–) secretors. The product defined by anti-Le^d has been identified as the Type 1 oligosaccharide to which Fuc has been added at the H-active site. Anti-Le^d should more correctly be called anti-Type 1 H. The material that reacts with anti-Le^c seems to be the Type 1 chain with no added Fuc molecules. No examples of anti-Le^d have been found in humans but both anti-Le^c and anti-Le^d have been successfully produced in goats injected with saliva from Le(a–b–) nonsecretors and Le(a–b–) secretors of H, respectively.[43]

Transfusion Practice

Lewis antigens readily adsorb to and elute from rbc membranes. Transfused rbcs shed their Lewis antigens and assume the Lewis phenotype of the recipient within a few days of entering the circulation. Lewis antibodies in a recipient's serum are readily neutralized by Lewis blood group substance in donor plasma. For these reasons, it is exceedingly rare for Lewis antibodies to cause hemolysis of transfused Le(a+) or Le(b+) rbcs. However, antibodies that cause hemolysis in vitro or that give strong reactions in the IAT phase of the crossmatch have been as-

sociated with posttransfusion hemolysis.

It is not considered necessary to type donor blood for the presence or absence of Lewis antigens before transfusion or when crossmatching. Reactions obtained in the crossmatch with anti-Le^a or anti-Le^b provide a good index of transfusion safety.[44,45] Some workers have used plasma containing Lewis substances to neutralize Lewis antibodies in recipients before transfusing Lewis positive blood.[4] Such a practice should be avoided since it increases the risk of exposure to transfusion-transmitted infectious agents. Many transfusion specialists regularly give Le(a–b+) blood, compatible by routine crossmatch, to patients with anti-Le^a.

Lewis Antigens in Children

Rbcs from newborn infants usually fail to react with both human anti-Le^a and anti-Le^b and, thus, are considered to be Le(a–b–). Some can be shown to carry small amounts of Le^a when tested with potent monoclonal or goat anti-Le^a reagents.[22] Reliable Lewis grouping of young children may not be possible, as test reactions may not reflect the correct phenotype until approximately 6 years of age. Among children, the incidence of Le(a+) rbcs is high and that of Le(b+) rbcs low. The phenotype Le(a+b+) may be observed as a transient phase in children whose phenotypes as adults will be Le(a–b+).

Cord rbcs are agglutinated by anti-Le^x sera that agglutinate the Le(a+b–) and Le(a–b+), but not Le(a–b–), rbcs of adults.[46] In serologic tests, these sera behave as if they are inseparable forms of anti-Le^a and Le^b. They define a determinant that has been called Le^x, and that is present on the majority of cord rbcs and on the Le(a+) or Le(b+) rbcs of adults. Many serologists have suggested anti-Le^x

may represent a more potent or more avid form of anti-Le^a.

The I/i Antigens

The unexpected antibodies most frequently encountered when serologic tests are performed at room temperature are those directed at the I and i antigens. They reside in the subterminal portions of the oligosaccharides that eventually are converted to H and A or B antigens. I and i structures are found on membrane-associated glycoproteins and glycosphingolipids. The Type 1 and Type 2 oligosaccharide chains include multiple β-GlcNAc(1→3)β-Gal(1→4) units.[47] The i antigen appears when two of these disaccharide units are linked in a straight chain oligosaccharide. Many of these linear chains are modified on the rbcs of adults by the addition of branched structures consisting of β-Gal(1→4)β–GlcNAc linked in β(1→6) to a galactose internal to the repeating sequence. I specificity results when the branched structure appears. The heterogeneity that is observed in serologic tests with different anti-I sera may reflect the fact that different antibodies recognize different portions of the branched oligosaccharide chain. Fetal rbcs are rich in i antigen. They carry few branched oligosaccharides and, therefore, have a poorly developed I antigen. During the first 2 years of life, the I antigen gradually develops at the expense of i. The rbcs of most adults are strongly re-

active with anti-I and only weakly or nonreactive with anti-i. (See Table 10-6.) Rare adults have rbcs that are I–. They usually have anti-I as an alloantibody in their sera, but the antibodies may be so weak in some cases as to require enzyme techniques for their detection.

Antibodies to I/i

Anti-I is usually identified by its failure to react with rbcs from cord bloods or from I-negative adults. If tests are performed at 4 C, many I+ people can be shown to have autoanti-I in their sera. Anti-I is a common autoantibody, but it usually occurs as a cold-reactive agglutinin having a narrow thermal range and a low titer (less than 64 at 4 C). Anti-I assumes pathologic significance in cases of cold antibody (agglutinin) syndrome (CAS), in which it behaves as a complement-binding antibody with a high titer and wide thermal range. Autoanti-i is less often implicated in cases of CAS than anti-I. On rare occasions, anti-i may be seen as a relatively weak cold autoagglutinin reacting only at 4-10 C. Patients with infectious mononucleosis often have transient anti-i in their sera.

As an aid to the identification of these antibodies, Table 10-6 shows the relative amounts of I and i antigens on different human rbcs. Table 10-7 provides exam-

Table 10-6. Amounts of I/i Antigens on Different Human Red Cells

	Antigen	
Phenotype	I	i
I$_{adult}$	Much	Trace
I$_{cord}$	Little	Much
i$_{adult}$	Trace	Much

Table 10-7. Serologic Behavior of the I Blood Group Antibodies With Saline Red Cell Suspensions

		Anti-I	Anti-i
4 C	I$_{adult}$	4+	0−1+
	i$_{cord}$	0−2+	3+
	i$_{adult}$	0−1+	4+
22 C	I$_{adult}$	2+	0
	i$_{cord}$	0	2−3+
	i$_{adult}$	0	3+

ples that are meant to illustrate the serologic behavior of anti-I and anti-i at 4 C and 22 C. The strengths of reactions are purely relative and clear-cut differences in reactivity between the two are seen only with weaker examples of the antibodies. Titration studies may be needed to differentiate strong examples of the antibodies.

In some cases, positive reactions are obtained by the IAT with sera containing anti-I or anti-i. Rarely do these reactions indicate that the antibodies are reactive at 37 C. Most often these reactions occur because the antibodies bind complement during incubation. The complement remains bound to rbc surfaces although the activating antibody dissociates when the tests are incubated at 37 C. The problem can usually be avoided by either warming the serum and rbcs to 37 C before mixing them together and performing all phases of the IAT, including centrifugation and washing, at 37 C; or deleting the low ionic potentiator (if used) and substituting anti-IgG in place of polyspecific antihuman globulin.

Complex Reactivity

Antibodies such as anti-IH and anti-IP$_1$ probably recognize branched oligosaccharides that have been further modified by transferases for H and P$_1$, respectively. Anti-IH occurs quite commonly in the sera of A$_1$ people and, as would be expected, reacts quite strongly with rbcs that are strongly H+ as well as I+. A clue to the identity of anti-IH may be the observation that antibody detection tests performed with adult group O rbcs show agglutination, but crossmatches with A$_1$ rbcs or cold O rbcs are uniformly negative or only weakly reactive. Rbcs of group A$_1$, although I+, react poorly with anti-IH because their H antigen is weak. Anti-IH fails to react, or does so only poorly, with group O rbcs from cord blood or from adults of the i phenotype because, although the H antigen is present, I antigen is either absent or weak. Beck[48] provides additional discussion of I blood group antigens and antibodies.

The P Blood Group

The first antigen of the P blood group was discovered by Landsteiner and Levine in 1927, in the series of animal experiments that led also to the discovery of M and N. Originally called P, the name of the antigen was later changed to P$_1$. The designation P has since been reassigned to an antigen present on almost all human rbcs. The International Society for Blood Transfusion has recently made an effort to classify P antigens in a logical manner. (See Table 10-8.) The P blood group system has been renamed P1. The definitive antigen in this system is P$_1$. P, P^k and Luke (LKE) antigens have been assigned to the globoside collection of antigens. Another antigen, p, has

Table 10-8. Phenotypes and Frequencies in the P Blood Group

| | Reactions With Anti- | | | | Phenotype Frequency % | |
P$_1$	P	P^k	PP$_1$P^k	Phenotype	Whites	Blacks
+	+	0	+	P$_1$	79	94
0	+	0	+	P$_2$	21	6
0	0*	0	0	p		
+	0	+	+	P$_1^k$	All extremely rare	
0	0	+	+	P$_2^k$		

*Usually negative, occasionally weakly positive.

not yet been assigned to a system.[49,50] Rbcs lacking P_1, but shown to possess P, are of the P_2 phenotype. P_1 is present on the rbcs of approximately 80% of Whites and 94% of Blacks. Another antigen of this system is P^k.

P blood group antigens are built through the addition of sugars to precursor glycosphingolipids, a process thought to be analogous to the development of the A, B and H antigens. P^k determinants are formed when Gal is added in $\alpha(1{\to}4)$ linkage to the terminal Gal residues of lactosylceramide (also called ceramide dihexoside or CDH).[51] Subsequently, this structure can be converted to P antigen (globoside) by the addition of GalNAc. Neither P^k nor P serve as substrate for P_1. Instead, Gal is added in $\alpha(1{\to}4)$ linkage to a different structure called paragloboside to form P_1. Paragloboside is the precursor on which cellular A, B, H, I and i antigens are also found. By adding NeuNAc to the terminal galactose in $\alpha(2{\to}3)$, the p antigen results. It is thought the gene specifying the responsible transferase is independent of the P system. The biochemical structures of the P blood groups, compiled by Anstall and Blaycock,[50] are shown in Fig 10-5.

Rare Phenotypes

Several rare phenotypes are associated with the P blood groups and these are shown in Table 10-8. The P^k phenotype occurs when the P^k antigen is not converted to P. Persons whose rbcs have P^k instead of P consistently make a strong alloanti-P that reacts in tests with P_1+P+ (P_1 phenotype) and P_1–P+ (P_2 phenotype) rbcs. The biphasic hemolysin of paroxysmal cold hemoglobinuria (PCH) is often, but not always, of this specificity. Unlike the IgM anti-P of P^k persons, the autoanti-P found in people with PCH is IgG in nature.

Very rare people lack P_1, P and P^k. Their rbcs are said to be of the p phenotype. Characteristically, a potent hemolytic IgM antibody with anti-P_1+P+P^k specificity is found in their serum. The antibody, formerly called anti-Tj[a], has caused HTRs and, occasionally, HDN. There is a curious association between anti-P_1+P+P^k and abortions occurring early in pregnancy in p women.[52,53] Race and Sanger[21] cite an accumulation of data to support the association, although it is not clear that the maternal antibody, itself, causes early fetal death.

Anti-P_1

The sera of P_2 persons commonly contain anti-P_1. In fact, if sufficiently sensitive techniques are applied, it is likely that anti-P_1 would be detected in the serum of virtually every P_2 person. The antibody reacts optimally at 4 C but may occasionally be detected at 37 C. As anti-P_1 is nearly always IgM, it does not cross the placenta and has not been reported to cause HDN. Anti-P_1 has rarely been reported to cause hemolysis in vivo.[54]

The strength of the P_1 antigen varies among different rbc samples, and antigen strength has been reported to diminish when rbcs are stored.[4,19] These characteristics sometimes create difficulties, both in testing rbcs for the antigen and in the identification of the antibody. Anti-P_1 blood typing reagents are usually sufficiently potent to detect weak forms of the antigen. An antibody that is weakly reactive on room temperature testing can often be shown to have anti-P_1 specificity by lower incubation temperatures or using enzyme-treated rbcs. Hydatid cyst fluid or P_1 substance derived from pigeon eggs inhibits the activity of anti-P_1. Inhibition may be a useful aid to the identification of anti-P_1, especially if the antibody is present in a serum with antibodies of other specificities.

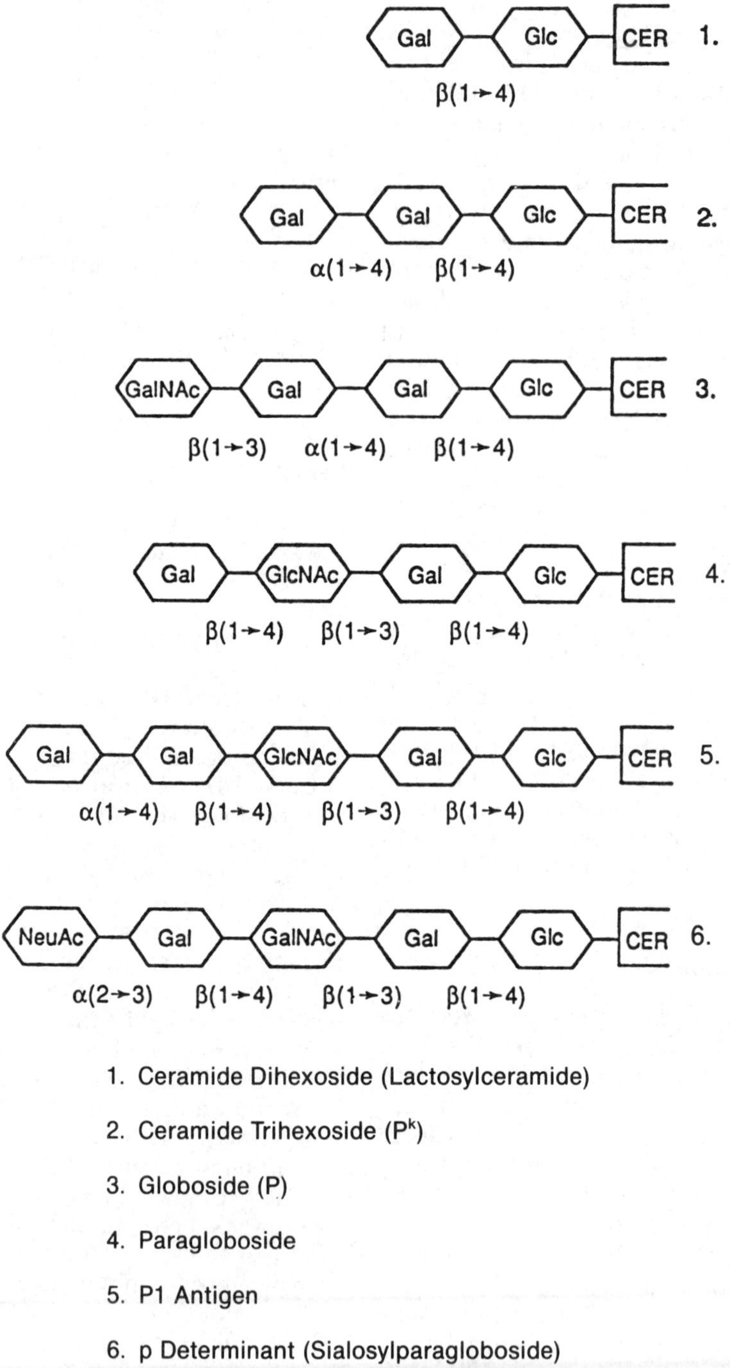
Gal
Glc
CER
1.
β(1→4)
Gal
Gal
Glc
CER
2.
α(1→4)
β(1→4)
GalNAc
Gal
Gal
Glc
CER
3.
β(1→3)
α(1→4)
β(1→4)
Gal
GlcNAc
Gal
Glc
CER
4.
β(1→4)
β(1→3)
β(1→4)
Gal
Gal
GlcNAc
Gal
Glc
CER
5.
α(1→4)
β(1→4)
β(1→3)
β(1→4)
NeuAc
Gal
GalNAc
Gal
Glc
CER
6.
α(2→3)
β(1→4)
β(1→3)
β(1→4)
1. Ceramide Dihexoside (Lactosylceramide)
2. Ceramide Trihexoside (P^k)
3. Globoside (P)
4. Paragloboside
5. P1 Antigen
6. p Determinant (Sialosylparagloboside)

Figure 10-5. Biochemical structures of P antigens (adapted from Anstall and Blaycock[50]).

References

1. Watkins WM, Morgan WTJ. Possible genetical pathway for the biosynthesis of blood group mucopolysaccharides. Vox Sang 1959;4:97-119.
2. Steane S. Proteins, lipids, carbohydrates and nucleic acids. In: Pierce S, Steane S, eds. Biochemistry for blood bankers: Selected topics. Arlington, VA: American Association of Blood Banks, 1983:43-66.
3. Mourant AE, Kopec AC, Domaniewska-Scoczak K. The distribution of the human blood groups and other polymorphisms. 2nd ed. London: Oxford University Press, 1976.
4. Mollison PL, Engelfriet CP, Contreras M. Blood transfusion in clinical medicine. 9th ed. Oxford: Blackwell Scientific Publications, 1993.
5. Watkins WM. The glycosyltransferase products of the A, B, H and Le genes and their relationship to the structure of the blood group antigens. In: Mohn JF, Plunkett RW, Cunningham RK, Lambert RM, eds. Human blood groups. Basel: Karger, 1977:134-42.
6. Larsen RD, Enst LK, Nair RP, Low JB. Molecular cloning sequence, and expression of a human GDP-L-fucose: β-D-galactose 2-α-L-fucosyltransferase cDNA that can form the H blood group antigen. Proc Natl Acad Sci USA 1990;87:6674-8.
7. Oriol R, Danilovs J, Hawkins BR. A new genetic model proposing that the Se gene is a structural gene closely linked to the H gene. Am J Hum Genet 1981;33:421-31.
8. Mulet C, Cartron JP, Badet J, Salmon C. Activity of α-2-L-fucosyltransferase in human sera and red cell membranes. A study of common ABH blood donors, rare "Bombay" and "Parabombay" individuals. FEBS Lett 1977;84:74.
9. Hakomori SI. Blood group ABH and Ii antigens of human erythrocytes: Chemistry, polymorphism and their developmental change. Semin Hematol 1981;18:39-47.
10. Watkins WM, Greenwell P, Yates AD, Johnson PH. Regulation of expression of carbohydrate blood group antigens. Biochimie 1988;70; 1597-611.
11. Clausen H, Hakomori S. ABH and related histo-blood group antigens; immunochemical differences in carrier isotypes and their distribution. Vox Sang 1989;56:1-20.
12. Anstee DJ. Blood-group active surface molecules of the human red blood cell. Vox Sang 1990;58:1-20.
13. Bermeman Z, van Bockstaele DR, Uyttenbroeck WM, et al. Flow cytometric analysis of erythrocyte blood group A antigen density profiles. Vox Sang 1991;61:265-74.
14. Clausen H, Levery SB, Nudelman E, et al. Repetitive A epitope (type 3 chain A) defined by group A1-specific monoclonal antibody TH-1: Chemical basis of qualitative A1 and A2 distinction. Proc Natl Acad Sci USA 1985;82:1199-203.
15. Goldstein J. Conversion of ABO blood groups. Transfus Med Rev 1989;3:206-12.
16. Yamamoto F, Clausen H, White T, et al. Molecular genetic basis of the histo-blood group ABO system. Nature 1990;345:229-32.
17. Yamamoto F, Hakomori S. Sugar-nucleotide donor specificity of histo-blood group A and B transferases is based on amino acid substitutions. J Biol Chem 1990;265:19257-62.
18. Salmon C, Cartron JP, Rouger P. The human blood groups. New York: Masson Publishing, USA, 1984.
19. Beattie KM. Discrepancies in ABO grouping. In: A seminar on problems encountered in pretransfusion tests. Washington, DC: American Association of Blood Banks, 1972:129-65.
20. Grundbacher FJ. Changes in the human A antigen of erythrocytes with the individual's age. Nature 1964;204:192-4.
21. Race RR, Sanger R. Blood groups in man. 6th ed. Oxford: Blackwell Scientific Publications, 1975.
22. Rolih SD. New frontiers in serologic testing. In: Wallas CH, McCarthy LJ, eds. New frontiers in blood banking. Arlington, VA: American Association of Blood Banks, 1986:127-33.
23. Toivanen P, Hirvonen T. Iso- and heteroagglutinins in human fetal and neonatal sera. Scand J Haematol 1969;6:42-8.
24. Code of federal regulations. Title 21 CFR, part 660.26. Washington, DC: US Government Printing Office, 1992. (Revised annually.)
25. Widmann FK, ed. Standards for blood banks and transfusion services. 15th ed. Bethesda, MD: American Association of Blood Banks, 1993.
26. Yates AD, Feeney J, Donald ASR, Watkins WM. Characterisation of a blood group A-active tetrasaccharide synthesized by a blood-group B-gene-specified glycosyltransferase. Carborhydr Res 1984;130:251-60.
27. Beck ML, Yates AD, Hardman J, Kowalski MA. Identification of a subset of group B donors reactive with monoclonal anti-A reagent. Am J Clin Pathol 1989;92:625-9.
28. Judd WJ, Butch SH. Streamlining serological testing. In: Smith DM, Judd WJ, eds. Blood banking in a changing environment. Arlington, VA: American Association of Blood Banks, 1984:15-39.
29. Moulds JM. Polyagglutination: Overview and resolution. In: Beck ML, Judd WJ, eds. Polyagglutination. Washington, DC: American Association of Blood Banks, 1980:1-22.
30. Beck ML. Blood group antigens acquired de novo. In: Garratty G, ed. Blood group antigens

and disease. Arlington, VA: American Association of Blood Banks, 1983:45-66.

31. Judd WJ. Microbial-associated forms of polyagglutination (T, Tk and acquired B). In: Beck ML, Judd WJ, eds. Polyagglutination. Washington, DC: American Association of Blood Banks, 1980:23-54.

32. Barber M, Dunsford I. Excess blood-group substance A in serum of patient dying with carcinoma of stomach. Br Med J 1959;1:607.

33. Pierce S. Anomalous blood bank results. In: Trouble-shooting the crossmatch. Washington, DC: American Association of Blood Banks, 1977: 85-114.

34. Judd WJ, Steiner EA, Oberman HJ. Reverse and typing errors due to prozone: How safe is the immediate spin crossmatch? (abstract). Transfusion 1987;27:527.

35. Beck ML, Kowalski MA, Kirkegaard JR, Korth JL. Unexpected activity with monoclonal anti-B reagents. Immunohematology 1992;8:22-3.

36. Judd WJ. Methods in immunohematology. Miami, FL: Montgomery Scientific Publications, 1988.

37. Reid M. Autoagglutination dispersal utilizing sulphydryl compounds. Transfusion 1978;18: 353-5.

38. Bhatia HM, Sathe MS. Incidence of "Bombay" (O_h) phenotype and weaker variants of A and B antigens in Bombay (India). Vox Sang 1974; 27:524-32.

39. Davey RJ, Touralt MA, Holland PV. The clinical significance of anti-H in an individual with the Oh (Bombay) phenotype. Transfusion 1978; 18:738-42.

40. Messeter L, Brodin T, Chester MA, et al. Immunochemical characterization of a monoclonal anti-Le[b] grouping reagent. Vox Sang 1984; 46:66-74.

41. Longworth C, Rolih S, Moheng M, et al. Mouse monoclonal anti-Le[a] and anti-Le[b] as routine grouping reagents (abstract). Transfusion 1985; 25:446.

42. Gunson HH, Latham V. An agglutinin in human serum reacting with cells from Le(a–b–) nonsecretor individuals. Vox Sang 1972; 22:344-53.

43. Potapov MI. Production of immune anti-Lewis sera in goats. Vox Sang 1972;30:211-3.

44. Waheed A, Kennedy MS, Gerhan S. Transfusion significance of Lewis system antibodies: Report on a nationwide survey. Transfusion 1981;21:542-5.

45. Issitt PD. Antibodies reactive at 30 C, room temperature and below. In: Clinically significant and insignificant antibodies. Washington, DC: American Association of Blood Banks, 1979:13-28.

46. Arcilla MC, Sturgeon P. Le[x], the spurned antigen of the Lewis blood group system. Vox Sang 1974;26:425-38.

47. Feizi T. The blood group Ii system: A carbohydrate antigen system defined by naturally monoclonal or oligoclonal autoantibodies of man. Immunol Commun 1981;10:127-56.

48. Beck ML. The I blood group collection. In: Moulds JM, Woods LL, eds. Blood groups: P, I, Sd[a] and Pr. Arlington, VA: American Association of Blood Banks, 1991:23-52.

49. Lewis M, Anstee DA, Bird GWG, et al. Blood group terminology 1990. From the ISBT working party on terminology for red cell surface antigens. Vox Sang 1990;58:154-69.

50. Anstall HB, Blaycock RC. The P blood group system: Biochemistry, genetics and clinical significance. In: Moulds JM, Woods LL, eds. Blood groups: P, I, Sd[a] and Pr. Arlington, VA: American Association of Blood Banks, 1991:1-19.

51. Naiki M, Marcus DM. An immunochemical study of human blood group P_1, P and P[k] glycosphingolipid antigens. Biochemistry 1975;14:4837-41.

52. Levene C, Sela R, Rudolphson Y, et al. Hemolytic disease of the newborn due to anti-PP_1P[k] (anti-Tj[a]). Transfusion 1977;17:569-72.

53. Levine P. Comments on hemolytic disease of the newborn due to anti-PP_1P[k] (anti-Tj[a]). Transfusion 1977;17:573.

54. Chandeysson PL, Flyte MW, Simpkins SM, Holland PV. Delayed hemolytic transfusion reaction caused by anti-P_1 antibody. Transfusion 1981;21:77-82.

11

Rh and LW Blood Groups

Introduction

The Rh system is complex, and certain aspects of its genetics, nomenclature and antigenic interactions are unsettled. The aim in this chapter will be to concentrate on commonly encountered observations, problems and solutions, without exhaustive theoretical considerations. More information can be found in the literature listed at the end of this chapter.

Rh Positive and Rh Negative

The unmodified descriptive terms Rh+ and Rh− refer to presence or absence of the red cell antigen D. An earlier name for D, Rh_0, has fallen largely into disuse, but remains of historical interest. To minimize confusion, the CDE nomenclature of Fisher and Race is used almost exclusively in this chapter, but sometimes it is necessary to use a combination of CDE and the Rh-Hr terminology of Wiener to facilitate understanding. Table 11-1 gives the equivalent names and may be used when needed for reference.

Discovery of D

The first human example of the antibody directed at the D antigen was reported in 1939 by Levine and Stetson,[5] who found it in the serum of a woman whose fetus had fatal hemolytic disease of the newborn. In 1940, by immunizing guinea pigs and rabbits with the rbcs of Rhesus monkeys, Landsteiner and Wiener[6] raised an antibody that agglutinated the rbcs of approximately 85% of humans tested. They called the corresponding determinant the *Rh factor*.

The clinical importance of the Rh factor was recognized the same year, when Levine and Katzin[7] found several postpartum women whose sera contained similar antibodies, at least one of which gave reactions that were parallel to those of the animal anti-Rhesus sera. Also in 1940, Wiener and Peters[8] observed examples of human anti-Rh in Rh− patients who had received ABO-compatible transfusions of Rh+ blood. Later evidence established that the antigen detected by animal anti-Rhesus and human anti-D are not identical, but by that time the Rh blood group system had already received its name.

Clinical Significance

The D antigen is, after A and B, the most important rbc antigen in transfusion practice. Persons whose rbcs lack the D antigen do not regularly have anti-D in their serum. Formation of the antibody almost always results from exposure, through either transfusion or pregnancy, to rbcs possessing the D antigen. A high proportion of D− subjects so exposed will produce anti-D. The immunogenicity of D (ie, the likelihood of its provoking an antibody if introduced into a D− recipient) is greater

Table 11-1. Equivalent Notations in the Rh Blood Group System

Numerical Designation	CDE	Rh-Hr	Other	Numerical Designation	CDE	Rh-Hr	Other
Rh1	D	Rh_0		Rh26	"c-like"		Deal
Rh2	C	rh'		Rh27	cE	rh*	
Rh3	E	rh"		Rh28		hr^H	Hernandez
Rh4	c	hr'		Rh29			total Rh
Rh5	e	hr"		Rh30	D^{Cor}		Go^a
Rh6	ce,(f)	hr		Rh31		hr^B	
Rh7	Ce	rh_i		Rh32‡			Troll
Rh8	C^w	rh^{w1}		Rh33			
Rh9	C^x	rh^x		Rh34		Hr^B	Bastiaan
Rh10	ce^s	hr^v	V	Rh35			1114
Rh11	E^w	rh^{w2}		Rh36			Be^a
Rh12	G	rh^G		Rh37			Evans§
Rh13	†	Rh^A		Rh39	"C-like"		
Rh14	†	Rh^B		Rh40			Targett (Tar)
Rh15	†	Rh^C		Rh41	"Ce-like"		
Rh16	†	Rh^D		Rh42	Ce^s	rh^s	Thornton
Rh17		Hr_0		Rh43			Crawford
Rh18		Hr		Rh44			Nou
Rh19		hr^s		Rh45			Riv
Rh20	e^s		VS	Rh46			Sec
Rh21	C^G			Rh47			Dav
Rh22	CE	rh*	Jarvis	Rh48			JAL
Rh23	D^w		Wiel				
Rh24	E^T						

The table is compiled from the findings of the ISBT Working Party on Terminology for Red Cell Surface Antigens[1,2]
*The Rh-Hr designations for Rh22 and Rh27 were the subject of a personal communication from Dr. A.S. Wiener (1972).
†Categories I through VII of Tippett and Sanger[3,4] include these subdivisions of the D antigen, but the notations are not directly comparable.
‡Rh32 is a low-incidence antigen that is a product of the predominantly Black gene $\overline{R}^N$, the other products of which include a reduced expression of C and e. The antibody that defines Rh32 should never be called "anti-$\overline{R}^N$."
§Rh37 is the low-incidence antigen Evans, which occurs in association with the · D · haplotype. This is similar to –D–, except for the presence of the Evans antigen and a lesser exaltation of D activity.
Rh25 and Rh38 are no longer used. LW and Duclos are antigens produced by genes independent of Rh. The antigens are associated with Rh only at the phenotypic level.

than that of virtually all other rbc antigens studied with the exception of A and B. It has been reported that the majority (>80%) of D– persons who receive a single unit of D+ blood can be expected to develop anti-D.[9,10] Accordingly, the blood of all recipients and donors is routinely tested for D, so that D– recipients can be identified and given D– blood.

Soon after anti-D was discovered, family studies showed that the D antigen is genetically determined, and that the gene controlling its production is an autosomal dominant. The *Rh* genes have been shown to reside on chromosome 1.[11-13] With only a few interesting exceptions, persons who have the gene for D will have the antigen detectable on their rbcs.

Other Important Antigens

More frequent and sophisticated pretransfusion testing, as well as investigations of transfusion reactions, soon revealed antibodies that identified antigens showing an association with D. By the mid-1940's, four additional antigens had been recognized as belonging to what is now called the Rh system[14-17]; subsequent new discoveries have brought the total of Rh-related antigens to nearly 50 (Table 11-1). The reader should be aware that these exist, but the five principal antigens (D, C, E, c, e) and their specific antibodies are likely to account for more than 99% of clinical problems with respect to Rh.

After D, the next four antigens to be recognized were C, E, c and e. The association of these antigenic factors suggests that immunologic activity of Rh arises from surface material with several determinant areas. Some antigenic associations include D and some do not. Combinations that do not include D nevertheless possess activity at other sites. The composition of these antigenic configurations is genetically determined. In terms of the five main antigens under discussion, a single gene (or gene complex) will determine the production or nonproduction of D, together with the production of either C or c and E or e. Many variations or combinations have been recognized and investigated, but these five antigens and the comparatively common antibodies that characterize them are the backbone of the Rh blood group system.

Inheritance and Nomenclature

Genes and Dosage

The genes that determine the Rh antigens are transmitted as discrete units (Wiener) or as haplotypes (Fisher and Race). It is convenient to think of an Rh haplotype as a single "gene" composed of nucleotide sequences within the gene that encode multiple individual epitopes. A person can be thought of as inheriting one *Rh* gene from each parent. If these are identical the individual is homozygous for that gene and all the products of the gene will be expressed in double dose on that person's rbcs. When the genes inherited from each parent are not identical, the person is heterozygous for two different genes and, since the *Rh* genes are codominant, the products of both will be expressed on that person's rbcs. Antigens that are products of genes from both parents will be present in double dose, while those produced by only one of the pair of genes will be present in single dose. In this context, the terms *homozygous* and *heterozygous* may be used in reference to an imagined sublocus. Thus, to be "homozygous for *D*" means that the person's two *Rh* genes both code for the production of D, not necessarily that both *Rh* genes are the same.

Recent studies have suggested the presence of two *Rh* genes per haploid genome at the Rh locus of D+, but not D– persons. For further discussion of recent findings see Biochemical Considerations.

Serologic Reactivity

Testing rbcs with specific Rh antibodies gives reaction patterns that do not consistently parallel antigen dose. This is due to variables in concentration of the test rbcs and the fact that the expression of the antigens is sometimes influenced by interaction between the two encoding genes, or interaction between subloci of the same gene. This subject is treated in greater detail in Chapter 9.

Since attempts to isolate the Rh antigens for chemical study have met with only limited success, it is not yet clear how genetic information is translated into serologically demonstrable characteristics. Several models have been proposed to explain the production of Rh antigens. Rosenfeld et al[18] described a genetic model that consisted of four sets of operator and structural genes. Production of the Rh antigens, encoded by the structural genes, is directly influenced by the operator genes. A different hypothesis, put forth by Giorno,[19] suggests that Rh antigen production is influenced by discontinuous genes consisting of introns (noncoding gene segments) and exons (coding) gene segments. Tippett[20] has proposed yet another model that takes into consideration known Rh biochemical data. Tippett's hypothesis is that the presence or absence of Rh antigens is determined by the alleles residing at two structural loci, called D and $CcEe$. The reader who is interested in further details on these proposed pathways should consult the reviews by Wilkinson[21] and Issitt.[22]

Terminology

Three systems of nomenclature have been used to express genetic and serologic information about the Rh system.

System Notations

The Rh-Hr terminology derives from the work of Wiener,[23] who believed that the immediate gene product is a single entity he called an *agglutinogen*. According to Wiener's concept, each agglutinogen is characterized by numerous individual serologic specificities called *factors*, each of which is recognized by its own specific antibody. What Wiener called *factors* are now called epitopes.

CDE terminology was introduced by British workers Fisher and Race,[24] who postulated three closely linked loci. The same letter designation is used for both gene and gene product, except that, by convention, the symbols for genes are always printed in italics.

Rosenfield and coworkers[18,25] proposed a system of nomenclature based simply on serologic observations. The symbols were not intended to convey genetic information, but merely to facilitate the recording of phenotypic data. Antigens are numbered, generally in order of their discovery or of their assignment to the Rh system, and their presence on the rbcs is designated by the use of the appropriate numbers following the prefix Rh and a colon. A negative symbol preceding a number indicates the absence of that antigen.

It is useful to be familiar with both the CDE and Rh-Hr nomenclatures, and it may be helpful to have some knowledge of the numerical system listed in Table 11-1. Table 11-2 shows the most

Table 11-2. Frequencies of the Principal Rh Genes (or Gene Complexes)

Haplotype	Fisher-Race Terminology Gene Combination	Antigenic Specificities	Frequency in US Population Whites	Blacks	Native Americans	Orientals
R^1	CDe	C,D,e	0.42	0.17	0.44	0.70
r	cde	c,e	0.37	0.26	0.11	0.03
R^2	cDE	c,D,E	0.14	0.11	0.34	0.21
R^o	cDe	c,D,e	0.04	0.44	0.02	0.03
r′	Cde	C,e	0.02	0.02	0.02	0.02
r″	cdE	c,E	0.01	0.00	0.06	0.00
R^z	CDE	C,D,E	0.00	0.00	0.06	0.01
r^y	CdE	C,E	0.00	0.00	0.00	0.00

All figures were calculated from Mourant et al[26] and represent averages of several series in each case. Those for Native Americans are averaged from a total of 15 series and, in view of large regional variations, may be misleading.

common combinations of antigens determined by allelic gene complexes. Table 11-3 shows the reaction patterns of various rbcs tested with antibodies to the five principal antigens, together with the descriptive terms used for phenotype in three systems of nomenclature.

Phenotypic Notations

For informal designation of phenotype, particularly in conversation, many workers use a shorthand system based on Wiener's Rh-Hr notations and used by the English in the 1940's. These do not fit into any nomenclature, but they convey information in a convenient and efficient fashion. In Wiener's terminology, genes were designated by single italic letters: R for genes that include $Rh_o(D)$ among their products and r for genes that do not encode D, with various superscript symbols (R^1, R^2, R^o, R^z, r', r'', r and r^y) to denote the different alleles. The gene products were designated by Roman type Rh and rh with subscripts to indicate the haplotype from which they evolved. Again, a capital letter R was used when the gene

product included $Rh_o(D)$. The symbols for individual antigens were Roman characters in boldface type, with **Rh_o** representing D and **rh′**, **rh″**, **hr′** and **hr″** representing C, E, c and e, respectively.

The shorthand phenotype notations employ single letters R and r in Roman type (for the haplotype producing or not producing D, respectively), with subscripts, or occasionally superscripts, to indicate antigenic combinations. These subscripts are based approximately on the notations shown in the first column of Table 11-2. Thus R_1 indicates C, D and e together; R_2 indicates c, D and E; r indicates c and e; R_o indicates c, D and e; and so on. In Table 11-3, the shorthand notations for the first six phenotypes would be R_1r, R_1, R_1R_2, R_o, R_2r and R_2.

Phenotype and Genotype

In clinical practice, five blood typing reagents are readily available (anti-D, -C, -E, -c and -e). Routine pretransfusion studies include only tests for D. Other reagents are used principally in the resolution of antibody problems or in fam-

Table 11-3. Determination of Some Rh Phenotypes From the Results of Tests With the Five Principal Rh Blood Typing Reagents

		Reagent			Phenotypes in Three Nomenclatures		
Anti-D	Anti-C	Anti-E	Anti-c	Anti-e	Rh-hr*	CDE	Numerical
+	+	0	+	+	R_1r	CcDe	Rh:1,2,$-$3,4,5
+	+	0	0	+	R_1	CDe	Rh:1,2,$-$3,$-$4,5
+	+	+	+	+	R_1R_2	CcDEe	Rh:1,2,3,4,5
+	0	0	+	+	R_0	cDe	Rh:1,$-$2,$-$3,4,5
+	0	+	+	+	R_2r	cDEe	Rh:1,$-$2,3,4,5
+	0	+	+	0	R_2	cDE	Rh:1,$-$2,3,4,$-$5
+	+	+	0	+	R_zR_1	CDEe	Rh:1,2,3,$-$4,5
+	+	+	+	0	R_zR_2	CcDE	Rh:1,2,3,4,$-$5
+	+	+	0	0	R_z	CDE	Rh:1,2,3,$-$4,$-$5
0	0	0	+	+	r	ce	Rh:$-$1,$-$2,$-$3,4,5
0	+	0	+	+	$r'r$	Cce	Rh:$-$1,2,$-$3,4,5
0	0	+	+	+	$r''r$	cEe	Rh:$-$1,$-$2,3,4,5
0	+	+	+	+	$r'r''$	CcEe	Rh:$-$1,2,3,4,5

*Shorthand terminology

ily studies. The assortment of antigens detected on a person's rbcs constitutes that person's Rh phenotype. Since any one antigen may derive from any of several different haploid genomes, identifying antigens does not always allow deduction of genotype with certainty. Presumptions regarding the most probable genotype rest on knowledge of the frequency with which particular antigenic combinations derive from a single haploid genome complex. Inferences about genotype are useful in population studies and in the investigation of disputed parentage. Such analyses are also used to predict whether the sexual partner of a woman with Rh antibodies is likely to transmit the genes that will result in offspring negative for the particular antigen.

Unique Problem of D

In order to determine whether a person has genes that encode C, c, E and e, test the rbcs for the presence of each of these antigens. If the rbcs test positive for C and c or E and e, it can be assumed that they are from a person who possesses the corresponding genes. If the rbcs carry only C or c, or only E or e, it is most likely that the person is homozygous. This can sometimes be proved in titration studies because the amount of antigen on the rbcs of homozygotes is greater than when only a single copy of the gene exists (a characteristic referred to as dosage). Tests for the D antigen can only be used to determine its presence or absence. If D is absent, it is normally correct to assume that the person tested possesses two genes that code for membrane structures lacking D. If D is present there is no simple serologic technique to establish whether two genes are present that code for D, or whether the antigenic material is the product of only one such gene. No antibody has been found that

reacts specifically with a product common to all genes that code for haplotypes lacking D, and dosage studies utilizing titrations of anti-D do not give reliable information.

Position Effect

Position effect reflects interaction between genes. If the interaction is between genes on the same chromosome, or between their products, it is called a "*cis* effect." If a gene or its product interacts with one on the opposite chromosome, it is called a "*trans* effect." Examples of both effects were first reported in 1950 by Lawler and Race,[27] who noted as a *cis* effect that the E antigen produced by the *cDE* (R^2) gene is quantitatively weaker than E produced by *cdE* (r''). They noted as *trans* effects that both C and E are weaker when they result from the genotype CDe/cDE (R^1R^2) than when the genotypes are *CDe/cde* (R^1r) or *cDE/cde* (R^2r), respectively.

Homozygous and Heterozygous Expression of D

All D− persons lack the gene that encodes D. Most D− persons are homozygous for the gene *r*, which produces c and e. Less often, a person who lacks the *D* gene may have a gene that produces C or E, described as *r'* and *r''*, respectively. The gene that produces both C and E (r^y) is quite rare. In any event, the determination of genotype is relatively simple when the rbcs are D−. In the case of D+ blood, however, the determination of genotype is considerably more difficult. Since there is no consistently reliable serologic method to distinguish between rbcs with D antigen resulting from one gene and those that have D as a product of two genes, a person whose rbcs are D+ can be assigned a genotype only by inference from the frequencies with which the individual Rh haploid gene complexes occur in the population (see Table 11-2). Differences in strength of reactions among D+ persons have been noted but they are not due to the zygosity of D. Such differences are due to other factors that may include rbc concentration or whether the rbcs are R_1, R_2, R_0, etc. R_2 rbcs tend to react more strongly with anti-D than rbcs of other common Rh phenotypes.

Effect of Race

A person whose rbcs are of the phenotype CDe is most likely to have the genotype R^1R^1 (*CDe/CDe*), in which case a gene encoding D will be passed to all offspring. A less likely alternative, since the haplotype r' is infrequent in most populations, is that the person's genotype is R^1r' (*CDe/Cde*). The racial origin of the person concerned should influence deductions about genotype because the frequencies of *Rh* genes differ by race. For example, a White person with the phenotype cDe would probably be R^0r (*cDe/cde*) because r is much more common than R^0 among Whites; but a Black person of the same phenotype would be almost equally likely to be R^0R^0 (*cDe/cDe*) as R^0r (*cDe/cde*).

Effect of Gene Frequency

A person of the phenotype CcDEe (line 3 of Table 11-3) could have any one of several genotypes. The genotype most likely to produce this phenotype in any population is R^1R^2 (*CDe/cDE*), as R^1 and R^2 are common. Since both genes encode D, the inference usually made in this situation is that the person is homozygous at the *D* sublocus, although actually heterozygous for the R^1 and R^2 genes. Some less likely alternatives could mean that the person is heterozygous at the *D* sublocus. For example, the true genotype could be R^1r'' (*CDe/cdE*), R^2r' (*cDE/Cde*) or R^zr (*CDE/cde*), but r', r'' and

R^z are uncommon in all populations. An even less likely possibility is R^0r^y (*cDe/CdE*).

Table 11-4 gives the frequencies of the more common genotypes in D+ persons. The figures given are for Whites or Blacks. In other racial groups the likelihood of being heterozygous for D is reduced because, as shown in Table 11-2, genes that code for the absence of D are even less frequent than among Blacks.

Weak Expression of D

Not all D+ rbc samples react equally well with every anti-D blood grouping reagent. Most D+ rbcs show clear-cut macroscopic agglutination after centrifugation of rbcs with serum, and can readily be classified as D+. Red cells that are not immediately agglutinated cannot as easily be classified as D– because some D+ rbcs may not be directly agglutinated by anti-D. The rbcs are D+ because the D antigen is present, but additional testing may be required to demonstrate the presence of a weakly expressed D antigen. Weak reactivity with anti-D sera has, in the past, been designated by the collective term D^u. This term has fallen into disfavor, since D^u has also been used to refer to a test, rather than an antigen. Red cells that carry weak forms of D are, by today's convention, more correctly called weak D blood. The phenotype can be written as D+w.

Weak D Due to Transmissible Gene

D+w phenotypes can arise from several different genetic circumstances. Some *Rh* genes appear to encode a weakly reactive D antigen. This characteristic, which appears to be essentially quantitative, follows the regular pattern of Mendelian dominant inheritance and is fairly common in Blacks, often appearing as the product of an unusual R^0 (*cDe*) gene.

Table 11-4. Frequencies of the More Common Genotypes in D-Positive Individuals

Phenotype	Genotype		Genotype Frequency %*		Likelihood of Zygosity for D %			
					Whites		Blacks	
CDE	CDE	Rh-hr	Whites	Blacks	Homo-	Hetero-	Homo-	Hetero-
	CDe/cde	R^1r	31.1	8.8				
CcDe	*CDe/cDe*	R^1R^o	3.4	15.0	10	90	59	41
	Cde/cDe	$r'R^o$	0.2	1.8				
CDe	*CDe/CDe*	R^1R^1	17.6	2.9	91	9	81	19
	CDe/Cde	R^1r'	1.7	0.7				
cDEe	*cDE/cde*	R^2r	10.4	5.7	10	90	63	37
	cDE/cDe	R^2R^o	1.1	9.7				
cDE	*cDE/cDE*	R^2R^2	2.0	1.2	87	13	99	1
	cDE/cdE	R^2r''	0.3	<0.1				
	CDe/cDE	R^1R^2	11.8	3.7				
CcDEe	*CDe/cdE*	R^1r''	0.8	<0.1	89	11	90	10
	Cde/cDE	$r'R^2$	0.6	0.4				
cDe	*cDe/cde*	R^or	3.0	22.9	6	94	46	54
	cDe/cDe	R^oR^o	0.2	19.4				

*Calculated from the gene frequencies given in Table 11-2. For the rare phenotypes and genotypes not shown in this table consult the reference books listed at the end of this chapter.

Transmission of a gene for weakened D is considerably less common in Whites. When it occurs it is more often the product of an unusual R^1 (*CDe*) or R^2 (*cDE*) gene, either of which is considerably more common among Whites than R^o.

Most of these genetically determined weak D antigens either fail to react, or produce very weak reactions, in direct agglutination tests with the majority of anti-D, but are usually readily detected when the same reagents are used in an antiglobulin procedure.

Weak D as Position Effect

Perhaps the best-known example of position effect (discussed previously) is weakening of the D antigen by "*C* in *trans*." The observation that rbcs representing the genotype *CDe/Cde* (R^1r') appear to show weakened expression of D was explained

in 1955 by Ceppellini and his associates[28] as being due to the effect of C in the *trans* position on the expression of genes on the opposite *Rh* chromosome. Similar depression of D is seen when other *Rh* genes are accompanied by *Cde*. For example, rbcs resulting from *CDe/cde* have the same antigens as those resulting from *Cde/cDe*, but the D antigen is often perceptibly weaker in the latter case.

This kind of weak D antigen has previously been referred to as *gene interaction D^u*, or *high-grade D^u*, and it seems likely that this was the kind of weak D phenotype observed by Stratton when he coined the term D^u on observing variable reactivity with anti-D sera in 1946.[29] Stratton's study was carried out exclusively with saline-reactive anti-D, which sometimes gives negative reactions with rbcs belonging to this class of weak D. Potentiators incorporated into reagents now used for most D typing tests may enhance reactions to such a degree that these rbcs produce normal (rather than weaker) reactions, and thus go unrecognized. A similar minor depression of D antigen reactivity is sometimes associated with the presence of a low-incidence antigen called Targett (Tar, Rh40).[30] The weak D phenotype as a manifestation of the partial D phenotype is discussed later in this chapter.

Significance of Weak D in Donors

The widely held belief that D+w blood should not be administered to D− recipients rests on the possibility that, since D+w rbcs are D+, albeit weakly so, they may elicit an immune response to D. The possibility of such a response may be more apparent than real, as the weak form of the D antigen seems to be substantially less immunogenic than "normal" D. Experimental transfusion of 68 units of D+w blood into 45 D− recipients (15 of whom were admittedly receiving immunosuppressant therapy) failed to stimulate the production of a single example of anti-D, although one person in the series made anti-E and a second made anti-K.[31] It now seems probable that an earlier report[32] of "anti-CD" produced in response to CD^u e rbcs may in reality have described anti-G (see below).

A more important consideration than the potential immunogenicity of weakened D could be the fact that D+w rbcs may suffer accelerated destruction if introduced into the circulation of a recipient whose serum already contains anti-D. A severe hemolytic transfusion reaction has been reported in these circumstances,[33] and a case of hemolytic disease of the newborn occurred in a D+w infant whose D− mother had been immunized by the cells of a D+ fetus during an earlier pregnancy.[34]

Categories of Partial D

The concept that the D antigen is a structure composed of a number of genetically determined epitopes was devised to explain the fact that some people with D+ rbcs produced anti-D that was nonreactive with their own rbcs. Wiener and Unger[35,36] proposed that the D antigen on normal D+ rbcs includes all the epitopes of the structure, to which they gave the designation "Rh_o-associated cognate specificities: Rh^A, Rh^B, Rh^C and Rh^D." In rare cases, one or more of these epitopes may be missing from D+ red cells. Most red cells of this type show strong positive reactions when tested with anti-D. Others may react weakly with anti-D. These should still be classified as D+. Rbcs lacking parts of the D antigen complex have been referred to as "D mosaic" or "D variant." More correct terminology would indicate that such rbcs are deficient in epitopes of D, hence the term "partial D."

Rbcs lacking part of the D antigen may appear phenotypically similar to those that arise due to the inheritance of a weak *D* gene except in tests with certain anti-D. The important distinction between the two D types is that the D antigens of the epitope-deficient types are *qualitatively* different from normal, whereas D due to genes that encode weak D differs from normal D quantitatively. Individuals of the D− epitope-deficient phenotypes, since their rbcs lack portions of D, sometimes respond to a transfusion of Rh+ blood or to a fetal-maternal hemorrhage from a D+ fetus by producing antibodies directed at the portions of the D antigen not present on their own rbcs. When this occurs the antibody is indistinguishable from anti-D, except that it is nonreactive with the patient's own D+ rbcs and with others that lack the same components. Not all persons who are D+ and produce an apparent anti-D should be assumed to have rbcs that are epitope deficient. As an example, weakly reactive anti-LW can react with D+ but not D− rbcs. Thus, a D+ person who has produced a weakly reactive anti-LW may be indistinguishable on initial serologic testing from a D+ who has made anti-D to missing epitopes. (See section on The LW Antigen.) Anti-LW can be differentiated from anti-D in tests with sulfhydryl-treated rbcs. The LW antigen is destroyed by sulfhydryl reagents.

Tippett and Sanger[3,4] divided these uncommon D+ phenotypes into seven numbered categories, I through VII. Category I has since been dropped, while categories III, IV and V have been subdivided in the light of further serologic evidence.[3] The reader who is interested in a review of the D antigen categories is referred to Tippett.[20] The classifications described by Tippett and those of Wiener and Unger[36] are not irreconcilable.

Significance of Weak D in Recipients

The status of a transfusion recipient whose red cells carry weak D is sometimes a topic of debate. Theoretically, such a patient, being D+, can receive Rh+ blood without the risk of being immunized. Yet if the D+w status of the rbcs should mean that they lack one part of the D epitopes, the possibility exists that transfusion of Rh+ blood could elicit production of a form of anti-D. This possibility exists equally for persons whose rbcs react strongly with anti-D reagents even though they represent an epitope-deficient type.

AABB *Standards for Blood Banks and Transfusion Services*[37] requires that donor blood samples shall be tested using a method designed to detect weak D (D^u) and labeled as D+ if the test is positive. Once labeled as D+, the units do not need to be retested on receipt at another facility. Since antiglobulin tests for D

need not be performed on recipient samples, some weak D patients may be recorded as D− and will be given Rh− blood. This situation occurs infrequently in today's blood transfusion service. The potency of the anti-D blood grouping reagents now available type most patients with weak D as D+. For this reason, many workers have stopped testing patients by the antiglobulin test for D. So few are found that the saving of Rh− blood does not justify the effort. Some workers believe that it is safer to give Rh− blood to patients whose rbcs are not directly agglutinated by anti-D. On the other hand, others consider this practice wasteful of Rh− blood, and regularly issue Rh+ blood for recipients with weakened D. If D+w patients are to receive Rh+ blood, it is important to safeguard against careless or incorrect interpretation of tests for D. Rh− recipients erroneously classified as D+ by the antiglobulin test for D and given Rh+ blood run the risk of immunization to D. Precautions to be taken might include testing with two anti-D sera and requiring that both give unequivocal positive reactions in the indirect antiglobulin test before the patient is classified as D+ by the antiglobulin test. These tests must not be examined microscopically, as it is safer in case of any doubt to assume that the patient is D−. (See Chapter 18 for discussion of microscopic examination of antiglobulin tests for D in prenatal and postpartum blood specimens.)

Weak D persons, whose antigens are detected only in antiglobulin tests, will be classified as Rh+ at the time of blood donation (since such tests must be performed on donor blood) but may be classified as Rh− as a potential transfusion recipient (where antiglobulin testing is not required). This presents special problems in autologous donations where the patient's own blood has been labeled as Rh+. In this case, confirmation of the patient's D status by antiglobulin testing will resolve the apparent discrepancy between recipient and donor D types.

Other Rh Antigens

Close to 50 Rh antigens have been identified, but most of these are rarely encountered in routine blood transfusion therapy. Table 11-1 lists the antigens sufficiently well-characterized to have been allocated names and/or numbers. The advantages of a numerical system of nomenclature are obvious at these esoteric levels. A few of the antigens and some of the phenotypes deserve additional comments. The interested reader should refer to books listed at the end of this chapter, or to the papers of Rosenfield and colleagues[18,25,38] for references other than those given.

Cis Product Antigens

The material on the rbc surface that displays Rh activity has numerous possible antigenic subdivisions. Each gene or gene complex determines a series of interrelated surface structures, of which some portions are more likely than others to elicit an immune response. The products of the gene R^1 (CDe) possess antigenic activity defined as D, C and e. They also include Ce (rh$_i$) a cis product that almost always accompanies C and e when they are encoded by the same haplotype. Red cells having C and e encoded by different haplotypes, as for example in a person of the genotype $R^z r$ (CDE/cde), do not have the Ce antigen. Similar cis product antigens exist for c and e determined by the same haplotype (the antigen called ce or f), for c and E (cE) and for C and E (CE).

Although antibodies directed at cis product antigens are encountered infrequently, it would not be correct to consider them rare. Such antibodies may be concealed within sera containing anti-

bodies of the more obvious Rh specificities; only adsorption with rbcs of selected phenotypes would demonstrate their presence. Anti-f(ce) may be present, for example, as a component of some anti-c and anti-e sera. Its presence would be of little practical significance, since the additional antibody should not confuse the reaction patterns given by anti-c and anti-e. It is exceedingly rare for rbcs to be c– (or e–) and at the same time be f+. An example of this rare event results from one form of the very uncommon gene cD–, which is known to produce c and a weak ce antigen but no e.[39]

Serologic Significance

Many examples of human polyclonal anti-C used as reagent antisera contain as their predominant component anti-Ce (more often called anti-rh$_i$). If the rbcs being tested possess C as a product of R^z (CDE) or r^y (CdE), reagent "anti-C" consisting largely of anti-Ce would give weaker than normal reactions that might lead to a negative interpretation. Since the rbcs most likely to be used for the positive control for anti-C are e+ as well as C+ (ie, CDe/cde, CDe/cDE or Cde/cde), a reassuringly strong reaction would be observed in the control test. The reaction with C+Ce– rbcs, by contrast, would be significantly weaker, take longer to develop or, in the worst case, be negative. This situation could lead to a false-negative test result, and to the possibility of a serious misinterpretation in investigating disputed parentage. The remedy is to confirm negative anti-C results with particular care when the test rbcs are E+ and, when possible, to use C+e– rbcs as a control. Unfortunately, such cells (ie, R_zR_2) are rather rare; only infrequently are they included as parts of panels of cells distributed by some reagent manufacturers. Weak expression of C is also a feature of some phenotypes that occur predominantly in

Blacks, often accompanied by atypical expression of e (see later discussion).

When correctly identified, antibodies specific for *cis* product antigens can be useful in determining genotypes. For example, if tests are limited to the five basic Rh blood grouping reagents, the rbcs of a *CDE/cde* person are phenotypically identical to those of a *CDe/cDE* person. The use of anti-f could assist with the differentiation between the two because the former rbcs would be f+ and the latter f–. A pure example of anti-Ce would be equally informative in this situation, as it would give reactions opposite to those of anti-f.

Deletions

Rare genes exist that either fail to encode Rh material or encode Rh material lacking activity at the E/e site, or at the sites of both C/c and E/e. Some portions of the surface configuration are not detectable, leaving D (or C/c and D) as the only remaining site(s). The haplotypes $C^W D-$, $(C)D^{IV}-$, $cD-$, $-D-$, $\cdot D\cdot$ and $---$ have all been reported but are exceedingly uncommon.

Red cells that lack C/c and/or E/e antigens may show exceptionally strong D activity, an observation that may allow such rbcs to be recognized during routine testing. The –D– phenotype may be identified in the course of studies to investigate an unexpected antibody in the person's serum. The specificity of the antibody may be complex, since the subject's rbcs lack many Rh antigens other than D. A single antibody with anti-Hr$_0$ (anti-Rh17) specificity is often made by persons of this rare phenotype, although some such sera have been reported to contain apparently separable specificities, such as anti-e. The $\cdot D\cdot$ phenotype is similar in most respects to –D–, except that the D antigen is not exalted to the same degree. $\cdot D\cdot$ rbcs may be agglutinated weakly by some examples of sera from immunized Rh deletion persons since those sera contain, in addition to anti-Rh17, anti-Rh47. The $\cdot D\cdot$ gene encodes Rh47. A distinguishing characteristic of $\cdot D\cdot$ rbcs is that they possess a low-incidence antigen known as Evans (Rh37).[40,41]

The Antigen G and Cross-Reactions

The G antigen cannot be fitted neatly into the concept of three antigenic regions. G is almost invariably present on rbcs possessing either C or D, so that antibodies against G appear superficially to be anti-C+D. The anti-G activity cannot, however, be separated into anti-C and anti-D. The fact that G appears to exist as an entity common to C and D explains the fact that D– persons immunized by C–D+ rbcs sometimes appear to make anti-C plus D. It may also explain why D– persons who are exposed to C+D– red cells may develop antibodies appearing to contain an anti-D component.

Rare rbcs have been described that possess G but lack D altogether and show greatly diminished, altered or absent expression of C(– –eG).[42] The D–G+ phenotype also occurs in Blacks, but is evidently not quite the same as when it occurs in Whites.[43] Red cells also exist that express at least a part of D but lack G entirely.[44-46]

Variant Antigens

There must be innumerable subtle differences in composition among various *Rh* gene products. Although red cells from most people give straightforward reactions with common antibodies, those from some give atypical reactions, and others stimulate the production of antibodies that do not react with rbcs of common Rh phenotypes. It has been convenient to consider C and c, and E and e, as antithetical antigens at specific surface sites. This scheme can be expanded to include variant antigens that seem to reside at the same site, but are determined by genes encoding for products distinct from the common Rh determinants. Such antigens may represent epitopes of a larger entity.

Most people have red cells with all epitopes of the Rh antigens. However, others may lack some of the epitopes of certain Rh antigens, such as D, C, V, VS, Hr and Hr_o.[47] For example, several distinct forms of the e antigen have been identified, such as hr^S and hr^B. Red cells lacking one or both of these epitopes are frequently found in Blacks. Diminished C and markedly diminished e activity are among the features of products of the $\overline{R}^N$ gene, which also encodes a low-incidence antigen, Rh32. Genes that encode weakly expressed antigens may be designated by parentheses—eg, (C)D(e). Among Whites, a weakened e antigen is among the products of genes that encode the Rh33 and the Rh36 (Berrens, Be^a) antigens.

Antigens that behave on most occasions as if they had an antithetical relationship to C/c or E/e have been found, mainly in Whites. The most common is C^w, which occurs in 2% or more of some White populations. Table 11-1 lists many of the separate antigens that have been found to belong to the Rh system and have contributed to the advancing complexity of the system and its nomenclature.

Biochemical Considerations

The quantitative expression of Rh epitopes present on rbcs varies with the Rh phenotype. For example, R_1 rbcs are believed to carry 14,500-19,500 D sites, 46,000-56,500 C sites and 18,000-24,500 e sites. R_2 rbcs are believed to carry 16,000-33,500 copies of D, 25,500 of E and 70,000-85,000 copies of c. Early attempts at the isolation of the Rh protein(s) produced conflicting data. (For an in-depth discussion regarding these attempts at isolation the reader is referred to the literature.[22,48,49]) In the late 1980's, biochemical data collected by Bloy et al[50] suggested that common Rh haplotypes encoded three distinct nonglycosylated polypeptide chains carrying D, C/c and E/e epitopes, respectively. The 30-32 kDa Rh proteins described by these authors were unusual in several aspects. First, and most surprising, the polypeptides did not appear to carry carbohydrate residues. This is an unusual finding since all other proteins known to carry blood group antigens have been glycosylated. Second, the Rh polypeptides exhibited a high degree of hydrophobicity. It has been suggested that the polypeptides traverse the rbc membrane up to 13 times, with only short segments of amino acids extending outside the rbc or at the cytoplasmic (interior) membrane surface. (See Fig 11-1.) Third, the proteins shared the same N-terminal amino acid sequence. How many genes encode these proteins is not yet known.

The complete primary structure of one Rh polypeptide has recently been deduced from sequence analysis of its mRNA, but basis for the D, Cc and Ee specificities was not established.[51] The Rh polypeptides probably reside in the rbc membrane as part of a larger membrane complex that includes other membrane glycoproteins. Evidence for such a complex has only been deduced indirectly.

The Rh proteins may affect the expression or orientation of other proteins. For example, glycoproteins that carry the U, LW, and Fy5 antigens are missing from Rh_{null} rbcs (rbcs devoid of Rh antigens). Colin et al[52] used Southern blot analysis of genomic DNA derived from donors of different Rh phenotypes to determine how many genes encode the three Rh-related proteins. These workers

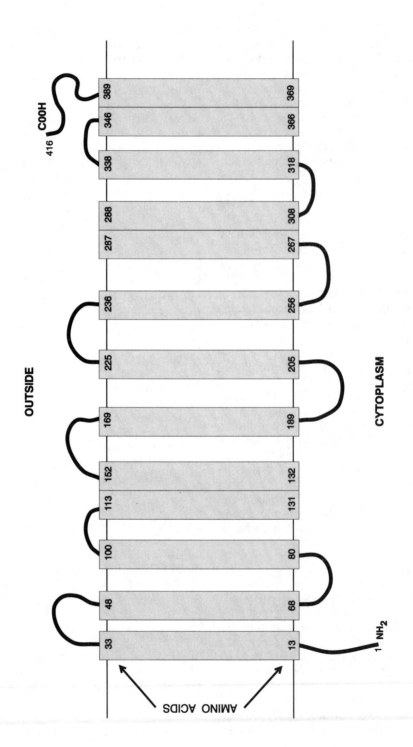

Figure 11-1. Proposed molecular structure of the Rh polypeptide.[51]

found two struc-tural genes present within the Rh locus of D+ persons. The organization of the two genes was identical in all D+ genomes whether or not they expressed C or c and E or e antigens. One of the two genes was completely missing in D– persons. The authors have therefore suggested that one gene encodes the D protein and that in its absence the D– phenotype arises. This would explain why no d antigen or anti-d antibodies have been found because d is not allelic to D. The second gene, a CcEe gene, governs the appearance of C, cE and/or e. According to the genetic model proposed by these authors, the phenotypes such as cD– and –D–, referred to as deletion phenotypes, actually might arise through single genetic events, such as point mutations, rather than deletion of genetic material.

The LW Antigen

As work progressed on the Rh system, evidence accumulated that the antigen identified by some of the animal antisera of Landsteiner and Wiener[6] were not, after all, identical to that defined by the human antibody reported by Levine and Stetson.[5] Specificity appeared at first to be similar because D+ rbcs gave significantly stronger reactions with the animal antisera than D– rbcs, which were accordingly interpreted as negative by the original investigators. It is now recognized that the antigen identified on Rhesus monkey rbcs is present on nearly all human rbcs, although D– rbcs from adults have comparatively weak reactivity.[53] Umbilical cord rbcs, both D+ and D–, are strongly reactive. Since the term Rh was so firmly established for the system of antigens first defined by human anti-D, Levine and his associates[54,55] suggested the name LW, in honor of Landsteiner and Wiener, for the antigen

characterized by the original rabbit anti-Rhesus sera. The LW genes have been assigned to chromosome 19.[56]

LW Phenotypes

Rare persons exist whose rbcs lack the LW antigen, yet have normal Rh antigens, with or without D. These persons can form alloanti-LW,[55] and this antibody shows the same graded reactivity with D+ and D– rbcs as the animal antisera. The notations LW_1 and LW_2 were adopted (quite improperly, it turned out) to describe, respectively, the strong LW reactivity of D+ rbcs and the comparatively weaker LW reactivity of adult D– rbcs. The notation LW_3 was used to describe the phenotype of persons who made anti-LW and whose rbcs did not react with the antibody, and LW_4 was applied to describe the phenotype of the one LW–proposita (Mrs. Big.) whose serum contained a potent form of anti-LW that agglutinated LW_3 rbcs,[57] as well as LW_1 and LW_2 cells. Mrs. Big.'s LW– status was originally recognized when her blood was investigated after her newborn infant was found to have a weakly positive DAT and her serum was found to contain potent anti-LW with a titer of 32,000 against D+ and 400 against D– rbcs.[58]

Anti-LW has sometimes been identified in sera from LW+ people,[59,60] whose rbcs, at the time of antibody formation, were either transiently LW– or showed feeble reactivity with anti-LW sera. In these cases the normal LW+ status of the rbcs has been observed to return as the antibody disappears.

Antithetical LW Antigens

In 1981, a new blood group antigen called Ne^a was reported, with an incidence of approximately 5% in the Finnish population.[61] Anti-Ne^a showed variation in strength of reactivity similar to that of anti-LW,[62] suggesting a relationship between Ne^a and LW. With Ne(a+) rbcs from adults, agglutination was consistently stronger if the D antigen was present than if it was absent; and Ne(a+) cord blood rbcs showed strong agglutination irrespective of D status. Tests on blood from 11 unrelated LW$_3$ persons showed that all were Ne(a+), and family studies confirmed that LW and Ne^a are products of allelic genes. Accordingly, Sistonen and Tippett[63] proposed that the names of the antigens should be changed to reflect the proved relationship. Thus, the antigen formerly called LW becomes LW^a and that formerly called Ne^a becomes LW^b.

The rbcs of Mrs. Big., the LW– proposita mentioned earlier whose rbcs had been classified as LW$_4$, were found to give negative reactions with anti-Ne^a as well as anti-LW; therefore, her rbcs are to be considered LW(a–b–), and her antibody may be thought of as anti-LW^{ab}. Red cells from persons with the transiently acquired form of LW– are also LW(a–b–), as are those of Rh$_{null}$ people, whose LW– state was formerly designated by the term LW$_0$. Sera from transiently LW– subjects may contain either anti-LW^a or anti-LW^{ab} for the duration of their LW(a–b–) status. The new terminology for LW phenotypes is shown in Table 11-5.

LW– blood may not be essential for transfusion to patients with anti-LW. D–, LW+ units have been successfully transfused to a patient whose LW antigen was transiently depressed and to patients who phenotypically were LW(a–b+).[64-66]

Genetic Independence

The genes determining LW^a and LW^b activity are not part of the Rh system. Genetic independence was established by studying families in which the gene responsible for the inherited LW– condition was shown to segregate independently of the Rh genes.[55,67] This independence has been confirmed in several of the Finnish families studied with anti-LW^a and anti-LW^b.[63] Phenotypically, however, the gene products are obviously related. Not only are both LW^a and LW^b activity always weaker in D– rbcs than in D+ rbcs of adults, but rbcs lacking demonstrable Rh antigens also lack LW^a and LW^b. The basis for the interaction is not clear. LW^a appears to require for its expression some product of Rh gene activity.

Other Observations on LW

The studies of Mallinson et al[68] suggest LW is carried on a glycoprotein. More molecules of anti-LW (either as anti-LW^a or anti-LW^b) are bound to D+ than D– rbcs. The differences in LW antigen concentration between D+ (4400) and D– (2835) rbcs contribute to difficulties often encountered in serologic tests with anti-LW^a or anti-LW^{ab}. These antibodies often behave as if they are mixtures of anti-D plus a weaker antibody. Reactions due to anti-LW sera can be differentiated from anti-D if thiol-treated rbcs are used.[69] One group of workers has reported that pronase destroys the LW antigens but has no effect on D.[70]

Table 11-5. LW Phenotypes and Genotypes

Old Phenotype		New Phenotype	New Genotype
LW+ in D+	LW$_1$	LW(a+b–) or LW(a+b+)	*LW^{a}LW^a*, *LW^{a}LW^b* or *LW^{a}LW*
LW+ in D–	LW$_2$	LW(a+b–) or LW(a+b+)	*LW^{a}LW^a*, *LW^{a}LW^b* or *LW^{a}LW*
Most LW –	LW$_3$	LW(a–b+)	*LW^{b}LW^b* or *LW^{b}LW*
LW – (Big.)	LW$_4$	LW(a–b–)	*LWLW*

Rh~null~ Syndrome and Rh~mod~

Genetic Constitution

The literature reports at least 43 persons in 14 families whose red cells appear to have no Rh antigens.[71] A number of others are also known but have not been reported. The term used to describe this phenotype is Rh_{null}. Numerous studies have revealed that it may be produced by two different genetic mechanisms. In the more common *regulator type* of Rh_{null}, the absence of a very common regulator gene, X^1, prevents expression of the person's perfectly normal genes at the Rh locus on chromosome 1. Such persons appear to transmit normal Rh genes to their offspring, in a manner roughly analogous to that in which the A or B genes are transmitted by people of the Bombay phenotype. These Rh_{null} subjects are thought to be homozygous for $X^o r$, a rare allele of $X^1 r$ that segregates independently of genes of the Rh system. In some cases, parents or offspring of people with the regulator type of Rh_{null} show overall depression of their Rh antigens; this finding is consistent with being heterozygous for a regulator gene.

The other form of Rh_{null} occurs in persons homozygous for an amorphic gene ($\bar{r}$) at the Rh locus itself. The gene appears to have no product detectable with Rh blood grouping reagents. In these cases, which are considerably rarer than the regulator type, parents and offspring are obligate heterozygotes for the amorph, and their phenotypes invariably reflect the presence of a single Rh haplotype, namely that inherited from the parent whose Rh antigens are normal. Thus, the rbcs of obligate $\bar{r}$ heterozygotes will never be both C+ and c+, nor E+ and e+.

Rbc Abnormalities

Whatever the genetic origin, rbcs lacking Rh antigens have membrane abnormalities that shorten their survival. Severity of hemolysis and anemia varies among affected persons, but stomatocytosis, shortened rbc survival and variably altered activity of other blood group antigens, especially S, s and U, have been consistent features.

Serologic Observations

A few Rh_{null} probands were recognized because their sera contained Rh antibodies, but some came to light when routine Rh phenotyping of their rbcs revealed the absence of Rh antigen activity. In three reported cases, the discovery resulted from deliberate testing for Rh antigens in patients who presented with hemolytic anemia. The antibodies produced by immunized Rh_{null} people have varied in specificity from apparently identifiable anti-e or anti-C to several examples that reacted with all rbcs tested except those of other Rh_{null} people. The specificity of this antibody is considered to be "anti-total Rh," which in the numerical nomenclature is identified as anti-Rh29.

Rh~mod~

The Rh_{mod} phenotype represents a less complete type of suppressed Rh gene expression. The genetic basis appears to be similar to that of the regulator Rh_{null}, and the name X^Q has been given to the unlinked recessive modifier gene thought to be responsible.[72] Unlike Rh_{null} rbcs, those classified as Rh_{mod} do not completely lack Rh and LW antigens. These show much reduced and sometimes varied activity, depending on the Rh system genes the proband possesses and on the potency and specificity of the antisera used in testing. Sometimes the Rh antigens are so weak as to require adsorption-elution techniques to demonstrate their presence. As in Rh_{null}, hemolytic anemia is a feature of the Rh_{mod} condition. It may be appropriate to think of the two abnormalities as being essentially similar and as differing only in degree.

Rh Antibodies in the Patient

Except for some examples of anti-E and anti-C^w that occur without known stimulus, most Rh antibodies result from immunization by pregnancy or transfusion. D is the most potent immunogen, followed by c and E.[73] Although a few examples of Rh antibodies give strong reactions as saline agglutinins, most react best in high-protein, antiglobulin or enzyme test systems. Even sera containing strong saline-reactive anti-D usually react to higher dilutions by the antiglobulin test. Some workers find enzyme techniques especially useful for detecting weak or developing Rh antibodies.

Detectable antibody levels usually persist for many years. When levels of circulating antibody fall below detectable thresholds, subsequent exposure to the antigen often results in a rapid secondary immune response. With exceedingly rare exceptions, of which the anti-CD serum Ripley is the example most often quoted, Rh antibodies do not bind complement when they combine with their antigens, at least to the extent recognizable by techniques currently used. The Ripley antibody is atypical of most Rh antibodies in that it shows a strong prozone when titrated by the bovine albumin test procedure.[74]

Dosage Effect

Anti-D seldom shows any difference in reactivity between rbcs that carry a double or single dose of the D antigen, although variably strong reactions may be observed with rbcs representing certain genotypes. For example, rbcs from an R_2 individual carry more D antigen sites than R_1 cells and may show higher titra-tion scores with anti-D. Dosage effect can sometimes be demonstrated with some antibodies directed at the E, c and e antigens and, occasionally, at the C antigen. Determining the number of antigen sites requires specialized techniques, such as radioisotope labeling, flow cytometry, immunoferritin localization or automated procedures.[75,76]

Concomitant Antibodies

Some Rh antibodies occur together. For example, an R_1 person who has made immune anti-E has almost certainly been exposed to c as well as E. Anti-c may be present in addition to anti-E, although its reactions can be substantially weaker such that they may not be detectable at the time the anti-E is found. This antibody combination may cause a delayed-type hemolytic reaction following transfusion of seemingly compatible E–c+ blood. It is not a sound principle to select, as a routine practice, donor blood negative for antigens against which the recipient *might* produce antibodies. However, a few workers feel the R_1 recipient with detectable anti-E is a case that merits special consideration. Since anti-c occurs frequently with anti-E in immunized people whose rbcs are E– and c–, some select blood of the patient's own R_1 phenotype for transfusion when the presence of anti-c cannot be demonstrated by the test procedures routinely used.

Serum that contains clearly detectable anti-c does not as consistently contain anti-E, as the patient can easily have been exposed to c without being exposed to E. Perhaps as many as one fifth of sera containing anti-c contain anti-E as well, but the presence of the second antibody is difficult to demonstrate unless an E+c– rbc sample is available for testing. Some commercial reagent rbc panels include an R_1R_z (CDe/CDE) rbc suspension for this purpose, but these rbcs are quite rare and it is difficult for manufacturers to procure them consistently. The issue is not important, however, as unsuspected anti-E in a serum known to contain anti-c is extremely unlikely to cause adverse serologic or clinical effects when c– donor units are selected for transfusion, precisely *because* the R_1R_z phenotype is so rare. To place matters in perspective, there is less clinical importance in definitively demonstrating anti-E in a serum known to contain anti-c than in identifying anti-Kp^a or anti-C^w, for example, as an unsuspected contaminant.

Rh Typing Tests

Routine rbc typing for donors and patients involves only the D antigen, with techniques to demonstrate the weak D antigen being required for donor blood. Tests for the other Rh antigens are performed when there are specific reasons for additional testing, such as identifying unexpected Rh antibodies, obtaining compatible blood for a patient with an Rh antibody, investigating disputed parentage or other family studies, selecting a panel of rbcs of different donors known to lack certain antigens or in attempting to determine whether a person is probably homozygous or heterozygous for *D*. In selecting blood for a recipient whose serum contains a comparatively weak Rh antibody, testing with potent blood grouping reagents may allow more reliable detection of antigen-negative rbcs than relying merely on a negative crossmatch. Testing the antibody-maker's own rbcs may help to provide confirmation of specificity, and will suggest which other Rh antibodies might develop.

Prudent Use of Resources

Routine testing for Rh antigens other than D is not recommended, except when there are clearly defined indications. Be-

sides the expenditure of time and money involved in unnecessary testing, excessive testing wastes scarce resources. Reagent anti-e sera, in particular, should be used sparingly, as there is sometimes a shortage of suitable raw material for their manufacture. In most cases it may be assumed without actual testing that rbcs negative for the E antigen are e+. This practice preserves precious supplies of anti-e for cases in which testing for the e antigen is specifically indicated, as it may be for E+ blood samples, or where there is good reason to suspect a deletion at the *E/e* sublocus.

Anti-D Reagents

High-Protein Reagents

Some anti-D reagents designated for use in slide, rapid tube or microplate tests contain high concentrations of protein (ie, 20-24%) and other macromolecular additives. Such reagents, nearly always prepared from pools of human sera, give rapid, reliable results when used in accordance with manufacturers' directions. Because the high molecular weight medium may cause spontaneous agglutination of rbcs coated with immunoglobulin, as in autoimmune conditions and hemolytic disease of the newborn, antisera with these additives may produce false-positive reactions. A D– patient whose rbcs were thus agglutinated spontaneously might receive transfusions of Rh+ blood and become immunized to D. To detect false agglutination due to high protein additives in the reagent, it is essential when typing patients to test the rbcs simultaneously against an immunologically inert reagent identical in formulation to the anti-D being used except lacking the antibody component. If aggregation of the rbcs occurs in the control test, the result of the anti-D test may not be valid. It will be possible in most cases to determine the D antigen status of the rbcs by further testing with other reagents, as detailed under "False Positives" later in this chapter.

The Control for High-Protein Reagents

Several circumstances may cause false-positive results in tests using high-protein reagents. Besides the above-mentioned spontaneous agglutination of immunoglobulin-coated rbcs, factors in the patient's own serum may affect the test, since unwashed rbcs suspended in their own serum or plasma are sometimes tested. Strong autoagglutinins, abnormal serum proteins that promote rouleaux formation, or antibodies directed at an additive in the reagent may each cause aggregation that can be mistaken for agglutination by anti-D. The best way to detect possibly invalid reactions in anti-D tests is to use, as the immunologically inert control reagent, the diluent used for manufacturing the particular anti-D reagent. This material contains the same additives present in high-protein anti-D except for anti-D, and can therefore be expected to potentiate spontaneous agglutination to the same degree as the anti-D itself.

Manufacturers offer their own high-protein diluents as control reagents; D typing performed on patients' rbcs with high-protein reagents must be controlled with this material. The nature and concentration of the additives differ significantly among different manufacturers' reagents. Using the control reagent from one manufacturer may not invariably detect all possible false-positive reactions due to components in another manufacturer's anti-D. Using 22% or 30% bovine albumin detects even fewer false positives,[77,78] since reagent bovine albumin solutions do not contain the other high molecular weight potentia-

tors present in high-protein reagents. Immunoglobulin-coated rbcs may not undergo spontaneous agglutination to the same degree in bovine albumin as in the reagent diluent.

Routine Testing for D

In the past, routine tests for the D antigen most often employed high-protein anti-D that could be used in slide, tube or microplate tests. More recently, low-protein chemically modified or monoclonal anti-D reagents have been substituted. Tube tests may employ rbcs suspended in saline, in serum or in plasma, but this should be confirmed by reading the manufacturer's directions before use. The recommended test procedure may vary somewhat among manufacturers.

Slide tests produce optimal results when a high concentration of rbcs and protein are combined at a temperature of 37 C. The viewing surface used to perform slide tests should be kept lighted at all times to maintain a temperature of 45-50 C, which permits rapid warming of the test mixture to 37 C. Because the slide test must be read within 2 minutes, the rbcs and serum on the glass slide must reach 37 C quickly. The slide test has the serious disadvantage that drying of the reaction mixture can cause aggregation of the rbcs that may be misinterpreted as agglutination. (For this reason, many serologists prefer to use a tube test.) The procedures for slide tests recommended by different manufacturers may not be precisely the same.

Microplate tests are performed similarly to tube tests but use very light suspensions of rbcs. Representative procedures of tube, slide and microplate tests are given in the Methods section of this manual. These procedures incorporate parallel tests performed with Rh control reagents to validate positive results obtained in tests with anti-D. If testing for the weak D antigen is indicated, an anti-globulin test for D must be performed. (See Method 2.9.)

A reliable test for weak D+ cannot be performed on a slide. If weak D+ rbcs are agglutinated in a slide test, the agglutination is invariably weaker than that seen with normal D+ rbcs. This distinction may not be recognized, however, unless the results of tests with the D+w cells are compared against those obtained with normal D+ rbcs tested in parallel. Rbcs demonstrating the stronger (gene interaction) form of D+w commonly give the same strength of reaction as normal D+ rbcs when tested with high-protein anti-D reagents, whether the test is performed on a slide or in a tube. As a result, this form of diminished D antigen most often passes for "normal" D. Accordingly, references to the D+w phenotype from this point will be confined to the form requiring an indirect antiglobulin test for its reliable detection.

Misleading Results

Causes of false reactions in Rh typing are dealt with comprehensively in the "Additional Considerations" section on p 253. Certain problems are unique to high-protein reagents, however, and it may be helpful to discuss these separately.

False Positives

1. Either immunoglobulin coating the patient's rbcs or factors in the patient's serum causing cellular aggregation can cause agglutination in the control tube containing immunologically inert reagent. Serum factors can be excluded by washing the rbcs thoroughly, using warm saline if the presence of cold agglutinins is known or suspected and then retesting the washed rbcs in a tube test. It is not necessary at this point to use a saline-reactive reagent. Retesting may be performed with the

original high-protein reagent, providing the manufacturer's directions state that the product is suitable for use with saline-suspended rbcs. The control test must again be performed concurrently. If the control test now gives a negative result and agglutination still occurs in the anti-D test, the rbcs are D+. If agglutination still occurs in the control test it is most likely that the rbcs are coated with immunoglobulin. In such cases, the rbcs may be tested with a saline-reactive reagent (see below).

2. If rbcs and anti-D are incubated together for too long before the test is read, the high-protein reagent may cause rouleaux to form. This may occur rapidly, particularly on a warm slide, as evaporation causes drying, which in turn increases the concentration of protein in the reaction mixture. Rouleaux may be mistaken for agglutination, so it is important not to exceed the manufacturer's recommendation to interpret the test within a fixed time period, usually 2 minutes.

False Negatives

1. Too heavy a rbc suspension in the tube test, or too weak a suspension in the slide test, may result in weak agglutination. To achieve the required 40-50% rbc suspension for the slide test, whole blood from a severely anemic patient may need to be concentrated by centrifuging and removing some of the plasma before testing.

2. Rbcs in a saline suspension may react poorly with some Rh reagents. Saline suspensions must not be used for the slide test.

3. Rbcs possessing comparatively weak expression of the D antigen may not react well within the 2-minute limit of the slide test, or upon immediate centrifugation in the tube test.

Low-Protein Reagents

Three kinds of low-protein saline-reactive Rh reagents are now available, and important differences exist among them. Rbcs with a positive DAT can usually be typed successfully with low-protein Rh reagents that contain saline-agglutinating antibodies and no additives that promote spontaneous agglutination of immunoglobulin-coated rbcs.

Manufacturers usually recommend a suitable concentration of bovine albumin when control tests are to be performed in parallel with low-protein D typing tests. Potentiators likely to enhance the spontaneous agglutination of DAT-positive rbcs are not normally used in low-protein saline-reactive reagents, but if such additives are present the fact should be stated in the "Reagent Description" section of the package insert.

Anti-D for the Saline Tube Test

Saline-reactive reagents prepared from predominantly IgM antibodies have always been relatively scarce because suitable raw material is difficult to obtain. Such reagents have been reserved for testing rbc samples that cannot be tested reliably with reagents containing a high concentration of protein. In contrast to the newer saline-reactive reagents, traditional saline tube test reagents require the test to be incubated at 37 C, usually for 15 minutes or longer, and they are unsuitable for slide tests. Reagents of this kind cannot be used for the indirect antiglobulin test, even when the rbcs being tested do not have a positive DAT, because IgM antibodies generally perform poorly in the IAT.

Chemically Modified IgG Antisera

The IgG antibodies in the raw material are converted to direct agglutinins by chemical reduction of their interchain disulfide bonds as described by Romans and colleagues.[79] This is usually achieved by treating the serum with a sulfhydryl compound, such as dithiothreitol or dithioerythritol. Pirofsky and Cordova[80] reported 2-mercaptoethanol to have the same effect on nonagglutinating antibodies as early as 1963, although this was later dismissed as being a nonspecific, nonimmunologic phenomenon.[81]

Chemical Considerations

Sulfhydryl reagents such as dithiothreitol can be used to convert IgG antibodies into direct agglutinins. These same agents have been used to abolish the activity of IgM antibodies. Sulfhydryl compounds cleave intersubunit disulfide bonds and, thus, depolymerize the larger IgM molecules, thereby nullifying the advantage of their greater size. In the case of IgG, mild reduction of the interchain disulfide bonds that link the heavy chains (see Fig 11-2) gives greater flexibility to the hinge region of the molecule. This greater flexibility allows the antigen-combining sites situated at the terminal end of each Fab portion to span a greater distance and agglutinate in a saline test medium rbcs possessing the corresponding antigen. Oxidation reverses the chemical reaction, so an alkylating agent is added to give permanence to the chemical modification. The reactants are removed by dialysis before final formulation of the blood grouping reagent, in a medium that usually includes bovine albumin at a protein concentration approximately equivalent to that of human serum.

Serologic Considerations

Saline-reactive reagents made from reduced and alkylated IgG antibodies show stronger reactivity than those prepared

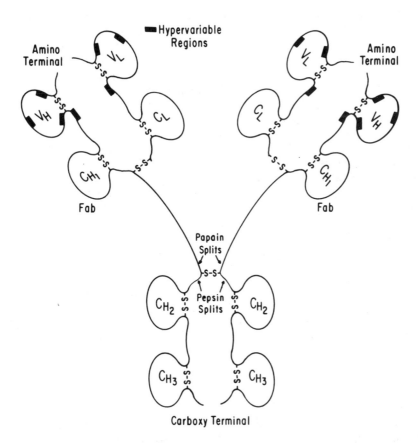

Figure 11-2. In chemically modified IgG molecules, the disulfide bonds shown holding the two heavy chains in close proximity undergo changes that allow greater separation of the chains, hence of the Fab portions of the molecule.

from IgM antibodies, and are usually suitable for tests performed on a slide. They are more abundantly available than the IgM kind, and may be confidently used routinely or when immunoglobulin coating precludes the use of high-protein anti-D on a red cell sample. These chemically modified anti-D are just as suitable as high-protein reagents for the antiglobulin D test although, naturally, an IAT test is not possible if the rbcs have a positive DAT. In such circumstances, a negative result in testing with either sort of saline-reactive anti-D merely indicates that the rbcs are *probably* D–. If the test sample is from a recipient, Rh– blood should be selected for transfusion.

Monoclonal Source Anti-D

Monoclonal anti-D reagents are made predominantly from IgM human monoclonal antibodies. The antibodies require no potentiators and agglutinate most D+ red cells of adults and infants in a saline system. They show stronger reactivity than IgG D typing reagents, including those of a chemically modified or high-protein nature. Nevertheless, monoclonal anti-D often fail to agglutinate red cells of partial D categories IV, VI and, in some instances, V. By blending in small amounts of polyclonal anti-D sera, the reagents can be made to react with partial D red cells in antiglobulin tests. The amount of polyclonal material added is strictly controlled by the reagent manufacturer. When too much polyclonal material is added, the reactivity of the monoclonal IgM component is reduced due to site blocking by IgG anti-D. Too little polyclonal anti-D results in a reagent that is less likely to detect partial D.

Licensed monoclonal/polyclonal blends can be used in slide, tube or microplate tests. They can be used as confidently as high-protein or chemically modified reagents in antiglobulin tests for weak D. Since they are prepared in a low-protein diluent, the reagents can be used to test rbcs with a positive DAT, provided those tests are not carried through to the antiglobulin phase.

Control for Low-Protein Reagents

Most reagents manufactured from chemically modified IgG and monoclonal IgM/polyclonal IgG antibodies are at a total protein concentration approximating that of human serum. False-positive reactions due to spontaneous agglutination of immunoglobulin-coated rbcs occur no more often with this kind of reagent than with other saline-reactive reagents. False-positive reactions may still occur, in any saline-reactive test system, if unwashed rbcs are tested and the sample contains cold autoagglutinins or a protein imbalance causing rouleaux. A suitable concurrent control to identify such false reactions could be observation of ABO grouping results. Absence of agglutination in either the anti-A or anti-B tube demonstrates absence of spontaneous agglutination, and no separate control test needs to be performed routinely. For rbc samples that show agglutination in all tubes (ie, give the reactions of group AB, D+), a concurrent control must be performed if the test rbcs are from a patient. A suitable control is to centrifuge the rbc suspension with its own serum, or with 6-8% bovine albumin at the same time the anti-D test is centrifuged. If the test is one of several requiring incubation before centrifugation, any test performed concurrently that gives a negative result serves as an adequate control. A separate control test is only required in the case of a rbc sample that gives positive reactions with all the Rh reagents (ie, D+C+E+c+e+).

Control for Medium-Protein Reagents

Some manufacturers have prepared reagents containing chemically modified IgG in a diluent having a level of protein between that of human serum and that of high-protein reagents. It is important not to confuse this type of reagent with the kind formulated in a low-protein diluent, as the higher protein concentration may cause spontaneous agglutination of at least some immunoglobulin-coated rbcs. The incidence of false reactions from this cause may be less than when a high-protein reagent is used, but a parallel control test with a suitably formulated control reagent is nevertheless required when testing patient samples. The need for a control will be stated in the manufacturer's instructions.

D Grouping in Hemolytic Disease of the Newborn

Since the rbcs of an infant suffering from HDN will be coated with immunoglobulin, a saline-reactive reagent is usually necessary for Rh testing. Occasionally, the rbcs may be so heavily coated with antibody that all antigen sites are occupied, leaving none to react with a saline-reactive antibody of appropriate specificity. This "blocking" phenomenon should be suspected if the infant's rbcs have a strongly positive DAT, yet give a negative result when tested with a saline-reactive reagent of the same specificity as the maternal antibody. Blocking occurs most commonly when the mother's antibody is anti-D, but it is usually possible to obtain the correct result with a saline anti-D after first eluting some of the maternal antibody from the cord rbcs at 45 C. (Refer to Method 2.14 for details and the precautions.) Elution liberates enough antigen sites to permit typing, but heat treatment of rbcs must be carried out cautiously because overexposure to heat may destroy Rh receptors.

Tests for Antigens Other Than D

Reagents are available to test for the other principal Rh antigens: C, E, c and e. These may be obtained either as low-protein (IgM, chemically modified, monoclonal) or as high-protein reagents. High-protein reagents of any specificity are prone to the same causes of false results as high-protein anti-D and therefore require a comparable control test. A negative reaction in the control for anti-D cannot be applied to tests for other Rh antigens, because results with anti-D are usually obtained after immediate centrifugation. However, tests for the other Rh antigens are usually incubated for a period at 37 C before being centrifuged and read. A valid control procedure must be performed concurrently with the test being controlled, using the same duration and conditions of incubation, and be interpreted together with the actual test.

Rh grouping reagents may show weak or negative reactions with rbcs possessing variant antigens. This is especially true of testing for the e antigen in Blacks,

among whom variants of e are relatively common. It is impossible to obtain anti-e reagents that react strongly and consistently with the various qualitative and quantitative variants of e that occur in persons of African descent. Variable reactivity with anti-C reagents may also be seen when testing the red cells of Blacks, and those of any race when the genes CDE or CdE are involved. Variant E and c antigens have been reported, but are considerably less common.

Precautions for Using Reagents

Whatever reagents are used, the manufacturer's directions must be carefully followed. The indirect antiglobulin technique must not be used unless the reagent is described explicitly by the manufacturer as suitable for this use. Reagents for the other Rh antigens derived from pools of human sera are more likely to contain antiglobulin-reactive contaminating specificities than is anti-D. Positive and negative controls should be tested in parallel with the test rbcs. Those selected for the positive control should be known to have a single dose of the antigen concerned, or be known to show weak reactivity with the reagent. If these reagents are used regularly, they should be included in the routine quality assurance program.

Additional Considerations in Rh Testing

The serologic problems associated with the use of high-protein anti-D apply equally to reagents of other specificities, and also to reagents made from chemically modified IgG if the formulation includes macromolecular additives or a total protein concentration much exceeding that of normal human serum. The following limitations are common to all Rh typing procedures, including those performed with high-protein reagents.

False-Positive Reactions

The following circumstances can produce false-positive cell grouping results.

1. The wrong reagent was inadvertently used. *The Code of Federal Regulations* 21 *CFR* 660.28(a)(1) permits a system of color-coding for the labels of certain blood grouping reagents. In the Rh system, color-coded labels may be used for high-protein and chemically modified reagents. For anti-D the approved color is grey; for anti-C, pink; for anti-E, brown; for anti-c, lavender; for anti-e, green; and for anti-CDE, orange. It is important, however, to read the label each time the reagent is used; label color or the location of the vial in a rack must not be relied upon to ensure selection of the correct reagent.

2. An unsuspected antibody of another specificity is present in the reagent. FDA regulations require that blood grouping reagents be tested by the manufacturer to ensure the absence of antibodies for antigens having an incidence of 1% or more in the general US population, but only by the test procedures recommended for use with the particular reagent. Use by a test method other than that described in the direction circular may give rise to false results.

   Antibodies for antigens having an incidence of less than 1% in the population may occasionally cause false-positive reactions, even when the manufacturer's directions are scrupulously followed. Though these antigens occur infrequently, antibodies to them are remarkably common, even in subjects who have no history of pregnancy or transfusions. Mixtures of several such antibodies are not rare, and it must be assumed that these arise through some stimulus other than exposure to human rbcs. There is evidence that this phenomenon occurs with greater frequency in sera from people who have produced an immune blood group antibody, and it is precisely these sera that are used to manufacture blood grouping reagents. It would not be reasonable to expect manufacturers to exclude from their products all antibodies directed at all low-incidence antigens. Fortunately, rbcs possessing these antigens are rarely encountered; for this reason, however, routine quality assurance programs offer no protection.

   In performing crucial antigen groupings, many workers routinely perform tests in duplicate, using reagents from different sources. This reduces the likelihood of a false classification, as discrepant reactions between two reagents of a given specificity would alert the serologist to the need for further testing. A major limitation of duplicate testing as a safeguard, however, is that reagents from different manufacturers are not necessarily prepared from antibody provided by different donors (in the case of polyclonal sera) or from different clones (monoclonal reagents). The scarcity of donors (or clones) producing acceptable titers of such relatively uncommon specificities as anti-C and anti-e, in particular, may lead to the same raw material being used by several manufacturers. In the case of polyclonal reagents, those produced by different manufacturers may thus contain the same contaminating antibody.

3. Polyagglutinable rbcs may be agglutinated by any reagent containing human serum. Although antibodies that agglutinate these surface-altered rbcs are present in most adult human sera,

they only rarely cause problems with reagents, as aging, dilution and various steps in the manufacturing process tend to eliminate these predominantly IgM antibodies. Polyagglutinability is more likely to become apparent in tests with ABO reagents than with Rh reagents, because ABO reagents are seldom diluted significantly in manufacture and a room temperature test is optimal for the reactivity of antibodies to polyagglutinable rbcs. The situation will usually be obvious when the results of rbc and serum tests for ABO disagree.

4. Autoagglutinins and abnormal proteins in the patient's serum may cause false-positive reactions when unwashed rbcs are tested. This cause of false reactions will usually be recognized through a discrepancy between rbc and serum grouping results in the ABO test. Should such a discrepancy be observed, retesting the rbcs after thorough washing in isotonic saline will in most cases give correct test results.

5. Reagent vials may become contaminated with bacteria, with foreign substances or with reagent from another vial. This can be prevented by using careful technique. Droppers should never be removed from more than one reagent at a time, and periodic inspection of the contents of vials for visual evidence of deterioration should become second nature. A point to remember with high-protein reagents is that bacterial contamination may not cause recognizable turbidity, as the refractive index of bacteria is similar to that of the material itself.

False-Negative Reactions

The following circumstances can produce false-negative rbc typing results.

1. The wrong reagent or some other similarly colored reagent was used, being mistaken for the required reagent. Vial labels should be checked carefully at each use. The reagents most likely to be mistaken for each other are antihuman globulin, bovine albumin, anti-D and its diluent control.

2. Blood typing reagent was not added to the tube (eg, to one of a long row of tubes). A good habit to cultivate is always to place the reagent in tubes first, checking each tube for the presence of the reagent before adding the rbc suspension.

3. A specific reagent fails to react with a variant form of the antigen. For example, anti-e sera may not react consistently with variant e antigens that are relatively common in Blacks. Less commonly, an anti-E serum may react weakly or not at all with the E^W antigen.

4. A reagent containing antibody that is predominantly directed at a *cis*-product Rh antigen may fail to give a reliably detectable reaction with rbcs carrying the individual antigens as separate gene products. This occurs most often with anti-C sera, which almost invariably give stronger reactions with C inherited as a product of R^1 or r' than when C is a product of R^z or r^y.

5. The manufacturer's directions were not followed, and the reagent was used incorrectly. For example, the wrong proportion of serum to rbcs was used, or incubation was at the incorrect temperature or for the wrong duration.

6. Unduly hard shaking in resuspending the red cell button after centrifugation may disperse weak agglutination.

7. Immunoglobulin in a reagent may have deteriorated due to contamination, improper storage or outdating. Chemically modified IgG antibody ap-

pears to be particularly susceptible to destruction by certain proteolytic enzymes, as might be produced by bacteria.

References

1. Issitt PD, Crookston MC. Blood group terminology: Current conventions. Transfusion 1984;24: 2-7.
2. ISBT Working Party on Terminology for Red Cell Surface Antigens. Blood group terminology. Vox Sang 1990;58:152-69.
3. Tippett P, Sanger R. Further observations on subdivisions of the Rh antigen D. Arztl Lab 1975;23:476-80.
4. Tippett P. Subdivisions of the Rh(D) antigen. Med Lab Sci 1988;45:88-93.
5. Levine P, Stetson RE. An unusual case of intragroup agglutination. JAMA 1939;113:126-7.
6. Landsteiner K, Wiener AS. An agglutinable factor in human blood recognized by immune sera for rhesus blood. Proc Soc Exp Biol NY 1940;43:223.
7. Levine P, Katzin EM. Isoimmunization in pregnancy and the variety of isoagglutinins observed. Proc Soc Exp Biol NY 1940;43:343-6.
8. Wiener AS, Peters HR. Hemolytic reactions following transfusions of blood of the homologous group, with three cases in which the same agglutinogen was responsible. Ann Intern Prn Med 1940;13:2306-22.
9. Diamond LK. Erythroblastosis fetalis or hemolytic disease of the newborn. Proc R Soc Med 1947;40:546-50.
10. Mollison PL, Englefreit CP, Contreras M. Blood transfusion in clinical medicine. 9th ed. Oxford: Blackwell Scientific Publications, 1993:225.
11. Ruddle F, Ricciuti FA, McMorris FA. Somatic cell genetic assignment of peptidase C and the Rh linkage group to chromosome No.1. Science 1972;176:1429-31.
12. Marsh WL, Chaganti RSK, Gardner FH, Mayer K, German J. Mapping human autosomes: Evidence supporting assignment of rhesus to the short arm of chromosome No.1. Science 1974; 183:966-8.
13. Povey S, Morton NE, Sherman SC. Report of the committee on the genetic constitution of chromosomes 1 and 2 (HGM8). Cytogenet Cell Genet 1985;40:67-106.
14. Race RR, Taylor GL. A serum that discloses the genotype of some Rh-positive people (letter). Nature 1943;152:300.
15. Race RR, Taylor GL, Cappell DF, McFarlane MN. Recognition of a further common Rh genotype in man. Nature 1944;153:52-3.
16. Levine P. On Hr factor and Rh genetic theory. Science 1945;102:1-4.
17. Mourant AE. A new rhesus antibody (letter). Nature 1945;155:542.
18. Rosenfield RE, Allen FH Jr, Rubinstein P. Genetic model for the Rh blood group system. Proc Natl Acad Sci USA 1973;70:1303-7.
19. Giorno R. Model for the Rh blood group system based on discontinuous gene structure. Vox Sang 1981;41:102-9.
20. Tippett P. Rh blood group system: The D antigen, high- and low-frequency Rh antigens. In: Vengelen-Tyler V, Pierce S, eds. Blood group systems: Rh. Arlington, VA: American Association of Blood Banks, 1987:25-54.
21. Wilkinson SL. Genetics and biochemistry of the Rh blood group system. In: Vengelen-Tyler V, Pierce S, eds. Blood group systems: Rh. Arlington, VA: American Association of Blood Banks, 1987:1-24.
22. Issitt PD. Biochemistry of the Rh blood group system. In: Vengelen-Tyler V, Judd WJ, eds. Recent advances in blood group biochemistry. Arlington, VA: American Association of Blood Banks, 1986:105-38.
23. Wiener AS. Genetic theory of the Rh blood types. Proc Soc Exp Biol NY 1943;54:316-19.
24. Race RR. The Rh genotypes and Fisher's theory. Blood 1948;3(suppl 2):27-42.
25. Rosenfield RE, Allen FH Jr, Swisher SN, Kochwa S. A review of Rh serology and presentation of a new terminology. Transfusion 1962;2:287-312.
26. Mourant AE, Kopec AC, Domaniewska-Sobozak K. The distribution of human blood groups and other polymorphisms. 2nd ed. London: Oxford University Press, 1976:351-505.
27. Lawler SD, Race RR. Quantitative aspects of Rh antigens. Proceedings of the International Society of Hematology 1950:168-70.
28. Ceppellini R, Dunn LC, Turri M. An interaction between alleles at the Rh locus in man which weakens the reactivity of the Rh_0 factor (D^u). Proc Natl Acad Sci USA 1955;41:283-8.
29. Stratton F. A new Rh allelomorph. Nature 1946;158:25.
30. Lewis M, Kaita H, Allerdice RW, et al. Assignment of the red cell antigen Targett (Rh40) to the Rh blood group system. Am J Hum Genet 1979;31:630-3.
31. Schmidt PJ, Morrison EG, Shohl J. The antigenicity of the Rh_0 D^u blood factor. Blood 1962;20:196-202.
32. Van Loghem JJ. Production of Rh agglutinins anti-C and anti-E by artificial immunization of volunteer donors. Br Med J 1947;ii:958-9.
33. Diamond LK, Allen FH Jr. Rh and other blood groups. N Engl J Med 1949;241:867-73.

34. Mollison PL, Cutbush M. La maladie hémolytique chez un enfant D^u. Rev Hématol 1949; 4:608-12.

35. Wiener AS, Unger LJ. Rh factors related to the Rh_o factor as a source of clinical problems. JAMA 1959;169:696-9.

36. Wiener AS, Unger LJ. Further observations on the blood factors Rh^A, Rh^B, Rh^C, and Rh^D. Transfusion 1962;2:230-3.

37. Widmann FK, ed. Standards for blood banks and transfusion services. 15th ed. Bethesda, MD: American Association of Blood Banks 1993.

38. Allen FH Jr, Rosenfield RE. Review of Rh serology. Eight new antigens in nine years. Hematologia 1972;6:113-20.

39. Tate H, Cunningham C, McDade MG, et al. An Rh gene complex $cD-$. Vox Sang 1960;5:398-402.

40. Contreras M, Armitage S, Daniels GL, Tippett P. Homozygous ·D·. Vox Sang 1979;36:81-4.

41. Contreras M, Stebbing B, Blessing M, Gavin J. The Rh antigen Evans. Vox Sang 1978;34:208-11.

42. Allen FH, Tippett PA. A new Rh blood type which reveals the Rh antigen G. Vox Sang 1958;3:321-30.

43. Kevy SV, Schmidt PJ, Leyshon WC. A second example of the blood type rhG. Vox Sang 1959; 4:257-66.

44. Stout TD, Moore BPL, Allen FH Jr, Corcoran P. A new phenotype D+G– (Rh:1,–12). Vox Sang 1963;8:262-8.

45. Shapiro M. Serology and genetics of a "new" blood factor: hr^H. J Forens Med 1964;11:52-66.

46. Zaino EC. A new Rh phenotype Rh_orh G-negative. Transfusion 1965;5:320-31.

47. Issitt PD. An invited review: The Rh antigen e, its variants, and some closely related serological observations. Immunohematology 1991; 7:29-36.

48. Issitt PD. The Rh blood group system 1988: Eight new antigens in nine years and some observations on the biochemistry and genetics of the system. Transfus Med Rev 1989;3:1-12.

49. Agre P, Cartron JP. Molecular biology of the Rh antigens. Blood 1991;78:551-3.

50. Bloy C, Blanchard D, Dahr W, et al. Determination of the N-terminal sequence of human red cell Rh(D) polypeptide and demonstration that the Rh(D),(c), and (E) antigens are carried by distinct polypeptide chains. Blood 1988;72:661-6.

51. Chérif-Zahar B, Bloy C, Le Van Kim C, et al. Molecular cloning and protein structure of a human blood group Rh polypeptide. Proc Natl Acad Sci USA 1990;87:6243-7.

52. Colin Y, Chérif-Zahar B, Le Van Kim C, et al. Genetic basis of the RhD-positive and RhD-negative blood group polymorphism as determined by Southern analysis. Blood 1991;78: 2747-52.

53. Beck ML. The LW system: A review and current concepts. In: Walker RH, ed. A seminar on recent advances in immunohematology. Washington, DC: American Association of Blood Banks, 1973:83-100.

54. Levine P, Celano MJ, Vos GH, Morrison J. The first human blood, – – –/– – –, which lacks the D-like antigen. Nature 1962;194:304.

55. Levine P, Celano MJ, Wallace J, Sanger R. A human "D-like" antibody. Nature 1963;198:596-7.

56. Sistonen P. Linkage of the LW blood group locus with the complement C3 and Lutheran blood group loci. Ann Hum Genet 1984;48:239-42.

57. Swanson JL, Azar M, Miller J, McCullough JJ. Evidence for heterogeneity of LW antigen revealed in a family. Transfusion 1974;14:470-4.

58. deVeber LL, Clark G, Hunking M, Stroup M. Maternal anti-LW. Transfusion 1971;11:33-5.

59. Chown B, Kaita H, Lowen D, Lewis M. Transient production of anti-LW by LW-positive people. Transfusion 1971;11:220-2.

60. Giles CM, Lundsgaard A. A complex serological investigation involving LW. Vox Sang 1967; 13:406-16.

61. Sistonen P, Nevanlinna HR, Virtaranta-Knowles K, et al. Ne^a, a new blood group antigen in Finland. Vox Sang 1981;40:352-7.

62. Sistonen P. A phenotypic association between the blood group antigen Ne^a and the Rh antigen D. Med Biol 1981;59:230-3.

63. Sistonen P, Tippett P. A "new" allele giving further insight into the LW blood group system. Vox Sang 1982;42:252-5.

64. Tregellas WM, Moulds JJ, South SF. Successful transfusion of a patient with anti-LW and LW positive blood (abstract). Transfusion 1978;18: 384.

65. Cummings E, Pisciotto P, Roth G. Normal survival of Rho(D) negative, LW(a+) red cells in a patient with allo-anti-LW^a. Vox Sang 1984;46: 286-90.

66. Chaplin H, Hunter VL, Rosche ME, Shirey RS. Long-term in vivo survival of Rh(D)-negative donor red cells in a patient with anti-LW. Transfusion 1985;25:39-43.

67. Swanson J, Matson GA. Third human "D-like" antibody or anti-LW. Transfusion 1964;4:257-61.

68. Mallinson GW, Martin PG, Anstee DJ, et al. Identification and partial characterization of the human erythrocyte membrane component(s) that express the antigens of the LW blood group system. Biochem J 1986;234:649-52.

69. Konigshaus GJ, Holland TI. The effect of dithiothreitol on the LW antigen. Transfusion 1984;24:536-7.

70. Lomas CG, Tippett P. Use of enzymes in distinguishing anti-LW^a and anti-LW^{ab} from anti-D. Med Lab Sci 1985;42:88-9.

71. Moulds JJ. Rh$_{nulls}$: Amorphs and regulators. In: Walker RH, ed. A seminar on recent advances in immunohematology. Washington, DC: American Association of Blood Banks 1973:63-82.

72. Chown B, Lewis M, Kaita H, Lowen B. An unlinked modifier of Rh blood groups: Effects when heterozygous and when homozygous. Am J Hum Genet 1972;24:623-37.

73. Giblett E. Blood group antibodies causing hemolytic disease of the newborn. Clin Obstet Gynecol 1964;7:1044-55.

74. Waller M, Lawler SD. A study of the properties of the rhesus antibody (Ri) diagnostic for the rheumatoid factor and its application to Gm grouping. Vox Sang 1962;4:591-606.

75. Masouredis SP. Quantitative and ultra-structural aspects of red cell membrane Rh antigens. In: Walker RH, ed. A seminar on recent advances in immunohematology. Washington, DC: American Association of Blood Banks, 1973:41-62.

76. Berkman EM, Nusbacher J, Kochwa S, Rosenfield RE. Quantitative blood typing profiles of human erythrocytes. Transfusion 1971; 11:317-32.

77. White WD, Issitt CH, McGuire D. Evaluation of the use of albumin controls in Rh typing. Transfusion 1974;14:67-71.

78. Reid ME, Ellisor SS, Frank BA. Another potential source of error in Rh-hr typing. Transfusion 1975;15:485-8.

79. Romans DG, Tilley CA, Crookston MC, et al. Conversion of incomplete antibodies to direct agglutinins by mild reduction: Evidence for segmental flexibility within the Fc fragment of immunoglobulin G. Proc Natl Acad Sci USA 1977;74:2531-5.

80. Pirofsky B, Cordova MR. Bivalent nature of incomplete anti-D (Rh$_o$). Nature 1963;197: 392-3.

81. Mandy WJ, Fudenberg HH, Lewis FB. On "incomplete" anti-Rh antibodies: Mechanism of direct agglutination induced by mercaptoethanol. J Clin Invest 1965;44:1352-61.

12

Other Blood Groups

In addition to the antigens discussed in Chapters 10 and 11, over 500 others can be detected on human rbcs. Some of these are found on other tissues. For example, those of the HLA system (see Chapter 13) are present on most human cells other than mature rbcs. Certain additional determinants are found only on human blood granulocytes or platelets. They deserve brief mention in this chapter since they may be of clinical significance in recipients who produce antibodies to them.

Antigens that are carried by a particular cell line of almost all persons are known as high-incidence or *public* antigens. Others, of low incidence, are sometimes called *private* antigens. Each of the known antigens described in this chapter was initially identified through the detection of its specific antibody in a serum. Tables listing phenotype frequencies among Whites and Blacks in the US population are given. Frequencies among other racial groups in the population are not given, as data are scanty and wide differences among groups of diverse Asian or Native American origins make generalizations about phenotypes inappropriate. A summary of the serologic behavior and characteristics of the major antibodies derived from human sources is shown in Table 12-1.

The MN Blood Groups

Anti-M and Anti-N

The M and N antigens (MNS1 and MNS2 in ISBT terminology[1]) were discovered in 1927, when Landsteiner and Levine obtained the antibodies defining them by immunizing rabbits with human rbcs.[2] Anti-M is detected frequently in human sera, usually occurring as a saline agglutinin in antibody tests performed at room temperature. Most examples of this antibody occur without an rbc-induced stimulus. Although anti-M sera are generally thought of as predominantly IgM, examples that are partly or wholly IgG are frequently found.[3] Thus, the ability to agglutinate M+ rbcs in a saline test is not necessarily an indication that a given example of anti-M is wholly IgM. As with the A and B antigens of the ABO system, the M antigen occurs in sufficient density on the rbcs that agglutination in a saline test may occur even when the antibody is wholly IgG. Some examples of anti-M manifest stronger agglutination if the pH of the test system is reduced to 6.5.[4]

Anti-M is rarely clinically significant, although examples that react at 37 C or at the antiglobulin phase of testing should be considered potentially significant. In a few exceptional cases, anti-M detect-

259

Table 12-1. Serologic Behavior of the Principal Antibodies of Different Blood Group Systems

Antibody	In-Vitro Hemolysis	Saline		Albumin		Papain/Ficin		Associated With	
		4 C	22 C	37 C	AGT	37 C	AGT	HDN*	HTR†
Anti-M	0	Most	Some	Few	Few	0	0	Few	Few
Anti-N	0	Most	Few	Occ.	Occ.	0	0	Rare	?
Anti-S	0	Few	Some	Some	Most	See text		Yes	Yes
Anti-s	0	0	Few	Few	Most	See text		Yes	Yes
Anti-U	0	0	Occ.	Some	Most	Most	Most	Yes	Yes
Anti-Luᵃ	0	Some	Most	Few	Few	Few	Few	No	?
Anti-Luᵇ	0	Few	Few	Few	Most	Few	Few	Mild	Yes
Anti-K	0		Few	Some	Most	Some	Most	Yes	Yes
Anti-k	0		Few	Few	Most	Some	Most	Yes	Yes
Anti-Kpᵃ	0		Some	Some	Most	Some	Most	Yes	?
Anti-Kpᵇ	0		Few	Few	Most	Some	Most	Yes	Yes
Anti-Jsᵃ	0		Few	Few	Most	Few	Most	Yes	?
Anti-Jsᵇ	0		0	0	Most	Few	Most	Yes	?
Anti-Fyᵃ	0		Rare	Rare	Most	0	0	Yes	Yes
Anti-Fyᵇ	0		Rare	Rare	Most	0	0	Yes	Yes
Anti-Jkᵃ	Some		Few	Few	Most	Some	Yes	Yes	Yes
Anti-Jkᵇ	Some		Few	Few	Most	Some	Most	Yes	Yes
Anti-Xgᵃ	0		Few	Few	Most	0	0	No report	
Anti-Diᵃ	0		Some	Some	Most	Some	Some	Yes	Yes
Anti-Diᵇ	0				Most	Some	Some	Yes	Yes
Anti-Ytᵃ	0		0	0	Most	0	Some	No	?
Anti-Ytᵇ	0				All			No report	
Anti-Doᵃ	0		0	0	Some	Some	Most	?	Yes
Anti-Doᵇ	0				All		All	No report	
Anti-Coᵃ	0		0	0	Some	Some	Most	Yes	?
Anti-Coᵇ	0		0	0	Some	Some	Most	No report	
Anti-Sc1	0				All			No report	
Anti-Sc2	0		Some	Some	Most	Most	Most	No report	

*Hemolytic disease of the newborn.
†Hemolytic transfusion reaction.
The reactivity shown in the table is based on the tube methods in common use. If tests are carried out by more sensitive test procedures (such as in capillary tubes, in microtiter plates or by the albumin layering method), direct agglutination (prior to the antiglobulin phase) may be observed more often with some antibodies. Blank spaces indicate a lack of sufficient data for generalization about antibody behavior.

able by the IAT has caused HDN and DHTRs.[5,6]

Anti-N, in contrast to anti-M, is comparatively rare. Examples are almost invariably IgG, and they typically behave like weakly reactive cold agglutinins. Some powerful and potentially significant IgG examples have been observed in a few persons of the rare phenotypes M+N– S–s–U– and M+N–S–s–U+ʷ. The presence of an anti-N-like agglutinating antibody in some hemodialysis patients, first reported in 1972,[7] was associated with the use of formaldehyde-sterilized dialyzer membranes.[8] The stimulus to antibody formation appears to be formaldehyde-induced alteration of the N and 'N' antigens.[9] 'N' is a structure present on both N+ and N– rbcs.

Antibodies Showing Dosage

The M and N antigens behave as products of paired allelic genes, in that they bear an obvious allelic relationship. With rare exceptions, rbcs type as M+N–, M–N+ or as M+N+. These phenotypes represent, respectively, homozygosity for *M*, homozygosity for *N* and heterozygosity for both genes. Some individual examples of anti-M and anti-N demonstrate dosage, showing significantly greater reaction strengths and higher titration scores against rbcs from homozygotes than against rbcs from heterozygotes. Examples of anti-M that react only with rbcs carrying a double dose of the M antigen are encountered frequently. Anti-N sera that react only with rbcs possessing a double dose of N are not often seen. In these cases, the specificities of the antibodies may not be immediately apparent from the reaction patterns obtained with a panel of rbcs. Reagent anti-M and anti-N rarely demonstrate dosage, having been selected and standardized to give good reactions with all rbcs possessing the relevant antigen, although with dilution dosage may become apparent.

Blood Grouping Reagents

Blood grouping reagents are available commercially for the detection of M and N antigens. Some are produced by immunizing rabbits with human rbcs. The resulting sera are pooled and then adsorbed to remove unwanted activity other than anti-M or anti-N. Reagents prepared from human antisera and mouse monoclonal antibodies and lectins are also available. The most widely used lectin reagent is the anti-N-like extract of *Vicia graminea* seeds. In most cases, reagents from these different sources will give concordant reactions, but occasional discrepancies may result from relatively subtle differences in specificity. Since almost all human rbcs carry some N antigen (for a reason that is explained later) anti-N reagents may react weakly with the rbcs of persons homozygous for the *M* gene. Interpretation of reactions with anti-M and anti-N reagents always requires special care, and it is particularly important that the manufacturer's instructions be followed carefully.

Variant Antigens

Unexpected phenotyping results may occur when variants of the M and N antigens are present.[10] For example, the M^g (MNS11) antigen, product of a very rare allele at the *MN* locus, reacts neither with anti-M nor with anti-N reagents. The rbcs of a person with the genotype M^gN will give the reactions M–N+, leading to the false conclusion that the genotype is actually *NN*. Similarly, the rbcs of a person of the genotype M^gM will give the reactions M+N–. Parentage can be falsely excluded if the M^gM and M^gN genotypes are interpreted as *MM* and *NN*, respectively. Anti-M^g occurs as a saline agglutinin in sera from persons who have had no rbc-induced stimuli.[5,11] However, the rarity of the M^g antigen makes the presence of anti-M^g obscure. It is found as a non-rbc-induced antibody in 1-2% of human sera, largely a matter of academic curiosity.

S, s and U Antigens

The antigens S (MNS3) and s (MNS4) are produced by a pair of allelic genes found at a locus closely linked to the *MN* locus. An example of linkage disequilibrium is seen in the fact that the gene complex that produces N with s is five times more common than that producing N with S.[5,11]

A small proportion of Blacks type as S– s–. In most cases, S–s– cells are also negative for a high-incidence antigen called U (MNS5), and persons of this phenotype may make anti-U when exposed to U+ rbcs. Although some S–s– rbcs are U+, the U antigen on these rbcs may be so weakly expressed that an adsorption/elution technique is needed to demonstrate its presence.

Table 12-2 shows the frequencies of the different phenotypes in the MN system.

Antibodies to S, s and U

Unlike anti-M and anti-N, antibodies to S, s and U usually occur following rbc stimulation. All are capable of causing HTRs and HDN. Although a few saline-reactive examples have been reported, antibodies to S, s and U are usually detected by the IAT. Anti-S occurs about as infrequently as anti-N. Anti-s is seen even less often, perhaps partly because the s– phenotype is less frequent than S–, but perhaps also because the s antigen is less immunogenic than S. Anti-U is found comparatively rarely, but should be considered when serum from a previously transfused or pregnant Black person contains antibody to a high-incidence antigen. It may not be possible to type the patient's rbcs for U, but the probability that they are U– can be established by proving they are S–s–.[11]

Biochemistry of MN System

GPA and M and N

Normal rbc membranes carry four distinct sialoglycoproteins (SGPs).[12] These are glycophorin A (synonyms: GPA, α SGP, MN SGP, PAS-1, PAS-2), glycophorin B (synonyms: GPB, δ SGP, Ss SGP, PAS-3), glycophorin C (synonyms: GPC, PAS-2′) and glycophorin D (GPD). GPD is assumed to be derived from GPC.

Antigens of the MN system are carried on GPA and GPB, molecules sensitive to cleavage at varying positions by certain proteases. (See Fig 12-1.) M and N antigens are found on GPA, of which approximately 500,000 copies are present on each rbc.[12] This structure has a molecular weight of 31,000 and consists of 131 amino acids, with approximately 60% of its total mass being composed of carbohydrate. It is a transmembrane molecule (ie, it traverses the membrane). Its carboxy terminal extends into the cytoplasm of the rbc, while a hydrophobic segment consisting of 23 amino acids is embedded within the lipid bilayer. An amino terminal segment extends into the extracellular environment.

Blood group antigen activity resides on the external segment, a sequence of approximately 70 amino acids with carbohydrate side chains attached within the first 50 residues of the amino termi-

Table 12-2. Phenotypes and Frequencies in the MNSs System

Reactions With Anti-						Phenotype Frequency %	
M	N	S	s	U	Phenotype	Whites	Blacks
+	0				M + N –	28	26
+	+				M + N +	50	44
0	+				M – N +	22	30
		+	0	+	S + s – U +	11	3
		+	+	+	S + s + U +	44	28
		0	+	+	S – s + U +	45	69
		0	0	0	S – s – U –	0	Less than 1
		0	0	(+)	S – s – U + w	0	Rare

less the appropriate rare rbcs are used in testing. The Wr[b] antigen has an antithetical relationship with Wr[a], which is produced by a gene that is independent from those of the MN system. However, Wr[b] is related at the biochemical level to GPA. Recent data suggest that Wr[b] may be an antigen formed by the association of band 3 rbc membrane protein with GPA.[12,14]

GPB and S, s and U

GPB is smaller, and there are fewer copies per rbc than GPA. Approximately 100,000 copies of this molecule are present, in contrast to 500,000 for GPA.[12] GPB carries S, s and probably U antigens and possesses, at the amino terminal, a segment consisting of 26 amino acids that duplicate the sequence of GPA[N]. This accounts for the presence of an 'N' antigen on almost all rbcs regardless of MN type. Those U– rbcs that lack GPB altogether lack not only S and s activity, but also lack 'N'. GPB of S+s– rbcs differs from that of S–s+ rbcs in an amino acid at position 29: methionine in S+s– and threonine in S–s+.[12]

Genes Encoding Glycophorins

The gene that produces GPA is called GYPA and the gene that encodes GPB is GYPB.[1] The similarities in amino acid sequences of GPA and GPB suggest GYPA and GYPB are derived from a common ancestral gene. It has been shown that GYPA and GYPB consist of 7 and 5 exons, respectively.[15] Both genes share >95% identical sequences from the 5′ flanking region to the region approximately 1 kilobase downstream from the exon encoding the transmembrane regions. In the homologous parts of the genes, GYPB lacks one exon due to a point mutation at the 5′ splicing site of the third intron. Following the homologous sequences, GYPA and GYPB differ significantly in the 3′ end sequences. It has

been proposed[15] that GYPA maintains close homology with an ancestral genomic structure. In contrast, GYPB has arisen from the acquisition of 3′ sequences that differ from those of GYPA.

The genes encoding the MN system antigens are located on chromosome 4 at 4q28-q31.

Pronounced SGP modifications occur in hybrid molecules considered to arise from unequal crossing over or gene conversion between GYPA and GYPB. Such hybrids have occasionally been noted to carry low-incidence antigens that are due to novel amino acid sequences.[16-19]

Some of the hybrid SGPs carry the amino-terminal portion of GPA and the carboxy-terminal portion of GPB and vice versa. Others have been recognized that appear to be a GPB molecule with a GPA insert. The low-incidence antigens Hil (MNS20), St[a] (Stones or MNS15), Dantu (MNS25) and Mur (MNS10) are associated with hybrid SGPs. The Dantu antigen occurs predominantly in Blacks.

Variant SGPs

The MN system includes a series of variant antigens. Though mainly of very low incidence, these may assume clinical significance on rare occasions. Many of the corresponding antibodies occur often as non-rbc-stimulated agglutinins. Antiglobulin-reactive examples have uncommonly been implicated in cases of HDN.

Reaction patterns with certain antibodies suggest that several low-incidence antigens of the MN system are serologically interrelated, forming the Miltenberger subsystem; some of these antigens appear to occur more commonly among Asians than in other population groups. Other low-incidence antigens have been assigned to the MN system by linkage data acquired through family studies. For some, recent biochemical data indicate that one or more amino acid substitutions, variation in the extent or type of glycosylation, or the existence of a hybrid SGP influence reactivity of the particular low-incidence determinant. Table 12-3 gives the amino acid sequences associated with variant antigens.

Proteolytic Enzymes

Since proteolytic enzymes such as ficin or papain cleave rbc membrane SGPs, reactivity with anti-M and anti-N is abolished by enzyme techniques commonly used in antibody detection or identification tests. (See Table 12-1.) This feature sometimes helps to identify these antibodies. The effects of various proteases on tests for the S and s antigens are less firmly established. Most investigators have found that papain or ficin destroy the reactivity of S+ rbcs with anti-S. However, depending on the enzyme solution employed, the reactivity of anti-s with s+ rbcs may be little affected by these enzymes.[20] A few examples of anti-S have been found to agglutinate U+ ficin- or papain-treated rbcs irrespective of their S antigen status. If enzyme-treated S–U– cells are tested, however, no agglutination occurs. As a consequence, these examples of anti-S could be mistaken for anti-U in an enzyme test system.[21] Although most examples of anti-U react equally with untreated and ficin- or papain-treated rbcs, examples of anti-U detecting an enzyme-sensitive determinant do exist.[22]

The effect of different enzymes on the expression of MN system antigens reflects the point at which the particular enzyme cleaves the antigen-bearing SGP and the position of the antigen relative to the cleavage site. (See Fig 12-1.)

Lutheran Blood Group System

The first example of anti-Lu^a (-Lu1) was found in 1945, in a serum that contained several other antibodies. The phenotypes of the Lutheran system, as defined by anti-Lu^a and anti-Lu^b (-Lu2), are shown in Table 12-4. The Lu(a–b–) phenotype is very rare and may arise from one of three distinct genetic circumstances. In the first, a presumably amorphic Lutheran gene *Lu* is inherited from both parents.[23] In the second, the negative phenotype is inherited as a dominant trait attributed to the independently segregating inhibitor gene *In(Lu)*, which prevents the normal expression of Lutheran and certain other blood group genes (notably *P^I* and *i*).[24] The third Lu(a–b–) phenotype is due to an X-borne suppressor, recessive in its effect.[25]

Lutheran system antibodies are not often encountered. Anti-Lu^a and anti-Lu^b are produced in response to pregnancy or transfusion, but have occurred in the absence of rbc stimulation. Lutheran antigens are poorly developed at birth, so it is not surprising that anti-Lu^a has not been reported as the cause of HDN. Neither has this antibody been associated

Table 12-4. Phenotypes and Frequencies in the Lutheran System in Whites

| Reactions With Anti- | | Phenotype | Phenotype |
Lu^a	Lu^b	Phenotype	Frequency %
+	0	Lu(a+b−)	0.15
+	+	Lu(a+b+)	7.5
0	+	Lu(a−b+)	92.35
0	0	Lu(a−b−)	Very rare

Insufficient data exist for the reliable calculation of frequencies in Blacks.

with HTRs. Anti-Lu^b has been reported to cause diminished survival of transfused rbcs and no or, at most, mild HDN. Most examples of anti-Lu^a and some anti-Lu^b will agglutinate saline-suspended rbcs possessing the relevant antigen, producing small to moderately sized, loosely agglutinated clumps of rbcs interspersed among many unagglutinated rbcs.[5] The mixed-field appearance is characteristic of reactions with some examples of anti-Lu^a.

The Lu^a and Lu^b antigens are destroyed by trypsin, chymotrypsin, pronase, 2-amino-ethylisothiouronium bromide (AET) and dithiothreitol (DTT). (See Methods 4.6 and 4.8.) These results, together with the results of immunoblotting experiments, suggest that these antigens are carried on glycoproteins that contain interchain or intrachain disulfide bonds.[26]

Associated Antigens

A series of high-incidence antigens [LU4, LU5, LU6, LU7, LU8, LU11, Much (LU12), Hughes (LU13), LU16 and LU17] have been assigned to the Lutheran system because the corresponding antibodies do not react with rbcs of the Lu(a–b–) phenotype derived from any of the three genetic backgrounds. Two low-incidence antigens, Mull (LU9) and LU14, have gained admission to the Lutheran system because of their apparent antithetical relationship to high-incidence antigens LU6 and LU8, respectively.

Au^a, an antigen of high incidence [80% of Whites are Au(a+)] and its antithetical partner, Au^b (incidence of 50%), have been recently shown to be part of the Lutheran system.[27,28] Thus, Au^a has been renamed LU18 and Au^b, LU19.

Gene Linkage and Chromosome Assignment

The *Lu* and *Se* (secretor) loci were shown to be linked in 1951, the first recorded example of autosomal linkage in man. The two loci have been assigned to chromosome 19 through their linkage with *C3*.

Biochemistry of Lutheran

Lutheran antigens are carried on two glycoproteins carrying both N-linked and O-linked oligosaccharides.[29,30] The antigens are destroyed by trypsin, α-chymotrypsin and thiol-reducing agents.[31] Tests performed with monoclonal anti-Lu^b have suggested the number of Lu^b antigen sites per rbc is low; approximately 600-1600 per Lu(a+b+) rbc and 1400-3800 per Lu(a–b+) rbc.[32]

Kell Blood Group System

The K (KEL1) antigen was first identified in 1946, because of an antibody that caused HDN. The gene responsible (*K*) is present in 9% of Whites and approximately 2% of Blacks. The existence of the expected allele (*k*) was confirmed when an antithetical relationship was established between K and the antigen detected by anti-k (-KEL2), which reacted with the rbcs of over 99% of the random population.[5] The Kell system antigens are represented at the rbc membrane in low density (K = 3500, k = 2000-5000 sites).

Anti-K and Anti-k

The K antigen is strongly immunogenic, and it is therefore not surprising that anti-K is frequently found in sera from transfused patients. In a few cases, anti-K has appeared as a saline agglutinin in sera from subjects never exposed to an rbc stimulus. Most examples detected are of immune origin and are reactive by the IAT; some bind complement. Some workers have suggested that examples of anti-K may react less well in tests that incorporate LISS solutions than in saline tests or tests that include albumin. Others, testing many examples of anti-K in low ionic systems, have not been able to show any differences in antibody reactivity. Anti-K has caused HTRs on numerous occasions, both immediate and delayed. Since over 90% of donors are K–, it is not difficult to find compatible blood for patients with anti-K. Anti-k has clinical and serologic characteristics similar to anti-K, but occurs much less frequently because only about one person in 500 lacks the k antigen.

Other Antigens

Other antithetical antigens of the Kell system include Kp^a (KEL3), Kp^b (KEL4) and Kp^c (KEL21)[33]; Js^a (KEL6) and Js^b (KEL7); KEL11 and KEL17; and, possibly, KEL14 and KEL24. These antigens, along with K and k, are inherited as if they are produced by alleles at closely linked loci, somewhat analogous to the situation that exists between the major antigens of the Rh system. Unlike findings in the Rh system, not all the theoretically possible genotype combinations have been recognized in the Kell system. For example, Kp^a and Js^a have never been found together on the same chromosome. Kp^a is predominantly a gene

found in Whites, and Js^a is found predominantly in Blacks. The haplotype containing K and Kp^a has also not been found. Table 12-5 shows some phenotypes of the Kell system. The table also includes the K_o phenotype, a null phenotype in which the rbcs lack all of the antigens of the system.

As in the Lutheran system, several high-incidence antigens have been assigned to the Kell system because the identifying antibodies were found to give negative reactions with K_o rbcs. For simplicity, the various other high-incidence and low-incidence Kell antigens are not included in the table.

Other Antibodies

Anti-Kp^a, anti-Kp^b, anti-Js^a and anti-Js^b are all much less common than anti-K, but show similar serologic characteristics and are considered clinically significant. Any of them may occur following transfusion or fetomaternal immunization. Their frequency is influenced by the immunogenicity of the particular antigen and by differences in the distribution of the relevant negative phenotypes among transfusion recipients and of the positive phenotypes among donors. (See Table 12-5.) These antibodies are rare, however, suggesting that the antigens

Table 12-5. Some Phenotypes and Frequencies in the Kell System

		Reactions With Anti-					Frequency %	
K	k	Kp^a	Kp^b	Js^a	Js^b	Phenotype	Whites	Blacks
+	0					K+k–	0.2	Rare
+	+					K+k+	8.8	2
0	+					K–k+	91	98
		+	0			Kp(a+b–)	Rare	0
		+	+			Kp(a+b+)	2.3	Rare
		0	+			Kp(a–b+)	97.7	100
				+	0	Js(a+b–)	0	1
				+	+	Js(a+b+)	Rare	19
				0	+	Js(a–b+)	100	80
0	0	0	0	0	0	K_o	Exceedingly rare	

are of low immunogenicity. Patients immunized to the high-incidence antigens k, Kp^b and Js^b, or to any high-incidence antigen, present a problem that may require assistance from a rare donor file if transfusion is required.

Anti-Ku (KEL 5) is the typical antibody of immunized K$_o$ persons. It appears to be directed at a single determinant. The antibody has not been separated into other Kell specificities.[34] However, anti-Ku may be present with antibodies to other Kell system antigens.

The Kx Antigen

Two proteins, encoded by different genes, have been associated with Kell system antigens.[35,36] One gene is autosomal, assigned to chromosome 7.[37] This gene gives rise to the 93-kD Kell protein. The other is X-linked, located on the short arm at Xp21. The normal X-linked allele, designated XK1, encodes a 37-kD protein that carries Kx. The Kx antigen is found in exalted amounts on K$_o$ red cells but only trace amounts on red cells of normal Kell phenotypes. The seeming reciprocal relationship between Kx and Kell antigen expression has suggested that Kx was a precursor of Kell system antigens. However, there is no biochemical evidence to support this theory.

The McLeod Phenotype

Red cells that lack Kx have shortened survival, decreased permeability to water, acanthocytic morphology, as well as markedly depressed expression of Kell system antigens.[38,39] This constellation of rbc abnormalities is called the McLeod phenotype, after the first subject in whom this syndrome was described. McLeod phenotype is perhaps a rather misleading term, since the antigens observed to be depressed in different people depend on the Kell genes present in the particular subject. Persons with McLeod rbcs

also have a poorly defined abnormality of the neuromuscular system characterized by persistently elevated serum levels of the enzyme creatine phosphokinase and, in older people, disordered muscular function. The McLeod phenotype may arise through deletion of the XK locus of chromosome X. The biochemical origins of the molecular lesion responsible for abnormal rbc morphology and osmotic fragility of McLeod rbcs are still unclear.

In a few instances the McLeod phenotype has been found in patients with chronic granulomatous disease (CGD). The granulocytes of these people can phagocytose microorganisms, but are unable to mobilize the enzyme pathways necessary to kill them. The McLeod phenotype associated with CGD appears to result from a deletion of part of the X chromosome, which includes the XK locus as well as X-CGD.

Other Phenotypes With Depressed Kell Antigens

K$_{mod}$ has been used to describe phenotypes characterized by weak expression of Kell system antigens.[40] Unlike McLeod rbcs, K$_{mod}$ rbcs (also referred to as Day[41] and Mullins[42] phenotypes) exhibit Kx antigen activity elevated even beyond that on K$_o$ cells. The Kell antigens often require adsorption/elution tests for detection. Some people of the K$_{mod}$ phenotype have made an anti-Ku-like antibody. The K$_{mod}$ phenotype is thought to arise through the inheritance of two recessive genes.

Red cells of persons with some Gerbich-negative phenotypes also exhibit depressed Kell phenotypes. Studies of persons of the Ge: –2, –3 and Ge: –2, –3, –4 (Leach) phenotypes have shown depression of at least some Kell system antigens. The depression may not be as great as that found in the McLeod phenotype.

A phenotype, defined as the Allen phenotype,[43] has been found in one family. A brother and sister in this family show enhanced expression of Kp^a, but depression of other Kell system antigens with the exception of the receptors defined by anti-KL(K20) and anti-Kx. The genetic background of the Allen phenotype remains unclear.

The *Kp^a* gene has been proven to modify the expression of *k* when in *cis* position. As a consequence, the k antigen of these red cells reacts more weakly than expected, and may appear as nonreactive with weaker examples of anti-k. The gene interaction can be recognized only under certain conditions; ie, when *K* is present on the opposite chromosome or when there is a *K$_o$* gene in *trans*. If serologic tests are performed properly, the *cis* modifying effect can also be seen when *Kp^a* is present on both chromosomes.

Biochemistry

The Kell system antigens are carried on a 93-kD glycoprotein that is found at a low density (only 2000-5000 copies/cell) on the rbc membrane.[36] Kell system antigens are inactivated by treating rbcs with sulfhydryl reagents, such as 2-ME, DTT or AET, which provides a useful method of artificially preparing rbcs lacking Kell system antigens as an aid to the identification of Kell-related antibodies. Treatment with sulfhydryl reagents may impair the reactivity of other antigens (LW, Do^a, Do^b, Yt^a and others), however, so the association of an antibody with the Kell system because of reduced reactivity with sulfhydryl-treated rbcs is only tentative. A reagent called ZZAP, a mixture of DTT and cysteine-activated papain,[44] also destroys Kell system antigens. (See Method 6.6.) The susceptibility of the Kell system antigens to sulfhydryl reagents suggested to serologists that disulfide bonds are essential for the maintenance of antigen activity. This hypothesis has been supported by recent biochemical characterization of Kell proteins derived from cloned cDNA.[45] The 2.5-kb gene sequence that was isolated predicts a 732 amino acid protein.

The 47 amino acids that form the N-terminal portion are located within the cytoplasm of the red cell. Twenty amino acids (at positions 48 to 67) form the transmembrane domain. The remaining 665 amino acids are at the external surface. These carry six glycosylation sites and 15 cysteine residues.[46] One additional cysteine is positioned within the transmembrane segment. The high number of cysteine residues indicates a good degree of folding of the Kell protein as disulfide linkages between cysteines are formed. Folding of the protein is probably necessary for antigen expression.

The Kell protein has structural similarities to a family of zinc-binding neutral endopeptidases.[45] It has most similarity with the common acute lymphoblastic leukemia antigen, a neutral endopeptidase on white cells.[45] Thus, Kell may be the first antigen that may be part of a red cell enzyme.

Duffy Blood Group System

The antigens Fy^a and Fy^b are encoded by a pair of codominant alleles. *Fy*, a third allele at this locus, has a high incidence among Blacks.[5] It produces no Fy^a or Fy^b antigens (Table 12-6). Blacks who are Fy(a–b–) are considered to be homozygous *FyFy*. A fourth allele in the system, *Fy^x*, encodes a weakened Fy^b antigen that may go undetected in *Fy^{a}Fy^x*, *FyFy^x* or *Fy^{x}Fy^x* persons unless powerful anti-Fy^b is used in testing, or unless adsorption/elution tests are performed with the rbcs.[5,47]

Table 12-6. Phenotypes and Frequencies in the Duffy System

Reactions With Anti-			Adult Phenotype Frequency %	
Fy^a	Fy^b	Phenotype	Whites	Blacks
+	0	Fy(a+b−)	17	9
+	+	Fy(a+b+)	49	1
0	+	Fy(a−b+)	34	22
0	0	Fy(a−b−)	V. rare	68

The *Fy* locus is located on chromosome 1, near the centromere. It is syntenic with the *Rh* locus. Their order is assumed to be: *PGD, Rh, PMG₁* and *Fy*.[47] Fy^a antigens are associated with a 35- to 43-kD membrane protein.[48] The protein is sensitive to destruction by enzymes such as ficin or papain.

Antibodies to Fy Antigens

Anti-Fy^a and anti-Fy^b cause both HDN and HTRs.[5] Anti-Fy^a is quite commonly encountered[47]; anti-Fy^b is considerably less common. These antibodies react best by the IAT. The antigen sites are destroyed by most proteases used in serologic tests, so anti-Fy^a and anti-Fy^b antibodies usually give negative reactions in enzyme test procedures.

Effect of Zygosity

Weak examples of anti-Fy^a or anti-Fy^b may give convincing reactions only with rbcs that have a double dose of the antigen. In White populations, rbcs that have only one of the two antigens are assumed to come from persons homozygous for the gene and to carry a double dose of the antigen. In Blacks, however, the *Fy* gene is so common that rbcs having only one of the two antigens are usually from persons heterozygous for *Fy*, and the active antigen is present only in single dose.

Rarely Encountered Antibodies

A White person of the Fy(a−b−) phenotype first made anti-Fy3, an exceedingly uncommon antibody that acts like a combination of anti-Fy^a and anti-Fy^b, although the specificities cannot be separated by adsorption and elution. Unlike anti-Fy^a and anti-Fy^b, anti-Fy3 reacts well with enzyme-treated Fy(a+) or Fy(b+) rbcs. Fy3 is considered to be an enzyme-resistant antigen present on all Fy(a+) and Fy(b+) rbcs but absent from Fy(a−b−) rbcs.

Two other rare antibodies have been described, both of which were reactive against papain-treated rbcs. One, anti-Fy4, reacts strongly with rbcs of the Fy(a−b−) phenotype, as well as with some Fy(a+b−) and some Fy(a−b+) rbcs from Blacks, but not with Fy(a+b+) rbcs. On this evidence, Fy4 is considered to be the product of an allele called *Fy* that, in the homozygous state, is responsible for the Fy(a−b−) phenotype in Blacks. The other antibody, anti-Fy5, is similar to anti-Fy3, except that it gives negative reactions with Fy:3;Rh$_{null}$ rbcs, as well as those of the Fy(a−b−) Blacks. This antibody was observed to react with the rbcs of a White Fy(a−b−) person, which provided a hitherto unrecognized distinction between the Fy(a−b−) phenotype so common in Blacks and the one so rare in Whites. It has been postulated that Fy5 is formed by the interaction of Rh and Duffy gene products.[49]

Fy(a−b−) red cells are resistant to invasion by the malarial parasite *Plasmodium knowlesi*, which infects monkeys. In West Africa, most Blacks are Fy(a−b−) and are resistant to *P. vivax* malaria; this would favor the natural selection of persons with the Fy(a−b−) phenotype in endemic areas. Discussions on the role of Duffy blood group antigens in malaria are available.[50]

Kidd Blood Group System

Anti-Jk^a and Anti-Jk^b

Anti-Jk^a was first recognized in 1951, in the serum of a woman who had given birth to a child with HDN.[5] Two years later, anti-Jk^b was found in the serum of a patient who had suffered a transfusion reaction. Both antibodies react best by the IAT, but saline reactivity is sometimes observed in freshly drawn specimens. These antibodies are often weak when first detected and some, perhaps because they are detected indirectly through the complement that they bind to rbcs, may become undetectable on storage. Even freshly drawn sera containing weak anti-Jk^a or anti-Jk^b may manifest a dosage effect, reacting only with rbcs expressing a double dose of the antigen.

Effects of Complement

Some workers report no difficulties in detecting anti-Jk^a and anti-Jk^b antibodies in low ionic tests that incorporate anti-IgG. Others feel that antiglobulin reagent containing an anticomplement component is needed for the reliable detection of these inconsistently reactive antibodies, while others feel rbcs carrying a double dose of Jk^a or Jk^b are needed in screening tests to reliably detect these antibodies. Anti-Jk^a and anti-Jk^b sera that have lost their reactivity during storage can sometimes be revived by adding fresh human serum as a source of complement, or by the use of an enzyme antiglobulin technique. Adding fresh serum, however, dilutes what may already be a weakly reactive antibody, and the procedure may not be successful if the anti-Jk^a or anti-Jk^b serum has become anticomplementary during storage.

A method that has proved satisfactory with some complement-dependent antibodies is the two-stage antiglobulin test of Polley and Mollison.[51] Red cells are first incubated with the test serum in the presence of EDTA, which allows antibody uptake but prevents complement from being bound. The rbcs are then washed and reincubated with antibody-free fresh human serum as a source of complement. After rewashing, a polyspecific antiglobulin reagent is added in the usual way.

Clinical Significance

Kidd system antibodies occasionally cause HDN, but this is usually mild. These antibodies are notorious, however, for involvement in severe HTRs, especially in delayed reactions, which occur when antibody, developing rapidly in an anamnestic response to antigens on transfused rbcs, destroys the still-circulating rbcs. In some reported cases, retesting the patient's pretransfusion serum has confirmed that the antibody was indeed undetectable in the original compatibility tests. Events of this kind highlight the importance of consulting previous records before selecting blood for transfusion; in some cases of delayed HTRs the antibody had previously been detected and identified.

Genes and Phenotypes

The four phenotypes defined by the reactions of anti-Jk^a and anti-Jk^b are shown in Table 12-7. The Jk(a–b–) phenotype is

Table 12-7. Phenotypes and Frequencies in the Kidd System

Reactions With Anti-			Adult Phenotype Frequency %	
Jk^a	Jk^b	Phenotype	Whites	Blacks
+	0	Jk(a+b–)	28	57
+	+	Jk(a+b+)	49	34
0	+	Jk(a–b+)	23	9
0	0	Jk(a–b–)	Exceedingly rare	

extremely rare except in some populations of Pacific Island origin. The phenotype can arise through two mechanisms. One is apparently the result of homozygosity for the silent *Jk* allele. A dominant inhibitor gene called *In(Jk)* has been responsible for the null phenotype in some families.[52] The dominant suppression of Kidd antigens is similar to the *In(Lu)* suppression of the Lutheran system. Sera from some rare *JkJk* persons have been found to contain an antibody that reacts with all Jk(a+) and Jk(b+) rbcs, but not with Jk(a–b–) rbcs. Although a minor anti-Jk[a] or anti-Jk[b] component is sometimes separable, most of the reactivity has been directed at an antigen called Jk3, which is considered to be present on both Jk(a+) and Jk(b+) red cells, in a manner analogous to that of Fy3 on Fy(a+) and Fy(b+) rbcs. Anti-Jk3 is most often rbc-stimulated in origin, but in one case an IgM example of the antibody was detected in a male Jk(a–b–) patient who had no history of transfusion.[53] Curiously, the man had a Jk(a–b–) sister who had been pregnant seven times but had produced no antibody.

Jk(a–b–) rbcs are resistant to lysis by 2 M urea.[54] Jk(a+b–), Jk(a–b+) or Jk(a+b+) rbcs swell rapidly after exposure to this solution and then rupture. In contrast, Jk(a–b–) rbcs shrink and do not lyse for long periods of time. The Jk blood group locus has been assigned to chromosome 18.[55]

Additional Pairs of Antithetical RBC Antigens

So far this chapter has been devoted to blood group systems of which the principal antibodies may be seen fairly frequently in the routine blood typing laboratory. Other systems of genetically determined antigens (Diego, Cartwright, Dombrock, Colton, Scianna) also exist and

the reader should be aware of them. Table 12-8 lists the phenotype frequencies for these systems among Whites. Antibodies directed at these antigens occur rarely, usually in sera containing multiple specificities, perhaps because an immune response to multiple antigens implies unusual susceptibility to producing blood group antibodies. The antigens themselves may be important in genetic investigations and population or family studies.

The phenotype frequencies in the Dombrock system are similar to those of Duffy, while those in the Cartwright and Colton systems parallel the incidences of K and k. The Diego system is useful as a racial marker, the Di[a] antigen being almost entirely confined to populations of Mongoloid origin, including Native Americans. All these antigens, and those of the Scianna system, appear to be less immunogenic than those of the other major blood group systems.

The Sex-Linked Blood Group Antigen Xg[a]

In 1962, an antibody was discovered that identified an antigen more common among women than among men. This would be expected of an X-borne characteristic, because females inherit an X chromosome from each parent, whereas males inherit X only from their mother. The antigen is called Xg[a], in recognition of its X-borne manner of inheritance. Table 12-9 gives the phenotype frequencies among White males and females.

Anti-Xg[a] is an uncommon antibody that usually reacts only by the IAT, although at least three examples are known that agglutinated saline-suspended rbcs. Enzymes most often used in serologic tests appear to alter the antigen, so negative reactions are to be expected in enzyme test systems. This antibody has not been implicated in

Table 12-8. Phenotype Frequencies in Other Blood Group Systems in Which Antithetical Antibodies Are Known

System	Reactions With Anti-		Phenotype	Phenotype Frequency % in Whites*
Diego	Di^a	Di^b		
	+	0	Di(a+b−)	0†
	+	+	Di(a+b+)	very rare†
	0	+	Di(a−b+)	100
Cartwright	Yt^a	Yt^b		
	+	0	Yt(a+b−)	91.9
	+	+	Yt(a+b+)	7.9
	0	+	Yt(a−b+)	0.2
Dombrock	Do^a	Do^b		
	+	0	Do(a+b−)	17.2
	+	+	Do(a+b+)	49.5
	0	+	Do(a−b+)	33.3
Colton	Co^a	Co^b		
	+	0	Co(a+b−)	89.3
	+	+	Co(a+b+)	10.4
	0	+	Co(a−b+)	0.3
	0	0	Co(a−b−)	very rare
Scianna	Sc1	Sc2		
	+	0	Sc:1,−2	99.7
	+	+	Sc:1,2	0.3
	0	+	Sc:−1,2	very rare
	0	0	Sc:−1,−2	very rare

*There are insufficient data for reliable calculation of frequencies in Blacks.
†The Di^a antigen has a much higher frequency in Orientals and Native Americans.

HDN or HTRs, but it is evidently capable of binding complement and one example has been reported as an autoantibody.[56] Anti-Xg^a may be useful for tracing the transmission of genetic traits associated with the X chromosome, although linkage with the *Xg* locus has been demonstrated for few traits to date.

High-Incidence RBC Antigens

Genetic Considerations

Persons who make alloantibody to a specific blood group antigen necessarily have

Table 12-9. Frequencies of the Xg(a+) and Xg(a−) Phenotypes in White Males and Females

Phenotype	Phenotype Frequency %	
	Males	Females
Xg(a+)	65.6	88.7
Xg(a−)	34.4	11.3

Frequencies are based on combined results of testing nearly 7000 random blood samples from populations of Northern European origin. There are insufficient data for reliable calculation of frequencies in Blacks.

Table 12-10. Antigens of High and Low Incidence

System/Collection Name	ISBT Symbol	Antigen	Frequency (%)
Gerbich	GE	Ge2	>99
		Ge3	>99
		Ge4	>99
		Wb	<1
		Ls^a	<1
		An^a	<1
		Dh^a	<1
Cromer	CROMER	Cr^a	>99
		Tc^a	>99
		Tc^b	<1
		Tc^c	<1
		Dr^a	>99
		Es^a	>99
		IFC	>99
		WES^a	<1
		WES^b	>99
		UMC	>99
Indian	IN	In^a	<1
		In^b	>99
Er	ER	Er^a	>99
		Er^b	<1

rbcs lacking that antigen. For this reason, antibodies directed at high-incidence antigens are rarely encountered. When they do occur, however, it may be exceedingly difficult to find compatible blood. Members of the patient's family, especially siblings, are usually the most promising sources of potential donors. Absence of a high-incidence antigen usually implies homozygosity for the rare recessive gene that encodes no antigen or an alternative antigen. Both parents of the patient are usually heterozygous for this gene, so there is one chance in four that each sibling will, like the patient, be homozygous for the rare gene and lack the high-incidence antigen. In the unlikely event that one of the parents is homozygous for the rare gene, the chance that any sibling will be homozygous increases to one in two. Tables 12-10 and 12-11 list some of the antigens of high incidence, defined as occurring in 92 to 99.9% or more of the general population.

Table 12-11. Some Antigens of High Incidence Not Assigned to a Blood Group System or Collection

Name	Symbol
August	At^a
	Vel
Joseph	Jo^a
	Ok^a
	MER2
Langeris	Lan
Sid	Sd^a
Fritz	Wr^b
Duclos	

Serologic Considerations

The antibodies corresponding to these antigens usually react best by the IAT, although a few examples of anti-Ge (Gerbich) and most anti-Vel may agglutinate saline-suspended rbcs. Despite its occurrence after known immunizing stimuli, anti-Vel is most commonly of the IgM type and has not been reported to cause HDN. The antibody has, however, been implicated in HTRs. Anti-Vel binds complement, and in-vitro hemolysis of incompatible rbcs is often seen when testing freshly drawn serum containing this antibody. Reactivity of anti-Vel is usually enhanced when enzyme-treated rbcs are used.

Of the antigens listed in Table 12-10, Gerbich (Ge) merits additional explanation. The Ge– phenotype is clearly heterogeneous,[57] because some antibodies identified as anti-Ge react with some rbcs described as Ge–.

Three types of Ge– phenotypes have been defined based on their reactions with anti-Ge2, -Ge3 and -Ge4.[57] (Ge1 is no longer in use as a term describing a Ge-related antigen.) Ge: –2, 3, 4 rbcs (Yus type of Ge–) will react with anti-Ge3 and -Ge4, but not with anti-Ge2. Ge: –2, –3, 4 rbcs (Gerbich type) are agglutinated by anti-Ge4 only. Ge: –2, –3, –4 rbc (Leach type) do not react with any Ge antibody. Ge: –2, –3, –4 rbcs lack glycophorin C (GPC) and glycophorin D (GPD). Such rbcs have been reported to have decreased mechanical stability.

GPC is encoded by *GYPC* located on chromosome 2.[58] This gene has four exons and may also encode GPD. Persons of the Ge: –2, 3, 4 (Yus) phenotype possess a *GYPC* gene that lacks exon 2. Those of the Ge: –2, –3, 4 (Gerbich) phenotype have a *GYPC* that lacks exon 3. The unusual genes of the Yus and Gerbich phenotypes encode abnormal proteins that can be detected on polyacrylamide gels.

Table 12-12 gives some of the differences between the Ge– phenotypes.[59,60]

Other RBC Antigens of Comparatively High Incidence

Serologic Behavior

Among the most frustrating problems encountered in testing sera for unexpected antibodies are those created by a group of antibodies formerly referred to as *high-titer, low-avidity* (HTLA) antibodies. These reactions are invariably observed in the antiglobulin phase of testing, but they are commonly weak, variable and sometimes irreproducible. Feeble reactions seen with undiluted serum often persist in serum subjected to considerable dilution; however, not all examples exhibit this pattern. This suggests that relatively unconvincing initial reactions reflect either low affinity of the antibodies or weak cellular expression of the antigens, rather than limited antibody concentration. These antibodies, although of debatable clinical significance, react with antigens having a fairly high

Table 12-12. Ge– Phenotypes

Phenotype	Antibody Produced
Ge: –2, 3, 4 (Yus type)	anti-Ge2
Ge: –2, –3, 4 (Gerbich type)	anti-Ge2 or anti-Ge3
Ge: –2, –3, –4 (Leach type)	anti-Ge2 or anti-Ge3

incidence in the population. When the antibody has been identified, blood can normally be issued without further delay. The corresponding antigens are listed in Table 12-13, together with their approximate frequencies in the population.

Antibodies to Cost (Cs^a, Cs^b), York (Yk^a), Knops (Kn^a, Kn^b), McCoy (McC^a, McC^b, McC^c, McC^d, McC^e, McC^f), Swain-Langley (Sl^a, Sl^b), Chido (Ch1-6), Rodgers (Rg1,2), JMH, Holley (Hy) and Gregory (Gy^a) were once part of the "HTLA" group.[62] Some workers consider anti-McC^c and -Sl^a to be one and the same. All antigens are of high incidence (92-99%) in the White population, with the exception of Cs^b, Kn^b, McC^b, McC^f and Sl^b.[62] McC^c and McC^e are found less frequently on the rbcs of Blacks.[62] Anti-Yk^a, -Ch, -Kn^a, -McC^a and -Sl^a (or -McC^c) are encountered frequently.

Knops/McCoy, Swain-Langley and York Antigens

The York, Knops, McCoy and Swain-Langley antigens are related at the structural level and have recently been shown to be part of complement receptor type 1 (CR1, CD35, C3b/C4b receptor).[63,64] CR1 receptors exhibit both size and expression polymorphisms. Thus, the number of CR1 receptors per rbc varies widely from person to person. Moulds et al[65] have shown that the variable reactions obtained with various anti-CR1-related sera are a direct reflection of the number of CR1 sites per rbc.

JMH, Hy and Gy^a Antigens

The JMH, Hy and Gy^a antigens are carried on proteins attached to phosphatidyl-inositol-glycan (GPI) anchors.[66,67] The GPI-anchored proteins are distinct from decay-

Table 12-13. Some Blood Group Antigens of Fairly High Incidence

Antigens	Phenotypes	Approximate Frequency % Whites	Blacks
Chido (Ch)	Ch +, Rg +	95	
and	Ch −, Rg +	2	
Rodgers (Rg)*	Ch +, Rg −	3	
	Ch −, Rg −	Very rare	
Cost (Cs^a)	Cs(a +), Yk(a +)	82.5	95.6
and	Cs(a +), Yk(a −)	13.5	3.2
York (Yk^a)	Cs(a −), Yk(a +)	2.1	0.6
	Cs(a −), Yk(a −)	1.9	0.6
Knops-Helgeson (Kn^a)	Kn(a +), McC(a +)	97	95
and	Kn(a +), McC(a −)	2	4
McCoy (McC^a)	Kn(a −), McC(a +)	1	1
	Kn(a −), McC(a −)	Rare	Rare
John Milton Hagen (JMH)	JMH +	99.9	
	JMH −	0.1	
Holley (Hy)	Hy +, Gy(a +)	>99	
and	Hy −, Gy(a + ^{w})		Rare
Gregory (Gy^a)	Hy −, Gy(a −)	Rare	

*Chido has been shown to have six subspecificities (1–6) and Rodgers has two known subspecificities (1, 2).[61]

accelerating factor (DAF), also a GPI-linked protein, involved in the regulation of complement activation. The Cromer-related antigens Cr^a, Tc^a, Tc^b, Tc^c, Dr^a, Es^a, WES^a, WES^b, IFC and UMC are carried on DAF.[68]

Some data suggest that some examples of anti-Hy may cause accelerated destruction of antigen-positive red cells.[62]

Ch and Rg Antigens

The Chido (Ch1-6) and Rodgers (Rg1,2) antigens are part of the C4 molecule of human complement,[69] and are not intrinsic to the rbc membrane. Ch and Rg antigens reside on the C4d fragment,[70] and many examples of the corresponding antibodies agglutinate saline suspensions of rbcs coated heavily with C4d.[71] Because C4 is present in human serum, anti-Ch and anti-Rg are neutralized by serum or plasma from persons positive for the relevant antigen; this is the majority of the population. Aids to the identification of these antibodies are that they agglutinate C4d-coated rbcs in a saline test system[71] and that most randomly selected sera neutralize their reactivity (see Methods 4.6 and 4.7). The antigens are destroyed by ficin and papain; thus, the antibodies fail to react in tests employing enzyme-treated rbcs.

The Sd^a Antigen

Sd^a (Sid) is another antigen of fairly high incidence that is widely distributed in mammalian tissues and body fluids.[72] The antigen is variably expressed on the rbcs of Sd(a+) individuals and may disappear transiently during pregnancy. The strongest expression of Sd^a has been observed on rbcs of the Cad phenotype, which are agglutinated by the lectin *Dolichos biflorus* and by many human sera.[73]

Antibody Behavior

Anti-Sd^a is most often detected when antiglobulin tests are examined microscopically, but most examples would be equally demonstrable if the rbc button in a saline agglutination test were examined microscopically after resuspension. Mixed-field agglutination is the characteristic reaction, with relatively small, tightly agglutinated clumps of rbcs present against a background of free rbcs. These agglutinates are refractile, so they often present a shining appearance when viewed microscopically. A single example of anti-Sd^a tested against different rbcs often gives agglutination reactions of different strengths.

RBC and Urine Reactivity

The frequency of Sd(a–) blood is generally considered to be around 9%, but weak positives are often difficult to distinguish from negatives. Among pregnant women, the incidence of the Sd(a–) rbc phenotype is variously reported to be from 30-75%. Urine from guinea pigs and from Sd(a+) humans inhibits the reactivity of anti-Sd^a, but urine from Sd(a–) people is noninhibitory. When populations are screened by urine testing, the true incidence of Sd(a–) appears closer to 4% than to 9%.

The inhibitory substance in guinea pig and in human Sd(a+) urine has been identified as a configuration of the Tamm and Horsfall urinary glycoprotein; the immunodominant sugar is N-acetylgalactosamine.[74] Urine can inhibit agglutination by antibodies other than anti-Sd^a, however, for nonimmunologic reasons such as salt concentration or pH. Urinary inhibition studies may not yield reliable results unless the urine sample is first adjusted for pH and then dialyzed against phosphate-buffered saline.[75] (See Methods 1.6 and 4.9.)

Clinical Significance

Although reported once as causing an HTR,[76] anti-Sd[a] is widely believed to have no clinical significance. However, rbcs of the rare Sd(a++) phenotype, or the even rarer Cad rbcs, may have decreased survival in the circulation of a patient whose serum contains potent anti-Sd[a].

Low-Incidence Red Cell Antigens

Many low-incidence rbc antigens have been recognized in addition to a growing number that have been assigned to the MN and Rh systems. Table 12-14 lists those that have been studied and shown to be inherited in a dominant manner. Antibodies specific for these low-incidence antigens react with so few random blood samples that they virtually never cause difficulties in selecting blood for transfusion. These antibodies are of interest to the serologist, however, because of the relatively high incidence with which they occur, often without an identifiable antigenic stimulus.

Significance of Antibodies

Antibodies to low-incidence antigens are encountered by chance in antibody screening or compatibility testing, when a screening rbc or a donor rbc selected for crossmatching happens to carry the corresponding antigen. Since routine antibody screening tests rarely detect such antibodies, the crossmatch affords the only opportunity to detect an incompatibility, should antigen-positive donor blood be selected for transfusion. The chance of choosing donor blood positive for that antigen, however, is quite remote.

Antibodies to low-incidence antigens may also be present as unsuspected contaminants in blood grouping reagents of human polyclonal source, and may

Table 12-14. Antigens of Low Incidence Not Assigned to a Blood Group System or Collection

Batty (By)*	Milne
Biles (Bi[a])	Moen (Mo[a])
Bishop (Bp[a])	NFLD
Bowyer (BOW)	Oldeide (Ol[a])
Box (Bx[a])	Os[a]
Christiansen (Chr[a])	Peters (Pt[a])
	Radin (Rd)*
ELO	Redelberger (Rb[a])
Froese (Fr[a])	Reid (Re[a])
HJK	Swann (Sw[a])
HOFM	SW1
Hey	Torkildsen (To[a])
Hughes (Hg[a])	Traversu (Tr[a])
JFV	VanVugt (Vg[a])
JONES	Waldner (Wd[a])
Jensen (Je[a])	Wright (Wr[a])*
Katagiri (Kg)	Wulfsberg (Wu)
Livesay (Li[a])	

The antigens occur with a frequency of 1 in 500 or less. *Antibodies to these antigens have been noted to arise in response to fetomaternal immunization and, in some cases, to have caused hemolytic disease of the newborn.

cause false-positive reactions if the rbcs tested carry the antigen. Replicate testing with reagents from different manufacturers may not eliminate this error, since the same donor may be the source of antibody-containing serum used by different manufacturers.

Occurrence and Behavior

In some cases, antibodies to low-incidence antigens are seen as saline agglutinins, but they can also occur as IgG antibodies reactive only at the antiglobulin phase of testing, even in persons lacking a history of exposure to rbcs. It is not uncommon for many of these antibodies to be present together in a single serum; multiple specificity is especially likely in sera from patients with AIHA. Indeed, whether or not there is clinical evidence of disease, autoantibodies in a serum are frequently accompanied by a mixture of alloantibodies directed at low-incidence antigens. These are usually separable from the autoantibody, and from each other, by adsorption using appropriate rbcs.

The Bg Antigens

Antibodies directed at certain leukocyte antigens sometimes cause confusing reactions in serologic tests with rbcs. The so-called Bg antigens are expressed to variable degrees on rbcs, with the result that reactions of differing strength are observed when a single serum containing "anti-Bg" is tested with different Bg+ red cells. Reactivity is most commonly observed in the IAT, but sufficiently potent anti-Bg sera may cause direct agglutination of rbcs with unusually enhanced expression of the Bg antigens.

At least three separate antigens have been recognized, called Bg^a, Bg^b and Bg^c, but confident and precise classification is made difficult by the weak expression of these antigens on some rbcs, and by multiple specificities among different examples of the Bg antibodies. These antibodies may also occur as unsuspected contaminants in blood grouping sera, where they may cause false-positive reactions with cells having unusually strong expression of the corresponding Bg antigen. The rbc antigen Bg^a corresponds with the leukocyte antigen HLA-B7; Bg^b with HLA-B17; and Bg^c with HLA-A28. A fourth antibody in some antileukocyte sera has been shown to react with the rbcs of persons with the leukocyte antigen HLA-A10. Bg-related antigens are denatured by chloroquine diphosphate and a solution of glycine-HCl/EDTA. (See Methods 2.15 and 2.16.)

Determinants of Other Cellular Elements of Human Blood

Granulocyte Antigens

The procedures used to demonstrate antigens on granulocytes differ from red cell typing tests. Agglutination tests in tube, capillary or microplate tests use heat-inactivated serum in the presence of EDTA. For nonagglutinating antibodies, useful procedures are surface-binding tests utilizing either fluorescein-labeled antiglobulin serum or an enzyme-linked immunoglobulin for detection. A granulocytotoxicity test comparable to lymphocytotoxicity procedures has been developed for the detection of HLA antigens on granulocytes. Certain functional assay procedures have also been developed, but these are technically difficult to perform and are beyond the scope of most blood transfusion service laboratories. Details, test procedures and references are given by Thompson and Severson.[77]

Antigens Shared With Lymphocytes and Other Tissues

The HLA antigens exist on most tissue cells. (See Chapter 13.) Some may be demonstrated on granulocytes by leukoagglutination with suitable antisera. Sera containing strong and specific lymphocytotoxic antibodies may, however, give negative reactions with granulocytes, even by granulocytotoxicity tests.

Antigens of Mature Granulocytes

Leukoagglutination or immunofluorescence techniques have sometimes demonstrated antibodies specific for several determinants present only on mature granulocytes in the sera of persons with immune neutropenia. These include NA1 and NA2, which are thought to be reciprocally related; NB1 and NB2, products of a second locus; NC1, ND1 and NE1; 9a; and a series of related antigens called *human granulocyte antigens* (HGA) HGA-3a, -3b, -3c, -3d and -3e. Antibodies to the HGA-3 series of antigens are sometimes associated with febrile transfusion reactions as well as immune neutropenia. The HGA-3 antibodies are not reactive as agglutinins. Original references to the antigens listed are cited by Thompson and Severson[77]; an additional discussion of neutrophil antigens and their significance is presented by McCullough et al.[78]

The antigens 5a and 5b appear to be independent of other systems. They are considered to be products of allelic genes, and antibodies directed at them are usually detected by agglutination methods. Such antibodies occasionally occur in women after pregnancy and may be associated with febrile transfusion reactions.

Platelet Antigens

Platelet antigens are carried in greatest density on, but are not restricted to, platelets.[79,80] Testing for platelet antibodies may be of little benefit for the majority of patients, but can be useful as an adjunct to HLA matching in selecting compatible platelets for recipients with alloantibodies directed at platelet antigens. Platelet-specific alloantigens are immunogens in posttransfusion purpura (PTP) and neonatal alloimmune thrombocytopenic purpura (NATP). Sensitization to HPA-1a (Pl^{A1}) accounts for more than 75% of cases of NATP and PTP.[80] Antibodies to HPA-5b, -4a, -4b and -3a (Br^a, Pen^a, Pen^b and Bak^a, respectively) have also been implicated in NATP.

Glycoproteins GPIa, Ib, Ic, IIa, IIIa, IIIb and IX have been identified as parts of the platelet membrane.[81] Figure 12-2 shows how GPIa, IIa and IIIa each

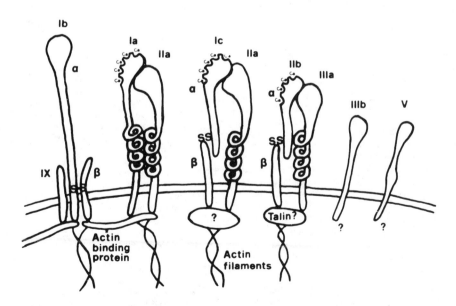

Figure 12-2. Schematic drawing of the major platelet membrane glycoproteins indicating known or suspected complexes, disulfide bonds between chains, calcium-binding domains and interactions with cytoskeletal components.[81]

Table 12-15. Nomenclature and Phenotype Frequency of Human Platelet Antigens[82, 83]

Antigen System	Glycoprotein (GP) Location	Other Names	Antigens	Other Names	Phenotype Frequency (%) White*	Japanese†
HPA-1	GPIIIa	Zw, PlA	HPA-1a	Zwa, PlA1	97.9	99.9
			HPA-1b	Zwb, PlA2	26.5	3.7
HPA-2	GPIb	Ko, Sib	HPA-2a	Kob	99.3	NT‡
			HPA-2b	Koa, Siba	14.6	25.4
HPA-3	GPIIb	Bak, Lek	HPA-3a	Baka, Leka	87.7	78.9
			HPA-3b	Bakb	64.1	NT
HPA-4	GPIIIa	Pen, Yuk	HPA-4a	Pena, Yukb	99.9	99.9
			HPA-4b	Penb, Yuka	0.2	1.7
HPA-5	GPIa	Br, Hc, Zav	HPA-5a	Brb, Zavb	99.2	NT
			HPA-5b	Bra, Zava, Hca	20.6	NT

*Calculated from data in the literature.
†Data provided by H.Saji (Japanese Workshop data).
‡Not tested.

consist of single polypeptide chains that carry several intrachain disulfide bonds. Ib, Ic and IIb proteins are composed of one large (alpha) chain linked via disulfide bridges to a smaller (beta) chain. Platelet-specific antigens associated with the surface glycoproteins are listed in Table 12-15.

References

1. Lewis M, Anstee DJ, Bird GWG, et al. Blood group terminology 1990. From the ISBT working party on terminology for red cell surface antigens. Vox Sang 1990;58:152-69.
2. Landsteiner K, Levine P. A new agglutinable factor differentiating human blood. Proc Soc Exp Biol 1927;24:600-3.
3. Smith ML, Beck M. The immunoglobulin structure of human anti-M agglutinins. Transfusion 1988;23:113-8.
4. Beattie KM, Zuelzer WW. The frequency and properties of pH-dependent anti-M. Transfusion 1965;5:322-6.
5. Race RR, Sanger R. Blood groups in man. 6th ed. Oxford: Blackwell Scientific Publications, 1975.
6. Alperin JB, Riglin H, Branch DR, et al. Anti-M causing a delayed transfusion reaction. Transfusion 1983;23:322-4.
7. Howell ED, Perkins HA. Anti-N-like antibodies in the sera of patients undergoing chronic hemodialysis. Vox Sang 1972;23:291-9.

8. Harrison PB, Jansson K, Kronenberg H, et al. Cold agglutinin formation in patients undergoing hemodialysis. A possible relationship to dialyzer reuse. Aust NZ J Med 1975;5:195-7.
9. Dahr W, Moulds J. An immunochemical study on anti-N antibodies from dialysis patients. Immunol Commun 1981;10:173-83.
10. Metaxas MN, Metaxas-Bühler M. Rare genes of the MNSs system affecting red cell membranes. In: Mohn JL, Plunkett RW, Cunningham RK, Lambert RM, eds. Human blood groups. Basel: Karger, 1977:344-52.
11. Issitt PD. The MN blood group system. Cincinnati: Montgomery Scientific Publications, 1981.
12. Dahr W. Immunochemistry of sialoglycoproteins in human red cell membranes. In: Vengelen-Tyler V, Judd WJ, eds. Recent advances in blood group biochemistry. Arlington, VA: American Association of Blood Banks, 1986:23-66.
13. Ellisor S. Action and application of enzymes in immunohematology. In: Bell CA, ed. A seminar on antigen-antibody reactions revisited. Arlington, VA: American Association of Blood Banks, 1982:133-74.
14. Telen MJ, Chasis JA. Relationship of the human erythrocyte Wrb antigen to an interaction between glycophorin A and band 3. Blood 1990;76:842-8.
15. Kudo S, Fukuda M. Structural organization of glycophorin A and B genes: Glycophorin B gene evolved by homologous recombination at *Alu* repeat sequences. Proc Natl Acad Sci USA 1989;86:4619-23.
16. Contreras M, Green C, Humphreys J, et al. Serology and genetics of an MNSs-associated antigen, Dantu. Vox Sang 1984;46:377-86.

17. Tanner MJA, Anstee DJ, Mawby WJ. A new human erythrocyte variant (Ph) containing an abnormal membrane sialoglycoprotein. Biochem J 1980;187;493-500.

18. Unger P, Procter JL, Moulds JJ, et al. The Dantu erythrocyte phenotype of the NE variety. II. Serology, immunochemistry, genetics and frequency. Blut 1986;55:33-43.

19. Huang CH, Blumenfield OO. Molecular genetics of human erythrocyte Mi. III and Mi. VI glycophorins. J Biol Chem 1991;266:7248-56.

20. Issitt PD, Jerez G. Adsorption of unwanted antibodies from sera containing MNS or Duffy group antibodies without the need for selecting "appropriately negative" cells. Transfusion 1955;6:155-9.

21. Case J. The behavior of anti-S antibodies with ficin-treated human red cells. In: Abstracts of volunteer papers. 30th Annual Meeting of the American Association of Blood Banks. Washington, DC: American Association of Blood Banks, 1977:36.

22. Issitt PD, Marsh WL, Wren MR, et al. Heterogeneity of anti-U demonstrable by the use of papain-treated red cells. Transfusion 1989;29:509-13.

23. Brown F, Simpson S, Cornwall S et al. The recessive Lu(a–b–) phenotype. A family study. Vox Sang 1974;26:259-64.

24. Taliano V, Guevin RM, Tippett P. The genetics of a dominant inhibitor of the Lutheran antigens. Vox Sang 1973;24:42-7.

25. Norman PC, Tippett P, Beal RW. An Lu(a–b–) phenotype caused by an X-linked recessive gene. Vox Sang 1986;51:49-52.

26. Anstee DJ. Blood group active components of the human red cell membrane. In: Garratty G, ed. Red cell antigens and antibodies. Arlington, VA: American Association of Blood Banks, 1986:1-15.

27. Daniels G. Evidence that Auberger blood group antigens are located on the Lutheran glycoproteins. Vox Sang 1990;58:56-60.

28. Zelinski K, Kaita H, Coghlan G, Philipps S. Assignment of the Auberger red cell antigen polymorphism to the Lutheran blood group system: Genetic justification. Vox Sang 1991;61:275-6.

29. Daniels G, Khalid G. Identification, by immunoblotting, of the structures carrying Lutheran and para-Lutheran blood group antigens. Vox Sang 1989;57:137-41.

30. Parsons SF, Mallinson G, Judson PA, et al. Evidence that the Lu^b blood group antigen is located on red cell membrane glycoproteins of 85 and 78 kd. Transfusion 1987;27:61-3.

31. Daniels G. The Lutheran blood group system: Monoclonal antibodies, biochemistry and the effect of In(Lu). In: Pierce SP, MacPherson CR, eds. Blood group systems: Duffy, Kidd and Lutheran. Arlington, VA: American Association of Blood Banks, 1988:119-47.

32. Merry AH, Gardner B, Parsons SF, Anstee DJ. Estimation of the number of binding sites for a murine monoclonal anti-Lu^b on human erythrocytes. Vox Sang 1987;53:57-60.

33. Gavin J, Daniels GJ, Yamaguchi H, et al. The red cell antigen once called Levay is the antigen Kp^c of the Kell blood group system. Vox Sang 1979;36:31-3.

34. Daniels G. The Kell blood group system: Genetics. In: Laird-Fryer B, Daniels G, Levitt J, eds. Blood group systems: Kell. Arlington, VA: American Association of Blood Banks, 1990:1-36.

35. Pehta JC, Redman CM, Marsh WL. Biochemistry of the Kell blood group. In: Laird-Fryer B, Daniels G, Levitt J, eds. Blood group systems: Kell. Arlington, VA: American Association of Blood Banks, 1990:69-76.

36. Marsh WL, Redman CM. The Kell blood group system: A review. Transfusion 1990;30:158-66.

37. Zelinski T, Coghlan G, Myal Y, et al. Genetic linkage between the Kell blood group system and prolactin-inducible protein loci: Provisional assignment of KEL to chromosome 7. Ann Hum Genet 1991;55:137-40.

38. Redman CM, Marsh WL, Scarborough A, et al. Biochemical studies on McLeod phenotype red cells and isolation of Kx antigen. Br J Haematol 1988;68:131-6.

39. Rouger P. Defects of McLeod red blood cells and association with disease. In: Laird-Fryer B, Daniels G, Levitt J, eds. Blood group systems: Kell. Arlington, VA: American Association of Blood Banks, 1991:77-88.

40. Marsh WL, Redman CM. Recent developments in the Kell blood group system. Transfus Med Rev 1987;1:4-20.

41. Brown A, Berger R, Lasko D, et al. The Day phenotype: A "new" variant in the Kell blood group system. Bl Transf Immunohaematol 1982;25:619-27.

42. Peloquin P, Yochum G, Hagy L, et al. The Mullins phenotype: Another rbc phenotype characterized by weak Kell antigens (abstract). Transfusion 1988;28:19S.

43. Norman PC, Daniels GL. Unusual suppression of Kell system antigens in a healthy blood donor. Transfusion 1988;28:460-2.

44. Branch DR, Petz LD. A new reagent (ZZAP) having multiple applications in immunohematology. Am J Clin Pathol 1982;78:161-7.

45. Marsh WL. Molecular biology of blood groups: Cloning the Kell gene (editorial). Transfusion 1992;32:98-101.

46. Marsh WL, Lee S, Zambas E, Redman CM. Molecular cloning of Kell (abstract). Transfusion 1991;31:44S.

47. Beattie KM. The Duffy blood group system: Distribution, serology and genetics. In: Pierce SR, MacPherson CR, eds. Blood group systems: Duffy, Kidd and Lutheran. Arlington, VA: American Association of Blood Banks, 1988:1-25.

48. Hadley TJ, David PH, McGuinniss MH, et al. Identification of an erythrocyte component carrying the Duffy blood group Fy^a antigen. Science 1984;223:597-9.

49. Colledge KI, Pezzulich M, Marsh WL. Anti-Fy5, an antibody disclosing a probable association between the Rhesus and Duffy blood groups. Vox Sang 1973;24:193-9.

50. Valko D. The Duffy blood group system: Biochemistry and role in malaria. In: Pierce SR, MacPherson CR, eds. Blood group systems: Duffy, Kidd and Lutheran. Arlington VA: American Association of Blood Banks, 1988: 27-52.

51. Polley MT, Mollison PL. The role of complement in the detection of blood group antibodies. Special reference to the antiglobulin test. Transfusion 1961;1:9-11.

52. Okubo Y, Yamaguchi H, Nagao N, et al. Heterogeneity of the phenotype Jk(a−b−) found in Japanese. Transfusion 1986;26:237-9.

53. Arcara PC, O'Connor MA, Dimmette RM. A family with three Jk(a−b−) members (abstract). Transfusion 1969;9:282.

54. Heaton DC, McLoughlin K. Jk(a−b−) red blood cells resist urea lysis. Transfusion 1982;22:70.

55. Geituik GA, Høyheim B, Gedde-Dahl T, et al. The Kidd (Jk) blood group locus assigned to chromosome 18 by close linkage to DNA-RFLP. Hum Genet 1987;77:205-9.

56. Yokoyama M, Eith DT, Bowman M. The first example of auto anti-Xg^a. Vox Sang 1967;12: 138-9.

57. Reid ME. Hybrid sialoglycoproteins, Gerbich, Webb and Cad blood group determinants. In: Vengelen-Tyler V, Judd WJ, eds. Recent advances in blood group biochemistry. Arlington, VA: American Association of Blood Banks, 1986:67-103.

58. Mattei MG, Colin Y, Le Van Kim C, et al. Localization of the gene for human erythrocyte glycophorin C to chromosome 2.q14-21. Hum Genet 1986;74:420-2.

59. Unger PJ. The Gerbich blood groups: Distribution, serology and genetics. In: Unger P, Laird-Fryer B, eds. Blood group systems: MN and Gerbich. Arlington, VA: American Association of Blood Banks, 1989:59-72.

60. Reid M. Biochemistry and molecular cloning analysis of human red cell sialoglycoproteins that carry Gerbich blood group antigens. In: Unger P, Laird-Fryer B, eds. Blood group systems: MN and Gerbich. Arlington, VA: American Association of Blood Banks, 1989:73-103.

61. Giles CM. Antigenic determinants of human C4, Rodgers and Chido. Exp Clin Immunogenet 1988;5:99-114.

62. Rolih S. A review: Antibodies with high-titer, low-avidity characteristics. Immunohematology 1990;6:59-67.

63. Moulds JM, Nickells MV, Moulds JJ, et al. The C3b/C4b receptor is recognized by the Knops, McCoy, Swain-Langley, and York blood group antisera. J Exp Med 1991;171:1159-63.

64. Rao N, Ferguson DJ, Lee SF, Telen MJ. Identification of human erythrocyte blood group antigens on the C3b/C4b receptor. J Immunol 1991;146:3502-7.

65. Moulds JM, Moulds JJ, Brown M, Atkinson JP. Antiglobulin testing for CR1-related (Knops/McCoy/Swain-Langley/York) blood group antigens: Negative and weak reactions are caused by variable expression of CRI. Vox Sang 1992; 62:230-5.

66. Bobolis KA, Moulds JJ, Telen MJ. Isolation of the JMH antigen on a novel phosphatidylinositol-linked human membrane protein. Blood 1991;79:1574-81.

67. Spring FA, Reid ME. Evidence that the human blood group antigens Gy^a and Hy are carried on a novel glycophosphatidylinositol-linked erythrocyte membrane glycoprotein. Vox Sang 1991;60:53-9.

68. Telen MJ. Phosphatidylinositol-linked red blood cell membrane proteins and blood group antigens. Immunohematology 1991;7:65-72.

69. O'Neill GJ, Yang SY, Tegoli J, et al. Chido and Rodgers blood groups are antigenically distinct components of human complement C4. Nature 1978;273:668-70.

70. Tilley CA, Romans DG, Crookston MC. Localization of Chido and Rodgers determinants of the C4d fragment of human C4. Nature 1978;276:713-5.

71. Judd WJ, Kraemer K, Moulds J. The rapid identification of Chido and Rodgers antibodies using C4d-coated red blood cells. Transfusion 1981;21:189-92.

72. Morton JA, Pickles MM, Terry AM. The Sd^a blood group antigen in tissues and body fluids. Vox Sang 1970;19:472-82.

73. Cazal P, Monis M, Caubel J, Brives J. Polyagglutinabilité héréditaire dominante: Antigen privé (Cad) correspondent à une anticorps public et à une lectine de *Dolichos biflorus*. Rev Fr Transfus 1968;11:209-21.

74. Soh CPC, Morgan WTJ, Watkins WM, Donald ASR. The relationship between the N-acetylgalactosamine content and the blood group Sd^a activity of Tamm and Horsfall urinary glycoprotein. Biochem Biophys Res Comm 1980; 93:1123-39.

75. Judd JW. Urines for inhibition (Letter). Transfusion 1983;23:404-5.

76. Peetermans ME, Cole-Dergent J. Haemolytic transfusion reaction due to anti-Sd^a. Vox Sang 1970;18:67-70.

77. Thompson JS, Severson DC. Granulocyte antigens. In: Bell CA, ed. A seminar on antigens in blood cells and body fluids. Washington, DC: American Association of Blood Banks, 1980: 151-87.

78. McCullough J, Clay M, Kline W. Granulocyte antigens and antibodies. Transfus Med Rev 1987;1:150-60.

79. Kunicki TJ, Furihata K, Bull B, Nugent DJ. The immunogenicity of platelet membrane glycoproteins. Transfus Med Rev 1987;1:21-33.

80. Kunicki T. Human platelet antigen systems. In: Smith DM, Summers SH, eds. Platelets. Arlington, VA: American Association of Blood Banks, 1988:15-53.

81. Clemetson KJ. Glycoproteins of the platelet plasma membrane. In: George JN, Nurden AT, Phillips DR, eds. Platelet membrane glycoproteins. New York: Plenum Press, 1985:51-86.

82. Von dem Borne AEGKr, Decary F. Nomenclature of platelet-specific antigens. Transfusion 1990;30:477.

83. Mueller-Eckhart C, Kiefel V, Sansoto S. Review and update of platelet alloantigen systems. Transfus Med Rev 1990;4:98-109.

13

The HLA System

Introduction

The HLA system includes a complex array of genes and their molecular products that are important in immune regulation, transplantation and transfusion. The antigens of the HLA system are determined by genes present in the major histocompatibility complex (MHC) on the short arm of chromosome 6. These genes contribute to recognition of nonself, to the immune responses to new antigens and to coordination of cellular and humoral immunity. The HLA gene products are glycoprotein antigens found on the surface membranes of all nucleated cells of the body, including those of solid tissues, lymphocytes, granulocytes, monocytes and platelets. In contrast to such cells, mature red cells usually lack HLA antigens demonstrable by conventional methods, but immature, nucleated red cells exhibit HLA reactivity. Antigens of the HLA system have been variously designated histocompatibility locus antigens, human leukocyte antigens, transplantation antigens and tissue antigens.

HLA antigens and antibodies are important in a number of complications of blood transfusion therapy including immune-mediated platelet refractoriness, febrile nonhemolytic (FNH) transfusion reactions and posttransfusion graft-vs-host disease (GVHD). In addition, the HLA system is second in importance only to the ABO antigens in influencing the survival of transplanted solid organs. Immunologic recognition of differences in HLA antigens is probably the first step in the rejection of transplanted tissue. Typing for HLA antigens is of great value in parentage testing and has been used to study susceptibility to certain diseases. Several introductory texts are available for those wishing to learn more about HLA.[1-4]

History

Delineation of the first human leukocyte antigen began in the 1950's when several investigators independently described leukoagglutinating antibodies in the sera of patients immunized by blood transfusion[5] or pregnancy.[6] Further studies revealed that these leukoagglutinins defined a series of polymorphic, genetically determined antigens.[7,8] By the early 1960's, an association between human leukoagglutinating antibodies and tissue transplantation was inferred from observations of accelerated skin graft rejection in recipients who were preimmunized with peripheral blood leukocytes from the prospective donor.[9] A major technical advance occurred in 1964 with the introduction of the microlymphocytotoxicity test.[10] A modified form of the original lymphocytotoxicity test is in common use today. The greater interlaboratory reproducibility achieved by microlymphocytotoxicity testing and international workshops paved the way for a World Health Organization (WHO) Terminology Committee to standardize HLA nomenclature in 1967. As increasing numbers of very specific antisera became available and as understanding of the genetics of the system improved, nomenclature has been logically expanded and systematized.[11] The current classification of HLA antigens is outlined in Table 13-1.

Table 13-1. Table of HLA Specificities (WHO Report, 11th Workshop, Tokyo, 1991)[11]

A	B		C	D	DR	DQ	DP
A1	B5	B49(21)	Cw1	Dw1	DR1	DQ1	DPw1
A2	B7	B50(21)	Cw2	Dw2	DR103	DQ2	DPw2
A203	B703	B51(5)	Cw3	Dw3	DR2	DQ3	DPw3
A210	B8	B5102	Cw4	Dw4	DR3	DQ4	DPw4
A3	B12	B5103	Cw5	Dw5	DR4	DQ5(1)	DPw5
A9	B13	B52(5)	Cw6	Dw6	DR5	DQ6(1)	DPw6
A10	B14	B53	Cw7	Dw7	DR6	DQ7(3)	
A11	B15	B54(22)	Cw8	Dw8	DR7	DQ8(3)	
A19	B16	B55(22)	Cw9(w3)	Dw9	DR8	DQ9(3)	
A23(9)	B17	B56(22)	Cw10(w3)	Dw10	DR9		
A24(9)	B18	B57(17)		Dw11(7)	DR10		
A2403	B21	B58(17)		Dw12	DR11(5)		
A25(10)	B22	B59		Dw13	DR12(5)		
A26(10)	B27	B60(40)		Dw14	DR13(6)		
A28	B35	B61(40)		Dw15	DR14(6)		
A29(19)	B37	B62(15)		Dw16	DR1403		
A30(19)	B38(16)	B63(15)		Dw17(w7)	DR1404		
A31(19)	B39(19)	B64(14)		Dw18(w6)	DR15(2)		
A32(19)	B3901	B65(14)		Dw19(w6)	DR16(2)		
A33(19)	B3902	B67		Dw20	DR17(3)		
A34(10)	B40	B70		Dw21	DR18(3)		
A36	B4005	B71(70)		Dw22			
A43	B41	B72(70)		Dw23	DR51		
A66(10)	B42	B73					
A68(28)	B44(12)	B75(15)		Dw24	DR52		
A69(28)	B45(12)	B76(15)		Dw25			
A74(19)	B46	B77(15)		Dw26	DR53		
	B47	B7801					
	B48						

Bw4:   B5, B5102, B5103, B13, B17, B27, B37, B38(16), B44(12), B47, B49(21), B51(5), B52(5), B53, B57(17), B58(17), B59, B63(15), B77(15)

Bw6:   B7, B703, B8, B14, B18, B22, B35, B39(16), B3901, B3902, B40, B4005, B41, B42, B45(12), B46, B48, B50(21), B54(22), B55(22), B56(22), B60(40), B61(40), B62(15), B64(14), B65(14), B67, B70, B71(70), B72(70), B73, B75(15), B76(15), B7801

Genetics of the Major Histocompatibility Complex

The HLA antigens reside on cell surface glycoproteins that are products of closely linked genes present at region p21.3 of the short arm of chromosome 6 (see Fig 13-1). This region of DNA is referred to as the MHC and is usually inherited en bloc as a haplotype. Each locus has multiple alleles with codominant expression of the products from each chromosome. The HLA system constitutes one of the most polymorphic genetic systems known in humans.

The HLA-A, HLA-B and HLA-C genes are responsible for the corresponding Class I HLA antigens. The HLA-DR, HLA-DQ and HLA-DP gene cluster codes for the production of corresponding Class II antigens. Located between the Class I and Class II genes is a group of genes coding for HLA Class III molecules. These include genes coding for the production of the complement proteins C2, Bf, C4A, C4B, as well as genes coding for a steroid enzyme (21-hydroxylase) and a cytokine (tumor necrosis factor).

Although the HLA Class I region consists of the classical genes HLA-A, HLA-B and HLA-C, other gene loci exist including HLA-E, HLA-F, HLA-G and HLA-H.[13] These genes either express proteins that are nonfunctional or are unable to express a protein product as a result of internal deletions. Genes that are unable to express a protein product are termed pseudogenes and likely represent an evolutionary dead end. DNA analysis of the HLA-C gene region reveals that this locus probably arose from the HLA-B region by gene duplication.[14]

The genetic organization of the MHC Class II region (HLA-D region) is more complex.[12,13] HLA Class II proteins consist of one alpha (α) chain and one beta (β) chain. There are 16 loci that code for either α or β chains of the Class II MHC proteins. (See Fig 13-1.) The HLA-DR gene cluster consists of four β chains and one α chain. One of the four β genes (B2) is a pseudogene. The proteins coded

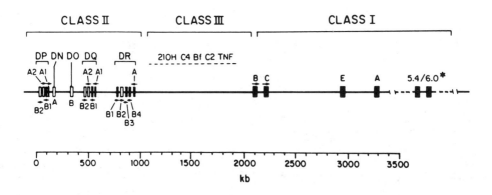

Figure 13-1. The MHC on chromosome 6. The Class I, Class II and Class III gene clusters are shown. Dark rectangles represent loci coding for proteins that are known to be expressed. Clear rectangles represent loci that are not expressed. Loci 6.0 and 5.4 refer to HLA-E and HLA-F, respectively. The Class III region contains complement genes (C2, Bf, C4), the 21-hydroxylase gene (21OH) and the gene for tumor necrosis factor (TNF).[12]

by the A gene and the B1 gene carry HLA-DR1 through HLA-DRw18. The products of the A gene and the B3 gene express HLA-DRw52; while the products of the A gene and the B4 gene express HLA-DRw53. The HLA-DQw1 through DQw9 antigens are expressed on the glycoproteins coded by the DQA1 and DQB1 genes in the DQ gene cluster. The other genes of the DQ cluster are pseudogenes and thus have no protein product. A similar organization is found in the HLA-DP gene cluster. The MHC Class III region contains four complement genes, which are generally inherited as a unit termed a complotype. There are more than 10 different complotypes inherited in humans.[15] Two of the Class III genes, C4A and C4B, code for variants of the C4 molecule. These variants have distinct protein structure and function, and carry antigenic determinants expressed on the surface of red cells. The C4A molecule carries the Rodgers antigen and the C4B molecule carries the Chido antigen.

The MHC demonstrates a number of genetic principles. Each person has two chromosomes and, thus, two MHC haplotypes, each inherited from one parent. Since the genes are autosomal and codominant, the phenotype represents the combined expression of both haplotypes. Figure 13-2 illustrates inheritance of haplotypes. Each child receives one chromosome, hence one haplotype, from each parent. Since each parent has two different number 6 chromosomes, four different combinations of haplotypes are possible in the offspring (in the absence of recombination). This inheritance pattern is an important factor in finding compatible related donors for transplantation. The chance that two siblings will be HLA identical is, therefore, 25%. The chance that any one patient with "n" siblings will have at least one HLA identical sib-

ling is $1-(3/4)^n$. Although each chromosome will express its gene products, some individuals may test positive for only one antigen at a given locus. In such a case the missing antigen is referred to as a "blank." A blank may occur when the individual expresses an antigen for which the appropriate antisera are not available, when the individual is homozygous for the relevant gene at that locus, when a null gene is present or when a technical failure (false-negative) occurs. When describing a phenotype, a blank is often written as "x," "y" or "–" (eg, A1,x;B7,40 or A1,–;B7,40). Family studies are required to determine the correct genotype.

The genes of the HLA region occasionally demonstrate chromosome crossover, in which segments containing linked genetic material are exchanged between the two chromosomes during gametogenesis. See Fig 9-1. These recombinants are then transmitted as new haplotypes to the offspring. Crossover frequency is directly related to the distance between genes. The HLA-A and HLA-B loci, for example, are close together and the crossover rate is only 0.8%. The possibility of recombination must be considered in family studies and in parentage testing.

Alleles of the MHC system exhibit linkage disequilibrium, a phenomenon in which certain alleles occur together in the same haplotype more often than would be expected by chance. See Chapter 9. Expected HLA haplotype frequencies are calculated by multiplying the frequencies of the genes together. Certain allelic combinations occur with increased frequency in different racial groups, and constitute common haplotypes in those populations. For example, in Caucasians, the overall frequency of the gene coding for HLA-A1 is 0.15 and for the gene coding for HLA-B8 is 0.10; therefore, 1.5% (0.15×0.10) of all Caucasian HLA haplotypes would be expected to contain genes coding for both HLA-A1 and HLA-B8 if these were randomly distributed. The actual frequency of the A1 and B8 combination, however, is 7-8% in the Caucasian population as a result of linkage disequilibrium. Linkage disequilibrium in the HLA system is important in studies of parentage, because haplotype frequencies in the relevant population make transmission of certain gene combinations more likely than others.

Biochemistry, Tissue Distribution and Structure

The HLA antigens are heterodimeric cell surface glycoproteins that are divided into two classes according to biochemical structure.[16] Class I antigens (HLA-A, -B and -C) have a molecular weight around 56,000 daltons and consist of two chains: a glycoprotein heavy chain (α) and a light chain (β_2 microglobulin). See Fig 13-3. The α chain is attached to the cell membrane; β_2 microglobulin is not.

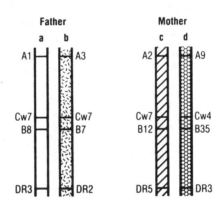

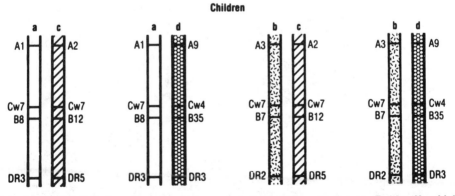

Figure 13-2. The linked genes on each chromosome constitute a haplotype. To identify which haplotypes a person possesses, one must know the antigens present and also the inheritance pattern in the specific kindred. The observed typing results of the father in this family are interpreted into the following phenotype: A1,3;B7,8;Cw7,-;DR2,3. The observed results plus the family study reveal the haplotypes of the father to be: a=A1,Cw7,B8,DR3 and b=A3,Cw7,B7,DR2. Offspring of a single mating pair must have one of only four possible combinations of haplotypes, assuming there has been no crossing over.

β_2 microglobulin (chromosome 12) associates with the α chain but is not covalently bound to it. The α chain consists of three amino acid domains, the outer two of which contain variable regions representing the various Class I alleles. Class I molecules are found on virtually all body tissue cells. However, only vestigial amounts remain on mature red cells, with certain allotypes better expressed than others. HLA antigens on red cells were independently recognized as alloantigens by red cell serologists and were designated as Bennett-Goodspeed (Bg) antigens. Bg^a is HLA-B7; Bg^b is HLA-B17; and Bg^c is HLA-A28. Platelets express primarily HLA-A and HLA-B antigens. HLA-C antigens are weakly present and Class II antigens are not expressed on platelets.

Class II antigens (HLA-DR, -DQ and -DP) have a molecular weight of approximately 63,000 daltons and consist of two dissimilar glycoprotein chains designated α and β.[17] Each chain consists of two extramembranous amino acid domains and the outer domains of each molecule contain the variable regions corresponding to the Class II alleles. Although Class I antigens are expressed on all nucleated cells of the body, the expression of Class II antigens is more restricted. Class II antigens are found on B lymphocytes, activated T lymphocytes, monocytes, macrophages, dendritic cells, early hematopoietic cells, endothelial cells and some tumor cells.

X-ray crystallographic analysis of purified HLA antigens has revealed a characteristic three-dimensional structure of these molecules.[18] See Fig 13-4. The outer domains, which contain the regions of amino acid variability and the antigenic epitopes of the molecules, form a structure known as the "peptide binding groove." Different HLA gene products, each with a unique amino acid sequence, form unique binding grooves, each able to bind different classes of peptides. The peptide binding groove is critical for the functional aspects of HLA molecules. See Biological Function.

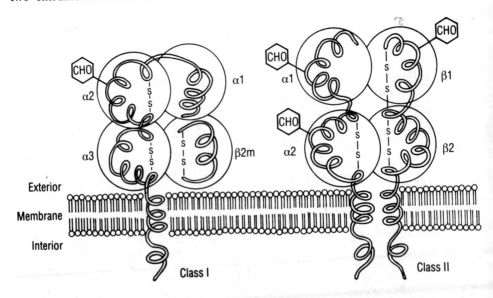

Figure 13-3. Stylized diagram of Class I and Class II MHC molecules showing α and β polypeptide chains, their structural domains and attached carbohydrate units.

Nomenclature

Table 13-1 lists identified HLA specificities. For each HLA locus there are multiple alleles, each corresponding to a different antigen. The extreme polymorphism of the HLA system derives from the existence of multiple alleles at several loci. It is estimated that more than 100 million different phenotypes can result from all combinations of alleles in HLA. An individual's extended haplotypes are nearly unique.

Established HLA antigens are designated by a number following the letter that denotes the HLA series (eg, HLA-A1 or HLA-B8). Provisional antigenic specificities that have not yet been fully confirmed carry the prefix "w" for "workshop," eg, HLA-Dw7. When identification of the antigen becomes definitive, the WHO Terminology Committee drops the "w" from the designation. The WHO Terminology Committee meets every few years to update the nomenclature by either dropping the "w" designations or by recognizing new specificities or genetic loci. The numerical designations for the HLA-A and HLA-B specificities are not in sequence because numbers were assigned before the existence of the two major gene loci, HLA-A and HLA-B, was recognized. All C locus antigens (including established antigens) retain the "w" prefix so as not to confuse their nomenclature with that of the complement system.

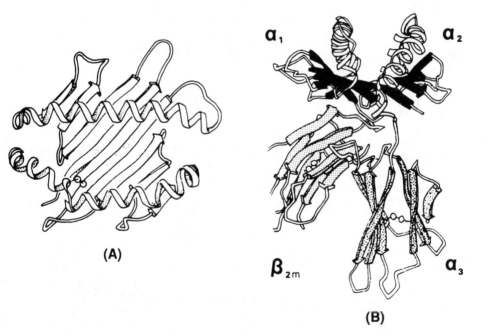

(A)

α_1 α_2

β_{2m} α_3

(B)

Figure 13-4. Three dimensional schematic representation of an HLA molecule. (A) The molecule is shown projecting out of the page. The central groove is shown without peptide present. (B) The molecule is shown with the membrane proximal immunoglobulin-like domains (α_3, β_{2m}) at the bottom and the polymorphic α_1 and α_2 domains at the top. The peptide binding groove is shown on edge at the top center.[18]

Shared Determinants: Splits, Cross-Reactive Groups and Public Antigens

As the specificity of HLA typing sera became increasingly refined, it was found that some antigens shared common epitopes. Antibodies to these common epitopes identified antigens common to a group, with individual members of the group identified by more precise antisera. Thus, antigen groups could be "split" into individual specificities. For example, HLA-B12 split into HLA-B44 and HLA-B45, each of which reacts with anti-HLA-B12 sera. Anti-HLA-B12 is said to be a more "broadly reacting" antibody. Red cell serologists will recognize that had anti-A,B been the first red cell antibody found, its specificity could later have been said to "split" into group A and group B. When an individual antigen that is a split of an earlier recognized antigen is referenced, the parent antigen is often included in parentheses as in HLA-B44(12).

In addition to "splits," HLA antigens and antigen groups share other common epitopes. Antibodies to these shared determinants often result in cross-reactions in serologic testing. The group of HLA antigens that exhibit such cross-reactivity is called a "*Cross REactive Group*" or CREG. For example, HLA-B44(12) and HLA-B45(12) are members of a CREG that includes HLA-B21 and HLA-B13. In practice this means that an anti-HLA-B12 is likely to show some reactivity (albeit a weaker strength of reaction) with cells that are positive for HLA-B21 or HLA-B13.

In addition to splits and CREGs, HLA cell surface proteins have public antigens that are common to many different HLA specificities.[19,20] Some of these public antigens are coded by separate exons with few alleles and generally represent the less variable portion of the HLA mol-

ecule located nearer to the cell surface. A similar situation exists with other cell surface glycoproteins [eg, M and N antigens sharing the public specificity known as the En(a) antigen] or with immunoglobulins (many different molecules sharing a common IgG heavy chain). Two well-characterized public antigens—HLA-Bw4 and HLA-Bw6—are found at the HLA-B locus. See Table 13-1. Each HLA Class I molecule carries one or the other of these two public antigens in addition to its individual antigen type ("private antigen"). For example, cells that are positive for HLA-B44(12) also test positive for HLA-Bw4. Several other public antigens have been recognized.[20] Public antigens are clinically important because studies suggest that patients exposed to foreign HLA antigens via pregnancy, transfusion or transplantation frequently make antibodies to public antigens.[19,20] A single antibody specificity, when made to a public antigen, can resemble the sum of multiple discrete alloantibodies.

Gene Nomenclature

As HLA antigens are being investigated by peptide mapping and nucleotide sequencing, an increasing number of HLA variant alleles is being identified, many of which share a common serologic phenotype. A uniform nomenclature for these alleles has been adopted.[11] The nomenclature takes into account the locus, the protein bearing the antigen, the major serologic specificity and the variant. For example, several unique variants of HLA-DR4 have been identified using isoelectric focusing, amino acid and nucleotide sequencing. The first HLA-DR4 variant is designated DRB1*0401. This designation gives the locus (DR), the protein (β_1 chain), an asterisk to represent that an allele name follows, the major serologic specificity

(04 for HLA-DR4) and the variant number (variant 01). For Class I variants, in which only one protein chain varies, the protein designation is dropped. Thus B*2704 represents the B27 allele, giving rise to the fourth unique variant of the HLA-B27 molecule.

Biological Function

As described in Chapter 7, MHC molecules are of central importance in the regulation of the immune response. Inside antigen-processing cells (APCs), MHC molecules follow a coordinated traffic pattern that brings them into contact with peptide antigens. Exogenous proteins are processed into small peptides, which are then transported to the cell surface by Class II molecules. In contrast, endogenous peptides are carried by Class I molecules.[21,22] Once on the cell surface, MHC molecules play a key role in intercellular communication for both the afferent and efferent limbs of the immune response.[23] MHC Class II molecules are important in the afferent limb of immunity, which is designed to recognize new antigens. Foreign proteins are engulfed by macrophage APCs that digest the proteins into smaller peptide fragments. As these fragments traverse the cells' endosomal system, they are deposited in the inner cleft of the peptide binding groove formed by HLA Class II molecules. The HLA Class II molecule is then transported to the cell surface where it displays the new foreign peptide. Helper T cells, whose T-cell antigen receptors match the peptide fragment and surrounding MHC Class II molecule, bind to the APC. Thus, APCs take up new antigens and then redisplay them in a context recognizable to T cells.

Class I MHC molecules are important in the efferent limb of immunity, which is designed to destroy cells bearing foreign antigens. In the case of viral infections, foreign viral peptides present within the cell are deposited in the binding groove of Class I MHC molecules and expressed on the cell surface. Cytotoxic T cells, whose T-cell antigen receptor matches the viral peptide fragment and surrounding MHC Class I molecule, bind to the infected cell. This matching results in activation of the T cell and cytotoxicity. Only cytotoxic T cells that share the *same MHC type* as the infected cell are capable of binding in a manner suitable for efficient cell cytotoxicity. This attribute is referred to as "MHC-restricted activity" or "MHC restriction." For example, hepatocytes infected with a hepatitis B virus express viral antigens deposited in the MHC groove of Class I MHC molecules on the cell surface. Host cytotoxic T cells recognize viral peptides and destroy the hepatocyte, creating inflammation (hepatitis) in the process.

Pregnancy, transfusion and transplantation are special immunologic circumstances in which the foreign antigens are in fact the donor MHC antigens themselves. Accumulated evidence suggests that the afferent limb (recipient recognition of the foreign tissue) depends on recipient exposure to donor cells bearing Class II antigens. However, the efferent limb (recipient immune response against the donor) is frequently directed against Class I donor antigens. This principle underlies the use of leukocyte-reduced blood components or ultraviolet light-treated components to alter Class II bearing cells and thus prevent sensitization to donor HLA antigens.[24]

Detection of HLA Antigens

Methods for the detection of HLA antigens fall into three groups: serologic assays, cellular assays and DNA assays.[12] Detailed procedures of commonly used assays are given in the Methods and in other publications.[25]

Serologic Assays

Lymphocytotoxicity

The standard technique used to detect HLA-A, -B, -C, -DR and -DQ antigens is the microlymphocytotoxicity test. Lymphocytes are used as targets because these antigens are expressed to varying degrees on lymphocytes and a relatively pure suspension of cells can be obtained from anticoagulated peripheral blood. Lymphocytes obtained from lymph nodes or spleen may also be used. HLA antisera of known specificity (typing sera) are placed in wells on a microdroplet test plate. HLA typing sera are obtained primarily from multiparous women who have been exposed during pregnancy to fetal cells bearing the father's HLA determinants. A concentrated suspension of lymphocytes (1-2 × 10^6 cells per mL) is added to each well. If the target lymphocytes possess the antigen corresponding to the antibody present in the antiserum, the antibody will bind to the cells. Rabbit complement is then added to the wells and, if sufficient antibody is bound to the lymphocyte membranes, complement is activated injuring the cell membranes (lymphocytotoxicity) and increasing their permeability. Cell injury is detected by dye exclusion: cells with intact membranes (negative reactions) exclude vital dyes; cells with permeable membranes (positive reactions) take up dye. The cells are examined for dye exclusion or uptake under phase contrast microscopy.

Since HLA-DR and HLA-DQ antigens are expressed on B cells and not on resting T cells, typing for these antigens usually requires that the initial lympho-cyte preparation be manipulated prior to testing to yield an enriched B-cell preparation. B cells can be separated from a mixed population of lymphocytes by several techniques including separation on nylon wool columns and separation by magnetic beads to which monoclonal anti-B cell antibodies have been bound.

The interpretation of serologic reactions requires skill and experience. Multiple controls are required and careful quality control of reagents is needed. In particular, the activity of the complement used to induce lymphocytotoxicity must be controlled. In addition, antigen assignments can only be made based on results obtained with multiple antisera, since few reagent antisera have sufficiently monospecific reliability to be used alone. The extreme polymorphism of the HLA system, the uneven distribution of antigens among different racial groups, the reliance on biologic antisera and living target cells, and the complexities introduced by splits, CREGs and public antigens all contribute to difficulties of accurate HLA typing.

Antibody Testing

The principle of the microlymphocytotoxicity test can be applied to analyzing test serum against target cells of known HLA phenotype. This is routinely done in HLA crossmatching in which the major crossmatch consists of recipient serum tested against unfractionated donor lymphocytes. A variation of the microlymphocytotoxicity test uses an antiglobulin reagent to increase the sensitivity of the test system. In this variation antibodies that recognize the kappa or lambda light chains of HLA antibodies may convert some noncytotoxic reactions into cytotoxic ones.[26] Care must be taken so that antiglobulin enhancement does not result in false-positive reactions. The antiglobulin test is not used in routine antigen typing, but is useful in enhancing the sensitivity of cross-match tests used for organ transplantation. Flow cytometry has also been used as an independent method to increase the sensitivity of the crossmatch.[27]

The degree of HLA alloimmunization can be assessed by testing the patient's serum against a panel of 30-60 or more different target cells. The percent of the panel cells to which the recipient has formed cytotoxic antibodies is referred to as the panel reactive antibody (PRA). Determination of the PRA is of great practical value in the investigation of suspected FNH transfusion reactions, in the workup of platelet refractoriness and in following patients who are awaiting cadaver solid organ transplants.

Cellular Assays

One-Way Mixed Lymphocyte Culture or Mixed Lymphocyte Reaction

The mixed lymphocyte culture (MLC) or mixed lymphocyte reaction (MLR) test is used to select living donors for organ transplantation. It is widely used in testing prior to bone marrow transplantation and prior to living related kidney transplantation. The test relies on the MLR, which can detect HLA differences that cannot be identified by serologic techniques. The MLR primarily detects differences at the HLA-D locus, a genetic region that includes HLA-DP, HLA-DQ and HLA-DR. In the MLR, lymphocytes from different individuals are cultured together. Cells from one source are designated as stimulator cells and cells from the other source are responder cells. Stimulator cells are irradiated at the beginning of the test to inhibit their ability to undergo DNA activation. During the coculture the responder cells have the opportunity to recognize and respond to foreign HLA-D region antigens present on the stimulator cells. The response is referred to as a "blastogenic response" in which the cells enlarge and undergo DNA division. At the end of the coculture period (usually 5-7 days) the degree of blastogenic response is quantitated by pulsing the culture with radioactive thymidine that is incorporated into the DNA of the responding cells. The greater the blastogenic response, the greater the uptake of thymidine by the responding cells.

Results of the MLR test are often expressed as the stimulation index (SI) and the relative response (RR). The SI represents the ratio of response to the stimulator cells over background. The RR expresses the result as a ratio of the response provoked by the stimulator to the response provoked by maximal stimulation from multiple unrelated stimulator cells. Values for SI and RR are used to assess the degree of Class II similarity between stimulator (organ donor) and responder (organ recipient).

HLA-D Typing and Homozygous Typing Cells

HLA-D types are defined by reactivity in the MLR. To assign an HLA-D type to an unknown cell, the test cell is cocultured with irradiated cells that are homozygous for D-region antigens. A negative MLR will occur in those cocultures in which the responding cell shares a D-region antigen with the cocultured homozygous typing cell. For example, a cell that fails to respond to a known HLA-Dw3 homozygous cell and a known HLA-Dw4 homozygous cell but that does respond to all other homozygous cells is an HLA-Dw3/HLA-Dw4 heterozygote. HLA-D typing can extend typing beyond that obtained with serologic techniques alone. For example, cells homozygous for DR2 and DQw1 may have either the Dw2 or Dw9 specificities.

Primed Lymphocyte Typing

Primed lymphocyte typing is a variation of MLC testing used for HLA-DP antigen typings. HLA-DP antigens generally do not provoke a sufficiently strong blastogenic response to be detected in a standard primary MLC test. The primed lymphocyte typing test requires the use of "immunologically primed" responder lymphocytes that are maintained in culture. If cells in a standard MLC are continued in culture for 9-14 days, the stimulator cells die and the responder cells, although still viable, cease to proliferate actively. These "primed" responder cells will undergo very rapid proliferation if again exposed to the DP antigens present on the original stimulating cell.

Cell-Mediated Lympholysis

The cell-mediated lympholysis (CML) test is used to define cytotoxic T-cell function, in which responding T cells directly kill the target cells.[28] Lymphocytes are first sensitized by 5 days of culture with irradiated stimulator cells. Next, the sensitized lymphocytes are incubated with ^{51}Cr-labeled target cells derived from the original sensitizing cell line. Upon contact with these ^{51}Cr-labeled cells, the sensitized responder cells attack and kill them by cell-mediated lympholysis. The endpoint is detected by measurement of ^{51}Cr release in the supernatant. CML studies have yielded important information about HLA antigens, MLC results and cytotoxic T-cell response.[28] CML response is strongest when the sensitizing and responding cells have different Class I and Class II antigens. Responder cells, provoked by recognition of Class II differences, lyse those target cells bearing different Class I antigens. Thus, CML testing can serve as an in-vitro model of the cellular immune response.

DNA Assays

In recent years, further definition of MHC genes and their products has been achieved through new techniques involving the use of the polymerase chain reaction (PCR) and allele-specific oligonucleotide (ASO) or sequence-specific oligonucleotide (SSO) probes. These methods can use minimal amounts of DNA starting material and amplify the region of DNA that codes for specific alleles. Using a complementary nucleotide probe for each known allele, the amplified DNA can be typed using labeled probes.[12,29] Typing for the HLA-$DQ\alpha$ genes by PCR may be of particular value in forensic applications in which only small amounts of the original material are available. The use of restriction fragment length polymorphisms, ASOs, SSOs and nucleotide sequencing has identified nucleotide differences among HLA gene regions that cannot be distinguished by other methods. As a result, the nomenclature for HLA genes and gene products has been revised as described above.

The HLA System and Transfusion

HLA system antigens and antibodies play an important role in a number of transfusion-related events. These include alloimmunization and platelet refractoriness, FNH transfusion reactions, transfusion-related acute lung injury and posttransfusion GVHD. HLA antigens are highly immunogenic. In response to pregnancy or transfusion, immunologically normal recipients are more likely to form antibodies to HLA antigens than to any other antigen system.

HLA Alloimmunization and Platelet Refractoriness

The incidence of HLA alloimmunization and platelet refractoriness among patients receiving repeated transfusion of cellular components is 30-60%.[30] The refractory state exists when transfusion of suitably preserved platelets fails to increase the recipient count. Platelet refractoriness may have an immune basis or be due to sepsis, high fever, disseminated intravascular coagulopathy, medications, hypersplenism, complement-mediated destruction or a combination of these.[31] See Chapter 17. Immune-mediated platelet refractoriness is usually caused by antibodies directed against HLA antigens, but antibodies to platelet-specific antigens may also be involved. HLA alloimmunization is provoked by residual leukocytes in blood components that bear HLA Class II antigens.[32] Once provoked, the recipient's immune response is generally directed against Class I antigens. Since platelets express Class I but not Class II antigens, blood platelets can be destroyed by an established HLA immune response but are less likely to provoke one. The threshold level of leukocytes required to provoke an HLA alloimmune response is unclear and likely varies among different recipients. Some studies have suggested that 5×10^6 may represent an immunizing dose.[33] Patients who have been previously sensitized by pregnancy or transfusion are likely to experience an anamnestic antibody response upon exposure to even lower numbers of allogeneic cells.

The HLA antibody response of transfused individuals may be directed against private alloantigens present on donor cells or against public alloantigens. The precise specificities are often difficult to determine. An overall assessment of the degree of alloimmunization can be obtained by measuring the PRA of the recipient's serum. Patients who are broadly alloimmunized (high PRA) and refractory to platelets are difficult to support with platelet transfusions. HLA-matched platelets, obtained by plateletpheresis, can be of benefit in approximately half of these refractory patients. Because of the limited availability of perfectly HLA-matched platelet donors, strategies for obtaining HLA-matched platelets vary. The use of partially mismatched donors based on serologically cross-reactive groups has been emphasized. See Table 13-2. However, selection of donors with HLA phenotypes that are serologically cross-reactive in vitro to that of the recipient may fail to provide an adequate transfusion response in vivo.[35] An alternative approach to the selection of donors is based on matching for public specificities rather than cross-reactive private antigens.[20] Matching for both HLA and platelet-specific antigens may further improve the success rate in refractory patients.[36]

Patients who may become alloimmunized and refractory should be HLA typed early in the course of their illness, when enough lymphocytes are present in the peripheral blood to obtain a reliable HLA type. It is very difficult to obtain enough cells for HLA typing after intensive chemotherapy.

Febrile Nonhemolytic Transfusion Reactions

HLA antibodies, as well as granulocyte and platelet-specific antibodies, have been implicated in the pathogenesis of FNH transfusion reactions.[37] These reactions may occur when recipient antibodies bind to donor antigens, resulting in the release of cytokines (eg, interleukin-1) capable of causing fever. Serologic investigation may require multiple tech-

Table 13-2. HLA-A and HLA-B Cross-Reactive Antigen Classification, Useful for Selection of Platelet Donors With "Minor" HLA Mismatches*

HLA-A Antigen	Cross-Reactive Specificities	HLA-B Antigen	Cross-Reactive Specificities
A1	A3,A11,A36	B5	B53,B35,B17,B15,B21,B18
A2	A28,A68	B7	B22,B27,B40,B42,B47
A3	A1,A11,A36	B8	B14,B16
A9	A23,A24,(A2)	B12	B21,B13
A10	A25,A26,A34,A11,A32	B13	B40,B12
A11	A1,A3,A26	B14	B8,B18
A19	A10,A34	B15	B35,B17,B53,B70,B5,B21
A25	A10,A26,A32,A34,A33	B16	B22
A26	A25,A10,A34,A11	B17	B15,B53,B70,B5,B35,B21
A28	A68,A69,A2,A33	B18	B5,B21,B15,B35,B14
A29	A30,A31,A19	B21	B12,B15,B53,B5,B17,B35
A30	A31,A32,A19,A10	B22	B7,B40,B41,B27,B16
A31	A30,A19,A10	B27	B7,B47,B40,B22
A32	A33,A74,A25,A19,A28	B35	B53,B15,B5,B17,B70,B21,B18
A33	A32,A74,A19,A28,A10	B40	B7,B13,B41,B42,B47
A34	A26,A10,A33,A32	B41	B40,B42,B7,B47,B13
A36	A1,A11,A3	B42	B7,B40,B41
A68	A28,A69,A2	B47	B27,B41,B40,B7
A69	A28,A68,A2,A33	B53	B35,B5,B15,B17,B70
A74	A32,A33,A19	B70	B15,B17,B53,B35,B5

*This table is an updated version by the original author of a previously published table (Duquesnoy[34]) prepared from subjective evaluation of literature reports and his own experience. Specificities are listed in descending order of approximate degree of cross-reactivity.

When selecting a donor for a patient with a mismatched B locus specificity, major consideration should be given to the Bw4/Bw6 assignments. They should be respected over all other considerations *if* the patient is homozygous for *Bw4* or *Bw6* (eg, B40 is preferred over B27 as the best match for B7 in a patient who has the B locus antigens B7, 8 since the patient is homozygous for *Bw6*). B40 is associated with Bw6 while B27 is Bw4 related. This rule applies *only* to patients who are homozygous for *Bw4* or *Bw6*.

niques and a panel of target cells from a number of different donors.[37] See Chapter 19.

Transfusion-Related Acute Lung Injury

In this unusual transfusion reaction, the recipient develops acute noncardiogenic pulmonary edema in response to transfusion. See Chapter 19. The exact pathogenesis is uncertain. Studies suggest that HLA antibodies present in donor blood may react with and fix complement on tissue antigens of the recipi-

ent.[38] It is possible that these antibodies bind directly to HLA antigens on the pulmonary capillary endothelium. Other studies in a canine model suggest a role for antigranulocyte antibodies.[39] Whatever the exact underlying mechanism, the result is pulmonary capillary leakage and lung edema.

Posttransfusion Graft-vs-Host Disease

The development of posttransfusion GVHD depends upon several factors, including the immunocompetence of the recipient, the number and viability of donor lymphocytes in the transfused product and the degree of HLA similarity between donor and recipient.[40] The observation of an unexpected increase in posttransfusion GVHD with the use of fresh directed donor blood components highlighted the role of the HLA system in GVHD.[41,42] Figure 13-5 demonstrates the situation in which the risk of GVHD is increased. Both parents share an HLA haplotype. Each child, therefore, has a one in four chance of inheriting the common haplotype from each parent. Child #1 is homozygous for the shared

parental HLA haplotype. If this child's blood were transfused to an unrelated recipient, there would be no consequence to the recipient. If, however, Child #1 were a directed donor for his/her parents or for sibling #3, then donor lymphocytes would not be recognized as foreign or eliminated by the recipient. However, these donor cells would recognize the recipient's environment as foreign. The donor cells would become activated, proliferate and attack the host. For this reason it is recommended that all directed cellular units from blood relatives be irradiated prior to transfusion.[43]

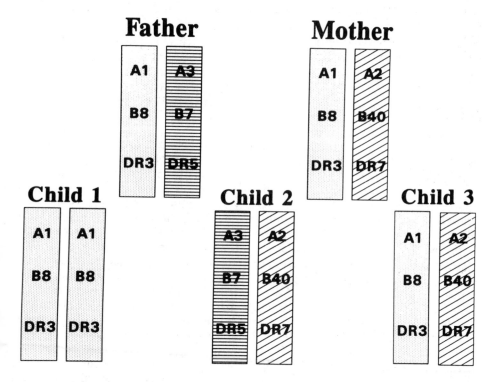

Figure 13-5. HLA haplotypes in a family at risk for transfusion-associated GVHD. In contrast to the family shown in Fig 13-2, each parent shares a common HLA haplotype, HLA-A1,B8,DR3. Child 1 is homozygous for the haplotype shared by the parents and by child 3. The lymphocytes of child 1 are capable of producing posttransfusion GVHD if transfused to either parent or to child 3.

Hemolytic Transfusion Reactions

HLA incompatibility has been implicated as a cause of shortened red cell survival in patients with HLA antibodies to antigens such as $Bg^a(B7)$, $Bg^b(B17)$ and $Bg^c(A28)$ that are expressed (weakly) on red blood cells.[44,45] See Chapter 12. Such an incompatibility may not be detected with conventional pretransfusion testing.

HLA Testing and Transplantation

HLA testing is an integral part of organ transplantation. The extent of testing differs for different types of transplants. Organ transplantation is also discussed in Chapter 6.

Bone Marrow Transplants

It has long been recognized that the HLA system represents an important transplant barrier for successful marrow transplantation. HLA similarity and compatibility of the donor to the recipient are required for engraftment. In addition, HLA similarity and compatibility of the recipient to the donor are required to prevent GVHD. Despite immunosuppressive conditioning regimens given to the recipient and despite T-lymphocyte depletion of the graft, some degree of rejection or GVHD remain common problems for allogeneic marrow transplant recipients. Candidate donors and recipients are tested for HLA-A, -B, -C, -DR and -DQ antigens. In addition, the MLR or DNA probe tests are performed on samples from the prospective donor and the recipient. Although sibling matched donors remain the standard choice for marrow transplant, there is increasing use of unrelated matched donors identified by computer search through the National Bone Marrow Donor Registry.

Kidney Transplants

ABO compatibility is the most important factor determining the immediate survival of kidney transplants. ABO-incompatible kidney transplants are at high risk for hyperacute rejection. An interesting exception to the requirement for ABO compatibility is the observation that A_2 donor kidneys appear to survive as well as O donor kidneys in group O recipients.[46] Since ABH antigens are expressed in varying amounts on all cells of the body, transplanted ABO-incompatible tissue comes into continuous contact with recipient ABO antibodies. Of particular importance is the expression of ABH antigens on vascular endothelial cells since the vascular supply in the transplant is a common site for rejection.

Both the recipient and the donor are ordinarily tested for ABO, HLA-A, -B and -DR antigens. HLA-C and -DQ testing is also usually performed. Prior to surgery a major crossmatch (recipient serum versus donor lymphocytes) is required. The AABB *Standards for Blood Banks and Transfusion Services* recommends that the crossmatch be done using a method with enhanced sensitivity relative to the routine microlymphocytotoxicity test. A variety of different crossmatch techniques exist. See section on Assays/Antibody Testing in this chapter and Methods 8.6 and 8.7. Because HLA antibody responses are dynamic, the serum used for the crossmatch is often obtained within 48 hours of surgery and is retained in the frozen state for any required subsequent testing. An incompatible major warm T-cell crossmatch is a contraindication to kidney transplantation since it predicts a high likelihood of hyperacute rejection.

The sera of patients awaiting cadaver donor kidney transplants are tested monthly for the degree of alloimmunization by determining the PRA. In addition, many organ banks will identify the specificities of HLA alloantibodies formed and avoid the corresponding antigen when allocating an available cadaver donor graft. The serum samples used for periodic PRA testing are usually frozen. Those samples with the highest PRA are sometimes used in addition to the preoperative sample for pretransplant crossmatching.

The approach to living related kidney transplants is different. When several possible donors are being considered for a living related kidney transplant, MLC testing between the recipient and the prospective donors is usually performed. Kidney transplants from recipient/donor pairs with low reactivity in the MLC test survive longer than those showing high reactivity.[47]

HLA matching of kidney donors and recipients contributes to the likelihood of long-term graft survival. See Figs 13-6 and 13-7. Matching is particularly valuable for alloimmunized recipients.

Other antigen systems play a less important role in kidney transplantation. There is some evidence that the Lewis system may be clinically important.[49] The vascular endothelial cell (VEC) antigen system is a poorly characterized tissue antigen system that may also play a clinically important role in the survival of vascular grafts.[50] Patients have been identified who have rejected ABO and HLA compatible kidney transplants and who appear to demonstrate anti-VEC an-

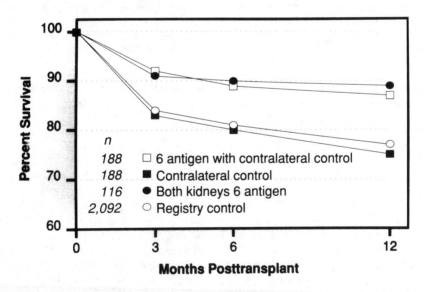

Figure 13-6. Effect of HLA matching on kidney graft survival[48] —comparison of the contralateral control graft survival. From 188 donors. One kidney was shipped to a 6-antigen matched recipient and the other went to an unmatched local recipient. A significantly higher graft survival was obtained with the 6-antigen matched kidney, despite longer cold ischemia times. As might be expected, the contralateral control kidneys had the same survival as the UCLA Registry controls that were also composed of nonshipped kidneys. There were 58 donors from whom both kidneys (116 kidneys) were shipped for 6-antigen matches (usually to different centers) and the graft survival was identical to the single 6-antigen matched kidney.

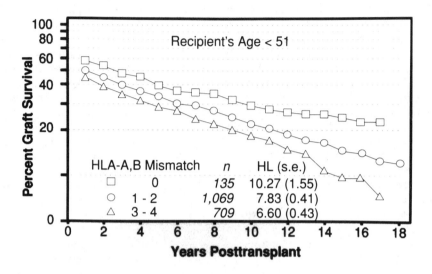

Figure 13-7. Effect of HLA matching on kidney graft survival[48]—the effect of HLA-A,B matching on long-term outcome. The number of transplants with no HLA-A,B mismatched antigens was small, but, overall, their graft survival rate was higher than those with incompatibilities. It should also be noted that HLA typing was still developing prior to 1975, and some of the specificities might have been missed. Despite this difficulty, there was a higher half-life of 10 years for 0-mismatched transplants as compared to 6.6 years for 3 or 4 antigens mismatched. HL(se) = half life (standard error).

tibodies in their serum. Blood mono-cytes may also carry VEC-like antigens. The use of monocytes in place of lymphocytes as target cells is being investigated as a method of studying VEC antigen-antibody reactions in vitro.

Other Solid Organ Transplants

For liver, pancreas, heart and heart/lung transplants, ABO compatibility remains the most important immunologic system for donor selection. HLA-A, -B and -DR testing is routinely done on both the donor and the recipient. A major lymphocyte crossmatch is also generally done. However, the degree of HLA matching between donor and recipient and the results of the crossmatch do not accurately predict the success of the transplant. Therefore, the crossmatch is not required prior to surgery and allocation of these organs

is not based on HLA matching but ABO compatibility is required.

Parentage Testing

HLA typing has proven extremely useful in parentage testing. Advantages of HLA typing in parentage testing include the following: 1) the HLA system is highly polymorphic, 2) the antigens are well developed at birth and 3) no single haplotype occurs with a high incidence in any population. HLA typing alone can exclude about 93% of falsely accused males.[51] With the addition of red cell antigen typing, the exclusion rate is 95%, rising to over 99% when typing for red cell enzymes and serum proteins are included.[52] The HLA system is also very powerful in calculations involving the probability that a specific person is the parent of a child.[53] HLA haplotype frequencies, rather than gene frequencies, are used in these calculations because linkage disequilibrium is so common in this genetic system. Care must be taken, however, to consider racial differences in haplotype frequencies. In addition, recombination events must be considered when haplotypes are scrutinized. HLA-A and -B gene products are the only antigens usually studied in parentage testing because tests for other antigens are expensive and/or difficult to interpret. Tests for red cell antigens, red cell enzymes, serum proteins or DNA probe analyses may all be used to supplement parentage information obtained by HLA typing.

HLA and Disease

Many factors determine susceptibility to disease. For some conditions, an association exists between HLA phenotype and occurrence of clinical disease. Several possible mechanisms could link the HLA system with disease, especially those in which immune response to microorganisms is known or suspected to be involved: 1) the genes that determine HLA antigens are the genes controlling the immune response, since the HLA molecules bind foreign antigens and thereby control their interactions with T cells; 2) some HLA antigens may be antigenically similar to certain viruses, possibly causing altered response to these viruses; and 3) some HLA antigens may provide receptors for certain viruses. Statistically significant associations have been noted between HLA antigens and a number of diseases.[54] The use of HLA profiles to identify individuals at risk represents no more than a statistical association except for monogenetic diseases caused by genes directly linked to HLA: 21-hydroxylase deficiency, idiopathic hemochromatosis and C2 or C4 deficiency. For these diseases there is an absolute association in individual families between transmission of these diseases and inheritance of certain HLA genes or haplotypes.

HLA typing is of only limited value in most diseases because the association is incomplete, often giving false-negative and false-positive results. The association in Caucasians of HLA-B27 and ankylosing spondylitis is instructive. The test is highly sensitive; more than 90% of Caucasian patients with ankylosing spondylitis possess the HLA-B27 antigen. On the other hand, specificity is low; only 20% of individuals with the B27 antigen will develop ankylosing spondylitis. Within affected families, the B27 antigen cannot be the only criterion for determining susceptibility to ankylosing spondylitis, since the association between disease and HLA type is not complete. In practice, HLA-B27 typing is most useful in differentiating ankylosing spondylitis from juvenile rheumatoid arthritis.

The degree of association between a given HLA type and a disease is often described in terms of a relative risk, based on the cross-product ratio of a 2 × 2 contingency table, as shown in Table 13-3. In this example, the relative risk value indicates that a person who is HLA-B27 positive is 149 times more likely to have ankylosing spondylitis than a person who is negative for the antigen.

Future research developments in HLA are likely to focus on increased understanding of the molecular biology of the MHC complex and the biologic function of the MHC in the immune response. The use of DNA techniques for HLA testing is likely to provide improved clinical testing for transplantation and more definition in parentage studies. Transfusion strategies designed to prevent HLA alloimmunization may result in a decreased demand for HLA-matched PCs.

Table 13-3. Analysis of 380 Individuals for Association Between Ankylosing Spondylitis and HLA-B27

		HLA-B27		
		+	−	
Ankylosing Spondylitis	+	a 158	b 12	170
	−	c 17	d 193	210
		175	205	380

Relative Risk formula

$$RR = \frac{ad}{bc} \text{ where}$$

a = patients with the antigen
b = patients without the antigen
c = healthy individuals (controls) with the antigen
d = healthy individuals (controls) without the antigen

Relative Risk = 30494/204 = 149

References

1. Mallory D, Hackel E, Fawcett K, eds. HLA techniques for blood bankers. Arlington VA: American Association of Blood Banks, 1984.
2. Fawcett K, ed. Histocompatibility testing: A self instructional course. Arlington, VA: American Association of Blood Banks, 1988.
3. Moulds JM, Fawcett KJ, Garner RJ, eds. Scientific and technical aspects of the major histocompatibility complex. Arlington, VA: American Association of Blood Banks, 1989.
4. Rodey G. HLA beyond tears. Atlanta: DeNovo, Inc, 1991.
5. Dausset J, Nenna A. Présence d'une leuco-agglutinine dans le sérum d'un cas d'agranulocytose chronique. Compt Rend Soc Bio 1952;146:1539-41.
6. Payne R, Rolfs MR. Fetomaternal leukocyte incompatibility. J Clin Invest 1958;37:1756-63.
7. Dausset J. Iso-leuco-anticorps. Acta Haematol 1958;20:156-66.
8. Payne R, Hackel E. Inheritance of human leukocyte antigens. Am J Hum Genet 1961;13:306-19.
9. Friedman EA, Retan JW, Marshall DC, et al. Accelerated skin graft rejection in humans preimmunized with homologous peripheral leukocytes. J Clin Invest 1961;40:2162-70.
10. Terasaki PI, McClelland JD. Microdroplet assay of human serum cytotoxins. Nature 1964;204:998-1000.
11. Bodmer JG, Marsh SGE, Albert ED, et al. Nomenclature for factors of the HLA system, 1991. Tissue Antigens 1992;39:161-73.
12. Beatty PG, Mickelson EM, Petersdorf EW, et al. Histocompatibility 1991. Transfusion 1991; 31:847-56.
13. Trowsdale J, Ragoussis J, Campbell RD. Map of the human MHC. Immunol Today 1991;12:443-6.
14. Lawlor DA, Zemmour J, Ennis PD, Parham P. Evolution of class I MHC genes and proteins: From natural selection to thymic selection. Ann Rev Immunol 1990;8:23-65.
15. Alper CA, Awdeh ZL, Rappeport J, et al. Complotypes in bone marrow transplantation. Transplant Proc 1985;17:440-1.
16. McCusker CT, Singal DP. The human leukocyte antigen (HLA) system: 1990. Transfus Med Rev 1990;4:279-87.
17. Fuller TC, Rodey GE. Specificity of alloantibodies against antigens of the HLA complex. In: Hackel E, Mallory D, eds. Theoretical aspects of HLA. Arlington, VA: American Association of Blood Banks, 1982:51-80.
18. Bjorkman PJ, Saper MA, Samraovi B, et al. Structure of the human class I histocompatibility antigen, HLA-A2. Nature 1987;329:506-12.
19. Konoeda Y, Terasaki PI, Wakisaka A, et al. Public determinants of HLA indicated by pregnancy antibodies. Transplantation 1986;41:253-9.
20. Rodey GE. Class I antigens: HLA-A, -B, -C and cross-reactive groups. In: Moulds JM, Fawcett KJ, Garner RJ, eds. Scientific and technical aspects of the major histocompatibility complex. Arlington, VA: American Association of Blood Banks, 1989:23-46.
21. Hackett CJ. Antigen presentation: Later for the rendezvous. Nature 1991; 349:655-6.
22. Brodsky FM, Guagliardi LE. The cell biology of antigen processing and presentation. Ann Rev Immunol 1991;9:707-44.
23. Carbone FR, Bevan MJ. Major histocompatibility complex control of T cell recognition. In: Paul WE, ed. Fundamental immunology, 2nd ed. New York: Raven Press, 1989:541-67.
24. Meryman HT. Transfusion-induced alloimmunization and immunosuppression and the effects of leukocyte depletion. Transfus Med Rev 1989;3:180-93.
25. Zachary AA, Teresi GA, eds. ASHI laboratory manual, 2nd ed. Lenexa, KS: American Society for Histocompatibility and Immunogenetics, 1990.

26. Fuller TC, Phelan D, Gebel HM, Rodey GE. The antigenic specificity of antibody reactive in the antiglobulin-augmented lymphocytotoxicity test. Transplantation 1982;34:24-9.

27. Scornik JC. Flow cytometry crossmatch. In: Zachary AA, Teresi GA, eds. ASHI laboratory manual, 2nd ed. Lenexa, KS: American Society for Histocompatibility and Immunogenetics, 1990:325-31.

28. Kristensen T, Madsen M, Johnsen HE. Cell-mediated lympholysis. In: Dick HM, Kissmeyer-Nielsen F, eds. Histocompatibility techniques. Amsterdam: Elsevier/North-Holland Biomedical Press, 1979:87-110.

29. Erlich HA, Bugawan TL. HLA class II gene polymorphisms: DNA typing, evolution, and relationship to disease susceptibility. In: Erlich HA, ed. PCR technology. New York: Stockton Press, 1989:193-208.

30. Heyman MR, Schiffer CA. Platelet transfusion to patients receiving chemotherapy. In: Rossi EC, Simon TL, Moss GS, eds. Principles of transfusion medicine. Baltimore: Williams and Wilkins, 1991:223-31.

31. Bishop JF, McGrath K, Wolf MM, et al. Clinical factors influencing the efficacy of pooled platelet transfusions. Blood 1988;71:383-7.

32. Claas FHJ, Smeenk RJT, Schmidt R, et al. Alloimmunization against the MHC antigens after platelet transfusions is due to contaminating leukocytes in the platelet suspension. Exp Hematol 1981;9:84-9.

33. Fisher M, Chapman JR, Ting A, Morris PJ. Alloimmunization to HLA antigens following transfusion with leukocyte-poor and purified platelet suspensions. Vox Sang 1985;49:331-5.

34. Duquesnoy RJ. Donor selection in platelet transfusion therapy of alloimmunized thrombocytopenic patients. In: Greenwalt TJ, Jamieson GA, eds. The blood platelet in transfusion therapy. New York: Alan R. Liss, 1978:231.

35. Dahlke MB, Weiss KL. Platelet transfusion from donors mismatched for crossreactive HLA antigens. Transfusion 1984;24:299-302.

36. Brand A, van Leeuwen A, Eernisse JG, van Rood JJ. Platelet transfusion therapy. Optimal donor selection with a combination of lymphocytotoxicity and platelet fluorescence tests. Blood 1978;51:781-8.

37. de Rie MA, van der Plas-van Dalen CM, Engelfriet CP, et al. The serology of febrile transfusion reactions. Vox Sang 1985;49:126-34.

38. Popovsky MA, Abel MD, Moore SB. Transfusion-related acute lung injury associated with passive transfer of antileukocyte antibodies. Am Rev Respir Dis 1983;128:185-9.

39. Seeger W, Schneider U, Kreusler B, et al. Reproduction of transfusion-related acute lung injury in an ex vivo lung model. Blood 1990; 76:1438-44.

40. Anderson K, Weinstein HC. Transfusion-associated graft-versus-host disease. N Engl J Med 1990;323:315-21.

41. Thaler M, Shamiss A, Orgad S, et al. The role of blood from HLA-homozygous donors in fatal transfusion-associated graft-versus-host disease after open heart surgery. N Engl J Med 1989;321:25-33.

42. Juji T, Takahashi K, Shibata Y, et al. Posttransfusion graft-versus-host disease in immunocompetent patients after cardiac surgery in Japan. N Engl J Med 1989;321:56.

43. Anderson K, Goodnough LT, Sayers M, et al. Variation in blood component irradiation practice: Implications for prevention of transfusion-associated graft-versus-host disease. Blood 1991;77:2096-102.

44. Everett ET, Kao K-J, Scornik JC. Class I HLA molecules on human erythrocytes. Transplantation 1987;44:123-9.

45. Panzer S, Mayr WR, Graninger W, et al. Haemolytic transfusion reactions due to HLA antibodies. Lancet 1987;1:474-8.

46. Breimer ME, Brynger H, Rydberg L, et al. Transplantation of blood group A2 kidneys to O recipients. Biochemical and immunological studies of group A antigens in human kidneys. Transplant Proc 1985;17:2640-3.

47. Bach FH, van Rood JJ. The major histocompatibility complex genetics and biology. N Engl J Med 1976;295:806-13, 872-8, 927-36.

48. Terasaki PI. Clinical transplants 1989. Los Angeles: UCLA Tissue Typing Laboratory, 1989:330,467.

49. Spitalnik S, Pfaff W, Cowles J, et al. Correlation of humoral immunity to Lewis blood group antigens with renal transplant rejection. Transplantation 1984;37:265-8.

50. Cerilli J, Clarke J, Doolin T, et al. The significance of a donor-specific vessel crossmatch in renal allografts. Transplantation 1988;46:359-62.

51. Walker RH, Meyers MA, Phillips LM. The probability of exclusion of the HLA-A, B system in North American whites and blacks in parentage tests. Transfusion 1987;27:75-9.

52. Walker RH, Pohl BA. Paternity testing with an absent mother: The probability of exclusion of red cell surface antigens, Gm, Hp, and HLA systems in North American whites and blacks. In: Mayr W, ed. Advances in forensic haemogenetics 2. Heidelberg: Springer-Verlag, 1988:597-9.

53. Walker RH. Analysis of parentage test case. In: Walker RH, ed. Inclusion probabilities in parentage testing. Arlington, VA: American Association of Blood Banks, 1983:443-88.

54. Dalton TA, Bennet JC. Autoimmune disease and the major histocompatibility complex: Therapeutic implications. Am J Med 1992;92:183-8.

14

Pretransfusion Testing

The purpose of pretransfusion testing is to select blood components that will have acceptable survival when transfused and will not cause clinically significant destruction of the recipient's own red blood cells (rbcs). AABB *Standards for Blood Banks and Transfusion Services*[1] states that the following procedures must be part of pretransfusion compatibility testing:

1. Positive identification of recipient and recipient's blood sample.
2. Review of transfusion service records for results of previous testing on samples from the recipient.
3. Tests on donor blood, as described in Chapter 1.
4. ABO and Rh typing of recipient's blood.
5. Antibody detection tests using the recipient's serum or plasma.
6. Selection of blood components of appropriate ABO and Rh types.
7. Tests with the recipient's serum or plasma and donor's rbcs, ie, a crossmatch.
8. Labeling of the components with the recipient's identifying information.

Transfusion is usually a beneficial and safe procedure. However, donor rbcs sometimes undergo accelerated destruction. Most hemolytic transfusion reactions result from errors in patient or sample identification,[2,3] but in some cases blood group antibodies exist that were not detected by standard serologic techniques.[4] Despite advances in blood group serology, pretransfusion testing will not detect all unexpected rbc antibodies in the recipient's serum or guarantee normal survival of transfused rbcs.[5] If performed properly, pretransfusion tests will:

1. Verify that blood components are ABO compatible.
2. Detect most clinically significant unexpected antibodies.

Transfusion Request Forms

Blood request forms must contain sufficient information for positive patient identification. *Standards*[1] states that the first and last names of the patient and an identification number unique to the patient must be on the form. Because blood is a drug, the name of the responsible physician should appear on the requisition form. Additional information such as sex and age of the patient, diagnosis, and transfusion and pregnancy history may be helpful in resolving problems should they occur. Blood request forms lacking the required information or containing illegible information are not acceptable.

Computer-transmitted requests are acceptable as long as the required information is complete. Telephone requests should be documented by subsequent submission of a properly completed blood request form. Personnel receiving telephone requests should note the caller's name and time the request is

309

received in addition to the patient's name and identification number.

Blood Sample

The collection of a properly labeled blood sample from the correct patient is critical to safe blood transfusion. The person who draws the blood sample must identify the patient in a positive manner by comparing the information on the request form with the information on the wristband. If there is a discrepancy between the two, the sample must not be collected. The phlebotomist must not rely on a bed tag, or on charts or records placed on the bed, nearby tables or equipment.

In the absence of a wristband, remind nursing staff that the patient must have a wristband to validate identification at the time of transfusion and ask that one be placed on the patient. When the patient's identity is unknown, use an emergency identification number on a temporary band. This number should be attached to the patient and blood samples and be cross-referenced with the patient's name and hospital identification number when they are known.

Preadmission laboratory testing poses a special problem for the blood bank if the patient's wristband is not kept on between the times of specimen collection and transfusion. A new specimen collected upon admission may be required in order to validate identification.

Labeling the Sample

Before leaving the bedside the phlebotomist must label the blood sample tubes with the patient's first and last names, identification number and the date of collection. Imprinted labels may be used if the information on the label is identical to that on the wristband and request

form. There must also be a way to identify the phlebotomist.[1] This can be done by having the phlebotomist initial or sign the label affixed to the tube or the requisition form.

Nature of Specimen

Serum or plasma may be used for pretransfusion testing.[1] Serum is preferred because, with plasma, small fibrin clots sometimes form, trapping test red cells that may be difficult to distinguish from true agglutination. Fibrin also can be a problem in nonanticoagulated samples that fail to clot, usually because the patient has been given heparin. In this situation, thrombin or protamine sulphate can be added to the sample. See Method 1.2. Anticoagulants, such as EDTA or citrate, chelate calcium and prevent complement activation. This should be considered if plasma is used in tests to detect antibodies demonstrable mainly through complement activation.

It is permissible to collect blood from an infusion line. Since residual intravenous fluid may interfere with serologic testing, the tubing should be flushed with saline and the first 5 mL of blood withdrawn discarded before collecting the sample.

Hemolyzed samples should not be used. Free serum hemoglobin may mask antibody-induced hemolysis. If there is no alternative to using serum containing hemoglobin, as with specimens from burn patients or those with acute hemolytic anemia, it is helpful to compare the size of the rbc button obtained in tests with the patient's serum against a control (saline or antibody-free serum) to see whether test rbcs have been lysed by the patient's serum.

Age of Specimen

Compatibility tests must be performed on blood samples collected within 3 days of red cell transfusions when the patient has been pregnant or transfused within the preceding 3 months or if the history is uncertain or unavailable.[1] It is important that the sample used for serologic tests represent the patient's current immunologic status. Recent transfusion or pregnancy may stimulate production of unexpected antibodies. Since it is not possible to predict when such antibodies will be demonstrable, a 3-day limit has been arbitrarily selected. Many laboratory directors prefer to set a 3-day limit on all specimens used for pretransfusion testing to avoid problems that might occur because of record-keeping errors or inaccurate history. Exceptions may be approved by the director when a patient has not been recently transfused or pregnant.

Specimens From Neonates

Requirements for samples from infants less than 4 months old are different and will be discussed in detail in Chapter 18. Briefly:
1. If there are no unexpected antibodies detected by initial tests and the infant receives no blood components containing unexpected clinically significant antibodies, antibody detection and crossmatching tests can be omitted throughout the neonatal period. The serum or plasma of either the mother or infant may be used for initial testing.
2. After the infant's ABO and Rh types have been determined, further ABO and Rh typing may be omitted, provided all red blood cells transfused are ABO compatible and are Rh negative or the child's original Rh type.

Confirming Sample Identity

When a sample is received in the laboratory, a qualified member of the staff must confirm that the information on the label and on the transfusion request form are identical. If there is any unresolved discrepancy, or doubt about the identity of the patient, a new sample must be obtained.[1] It is unacceptable for anyone to correct an incorrectly labeled sample. Each laboratory should establish policies and procedures in this regard.

Retaining and Storing Blood Samples

The recipient's blood specimen and a sample of the donor's rbcs must be sealed or stoppered and kept at 1-6 C for at least 7 days after each transfusion.[1] Donor rbcs may be from the remainder of the segment actually used in the crossmatch or a segment removed before issuing the blood. If the crossmatch segment is saved, it must be placed in a sealed or stoppered tube. Keeping the patient's and donor's samples makes it possible to do repeat or additional testing if the patient experiences a transfusion reaction.

Previous Records

Compatibility testing must include checking previous transfusion service records for the recipient's serologic history.[1] If the patient has been tested previously, results of current testing must be compared with the interpretation of previous testing. Concurrence between previous and current findings gives some assurance (but not proof) that there have been no identification errors and that tests have been correctly performed and interpreted. Discrepancies must be resolved before blood is issued.

Perhaps the most significant information to be obtained from the records is the existence of clinically significant antibodies active at 37 C. The specificity of antibodies detected previously should be compared with that of antibodies detectable currently. Even if the present antibody detection test is negative, the antiglobulin phase of the crossmatch is required for patients with a history of any clinically significant alloantibody.[1] Blood lacking the relevant antigens should be selected for transfusion even though rbcs possessing those antigens are serologically compatible at present.

Serologic Testing

The ABO and Rh types of the intended recipient must be determined before blood is issued for transfusion. In addition, if the patient is to receive WB, RBCs, (including washed or deglycerolized components), granulocytes or platelet concentrates containing more than 5 mL of red cells, the recipient's serum must also be tested for unexpected antibodies and for serologic compatibility with the donor's rbcs.[1]

Blood Grouping

To determine the ABO group of the recipient, the rbcs must be tested with anti-A and anti-B and the serum or plasma with A_1 and B rbcs. The techniques used and interpretation of results are described in Chapter 10 and the Methods. Any discrepant results should be resolved before blood is given. If the problem cannot be resolved before transfusion, the patient should receive group O rbcs, which are safest in an emergency situation.

The patient's rbcs must also be tested with anti-D. Routine testing for other Rh antigens is not recommended. Tests with anti-D must be controlled to avoid incorrectly concluding that an Rh– person is Rh+. See Chapter 11 for a discussion of Rh typing reagents and appropriate control techniques. If there is a problem in interpreting tests for D, the patient

should be given Rh– blood until the problem is resolved.

It is not necessary to determine whether a recipient's rbcs are of the weak D (D^u) phenotype because no harm results from giving these individuals Rh– blood. Omitting the weak D (D^u) test prevents misinterpretations arising from a positive direct antiglobulin test (DAT). In some laboratories the test for weak expression of D, the weak D (D^u) test, is done, especially if multiple transfusions are contemplated and/or there is a shortage of Rh– blood. Patients of the weak D (D^u) phenotype are Rh+ and can receive Rh+ blood. Only rarely will transfusion of Rh+ blood to a weak D (D^u) recipient evoke production of anti-D.[6]

Antibody Detection Tests

Clinically Significant Antibodies

Standards[1] states that the serum or plasma of a recipient must be tested against single-donor suspensions of group O reagent rbcs, not pooled rbcs. Such cells are selected to carry those blood group antigens necessary for detecting the most important clinically significant unexpected antibodies. Unexpected antibodies are those other than anti-A or anti-B. It is difficult to define "clinically significant" since the significance may depend on the specific clinical situation and on the condition of the patient. In general, an antibody is considered clinically significant if examples with that specificity are known to have caused hemolytic disease of the newborn, a hemolytic transfusion reaction or unacceptably short survival of transfused rbcs. Antibodies reactive at 37 C and/or in the antiglobulin test are more likely to be significant than those reactive only at room temperature or below. The antiglobulin phase of testing is required. In addition, IgG-coated rbcs must be used to detect false-negative antiglobulin tests due to inactivation of anti-IgG in the test sytem.

Practical Considerations

Performing antibody detection tests with reagent rbcs will often obviate the need to perform an antiglobulin crossmatch. Only tests for ABO incompatibility, such as immediate-spin (IS) tests, are required when properly performed antibody detection tests are nonreactive and there is no prior record of clinically significant unexpected antibodies.

Antibody detection tests may be done in advance of, or together with, a crossmatch between the patient's serum and donor rbcs. However, performing such tests before crossmatching not only facilitates implementation of IS crossmatch regimens, but also permits early recognition and identification of clinically significant antibodies, facilitating timely provision of blood for transfusion. The reagent rbcs used in the procedure (see below) are selected to express most clinically relevant antigens. They may also exhibit stronger expression of antigens than do donor rbcs. This facilitates detection of weakly reactive antibodies that might be missed in crossmatches, particularly those that manifest dosage (ie, react stronger with rbcs from homozygotes than with rbcs from heterozygotes). In addition, detecting and identifying an antibody permits screening of donor units for those that lack the relevant antigens, using potent reagent antisera.

Reagent Red Blood Cells

Group O rbcs suitable for antibody screening are available as commercially prepared products and are offered either as a set of two or three vials, each containing rbcs from a single donor, or as a pool of equal volumes of cells from two donors. The pooled cells may be used only for testing serum samples from donors. When testing serum samples from recipients, separate rbc samples are required to provide adequate sensitivity. The following antigens must be represented: D, C, E, c, e, M, N, S, s, P_1, Le^a, Le^b, K, k, Fy^a, Fy^b, Jk^a and Jk^b.[7] There is no requirement that other antigens be present, such as Lu^a, V or C^w, or that the rbcs have double-dose expression of antigens. However, some workers recommend that Jk(a+b–) rbcs be used to provide adequate detection of anti-Jk^a.[8] Reagent rbcs are suspended in a preservative solution. When not in use, they should be refrigerated. Aliquots may be washed and resuspended in saline or low-ionic strength saline (LISS) solution. They should not be stored in these wash solutions over 24 hours because the solutions may not be sterile. Also, some antigens, Fy^a in particular,[9] deteriorate rapidly in a low-ionic environment. Reagent rbcs may be as many as 9 weeks old at the expiration date. They should not be used for routine tests beyond this date because the strength of some antigens decreases on storage. The loss may be more pronounced on the rbcs of some donors than others.

Limitations of Antibody Detection Tests

Antibody screening tests cannot detect all antibodies of potential clinical significance. Antibodies reactive with low-incidence antigens are likely to be missed, as are those that manifest dosage. Some clinically significant antibodies manifest dosage, notably antibodies in the Rh, Duffy and Kidd systems. Therefore, it is desirable that donors of screening cells be apparently homozygous for the genes controlling expression of these antigens. Donors of the appropriate phenotypes are in short supply, and it is not always possible for manufacturers to provide reagent screening cells of the ideal phenotypes. The decision to use cells from three donors rather than two in an antibody screening procedure should be based on circumstances in an individual laboratory.

Crossmatching Tests

Unless the situation is urgent, the recipient's serum or plasma is usually tested with the donor's rbcs before WB and RBC components are given (ie, a major crossmatch is done). The sample from the recipient must be obtained and labeled as described on p 310, and the donor's rbcs must be from an originally attached donor segment.[1] For patients with clinically significant antibodies or a history of such antibodies, the methods used must include those that will demonstrate ABO incompatibility and must include an antiglobulin test. However, when no clinically significant antibodies are detected in antibody screening tests, and there is no history of such antibodies, the antiglobulin phase of the crossmatch is not required.[1] Rarely is a clinically significant unexpected antibody detected by the antiglobulin phase of the crossmatch when the antibody detection test is negative.[10,11] The policy to omit the antiglobulin phase of the crossmatch for patients who meet these criteria must be made by the medical director. Some points worth considering are:

1. The incidence of incompatible crossmatches when antibody detection tests are negative and the reasons for these results in the particular laboratory.
2. The sensitivity of the antibody detection procedure used in the laboratory.
3. The potential benefits of omitting a routine antiglobulin crossmatch in the laboratory, such as saving technologist time and reagents, and using blood effectively.

If clinically significant antibodies are detected in the screening procedure, the antiglobulin phase of the crossmatch is required. The tests to demonstrate ABO incompatibility are required at all times. The most important reason for doing a crossmatch is that it serves as a final check on ABO blood group compatibility.

It is not necessary to test the recipient's rbcs with the donor's serum or plasma (ie, perform a minor crossmatch). Antibody detection tests have already been done on samples from donors whose history indicates the likelihood of having clinically important antibodies. When antibodies are detected in a unit of blood, components are prepared that contain minimal amounts of plasma and the label indicates that the antibody screening test was positive.[1] The methods used for crossmatching may be the same as those used for antibody detection or they may differ.

Computerized Crossmatch

If a computer system has been validated on site to prevent the release of ABO-incompatible blood components, then it may be used prior to transfusion to detect ABO incompatibility instead of a serologic crossmatch provided that the following conditions have been met[1(p 25)]:

1. There have been two determinations of the recipient's ABO group as specified in B5.100. One determination must be made on a current sample. The second determination may be made on the same sample, a second current sample or by comparison with previous records.
2. The computer system contains the donor unit number, the component name, ABO and Rh types of the component, blood confirmatory test in-

terpretation and identification, and the ABO and Rh types of the recipient.

3. There is a method to ensure correct entry of data.

4. The system contains logic to alert the user to discrepancies between donor unit labeling and blood group confirmatory test interpretation and to ABO incompatibilities between recipient and donor unit.

Type and Screen

Type and screen is a policy in which crossmatched blood is not set aside for those patients undergoing surgical procedures that rarely require transfusion. Instead, the patient's blood sample is completely tested for ABO, Rh and unexpected antibodies, and is kept in the blood bank for immediate crossmatching, should this prove necessary. For procedures like cholecystectomy, hysterectomy, thyroidectomy and others, blood is so seldom needed that specific preoperative crossmatching is inappropriate. The blood bank must have appropriate donor blood available for all patients undergoing operations on a type and screen basis.[12,13]

If transfusion becomes necessary, ABO-, Rh-compatible blood can be safely released after immediate-spin crossmatch for patients with a negative antibody screen.[10,11] A crossmatch to demonstrate ABO compatibility should be completed before issue of the component, except in an emergency. If the patient does have blood group alloantibodies, donor blood known to lack the corresponding antigens must be available.

Autologous Control

Data published by Judd et al[14] indicate that performing an autologous control or DAT as part of routine pretransfusion testing may be of limited value, even when the patient has been recently transfused. *Standards* does not require an autologous control or DAT. See Chapter 16.

Selection of Units

ABO Group

Whenever possible, patients should receive blood components of their own ABO group. When this is not possible, components of alternative ABO groups may be selected. If the component to be transfused contains 5 mL or more of rbcs, the donor's rbcs must be ABO compatible with the recipient's plasma. For plasma-containing products, there is a possibility of damage to the recipient's rbcs. Ideally, therefore, the recipient's rbcs should be compatible with ABO antibodies in the donor's plasma. ABO blood group requirements for components and acceptable alternative ABO groups are summarized in Table 14-1.

Rh Type

Rh+ blood components should be selected for Rh+ recipients. Rh− units are also acceptable but, except in special circumstances, should be reserved for Rh− recipients. Rh− components should be selected for Rh− recipients to avoid immunizing the recipient to the D antigen. Occasionally, ABO-compatible Rh− components may not be available. In this situation there should be consultation with the blood bank medical director and the patient's physician, who may prefer postponing transfusion. However, if transfusion is urgently required, there may be no alternative. The risk of immunization (greater than 80% for the D antigen) may be less critical than the risk of delaying transfusion. Depending on the child-bearing potential of the patient it may be appropriate to administer

Table 14-1. Selection of Components When ABO Identical Donors Are Not Available

	Required Component Blood Type
Whole Blood	Must be identical to that of recipient.*
Red Blood Cells	Must be compatible with the recipient's plasma.
Granulocyte Concentrate	Must be compatible with the recipient's plasma.
Fresh Frozen Plasma	Should be compatible with the recipient's rbcs.
Platelet Concentrate*	All ABO groups acceptable; components compatible with recipient's rbcs preferred.
Single Donor Cryoprecipitate	All ABO groups acceptable.

*Since a large volume of plasma is administered, components compatible with the recipient's rbcs are preferred.

Rh Immune Globulin to a D– recipient of D+ blood components.[15] See p 397.

Blood Administered After Non-Group-Specific Transfusion

It is often desirable to return to transfusion of group-specific blood after administering blood of an ABO group other than the patient's own. Whether ABO group-specific blood can be given safely depends on the status of anti-A and/or anti-B in current samples of the recipient's blood.[16] When serum from a freshly drawn sample is compatible with rbcs of the patient's original ABO group, group-specific blood may be issued for transfusion. If the crossmatch is incompatible because of ABO antibodies, transfusion should be continued with rbcs of the alternative compatible ABO group.

If the change in blood group involved only the Rh system, the change back to Rh type-specific blood is simple, since antibodies are not expected to be present in the plasma of either recipient or donor. This situation may, however, be complicated if a patient has received blood of an Rh type other than his or her own before testing is done. This may make it difficult to determine the correct Rh type. The recipient's true Rh group can be established only by testing autologous cells from a sample collected before transfusion or autologous cells specially harvested posttransfusion.[17] See Method 2.17. If there is a question about the recipient's Rh type, it is best to transfuse Rh– blood.

Other Blood Groups

It is not necessary to routinely select units of blood on the basis of other blood groups. However, if the recipient has an unexpected antibody considered to be clinically significant, antigen-negative blood should be selected for crossmatching. If the antibody is weakly reactive or no longer demonstrable, it is necessary to use reagent antisera to screen donor units for the required antigen-negative phenotype. If, on the other hand, the antibodies react well with antigen-positive rbcs, a more economical approach is to screen units with the patient's serum, and then use blood grouping reagents to confirm that the compatible units lack the antigens in question. When commercial reagents are not available, patient or donor sera can be used, especially for low-incidence or uncommon antigens.

Techniques for Antibody Detection

The characteristics of ABO and Rh antibodies are described in Chapters 10 and 11. Table 12-1 summarizes the serologic behavior of antibodies of the other major blood groups.

Before deciding upon routine procedures for antibody detection, the blood bank director must decide which antibodies are considered significant. Once a procedure has been adopted, the method must be described in the SOP manual and each member of the staff must know and follow the directions as written.

There are numerous serologic techniques suitable for detection of blood group antibodies. To select blood for a recipient, it is best to use a method(s) that:

1. Will detect as many clinically significant antibodies as possible.
2. Will not detect clinically insignificant antibodies.
3. Will allow prompt delivery of blood to the recipient.

The test chosen should be of sufficient sensitivity to detect very low levels of antibody in a recipient's serum. This is important because transfusion of antigen-positive rbcs may result in rapid production of antibody with subsequent rbc destruction. The same procedure may be used for all categories of specimens, including pretransfusion obstetrical and donor screens. The methods selected for antibody detection and crossmatching tests may be the same or they may differ. For example, room temperature tests such as immediate-spin crossmatch may be preferred to detect ABO incompatibility but may not need to be included in antibody screening tests. Regardless of the procedures chosen, the antibody detection method must demonstrate clinically significant unexpected antibodies and must include the antiglobulin test. In addition the cross-match must be able to detect ABO incompatibility. See Methods 3.1 to 3.2.

Reading and Interpretation of Reactions

In serologic testing, the hemolysis or agglutination that constitutes the visible endpoint of an rbc antigen-antibody interaction must be observed accurately and consistently. Using a light source and optical aid (eg, an illuminated concave mirror) enhances the sensitivity and consistency. Since both hemolysis and agglutination are possible, the supernatant fluid should be observed for free hemoglobin immediately after centrifugation and then the rbcs gently dispersed to observe for agglutination. The manner in which cells are dislodged from the bottom of the tube affects detection of agglutination. The tube should be held at an angle so that the fluid cuts across the cell button as the tube is gently tilted. The reaction strength (or grade) should be determined when all cells have been resuspended. Overshaking may break up large agglutinates or disperse weakly cohesive agglutinates. The strength of agglutination or degree of hemolysis observed with each cell sample should be recorded as the test is read.

All personnel in a laboratory should use the same interpretations and notations and be consistent in grading reactions. Consistency in grading is especially important in antibody identification. Some laboratories prefer to use a scoring system to indicate reaction strength. See Method 1.9. Microscopic observation may be useful in distinguishing rouleaux from true agglutination and detecting specific patterns of agglutination characteristic of some antibodies, such as the mixed-field pattern seen with anti-Sd[a]. Routine microscopic observation is not required.

General Considerations

Labeling Tubes

Each tube used for serologic tests should be labeled with the recipient's initials (or other identifying information) and the donor unit number or reagent identification. The position of a tube in a rack or centrifuge head should not be used to identify the contents of a tube.

Volume of Serum

Instructions for most serologic procedures call for 2 drops of serum. Taswell and coworkers[4] presented data indicating that the volume dispensed in 2 drops may be insufficient to provide an optimal ratio of antibody to antigen in some cases. They found some alloantibodies detectable only when the volume of serum was increased to 3 or 4 drops. If antibody is present in low concentration, increasing the serum-to-rbc ratio will increase the amount of antibody uptake per cell.

Beattie[18] demonstrated tremendous variability in serum-to-rbc ratios resulting from differences in the internal measurements of Pasteur pipets and reagent droppers. Drops of serum dispensed from some disposable Pasteur pipets tend to be small and highly variable, while drops delivered from droppers in reagent vials tend to be large. It is important to standardize the volume of serum and rbcs used in routine test systems. This is particularly important for tests using low-ionic reagents (wash solutions and additives) that require equal volumes of serum and low-ionic reagent.

Cell Suspension

The rbcs used for crossmatching should be obtained from a sealed segment of tubing originally attached to the blood container. The cells should be washed once and resuspended to a 2-4% concentration in saline or LISS. Washing the donor's rbcs removes plasma and can prevent the formation of fibrin clots. Since the ratio of serum to cells markedly affects the sensitivity of agglutination tests, it is best to use the weakest cell suspension that can be observed easily for agglutination. Agglutination is dependent on a minimal number of antibody molecules per rbc. If too many cells are present in the serum-cell mixture, weak antibodies may be missed because too few antibody molecules are bound to each cell. Although suspensions of 2-4% are acceptable, many workers find that a 2% concentration gives the best results.

Saline Tests

The simplest serologic method is the saline technique in which serum is mixed with saline-suspended rbcs. The tube may be centrifuged immediately, incubated at room temperature or incubated at 37 C before centrifugation. ABO incompatibilities and antibodies reacting predominantly at room temperature, such as anti-M, -N, -P_1, -Le^a and -Le^b, are most often detected at this phase. Many workers use saline testing at room temperature for crossmatching to detect ABO incompatibility but have deleted it from antibody detection tests to avoid finding antibodies, active only at room temperature, that have little clinical significance. When saline tests are used for detection of clinically significant alloantibodies, the tubes are usually incubated at 37 C for 30 minutes. Centrifugation and observation after incubation may detect some antibodies (eg, potent anti-D, -K or -E) that can cause direct agglutination of rbcs. Also, some antibodies (eg, anti-Le^a, -Jk^a) may be detected by their lysis of antigen-positive cells during this phase. Most often, however, antibodies bind to the rbcs during incubation but are not demonstrable until the antiglobulin phase of testing.

If tests are incubated at both room temperature and 37 C, two sets of tubes are usually prepared. One set is incubated at room temperature, the other at 37 C to avoid positive antiglobulin reactions due to complement binding by cold agglutinins when polyspecific antihuman globulin is used. See Chapter 8 and Method 3.2.

Albumin-Enhanced Agglutination

Since 1945, bovine serum albumin solutions have been used to enhance sensitization and agglutination of rbcs by IgG antibodies.[19,20] Albumin can be used as an additive to the serum-cell mixture or can be layered on the cell button.[21] The additive technique is more frequently used in the United States, but the layering method is probably more sensitive for detecting direct agglutination by Rh antibodies or occasional examples of anti-Fy[a] and anti-K.[22] Polymerized albumin solutions enhance direct agglutination more effectively than unmodified albumin.[23,24]

In the 1960's, Stroup and MacIlroy[25] and Griffitts and coworkers[26] reported enhanced reactivity of many antibodies when albumin was included in the test system. Some of these antibodies were reactive in the antiglobulin phase after a shorter incubation time than when no albumin was included. These results suggested increased antibody uptake in the presence of albumin. Later it was shown that the effect of albumin itself is minimal on the first stage of the reaction. The increased antibody uptake reported earlier may have resulted from the low ionic strength of the albumin diluent.[27] The effect of ionic strength on antibody uptake is discussed below.

There is still controversy concerning the action of albumin in hemagglutination. For a discussion of the mechanisms involved the reader should see reviews by Steane[28] and Case.[22] See Method 3.1.2.

Low Ionic Strength Saline Tests

Allowing antigen-antibody reactions to occur in low ionic strength conditions shortens the incubation time required for the detection of most antibodies.[29-32] Antibody uptake, and consequently the degree of agglutination finally observed, are enhanced.[33] See p 167-9 for a discussion of physiochemical factors affecting the antigen-antibody reaction. LISS solutions can be prepared in the laboratory or can be purchased for use as wash solutions or additives. See Method 3.1.3.

Several important factors must be considered when using low ionic reagents. Adding additional serum to the test system increases the ionic strength of the mixture. The shortened incubation period and enhanced sensitivity in subsequent antiglobulin tests depend upon attainment of the desired ionic conditions. It is, therefore, important to adhere to the procedure recommended by the manufacturer or established in the individual laboratory by maintaining appropriate ratios of serum and LISS reagent. It may be convenient to prepare LISS-suspended screening cells sufficient for one working day, but these may be used only on the day of preparation since some antigens may deteriorate after prolonged incubation in LISS.

Polyethylene Glycol Tests

Polyethylene glycol (PEG) is a water soluble, neutral polymer that has also been shown to be an effective potentiator of antigen-antibody reactions.[34] Compared to albumin, PEG increases the rate of detection of clinically significant rbc antibodies, decreases detection of insignificant antibodies and may decrease the need for other serologic enhancement techniques.[35,36] See Method 3.1.4.

Antiglobulin Testing

The antiglobulin technique is required when testing samples from recipients for the presence of unexpected antibodies and, in some cases discussed above, for serologic compatibility with rbcs from donors. Chapter 8 contains an in-depth discussion of antiglobulin testing.

Either anti-IgG or a polyspecific antiglobulin reagent that contains anti-IgG and anti-C3d may be used for the antiglobulin phase of antibody detection and crossmatching. The polyspecific reagent, since it contains anti-C3d activity, will detect some rare antibodies demonstrable only because they activate complement. Some clinically significant antibodies detected by polyspecific, but not by anti-IgG, reagents have Kidd blood group specificity.[37] For some other antibodies, polyspecific antisera may also produce stronger reactions.[37,38] Consequently, some laboratory workers prefer using polyspecific antiglobulin reagent. See Chapter 8 for more information on the antiglobulin test.

The disadvantage of using antiglobulin reagents that contain anticomplement reactivity is that antibodies that are clinically insignificant, such as cold-reactive autoanti-I or -IH, are often detected. The director of the transfusion service may consider that the potential benefits of polyspecific reagents in detecting rare complement-dependent antibodies are not worth the amount of time expended in resolving problems caused by these antibodies. Each facility director should decide which reagent is best suited for that laboratory.

Enzyme Techniques

Enzyme techniques are more appropriately used for antibody identification than for antibody detection during pretransfusion testing. They are especially useful when increased sensitivity is desired, as in the investigation of delayed hemolytic transfusion reactions. However, if an enzyme method is used routinely for antibody detection it should never be the only technique employed because M, N, S, Fy^a, Fy^b and certain other antigens are usually destroyed so that antibodies to those antigens would not be detected.

Techniques employing proteolytic enzymes to enhance hemagglutination were first described in 1947.[39] Enzyme techniques strengthen the reactions seen with many antibodies, and there are a few blood group antibodies demonstrable only when enzyme techniques are used, notably in the Rh and Kidd systems. The exact mechanism by which enzymes enhance antibody reactivity is not clearly understood. The proposed mechanisms are discussed in a review by Ellisor.[40]

Several proteolytic enzymes (papain, bromelain, trypsin, ficin) are suitable for blood bank use. Papain and bromelain are usually added directly to a serum-cell mixture (one-stage technique); papain and ficin are used in a two-stage technique to treat the rbcs before serum is added. A one-stage technique is more convenient to perform but is less sensitive than a two-stage method. The reduced sensitivity of the one-stage method is due to the fact that serum proteins serve as substrate for the enzyme in addition to rbc proteins and, thus, there is less modification of the red cell membrane. A two-stage method, in addition to being more sensitive than a one-stage technique, has the additional advantage that the enzyme-modified cells can be tested before use to ensure that optimal treatment has been achieved. See Method 3.5.5. Reagent rbcs pretreated with enzymes are commercially available, but may also be prepared in the laboratory. Instructions for the preparation and use of papain and ficin are given in Methods 3.5.1 through 3.5.3. Due to the sensitive nature of enzyme test systems, it is important to follow the designated methods for use, either those of the manufacturer or those adopted in the laboratory in which solutions are prepared.

Low Ionic Polycation Tests

The manual Polybrene® test[41] (MPT) and the low ionic polycation (LIP) test[42] are rapid and sensitive methods to detect most blood group antibodies. Some antibodies, particularly those with Rh specificity, may be demonstrable only by these methods, but antibodies reacting with Kell blood group antigens react less well by these methods than by standard procedures. In general, examples of anti-K and anti-k react very weakly or not at all at the first stage of testing and are slightly less reactive in the antiglobulin phase than they are by saline, albumin or LISS antiglobulin techniques. The MPT and LIP procedures are based on the same principles. The required reagents are commercially available. Low ionic Polybrene® procedures are described in Methods 2.11 and 3.1.5.

Theoretical Considerations

Cationic polymers such as Polybrene® cause aggregation of normal rbcs, which can be dispersed with sodium citrate. However, sodium citrate does not disperse Polybrene®-induced aggregation of antibody-coated rbcs. In the manual Polybrene® procedure, rbcs are first incubated with serum under low ionic conditions at low pH to facilitate antibody

uptake. Aggregation of rbcs is then induced by Polybrene®. If antibody has coated the rbcs, immunoglobulin molecules form bridges between adjacent rbcs that persist after sodium citrate is added. The LIP procedure[42] uses protamine sulphate instead of Polybrene® and a buffered salt solution to disperse aggregation.

Suggested Procedures for Routine Crossmatching Tests

The methods used to test the recipient's serum with the donor's rbcs must demonstrate ABO incompatibility. The crossmatch procedure must demonstrate clinically significant antibodies and must include the antiglobulin test unless the prospective recipient has nonreactive antibody detection tests and has no history of having clinically significant antibodies.[1] The methods adopted for use in a laboratory will depend on whether the medical director has chosen to omit the antiglobulin phase of the crossmatch under permissible conditions. Suggested procedures for crossmatching, with and without an antiglobulin phase, are given below.

Demonstrating ABO Incompatibility

When the crossmatch is performed only to detect an ABO incompatibility between the recipient's serum and the donor's rbcs, Procedure A given in Table 14-2 is acceptable. Since the testing is done at room temperature, alloantibodies other than anti-A, anti-B or anti-A,B may be detected that were not detected in the antibody detection tests. See the section on interpretation for a discussion. Some workers have questioned the necessity of a room temperature crossmatch for detecting ABO errors.[43]

Table 14-2. Two Acceptable Crossmatch Procedures

Procedure A:*
1. Label 1 tube for each donor sample to be tested.
2. Add 2 drops of patient's serum to each tube.
3. Add 1 drop of 2-4% saline- or EDTA-saline-suspended donor rbcs to each tube.†
4. Centrifuge immediately,‡ read, grade and record results.

Procedure B:
1. Label 1 tube for each donor sample to be treated.
2. Add 2 drops of patient's serum to each tube.
3. Add 2 drops of 2% LISS-suspended donor rbcs to each tube.
4. Centrifuge immediately, read, grade and record results.§
5. Incubate at 37 C for 10-15 minutes.
6. Centrifuge, read, grade and record results.
7. Perform the antiglobulin test.
8. Confirm validity of negative tests with IgG-coated red cells.

---

*Acceptable method only if antibody detection tests are negative and the patient has no history of clinically significant antibodies.
†See Method 1.7.
‡Immediate-spin tests are acceptable. However, some workers incubate the tubes at room temperature for 5 minutes to improve the sensitivity of the test.
§Optional step in testing. Trudeau et al[37] have demonstrated that an immediate-spin crossmatch is not necessary for detection of ABO errors when LISS-suspended red cells are used for 37 C and antiglobulin testing.

Demonstrating ABO Incompatibility and Clinically Significant Antibodies

Procedure B outlined in Table 14-2 meets the requirements stated in *Standards* in all routine situations. Depending on workload and staffing it may be as convenient and cost-effective to include an antiglobulin test routinely as part of the crossmatch as to omit it. However, the antiglobulin phase of testing rarely uncovers clinically significant antibodies in a patient whose antibody screening test is negative.

Interpretation of Antibody Screening and Crossmatch Results

Negative Antibody Screen, Compatible Crossmatches

The vast majority of samples tested have a negative antibody screen and the cross-matches with donor's rbcs are compatible. However, such results do not guarantee the absence of antibody or normal rbc survival. A negative antibody screen, for example, does not necessarily mean that the serum contains no rbc antibodies, only that there are no antibodies that react with the screening cells by the techniques employed. A compatible crossmatch should be interpreted in a similar fashion.

If clinical circumstances are suspicious (eg, the patient fails to have the expected rise in hemoglobin) or other laboratory findings warrant additional investigation, the routine testing protocol should be expanded. For example, for patients in whom destruction of transfused cells is suspected, subsequently transfused units may need to be crossmatched with more sensitive techniques such as enzyme methods; these techniques may also be appropriate for investigation of the suspected transfusion reactions. In some cases, all the antibody may be bound to the transfused cells and an eluate will have to be tested to demonstrate the antibody causing rbc destruction. The DAT may or may not be positive, depending on the concentration of antibody. In other cases in-vivo rbc survival studies[5] or mononuclear phagocyte assays may be helpful in selecting compatible units.

Positive Antibody Screen, Incompatible Crossmatches

Alloantibodies, autoantibodies, problems with reagents (rbcs or additives) and rouleaux formation may cause the antibody screen, the crossmatch or both to be positive. If the antibody detection tests are positive, a crossmatch including an antiglobulin test must be done.[1] See Procedure B in Table 14-2. Whatever the cause, the problem should be identified before issuing blood for transfusion, unless the need for transfusion is urgent. If there is no time to identify the problem and locate serologically compatible blood, a transfusion service physician should advise the patient's physician of the potential risks involved in transfusion in such a case. Often the risk of death due to transfusing incompatible blood may be less than the risk of death due to depriving the patient of oxygen-carrying capacity.[44]

Alloantibodies

When unexpected alloantibodies are present, the antibody screening test will usually be positive; crossmatches may or may not be compatible depending on the frequency(ies) of the particular antigen(s) involved. The autologous control will be negative unless the patient has been recently transfused. When the screen is positive, it is necessary to:
1. Identify the specificity of the antibody(ies). See Chapter 15.

2. Use the appropriate blood group reagent to test rbcs from units found to be serologically compatible. Alternatively, units can be screened with blood group reagents first and then crossmatched with the recipient's serum. The decision to screen with the recipient's serum or reagents should be based on the strength with which the patient's serum reacts, the volume of serum available from the recipient and the availability and cost of the reagent. When antibodies have been identified in a patient's serum, testing with reagent antiserum is desirable because the reagent serum frequently reacts better than the patient's serum with donor rbcs having weak expression of the antigen. It is not necessary to confirm compatibility using reagent antisera if the patient's antibody is anti-M, -N, -P_1, -Le^a and/or -Le^b.[45,46]

3. Estimate the likelihood of finding compatible blood in available inventory and, if necessary because of the frequency distribution of the antigens, request assistance from the blood supplier or Rare Donor File.

If multiple antibodies or an antibody reacting with a high-incidence antigen is present, or if the antibody is present in very low concentration, it may not be possible to identify the antibody(ies) with available resources. If time permits, a sample can be sent to a reference laboratory for additional work. If the only antibody present reacts with a high-incidence antigen, siblings are the most promising source of compatible blood.

Alloantibody, Positive Autologous Control

An alloantibody may cause a positive reaction with autologous control cells in patients who have received blood or components within the preceding 2-3 months.

1. Alloantibody in the patient's serum may be reacting with transfused donor cells. Mixed-field agglutination is usually noted because only those cells positive for the antigen react with the antibody. These results are often found in patients experiencing delayed hemolytic transfusion reactions where antibody directed against the donor cells may be present in such low concentration that it is demonstrable only in an eluate prepared from the antigen-positive rbcs. See Methods Section 5. It is often necessary to use sensitive enhancement techniques to demonstrate antibody in the eluate or serum.

   Alloantibody reacting with circulating donor cells can be easily misinterpreted as autoantibody. It is important to differentiate the two because selection of blood for transfusion differs in the two situations. In most circumstances it is not necessary to attempt to find donor blood compatible with an autoantibody. In contrast, with alloantibodies it is important to identify the specificity and, if clinically significant, to transfuse blood that lacks the corresponding antigen. The patient's diagnosis and transfusion history may help in making the distinction, as well as the specificity of the antibody. If anti-Fy^a is eluted from the rbcs, for example, it would be most unlikely to be autoantibody. An antibody with apparent e specificity, however, might be either alloantibody or autoantibody.

2. There may have been alloantibody present in transfused plasma or injected plasma derivatives that may be reacting with the recipient's cells. Depending on the concentration of the antibody and its clinical significance, one might choose to give antigen-negative rbcs. If antibody is present in the serum, the antibody screen and crossmatches will probably be positive, and antigen-negative blood would be selected until the antibody is no longer demonstrable.

Cold-Reactive Autoantibodies

Potent cold-reactive autoantibodies may cause problems with ABO and Rh grouping, antibody detection, antibody identification and/or crossmatching. The most common specificity for autoantibody is anti-I, but transfusion of i_{adult} blood is unnecessary. The most important considerations are accurate determination of the patient's ABO and Rh types and determination of whether any alloantibodies are present. A detailed discussion of this problem is found in Chapter 16. Briefly,

1. Obtain rbcs free of autoantibody by collecting and maintaining the sample at 37 C until the serum and cells are separated. Wash the cells several times with warm saline. The saline-suspended cells should not agglutinate after centrifugation. If agglutination persists, washing with warm saline may not adequately remove the cold-reactive antibody. Treatment with dithiothreitol[47] (DTT) will disperse the cells. See Method 2.13. Use either washed or DTT-treated rbcs with controls for blood typing tests.

2. Obtain serum from a sample that has been allowed to clot at room temperature or in the refrigerator. Some of the autoantibody will be autoadsorbed from the serum.

3. Perform antibody detection and crossmatching tests strictly at 37 C using a prewarmed technique. See Method 3.2. Using an anti-IgG reagent for the antiglobulin test avoids detecting complement activated by cold-reactive antibody.

4. Perform autoadsorption techniques, if needed. This is unnecessary in most cases because using prewarmed testing and/or anti-IgG reagents eliminates most problems. Autoadsorption should not generally be performed in recently transfused patients, as circulating transfused rbcs may adsorb alloantibodies.

Warm-Reactive Autoantibodies

Warm-reactive autoantibodies rarely cause discrepancies in ABO grouping tests, but commonly do so in Rh tests if the reagent anti-D contains appreciable macromolecular additives. Using an anti-D reagent that contains a minimal amount of potentiator (eg, chemically modified anti-D) will give valid results in most cases; appropriate control tests must be performed concurrently. See Chapter 11. If autoantibody is present in the serum, antibody screening tests will be positive and crossmatches incompatible. See Chapter 16 for a complete discussion. To select blood for a patient with warm-reactive autoantibodies, test the serum, autoadsorbed if necessary, for the presence of alloantibodies with screening cells and donor's rbcs.

Rouleaux Formation

Rouleaux formation is a property of serum that causes all cells tested to appear agglutinated at room temperature and at 37 C. Because serum is removed by washing, rouleaux formation does not usually affect the antiglobulin test.

Classically, the flat surfaces of cells adhere to each other, giving "coin-like" stacks that are easily recognized. Rouleaux formation is most difficult to identify when the cells adhere in irregular clumps that resemble agglutination. To disperse rouleaux, add 1-3 drops of saline to the tube. Rouleaux formation tends to disperse, but antibody-mediated agglutination remains. See Method 3.3.

Reagent-Related Problems

Antibodies to a variety of drugs and additives can cause positive results in antibody screening and/or compatibility tests. When all the reagent rbcs are incompatible and all the donor rbcs are compatible, an antibody reactive with a substance in the rbc preservative solution should be suspected. In some cases the reagent rbcs will not react if they are washed with normal saline before testing, and testing can be completed with this minor modification.[48] Since preservative solutions vary from manufacturer to manufacturer, it may be helpful to use cells from another manufacturer if washing does not solve the problem.

If there is uniform agglutination of all rbcs, including the autologous rbcs, only in LISS tests (either additive or LISS-suspended rbc procedures), consider a LISS-potentiated autoantibody. LISS-additive reagents potentiate the reactivity of anti-I and anti-IH, while LISS-suspended rbcs enhance anti-Pr agglutinins. Use of anti-IgG, rather than a polyspecific antihuman globulin, is necessary when these unwanted reactions persist at the antiglobulin phase. Alternatively, saline-based procedures are less prone to yield unwanted reactions than LISS tests and can be used for antibody detection and crossmatching. A 20- to 30-minute incubation at 37 C is recommended for saline tests.

Some workers have observed anti-Jk^a-like reactivity in sera when using LISS containing methyl and propyl parabens as preservatives. These paraben-associated antibodies should be suspected when enzyme procedures used in antibody identification, which normally potentiate anti-Jk^a, are nonreactive. Another clue is a reactive LISS autologous control test in the absence of a positive

DAT, and the finding that the autologous rbcs are Jk(a+). Consultation with the reagent manufacturer is necessary to confirm the presence of parabens in the LISS reagent. Definitive studies include the preparation and use of LISS with and without parabens. See Method 3.1.3. Detection of anti-Jk[a]-like reactivity only with LISS + paraben provides conclusive evidence of this phenomenon.[49]

An antibody to thimerosal, which is used as a preservative in other LISS reagents, has also been described.[50] All crossmatches and tests with reagent rbcs and autologous cells will be positive. Using a procedure that does not include thimerosal will circumvent the problem. See the review by Pierce[48] for more information on reagent additives that cause anomalous serologic reactions.

Negative Antibody Screen, Incompatible Crossmatch

Some positive reactions occurring in the crossmatch but not in the antibody screen may be due to antibodies to antigens not present on the reagent rbcs used in the screening tests.[11] Alternatively, the donor rbcs may be coated with immunoglobulin, complement components or both. Depending on the phase of testing in which the incompatibility is detected, it may be necessary to do one or more of the following tests:

1. Repeat ABO grouping tests on the donor's sample.
2. Perform a DAT on the donor's rbcs.
3. Test the patient's serum with a panel of reagent rbcs or other selected rbcs exhibiting low-incidence antigens.

Crossmatch(es) Incompatible at Room Temperature

In the following situations the antibody screen may be negative but one (or more) of the crossmatches is (are) incompatible at room temperature:

1. Donor rbcs are ABO incompatible: In this situation the first thing to do is confirm the donor's ABO group. Labeling errors are more likely to cause this problem than technical errors. Most ABO antibodies present in a recipient's serum react strongly at room temperature and also at 37 C or in the antiglobulin test with most mislabeled A, B or AB rbcs. Rarely, a unit of blood from a donor whose rbcs have a weak expression of A or B antigens (eg, A_x) are incorrectly labeled as group O. In this case, the crossmatch with group O serum may be weakly incompatible only at the antiglobulin phase.

2. Anti-A_1 in the serum of A_2 or A_2B individuals: If room temperature testing is done, anti-A_1 will occasionally be encountered. Some, but not all, group A donor units may be incompatible. If the antibody reacts only at room temperature, it is not considered clinically significant; if it is reactive at 37 C, crossmatch-compatible blood should be given.[51]

3. Other alloantibodies reactive at room temperature: If the antibody detection protocol does not include a room temperature phase, antibodies such as anti-M may first be detected by a room temperature crossmatch. Performing tests with a reagent rbc panel at room temperature may facilitate identification of the antibody causing the incompatible crossmatch.

4. Polyagglutinable rbcs: All normal adult sera contain varying levels of naturally occurring antibodies (anti-T, -Tn, -Tk, -Cad, etc) that react with rbcs with abnormal surface structures, rendering them polyagglutinable. These antibodies are rarely a problem because most rbcs do not manifest the corresponding antigens.

Polyagglutinable cells, however, react with these antibodies either because they have acquired antigenic reactivity (T, Tn, Tk) or, more rarely, because the donor has inherited an unusual antigen (Cad).

Polyagglutinable donor rbcs may first be detected in the crossmatch. The problem might appear to result from an antibody to a low-incidence antigen because the recipient's serum is nonreactive with antibody screening cells, panel cells and all other donors' rbcs. The antibodies that recognize polyagglutinable rbcs are direct agglutinins that react best at room temperature so it is most common to see reactivity in the immediate-spin or room temperature phase of the crossmatch. Rabbit sera contain anti-T, anti-Tn, etc,[52] so these altered rbcs may react with antiglobulin reagents and the crossmatch may be incompatible at the antiglobulin phase.

Polyagglutinability often results from the action of bacterial enzymes. Cells from a healthy donor virtually never have this form of activation in vivo. Tn and Cad forms of polyagglutinability occur as often among donors as among patients, but are also very rare.

See Method 2.12 for a description of a procedure to recognize polyagglutinable rbcs. For more information the reader should see Beck and Judd.[53]

Crossmatch(es) Incompatible at the Antiglobulin Phase

If an antiglobulin test is part of the crossmatch procedure, some of the following situations may be encountered.

1. Donor rbcs have a positive DAT: Acceptable donors occasionally have rbcs that are coated with IgG and/or complement and cause incompatibility in the antiglobulin phase of the crossmatch. These units are not iden-

tified during processing since a DAT is not performed routinely. The problem can be quickly and easily identified by performing a DAT on the cells. The significance of a positive DAT in a normal donor is unknown. However, since the unit will be incompatible with the serum of all recipients, it should be returned to the donor center that supplied it.

2. Antibody reactive only with cells having strong expression of a particular antigen: A random donor's rbcs may have stronger expression of a particular antigen than do the screening cells, either because of dosage (eg, Rh, Kidd, Duffy antigens) or because of intrinsic variation in antigen strength (eg, P_1). If the patient's serum contains an antibody that reacts only with cells having strong expression of the antigen, the crossmatch may be positive and the antibody screen may be negative. The antibody can usually be identified by testing a full panel of rbcs since some of the panel cells are likely to have a double dose of the antigen in question. It may be necessary, however, to use a more sensitive technique for identification.

3. Antibody reactive with low-incidence antigen: Antibodies to some of the low-incidence antigens are relatively common. Anti-Wr^a, for example, may be present in as many as 1% of sera.[54] Low-incidence antigens may be present, unsuspected and unidentified, on either antibody detection cells or donor cells, causing unexpected positive reactions with sera containing these antibodies.

Positive Antibody Screen, Compatible Crossmatches

If all reagent rbcs are positive but many or all of the crossmatches are compatible, antibodies of one of the following specificities may be responsible:

Auto-Anti-H (-IH)

Group O cells have large amounts of H antigen; A_1 and A_1B cells have very little H. Serum containing auto-anti-H will agglutinate all group O reagent rbcs, but will not agglutinate A_1 and A_1B donor cells. Since A_2 cells have substantial amounts of H, a crossmatch with A_2 cells may be incompatible. Auto-anti-H found in A_1, A_1B and B sera is usually reactive only at room temperature and is not clinically significant. Most examples of apparent auto-anti-H can be shown actually to be -IH if group O cord blood rbcs or group O i_{adult} rbcs are available. Such antibodies are thought to recognize a product determined by both *H* and *I* genes. The same approach outlined above is required when selecting blood for transfusion to patients with auto-anti-IH.

Anti-Le^bH

This antibody reacts with Le(a–b+) rbcs that are group O, but not with A_1 or A_1B cells that are Le(a–b+). It is most often made by group A_1 or A_1B Le(a–b–) individuals. Anti-Le^bH is often reactive at room temperature but may be detected in the antiglobulin phase if the antihuman serum contains anticomplement reactivity. Compatible blood for transfusion can be found by screening random group A (or AB) units with the patient's serum. There is no need to type A_1 or A_1B units for Le^b.

Massive Transfusion

Massive transfusion is defined as infusion of a volume of blood approaching or exceeding replacement of the recipient's total blood volume within a 24-hour pe-

riod. This may occur unexpectedly in surgical and medical emergencies and/or in planned circumstances such as cardiac, vascular or liver surgery. Exchange transfusion of an infant is also a massive transfusion.

Following massive transfusion, there is such a small volume of the patient's blood left that complete crossmatching has limited benefit. The pretransfusion sample no longer represents currently circulating transfused blood and sensitive antiglobulin testing on the current specimen accomplishes virtually nothing.[55] It is only important to confirm ABO compatibility of subsequently transfused blood. Abbreviating the crossmatch is acceptable following massive transfusion, even when unexpected alloantibody is present in the patient's pretransfusion sample, provided that the donor blood is shown by testing with blood grouping reagents to lack the corresponding antigens. The procedures used in these situations should be selected by the blood bank director, should be in writing and should be followed consistently by all laboratory personnel.

Labeling and Release of Crossmatched Blood

A blood transfusion form indicating the recipient's name, identification number and ABO and Rh types must be completed for each unit of donor blood or component.[1] The form must also include:

1. Donor identification number.
2. Donor ABO and Rh types.
3. Interpretation of compatibility testing.
4. Identification of the person performing the tests.
5. The current status of serologic testing when blood must be issued before compatibility problems are resolved.

Before issuing a unit of blood, blood bank personnel must:

1. Securely attach to the unit of blood a label or tag that contains:
   a. The recipient's first and last names and identification number.
   b. The donor blood number assigned by the transfusing or collecting facility.
   c. An interpretation of the compatibility tests.
   d. Identification of the person performing the test.
2. Check the expiration date of the blood to avoid issuing an outdated component.
3. Inspect the unit to make certain it does not have abnormal color or appearance.
4. Indicate on an appropriate form the:
   a. Name of the individual issuing blood.
   b. Date and time blood was issued.
   c. Person to whom blood was issued or destination of unit.

Final identification of the recipient and the blood container rests with the transfusionist, who must identify the patient and donor unit and certify that identifying forms, tags and labels are in agreement. See p 418-19.

Release of Blood in Urgent Situations

When there is a desperate requirement for blood, the patient's physician must weigh the hazard of transfusing uncrossmatched or partially crossmatched blood against the risk of waiting while testing is completed. When blood is released before the crossmatch is completed, the records must contain a statement of the requesting physician indicating that the clinical situation was sufficiently urgent to require release of blood.[1] Such a statement does not absolve blood bank personnel from their responsibility to issue properly labeled donor blood of an ABO group compatible with the patient. When urgent release is requested:

1. Issue uncrossmatched blood and immediately begin compatibility testing procedures. Blood released should be:
   a. Group O rbcs if the patient's ABO group is unknown. It is preferable to give D– blood if the patient's Rh group is unknown, especially if the patient is female with the potential to bear children.
   b. ABO- and Rh-type compatible, if there has been time to perform ABO and D testing on the patient's current blood specimen. Previous records must not be used to determine which blood group to issue, nor may the patient's blood group be taken from other records such as cards, dog tags or driver's license.
2. Indicate in a conspicuous fashion on the attached tag or label that compatibility testing had not been completed at the time of issue.
3. Complete crossmatches promptly. If incompatibility is detected at any stage of testing, immediately notify the patient's physician and blood bank physician.

If the patient dies from a medical problem unrelated to the blood transfusion, it is not necessary to complete compatibility tests that may be pending. This decision rests with the physician responsible for the transfusion service. If there is any reason to suspect that transfusion aggravated the original problem or contributed to death, all testing should be completed.

Routine Surgical Blood Orders

Blood ordering levels for common elective procedures can be developed from previous records of blood use. For each of the procedures, the transfusion service can crossmatch the agreed-upon routine number of blood units.[11,56]

Since surgical requirements vary among institutions, the routine blood orders should be based on local transfusion utilization patterns.[1] The blood bank medical director, staff surgeons and anesthesiologists should agree on routine ordering levels, but there should be a way to modify the routine orders for patients with anemia, bleeding disorders or other conditions in which increased blood use is anticipated.[1] As with other circumstances that require rapid provision of blood, the transfusion service staff must be prepared to provide additional blood if an unexpected problem requires blood use greater than the routine level. Routine blood order schedules are successful only when there is cooperation and confidence among the professionals involved in setting and using the guidelines.

References

1. Widmann FK, ed. Standards for blood banks and transfusion services. 15th ed. Bethesda, MD: American Association of Blood Banks, 1993.
2. Honig CL, Bove JR. Transfusion-associated fatalities: Review of Bureau of Biologics reports 1976-1978. Transfusion 1980;20:653-61.
3. Schmidt PJ. The mortality from incompatible transfusion. In: Sandler SG, Nusbacher J, Schanfield MS, eds. Immunobiology of the erythrocyte. New York: Alan R Liss, 1980:251-61.
4. Taswell HF, Pineda AA, Moore SB. Hemolytic transfusion reactions—frequency and clinical and laboratory aspects. In: Bell CA, ed. A seminar on immune-mediated cell destruction. Washington, DC: American Association of Blood Banks, 1981:71-92.
5. Baldwin ML, Barrasso C, Ness PM, Garratty G. A clinically significant erythrocyte antibody detectable only by ^{51}Cr survival studies. Transfusion 1983;23:40-4.
6. Issitt PD. Serology and genetics of the Rhesus blood group system. Cincinnati: Montgomery Scientific Publications, 1979:34.
7. Code of federal regulations. Title 21, part 660, subpart D660.30-36. Washington, DC: US Government Printing Office, 1991. (Revised annually.)
8. Shulman IA, Nelson JM, Okamato M, Malone SA. Dependence of anti-Jk[a] detection on screening cell zygosity. Laboratory Medicine 1985;16:602-4.
9. Ellisor SS. The selection of reagent rbcs and antibody potentiating reagents. In: Considerations in the selection of reagents. Washington, DC: American Association of Blood Banks, 1979:83-91.
10. Oberman HA, Barnes BA, Steiner EA. Role of the crossmatch in testing for serologic incompatibility. Transfusion 1982;22:12-6.
11. Mintz PD, Haines AL, Sullivan MF. Incompatible crossmatch following nonreactive antibody detection test: Frequency and cause. Transfusion 1982;22:107-10.
12. Mintz PD, Nordine RB, Henry JB, Webb WR. Expected hemotherapy in elective surgery. NYS J Med 1976;76:532-7.
13. Boral LI, Henry JB. The type and screen: A safe alternative and supplement in selected surgical procedures. Transfusion 1977;17:163-8.
14. Judd WJ, Barnes BA, Steiner EA, et al. The evaluation of a positive direct antiglobulin test (autocontrol) in pretransfusion testing revisited. Transfusion 1986;26:220-4.
15. Pollack W, Ascari WQ, Crispen JF, et al. Studies on Rh prophylaxis II: Rh immune prophylaxis after transfusion with Rh-positive blood. Transfusion 1971;11:340-4.
16. Barnes A Jr, Allen TE. Transfusions subsequent to administration of universal donor blood in Viet Nam. JAMA 1968;204:695-7.
17. Mougey R. Red cell separation methods and their applications. In: Myers M, Reynolds A, eds. Micromethods in blood group serology. Arlington, VA: American Association of Blood Banks, 1984:19-35.
18. Beattie KM. Control of the antigen-antibody ratio in antibody detection/compatibility tests. Transfusion 1980;20:277-84.
19. Diamond LK, Denton RL. Rh agglutination in various media with particular reference to the value of albumin. J Lab Clin Med 1945;30:821-30.
20. Cameron JW, Diamond LK. Chemical, clinical and immunological studies on the products of human plasma fractionation. XXIX. Serum albumin as a diluent for Rh typing reagents. J Clin Invest 1945;24:793-801.
21. Case J. The albumin layering method for D typing. Vox Sang 1959;4:403-5.

22. Case J. Potentiators of agglutination. In: Bell CA, ed. Seminar on antigen-antibody reactions revisited. Arlington, VA: American Association of Blood Banks, 1982:99-132.

23. Jones JM, Kekwick RA, Goldsmith KLG. Influence of polymers on the efficacy of serum albumin as a potentiator of "incomplete" Rh agglutinins. Nature 1969;224:510-1.

24. Reckel RP, Harris J. The unique characteristics of covalently polymerized bovine serum albumin solutions when used as antibody detection media. Transfusion 1978;18:397-406.

25. Stroup M, MacIlroy M. Evaluation of the albumin antiglobulin technic in antibody detection. Transfusion 1965;5:184-91.

26. Griffitts JJ, Frank S, Schmidt P. The influence of albumin in the antiglobulin crossmatch. Transfusion 1964;4:461-8.

27. Leikola J, Perkins HA. Red cell antibodies and low ionic strength: a study with enzyme-linked antiglobulin test. Transfusion 1980;20:224-8.

28. Steane EA. Red blood cell agglutination: A current perspective. In: Bell CA, ed. Seminar on antigen-antibody reactions revisited. Arlington, VA: American Association of Blood Banks, 1982:67-98.

29. Elliot M, Bossom E, Dupuy ME, Masouredis SP. Effect of ionic strength on the serologic behavior of red cell isoantibodies. Vox Sang 1964;9:396-414.

30. Hughes-Jones NC, Polley MJ, Telford R, et al. Optimal conditions for detecting blood group antibodies by the antiglobulin test. Vox Sang 1964;9:385-95.

31. Low B, Messeter L. Antiglobulin tests in low-ionic strength salt solutions for rapid antibody screening and cross-matching. Vox Sang 1974;26:53-61.

32. Moore HC, Mollison PL. Use of a low-ionic-strength medium in manual tests for antibody detection. Transfusion 1976;16:291-6.

33. Fitzsimmons JM, Morel PA. The effects of red blood cell suspending media on hemagglutination and the antiglobulin test. Transfusion 1979;19:81-5.

34. Nance SJ, Garratty G. A new potentiator of red blood cell antigen-antibody reactions. Am J Clin Pathol 1987;87:633-5.

35. Wenz B, Apuzzo J. Polyethylene glycol improves the indirect antiglobulin test. Transfusion 1989;29:218-20.

36. Wenz B, Apuzzo J. Evaluation of the polyethylene glycol-potentiated indirect antiglobulin test. Transfusion 1990;30:318-21.

37. Howard JE, Winn LC, Gottlieb CE, et al. Clinical significance of the anti-complement component of antiglobulin antisera. Transfusion 1982;22:269-72.

38. Wright MS, Issitt PD. Anticomplement and the indirect antiglobulin test. Transfusion 1979;19:688-94.

39. Morton JA, Pickles MM. Use of trypsin in detection of anti-Rh antibodies. Nature 1947;159:779-80.

40. Ellisor SE. Action and applications of enzymes in immunohematology. In: Bell CA, ed. Seminar on antigen-antibody reactions revisited. Arlington, VA: American Association of Blood Banks, 1982:133-74.

41. Lalezari P, Jiang AF. The manual Polybrene® test: A simple and rapid procedure for detection of red cell antibodies. Transfusion 1980; 20:206-11.

42. Rosenfield RE, Shaikh SH, Innella F, et al. Augmentation of hemagglutination by low ionic conditions. Transfusion 1979;19:499-510.

43. Trudeau LR, Judd WJ, Butch SH, Oberman HA. Is a room-temperature crossmatch necessary for the detection of ABO errors? Transfusion 1983;23:237-9.

44. Grindon AJ. The decision to transfuse: Role of the immunohematology laboratory. Laboratory Medicine 1982;13:270-1.

45. Cronin CA, Pohl BA, Miller WV. Crossmatch compatible blood for patients with anti-P1. Transfusion 1978;18:728-30.

46. Waheed A, Kennedy MS, Gerhan S, Senhauser DA. Transfusion significance of Lewis system antibodies: Success in transfusion with crossmatch-compatible blood. Am J Clin Pathol 1981;76:294-8.

47. Reid ME. Autoagglutination dispersal utilizing sulphydryl compounds. Transfusion 1978; 18:353-5.

48. Pierce SR. Anomalous blood bank results. In: Dawson RB, ed. Trouble-shooting the crossmatch. Washington, DC: American Association of Blood Banks, 1976:85-114.

49. Judd WJ, Steiner EA, Cochran RK. Paraben-associated autoanti-Jkᵃ antibodies: Three examples detected using commercially prepared low-ionic-strength saline containing parabens. Transfusion 1982;22:31-5.

50. Shulman IA, Hasz LA, Simpson RB. Thimerosal dependent agglutination, a newly described blood bank problem. Transfusion 1982;22:241-3.

51. Mollison PL, Engelfriet CP, Contreras M, eds. Blood transfusion in clinical medicine, 9th ed. Oxford: Blackwell Scientific Publications, 1993:170-1.

52. Beck ML, Hicklin B, Pierce SR. Unexpected limitations in the use of commercial antiglobulin reagents. Transfusion 1976;16:71-5.

53. Beck ML, Judd WJ, eds. Polyagglutination. Washington, DC: American Association of Blood Banks, 1980.

54. Dunsford I. The Wright blood group system. Vox Sang 1954;4(OS):160-3.
55. Oberman HA, Barnes BA, Friedman BA. The risk of abbreviating the major crossmatch in urgent or massive transfusion. Transfusion 1978;18:137-41.
56. Friedman BA, Oberman HA, Chadwick AR, Kingdon KI. The maximum surgical blood order schedule and surgical blood use in the United States. Transfusion 1976;16:380-7.

15

Identification of Unexpected Alloantibodies

In contrast to *auto*antibodies (see Chapter 16), *allo*antibodies do not react with antigens present on the rbcs of the antibody producer. *Unexpected* alloantibodies are antibodies other than naturally occurring anti-A or -B. Such antibodies may be found in some 0.3-38% of the population, depending upon the selected group of patients or donors studied and the sensitivity of the test methods.[1,2] Immunization to "foreign" rbc antigens may result from pregnancy or transfusion, or following injection with immunogenic material. In some instances the immunizing event is unknown.

Once an unexpected antibody is detected, its specificity should be determined and its clinical significance assessed. A clinically significant antibody is one that shortens the anticipated survival of transfused rbcs or has been associated with hemolytic disease of the newborn (HDN). The degree of clinical significance varies, however. Some antibodies cause destruction of incompatible rbcs within a few hours or even minutes, while others decrease the anticipated survival by only a few days. Thus, documented experience with other examples of the same antibody specificity can be used in assessing the relative clinical significance of an antibody (see Table 12-1 for information on the significance of commonly encountered alloantibodies). Unfortunately, for some antibodies there are little or no data and decisions must be based on the premise that clinically significant antibodies are usually those active at 37 C and/or by the indirect antiglobulin test (IAT). That is not to say, however, that all antibodies active in vitro at 37 C and/or by the IAT are clinically significant.

Determining the specificity of antibodies encountered in pretransfusion testing is important in assessing the need to select antigen-negative blood for transfusion. Patients with clinically significant antibodies should, whenever practical, receive blood that has been found to lack the corresponding antigen using potent blood grouping reagents. In prenatal testing, knowing the specificity and immunoglobulin class of an antibody helps predict the likelihood of HDN. While it is not crucial to identify unexpected antibodies in donor blood, such testing is often done for the procurement of blood grouping reagents or teaching samples.

General Procedures

Blood Samples

An adequate quantity of test serum and rbcs is essential to the resolution of any serologic problem. As a source of serum, 10 mL of clotted blood is usually sufficient for identifying simple antibody

333

specificities. More serum may be required if multiple antibodies are present. An EDTA-anticoagulated blood sample is preferred for studies of autologous rbcs, to avoid problems associated with the in-vitro uptake of complement components by rbcs that may occur when clotted blood samples are used (see Chapters 8 and 16). NOTE: Throughout this chapter "serum" is used; however, either serum or plasma may be used in antibody identification tests (see Chapter 14).

Medical History

It is useful to know a patient's clinical diagnosis, number of pregnancies, transfusion history and recent drug therapy. A recent transfusion may necessitate the use of procedures such as reticulocyte enrichment to determine the blood type of the autologous rbcs (see Method 2.17). The known presence of autoantibodies, which are often associated with diseases of the lymphoreticular system or induced by drugs, will dictate the use of other procedures discussed in Chapter 16.

Methods

It is appropriate to test the serum under investigation at all test phases at which antibody activity was initially detected. However, additional antibodies may become apparent at different test phases, and the reactivity of some antibodies may be increased by extending incubation periods, increasing the serum-rbc ratio, lowering temperatures or by using enzyme or other enhancement techniques. (See Methods for Antibody Detection and Compatibility Testing, Section 3.)

There are considerable advantages in using enzyme techniques in antibody identification studies. The reactivities of some antibodies, such as Rh antibodies and complement-binding examples of anti-Le^a and anti-Jk^a, are enhanced in enzyme tests. In contrast, enzyme treatment denatures some blood group antigens, especially M, N, S, Fy^a and Fy^b.[3] Hemolysis, enhanced reactivity or loss of reactivity in enzyme tests are useful clues in antibody identification.

Reagent Red Cells

The serum under investigation should be tested by the desired techniques with a panel of eight or more group O reagent rbc samples of known blood group phenotype. Such panels may be obtained from commercial sources or may be made using rbcs from the local donor population. A list is provided with each commercially prepared panel that shows, in moderate detail, the phenotype of each rbc sample. To be functional, a reagent rbc panel must make it possible to identify with confidence those clinically significant alloantibodies that are most frequently encountered such as anti-D, -E, -K and -Fy^a. When a serum contains only one of these antibodies, the reagent rbc phenotypes should be such that the presence of most other common alloantibodies can be at least tentatively excluded. A distinct pattern of reactivity should be apparent for most examples of single alloantibodies; eg, all of the K+ samples should not be the only ones that are also E+. Further, so that chance alone can be excluded as the cause of an apparently definitive pattern, there must be sufficient rbc samples that lack, and sufficient rbc samples that carry, most of the antigens listed in Table 15-1.

Autocontrol

It is important to know how the serum under investigation reacts with the autologous rbcs. This helps determine whether alloantibody, autoantibody or

Table 15-1. A Reagent Red Cell Panel for Alloantibody Identification

Sample #	Rh Phenotype	C	Cw	c	D	E	e	K	Fya	Fyb	Jka	Jkb	P1	Lea	Leb	M	N	S	s
		Rhesus						**Kell**	**Duffy**		**Kidd**		**P**	**Lewis**		**MN**			
1	r'r	+	0	+	0	0	+	0	+	0	+	+	+	0	+	+	+	0	+
2	$R_1{}^w$	+	+	0	+	0	+	+	+	+	0	+	+	+	0	+	+	+	+
3	R_1	+	0	0	+	0	+	0	+	+	+	+	0	0	+	+	0	+	0
4	R_2	0	0	+	+	+	0	0	0	+	0	+	+	+	0	0	+	0	+
5	r"r	0	0	+	0	+	+	0	+	+	0	+	0	0	+	+	+	+	0
6	r	0	0	+	0	0	+	0	0	+	+	0	+	0	0	+	+	0	+
7	r	0	0	+	0	0	+	+	0	+	+	0	+	0	+	+	0	+	0
8	r	0	0	+	0	0	+	0	+	0	0	+	+	+	0	0	+	0	+
9	r	0	0	+	0	0	+	0	0	+	+	0	0	0	+	0	+	+	0
10	R_0	0	0	+	+	0	+	0	0	0	+	+	+	0	0	+	+	+	+

+ Denotes presence of antigen; 0 denotes absence of antigen.

both are present (see Table 15-2). Serum that reacts only with the reagent rbcs usually contains only alloantibody, whereas reactivity with both reagent and autologous rbcs suggests the presence of autoantibody, or autoantibody plus alloantibody. In a patient who is producing alloantibodies to antigens on recently transfused rbcs, the presence of donor rbcs coated with alloantibodies will result in a positive autocontrol, usually mixed field in hemagglutination tests. This may be misinterpreted as being due to autoantibody. A detailed history of recent transfusions should be obtained on all patients whose rbcs are coated with globulins in vivo (see Chapter 16).

The inclusion of an autocontrol in antibody identification studies, even if previously performed, is recommended. Repetition of this important test is not inappropriate, since it allows for concurrent comparison of reactions of the autologous and reagent rbcs.

The presence of a positive autocontrol may necessitate additional testing. Elution studies should be considered if the patient has been recently transfused, there is evidence of immune hemolysis and/or the results of serum studies prove inconclusive. For example, a weakly reactive alloantibody, reacting with most but not all Fy(a+) rbcs, may be present in the serum of a recently transfused patient whose rbcs manifest a positive autocontrol. In such an instance, it may be possible to confirm anti-Fy^a specificity by elution studies. Elution into a small fluid volume from a concentrated suspension of packed rbcs, in which each rbc is coated with a few antibody molecules, will often yield a potent eluate. In other instances, weak serum reactivity may be due to the presence of free autoantibody and a potent autoantibody will be revealed by elution.

Adsorption studies may be necessary to establish that autoantibodies are not masking the presence of coexisting alloantibodies. The need for such studies on transfusion candidates cannot be overemphasized (see Chapter 16). Proce-

Table 15-2. Patterns of Serum Reactivity

Reagent Red Cells	Autologous Red Cells	Interpretation
+	0	alloantibody
0	+	autoantibody*
+	+	autoantibody* or autoantibody* and alloantibody

*Alloantibodies in recently transfused patients may mimic autoantibodies.

dures for the detection of alloantibodies in the presence of cold-reactive autoantibodies include:

1. Prewarmed techniques, in which reagent rbcs and test serum are incubated at 37 C before they are mixed.
2. The use of anti-IgG rather than polyspecific antiglobulin serum (see p 176-8). This prevents the detection of complement components bound to reagent rbcs by cold-reactive autoantibodies and permits recognition of the vast majority of IgG alloantibodies.
3. Cold autoadsorption, using autologous rbcs at cold temperature to remove autoantibodies but not alloantibodies.
4. Heterologous adsorption with rabbit rbcs, to remove cold-reactive autoantibodies but not alloantibodies.

The first, second and fourth procedures are applicable when the patient has been recently transfused. Autoadsorption in these patients is inappropriate as the circulating transfused rbcs may be capable of adsorbing clinically significant serum alloantibodies. Procedures for the detection of concomitant alloantibodies in the presence of warm-reactive autoantibodies are discussed in detail on p 369-70 and in Methods 6.4 and 6.6.

Considerations in Interpreting Serologic Results

Alloantibodies of some blood group specificities often display consistent serologic characteristics (see Tables 10-5 and 12-1). In interpreting the results of serum studies, it is important to look for these characteristics, and to examine the phenotypes of both reactive and nonreactive rbc samples. The following should be considered:

1. What are the effects of temperature, suspending medium or proteolytic enzymes on the reaction with a particular rbc sample?
2. Is there any variation in the strength of agglutination observed among reactive rbc samples?
3. Is hemolysis present?
4. Are the autologous rbcs reactive or nonreactive?

The general serologic characteristics of blood group antibodies are given in Chapters 10, 11 and 12. With these data, and the results of tests against a reagent rbc panel, it is usually possible to identify an antibody, or to select additional reagent rbcs or procedures that can be used for conclusive identification. Table 15-3 includes an approach that may be used to interpret the results of alloantibody identification tests, and to select additional tests that are required for confirmation. These and other considerations are discussed more fully in the following sections.

Single Alloantibodies

It is usually easy to recognize the specificity of a single alloantibody that yields clear-cut positive and negative reactions with reagent rbc samples. For example, if a serum reacts with samples 4 and 5 of the reagent rbc panel shown in Table 15-1, anti-E is very likely to be present. Both reactive samples are E+ and all negative samples are E–. The reactions should be observed at a test phase that is characteristic of Rh antibodies. Antibodies that should react with antigens present on the E– samples can be excluded from consideration. For example, anti-K, if present, would react with samples 2 and 7. The presence of anti-E does not appear to mask the presence of other antibodies. Providing the autologous rbcs are E–, the identification of alloanti-E in this instance can be estab-

Table 15-3. A Sequential Approach to Resolving Alloantibody Problems

Autocontrol	Evaluate reactions of autocontrol. If negative, the presence of autoantibodies is excluded. If positive, consider autoantibodies and/or alloantibodies made in response to a previous, recent transfusion.
Reagent rbcs	Eliminate from initial consideration antibodies to antigens present on nonreactive samples.
Autologous rbcs	Eliminate from consideration antibodies to antigens present on autologous rbcs.
Enzyme-treated rbcs	Examine phenotypes (eg, S, Fy^a) of samples that react with untreated, but are nonreactive (or weaker) with enzyme-treated, rbcs. Eliminate from consideration antibodies (eg, anti-Rh) that, if present, should have reacted with antigens present on nonreactive enzyme-treated samples.
Reaction pattern	Examine reaction patterns at each test phase; keep in mind possible specificities involved; consider possible specificities relative to test phase and manner of reactivity (eg, direct agglutination with anti-P$_1$, hemolysis at 37 C with anti-Le^a, nonreactivity of anti-Fy^a with enzyme-treated rbcs).
Additional tests	Test sufficient red cell samples of appropriate phenotypes to obtain a p (probability) value less than 0.05 for each suspected antibody. Test serum against rbcs carrying a double-dose of antigens to which the serum may contain antibodies, if such rbcs were not among previously nonreactive samples.
	Test autologous rbcs with additional antisera (if necessary) to show absence of all antigens to which the serum contains antibodies.

lished using a single panel of reagent rbcs. Identification of single antibodies may not always be this simple. Some important considerations in antibody identification studies involving single antibodies are discussed below.

Reactions at an Unexpected Test Phase

An antibody may react in an unexpected manner. For example, most anti-S antibodies react only by the IAT. However, some directly agglutinate saline-suspended rbcs. While the test phase at which a serum reacts is suggestive of specificity, it is important to remember that exceptional examples will be encountered.

Variations in Antigen Expression

The reaction strengths of some antibodies vary from one rbc sample to another. This may be due to the phenomenon known as dosage, in which antibodies react preferentially with rbcs from homozygotes carrying a double dose of the antigen. Rbcs from individuals heterozygous for a gene may carry a single dose of antigen and may react weakly or be nonreactive. Many alloantibodies manifest dosage. This phenomenon is often found with antibodies in the Duffy, MN and Kidd systems. Some antigens (eg, I, P_1, Le^a and Sd^a) are expressed to varying degrees on rbcs from different adult donors. This expression is unrelated to zygosity; however, the antigenic differences can be demonstrated serologically.

Other antibodies, including those to I, Le^a, Le^b, Sd^a, Lu^a, Lu^b, Vel, Yt^a, Hy, McC^a, Yk^a, Cs^a, Ch and Rg antigens, react more weakly with cord rbcs than they do with rbcs from adults. Blood group antibodies may react less well with stored than with fresh rbcs. Some antigens deteriorate more rapidly than others and the rate of antigen deterioration varies among rbcs from different donors. The use of enhancement techniques often helps resolve problems associated with variations in antigen expression (see Methods 3.1.3, 3.1.4, 3.1.5 and 3.5.5).

No Discernible Specificity

In addition to variations in antigen expression, other factors may contribute to the difficulty in interpreting antibody identification test results. Antibodies such as anti-Bg that react with antigens on both leukocytes and rbcs often display nebulous reaction patterns that do not appear to fit any particular specificity. A rare cause is the incorrect grouping of reagent rbcs, resulting in a pattern of clear-cut reactive and nonreactive tests that cannot be interpreted.

In other instances a serum may react with an antigen not listed on the antigen profile supplied by the reagent manufacturer; Yt^b is one example. Even though serum studies yield clear-cut reactive and nonreactive tests, anti-Yt^b may not be suspected. In such circumstances it is often useful to ask the manufacturer for additional phenotype information. If the appropriate blood grouping reagent is available, reactive and nonreactive rbc samples, as well as the autologous rbcs, can be tested. These problems will often have to be referred to an immunohematology reference laboratory.

ABO Group of Test Red Cells

A serum may react with the majority or all of the group O reagent rbc samples, but not with rbcs of the same ABO phenotype as the autologous rbcs. This situation is seen most frequently with anti-H, -IH or -Le^{bH} antibodies. Group O and A_2 rbcs have large amounts of H antigen; A_1 and A_1B rbcs carry very little H (see Chapter 10). Serum containing anti-H or -IH will react strongly with group O reagent rbc samples, but autologous and donor group A_1 or A_1B rbcs may be weakly reactive or nonreactive. Similarly, anti-Le^{bH} reacts strongly with group O, Le(b+) rbcs, but may be nonreactive with Le(b+) rbcs from A_1 or A_1B individuals. In pretransfusion testing, such antibodies should be suspected when antibody detection studies using group O rbcs are strongly reactive, but serologically compatible A_1 or A_1B donor bloods can be obtained without difficulty.

Exclusion of Additional Antibodies

Although a serum displays a reaction pattern indicating a single antibody, it is important to remember that other antibodies may also be present. This should be a consideration even when the serum reacts uniformly with all rbc samples due to the presence of an antibody to a high-incidence antigen. In more routine situations it is easy to overlook additional antibodies, particularly if they are weakly reactive. Knowing the phenotype of the autologous rbcs may help predict the specificities of additional antibodies that might be present.

When necessary, tests with additional reagent rbcs (selected rbcs) should be performed. Such rbcs should be selected to enable the detection of antibodies to those antigens listed in Table 15-1. When practical, rbcs carrying a double dose of the relevant antigens are preferred. For example, if the serum of an S–s+, Fy(a–), Jk(a–), K– individual appears to contain anti-Jk^a, and Jk(a–) rbcs from S and Fy^a homozygotes were not among the samples initially tested, such rbcs should be used to exclude the presence of anti-S and anti-Fy^a. However, due to the rarity of k– rbcs, it may be impossible to exclude the presence of anti-K with Jk(a–), K+k– rbcs.

In the routine patient-care situation, it is not always necessary to exclude the presence of antibodies to antigens of relatively low incidence such as C^w, Kp^a and V. These antibodies are uncommon, and the corresponding antigens are present on the rbcs of less than 2% of the random population.

Special Considerations With Rh Antibodies

Some special considerations are necessary when certain Rh antibodies have been identified. If anti-E is identified in the serum of a transfusion candidate, the additional presence of anti-c should be considered. The Rh phenotype of the patient's rbcs should be determined. If they are of the R_1 phenotype (lacking c and E antigens), the anti-E will often be accompanied by anti-c.[4] Anti-c may be less reactive than the anti-E, and more sensitive methods such as enzyme techniques may be required to demonstrate its presence. Even when anti-c is not detectable, some workers select c–, E– blood for transfusion to R_1R_1 patients with anti-E, since anti-c is a common cause of delayed HTR. This practice is controversial. (See Chapter 11.)

The reverse situation causes less of a problem. If anti-c is identified, the additional presence of anti-E may not be determined unless rare R$_Z$R$_1$ rbcs are used. Note that Table 15-1 does not include such a sample, nor is it necessary to test all anti-c sera from transfusion candidates against R$_Z$R$_1$ rbcs. Failure to detect anti-E in the serum of an R_1 patient with anti-c does not pose a major transfusion hazard as almost all c-donor units also will be E–. Further, anti-E, if present, would be detected on the rare occasion that an R$_Z$R$_1$ donor unit might be selected for compatibility testing.

Phenotype of Autologous Red Cells

Once an alloantibody has been identified in a serum it is necessary to test the autologous rbcs for the corresponding antigen. This is an important confirmatory test. With rare exceptions, when an alloantibody is present in the serum, the corresponding antigen is absent on the autologous rbcs. For example, if the serum from an untransfused individual appears to contain anti-Fy^a but the autologous rbcs have a negative direct antiglobulin test (DAT) and type as Fy(a+), the data are clearly in conflict and further testing with additional reagent rbcs is necessary.

In recently transfused patients, the phenotype should be determined using a pretransfusion sample. Alternatively, the patient's own rbcs can be typed following separation from the transfused rbcs. Procedures for this are discussed in Methods 2.17 and 2.18. Even without separation, use of potent blood grouping reagents, appropriate controls and observing for mixed-field reactions can sometimes provide useful information.

Probability

For conclusive antibody identification, there must be sufficient reagent rbc samples tested that lack, and that carry, the antigen to which an antibody appears to display specificity. This is necessary to check that an observed pattern of reactivity is not due to chance alone. Table 15-4 shows the probabilities of various combinations of reactive and nonreactive tests, as calculated by Fisher's exact method for estimating probabilities. (See Method 4.1.)

The probability (p) values listed in Table 15-4 show the likelihood of a given set of results being due to chance alone. A p value of 0.05 means that an identical set of results would be obtained by chance once in 20 similar studies; the odds are 19 to 1 (95% probability) that the interpretation of the data is correct. For example, if a serum agglutinates three reagent rbc samples that are D+ and fails to agglutinate three that are D−, then p is 0.05; therefore, there is a 95% probability that the antibody is anti-D.

A p of 0.05 is the accepted minimum value at which an interpretation is considered statistically valid. Because of these statistical requirements in confirming antibody specificity, most reagent rbc panels are limited in their ability to provide conclusive identification of some blood group antibodies. For example, if a serum is tested against the panel of rbc samples shown in Table 15-1 and only sample 4 is nonreactive there is a 1 to 9 chance (p = 0.10) that the reactions are not due to anti-e. If, however, another e− sample was present in this panel and was also nonreactive, the p changes to 0.022. It is important to remember these unavoidable limitations when only a single panel of reagent rbcs is available for testing. It is often necessary to test additional rbc samples that lack moderately high-incidence antigens such as e, before conclusively assigning specificity to an antibody. Many workers use a standard approach of three posi-

Table 15-4. Probability Values

No. Tested	No. Positive	No. Negative	p
6	4	2	0.067
6	3	3	0.050
7	5	2	0.048
7	4	3	0.029
8	7	1	0.125
8	6	2	0.036
8	5	3	0.018
8	4	4	0.014
9	8	1	0.111
9	7	2	0.028
9	6	3	0.012
10	7	3	0.008
10	9	1	0.100
10	8	2	0.022
10	6	4	0.005
10	5	5	0.004

tives that react and three negatives that fail to react to meet this statistical requirement for each specificity identified.

Multiple Alloantibodies

When a serum contains two or more alloantibodies, it may be difficult to interpret the results of serum studies using a single panel of reagent rbcs. Multiple alloantibodies are usually present in one or more of the following ways:

1. The observed pattern of reactive and nonreactive tests does not fit that of a single antibody.
2. Reactions of variable strength are observed with rbc samples that cannot be explained on the basis of dosage.
3. Different rbc samples react at different test phases.
4. Unexpected reactions are obtained when attempts are made to confirm the specificity of a suspected single antibody. For example, if a serum suspected of containing anti-e is found to react with additional e− rbc

samples, it is possible that either another antibody is present or the suspected antibody is not really anti-e. In such a situation more e– rbc samples must be tested.

When multiple alloantibodies are present, an approach similar to that outlined in Table 15-3 can be used to determine the likely specificities involved, and to help decide what additional tests are necessary for conclusive identification. An example of how such an approach is applied is the following discussion of findings shown in Table 15-5. This case study concerns a serum containing anti-M, anti-Fy^a and anti-Jk^a. The resolution of this case is as follows:

1. *Evaluate reactions of autocontrol. If negative, the presence of autoantibodies is usually excluded. If positive, consider autoantibodies or alloantibodies made in response to a previous, recent transfusion.*

   The autocontrol is negative and autoantibodies are not considered. The antibodies present in the serum are most likely alloantibodies.

2. *Eliminate from initial consideration antibodies to antigens present on nonreactive reagent rbc samples.*

   Only sample 4 is nonreactive at all test phases. Thus, anti-c, -D, -E, -Fy^b,

-Jk^b, -P_1, -Le^a, -N and -s can all be provisionally excluded from consideration at this time. The findings with untreated rbcs may be due to a mixture of antibodies to a number of different antigens, including C, C^w, e, K, Fy^a, Jk^a, Le^b, M and S. Other specificities, not discernible from the rbc phenotypes provided, may also be present.

3. *Eliminate from consideration antibodies to antigens present on the autologous rbcs.*

   Alloantibodies, by definition, cannot usually be made against antigens present on the autologous rbcs. The phenotype of the autologous rbcs indicates that antibodies to c, D, e, P_1, Le^b, N and s antigens should not be present in the serum. There are, however, rare exceptions in which the corresponding antigen may be present in an altered form (eg, partial D with alloanti-D, see Chapter 11).

4. *Examine the phenotypes of rbc samples that react when untreated but are nonreactive (or weaker) with enzyme-treated rbcs.*

   The results of tests with enzyme-treated rbcs show that three additional samples (2, 5 and 8) fail to

Table 15-5. Example of Reactions Observed With Multiple Alloantibodies

Cell Number	C	C^w	c	D	E	e	K	Fy^a	Fy^b	Jk^a	Jk^b	P_1	Le^a	Le^b	M	N	S	s	LISS RT	LISS 37	LISS IAT	Ficin 37	Ficin IAT
1	+	0	+	0	0	+	0	+	0	+	+	+	0	+	+	+	0	+	1+	0	3+	0	4+
2	+	+	0	+	0	+	+	+	+	0	+	+	+	0	+	+	+	+	1+	0	2+	0	0
3	+	0	0	+	0	+	0	+	+	+	+	0	0	+	+	0	+	0	3+	2+	3+	0	4+
4	0	0	+	+	+	0	0	0	+	0	+	+	+	0	0	+	0	+	0	0	0	0	0
5	0	0	+	0	+	+	0	+	+	0	+	0	0	+	+	+	+	0	1+	0	3+	0	0
6	0	0	+	0	0	+	0	+	+	0	+	0	+	0	+	0	+	0	3+	2+	3+	*H	†
7	0	0	+	0	+	0	+	0	+	+	0	+	0	+	0	+	0	+	3+	2+	3+	*H	†
8	0	0	+	0	0	+	0	+	0	0	+	+	+	0	0	+	0	+	0	0	3+	0	0
9	0	0	+	0	0	+	0	+	+	0	0	0	+	0	+	+	0	+	1+	0	3+	*H	†
10	0	0	+	+	0	+	0	0	0	+	+	+	0	0	+	+	+	+		0	2+	0	4+
Auto	0	+	+	0	+	0	0			0	+	0	+	0	+	0	+		0	0	0	0	0

*denotes hemolysis   RT = Room temperature   IAT = Indirect antiglobulin testing
† = no cells left for testing   0 = no reaction   1-4 + = degree of agglutination

react at the antiglobulin phase, but these three rbc samples are reactive in the untreated state. All three samples are Fy(a+), and samples 2 and 5 are also S+; anti-Fy^a is a likely specificity, but anti-S cannot be excluded on the basis of these reactions.

5. *Eliminate from consideration antibodies that, if present, should have reacted with antigens present on the nonreactive enzyme-treated rbcs.*

Anti-C, anti-C^w and anti-K can now be eliminated from consideration. Sample 2 carries all three antigens, and is nonreactive in enzyme tests. Enhanced reactions with enzyme-treated rbcs would have been expected if Rh antibodies were present, and Kell system antigens are not adversely affected by ficin.

At this point in the investigation it is appropriate to consider that antibodies to Fy^a, Jk^a, M or S antigens may be present in the serum. These antigens are absent from the autologous rbcs. In order to ascertain which specificities may be involved it is necessary to:

6. *Examine reaction patterns at each test phase; keep in mind possible specificities involved; consider possible specificities relative to test phase and manner of reactivity.*

The results of tests in low ionic strength saline (LISS) at room temperature suggest the presence of anti-M. Reagent rbc samples 4, 8 and 9 are nonreactive and are M–N+. Samples that are M+N+ (1, 2, 5, 6 and 10) are weakly (1+) reactive, and samples 3 and 7 are M+N– and are strongly (3+) reactive. Further, only the two M+N– samples (3 and 7) are reactive in LISS tests at 37 C. This is a typical pattern of reactions of an anti-M showing dosage.

In the antiglobulin phase of testing with untreated rbcs, only sample 4 is nonreactive. Although this sample is the only one that is e–, anti-e has already been eliminated from consideration. The reactions at the antiglobulin phase also fit for a mixture of anti-Fy^a and anti-Jk^a, and it can be noted that the three samples that give a 2+ reaction (2, 5 and 10) probably carry only a single dose of either Fy^a or Jk^a. Three enzyme-treated Jk(a+b–) rbc samples (6, 7 and 9) are hemolyzed after incubation at 37 C. A distinct anti-Jk^a reaction pattern is observed in ficin IATs (considering that both hemolysis and agglutination are manifestations of an antigen-antibody reaction). The serologic findings, therefore, suggest the presence of anti-M, anti-Fy^a and anti-Jk^a in this serum. For conclusive identification, it is necessary to:

7. *Test sufficient rbc samples of appropriate phenotypes to obtain a p value less than 0.05 for each suspected antibody.*

A statistically valid interpretation of the data can be made for anti-M in room temperature tests and anti-Jk^a in ficin-antiglobulin tests. For anti-M, all three M– samples are nonreactive and all seven M+ samples are reactive; p = 0.008. For anti-Jk^a, there are six reactive Jk(a+) samples and four nonreactive Jk(a–) samples; p = 0.005. However, in the antiglobulin phase with untreated rbcs, three reactive Jk(a–) samples (2, 5 and 8) are Fy(a+) and the one nonreactive Jk(a–) sample (sample 4) is Fy(a–). The p value is only 0.25 for anti-Fy^a, and at least two more Fy(a–), Jk(a–) samples must be tested and found to be nonreactive to obtain a p of 0.05, before anti-Fy^a specificity can be confirmed. M–N+ rbcs may be required for these confirmatory studies, since it has yet to be established that the anti-M is solely reactive by direct agglutination tests.

8. *Test serum against rbcs carrying a double dose of antigens to which the serum may contain antibodies, if such rbcs are not among previously nonreactive samples.*

The presence of anti-S has not been excluded, and further tests with S+ rbcs that lack M, Fy^a and Jk^a antigens should be performed. S+s– rbcs should be included in these studies, if available.

While this sequential approach to resolving alloantibody problems necessitates that certain antibody specificities be excluded from initial consideration by the presence of the corresponding antigens on the nonreactive rbc samples, it is important to ensure that such exclusions are confirmed with rbcs carrying a double dose of the relevant antigens, if such rbcs are available. In this case, the phenotype of the autologous rbcs does not preclude the presence of anti-E, but sample 4, carrying a double dose of E, is nonreactive at all test phases.

9. *Test autologous rbcs with additional blood grouping reagents (if necessary) to show the absence of all antigens to which the serum contains antibodies.*

It may be necessary to test the autologous rbcs with additional reagents, to show that they lack all antigens corresponding to those antibodies that are present in the serum. If the approach shown in Table 15-3 has been followed, much of this testing will already have been performed; no further testing of the autologous rbcs is required for the case study presented in Table 15-5.

This case illustrates the value of performing tests with enzyme-treated rbcs, especially when multiple antibodies are present in a serum. Also, much valuable information can often be obtained early in the investigation if at least limited grouping of the autologous rbcs is performed concurrently with the serum studies. However, it must be stressed that not all problem cases can be resolved in this manner. Often, it is necessary to select additional procedures to determine the specificity of some antibodies or to exclude the presence of others. (See Method Sections 3 and 4.)

Antibodies to High-Incidence Antigens

An alloantibody to a high-incidence antigen should be suspected when all reagent rbc samples are reactive, but the autocontrol is nonreactive. These antibodies can often be identified with rbcs of selected rare phenotypes [eg, k– or Yt(a–)] and by testing the autologous rbcs with sera known to contain antibodies to high-incidence antigens. Knowing the serologic characteristics of the antibody and the race of the antibody producer will help in selecting additional reagents to be used. The following apply to antibodies against high-incidence antigens:

1. Reactivity in tests at room temperature is suggestive of anti-H, -I, -Tj^a (-PP$_1$P^k) or -Vel.

2. Lysis of reagent rbcs at 37 C is a characteristic of these antibodies and anti-Jk3.

3. Reduced or absent reactivity in enzyme tests is indicative of anti-Ch, -Rg or -JMH and is seen with some examples of anti-Yt^a and -Ge2 or -Ge3.

4. Weak nebulous reactions in the antihuman globulin (AHG) phase are often associated with anti-Kn^a, -McC^a, -Yk^a, -Cs^a and are also seen with complement-binding autoantibodies, such as anti-I or anti-IH, when polyspecific AHG reagents are used.

5. In Blacks, antibodies such as anti-U, -Sl[a], -Js[b], -Hy, -Tc[a], -Jo[a], -Cr[a] and -At[a] should be suspected, as individuals lacking these antigens are almost always Black.

Chapter 12 discusses serologic characteristics of antibodies reacting with high-incidence rbc antigens, and methods for evaluation of sera containing weak antibodies are given in Method Sections 3 and 4. Such problems will often have to be referred to an immunohematology reference laboratory. The patient's siblings are often the best source of serologically compatible blood for patients with antibodies to high-incidence antigens. Rare phenotypes lacking high-incidence rbc antigens usually occur in individuals homozygous for a rare blood group gene, one inherited from each parent. Offspring of the same parents are far more likely to have inherited the same two rare genes than someone from the random donor population. Rarely will blood from either parent also lack the same high-incidence antigen. For example, Lu(a–b–) phenotypes result from inheritance of the dominant *InLu* gene (see p 266). However, blood from both parents usually will carry only a single dose of the relevant antigen and, when transfusion is essential, can be considered preferable to random donor blood. The AABB Immunohematology Reference Laboratory Program, in collaboration with the AABB Rare Donor File, can be helpful in locating donors of the appropriate phenotypes when necessary (see Method 4.2). Autologous transfusion should also be considered for these patients if clinical situations allow.

Antibodies to Low-Incidence Antigens

When a serum sample reacts only with rbcs from a single donor unit, the possibility should be considered that the donor rbcs are ABO incompatible, have a positive DAT or are polyagglutinable. See p 326-7 for a discussion on rbc polyagglutination, and Chapter 16 for the investigation of a positive DAT.

Reactions between a serum and a single donor or reagent rbc sample may also be caused by antibodies to low-incidence antigens such as anti-Wr[a]. If rbcs known to carry low-incidence antigens are available, the serum may be tested against them. Conversely, the one reactive rbc sample can be tested with known examples of antibodies to low-incidence antigens. Multiple antibodies to low-incidence antigens are commonly found in the same serum, and the expertise and resources of an immunohematology reference laboratory may be required to confirm the suspected specificities. It is inappropriate to delay transfusion while such studies are undertaken. Some reference laboratories will not attempt to identify antibodies to low-incidence antigens, since they are often only of academic interest and staff are better used resolving problems of greater clinical importance. These antibodies should be investigated if found in the sera of pregnant women, to predict the possibility of HDN.

Anomalous Serologic Reactions

Antibodies to a variety of drugs and additives can cause positive results in antibody detection and identification tests. Antibodies against a preservative substance used in the preparation of reagent rbcs (eg, chloramphenicol, neomycin, tetracycline, hydrocortisone, lactose or EDTA) may cause agglutination of reagent rbcs suspended in the manufacturer's preservative solution.[5,6] Reactions rarely occur if the rbcs are washed with saline before testing, and the autologous control is nonreactive unless the autologous rbcs are suspended in the manufacturer's rbc diluent or a similar preservative. Antibodies to other reagent additives can cause agglutination of reagent, donor and autologous rbcs.

There are reports describing Jk^a antibodies that react with rbcs suspended in LISS diluents containing parabens as preservatives. Direct agglutination of Jk(a+) rbcs and reactivity in the antiglobulin phase of testing may occur when such antibodies are present. No anti-Jk^a reactivity is observed when other test procedures, such as saline or enzyme tests, are employed unless paraben is added to the reaction medium. The autologous Jk(a+) rbcs react to tests with LISS plus paraben to the same degree as reagent or donor rbcs, but a DAT will be nonreactive.

In yet other situations, the age of the test rbcs, or the fact that they have been washed in saline before use, may give rise to anomalous serologic reactions.[5] Antibodies to stored rbcs can cause agglutination of reagent rbcs by all techniques, and enhanced reactions may be observed in tests with enzyme-treated rbcs. Such reactivity is not affected by washing the rbcs in saline, and the autocontrol is usually nonreactive. No reactivity will be seen with tests on freshly collected rbcs (eg, from freshly drawn donor or autologous blood samples). For a detailed account of unusual phenomena that are encountered in antibody detection and compatibility studies, the review by Pierce[6] is recommended.

Selected Serologic Procedures

Enhancement Techniques

When a pattern of weak reactions fails to indicate specificity, or when the presence of an antibody is suspected but cannot be demonstrated, use of the following procedures may be helpful. An autocontrol should be included with each new test technique performed.

Enzyme Techniques

Tests with proteolytic enzymes are a useful addition to antibody identification studies. Treatment of rbcs with proteolytic enzymes enhances the reactivity of antibodies to antigens in the Rh, P, I, Kidd and Lewis blood group systems. Procedures for the preparation and use of proteolytic enzyme solutions are given in Methods 3.5 through 3.5.5.

Temperature Reduction

Some alloantibodies (eg, anti-M, -P$_1$) that react at room temperature react better at cold temperatures; specificity may only be apparent at or below 22 C. An autocontrol is especially important for tests at cold temperatures, because many sera contain cold-reactive autoantibodies.

Increased Serum-to-Cell Ratio

Increasing the volume of serum incubated with a standard volume of rbcs may enhance the reactivity of antibodies present in low concentration.[5] An acceptable procedure is to mix 5-10 volumes of serum with one volume of a 2-5% saline suspension of rbcs and incubate for 60 minutes at 37 C with periodic mixing to promote contact between rbcs and antibody molecules. The serum should be removed before washing rbcs for the antiglobulin test because the standard three to four wash phases may be insufficient to remove all unbound immunoglobulins. Additional wash phases are not recommended because bound antibody molecules may dissociate. NOTE: Be cautious when attempting to increase the serum-to-rbc ratio in LISS tests that require equal volumes of serum and LISS-suspended rbcs. (See Chapter 8.)

Increased Incubation Time

For some antibodies, particularly when saline or albumin media are employed, a 15-minute incubation period is insufficient to achieve equilibrium (see Chapter 7) and the observed reactions may be weak. Extending incubation to 60 minutes may improve reactivity and help clarify the observed pattern of reactions.

Alteration of pH

The reactions of certain antibodies, notably some examples of anti-M, are enhanced by decreasing the pH of the reaction medium to pH 6.5.[7] Thus, when anti-M specificity is suspected because only M+N– rbcs are agglutinated, tests with acidified serum may reveal a definitive anti-M pattern of reactivity. Decreasing the pH to 6.5 is achieved by the addition of one volume of 0.2 N HCl to nine volumes of serum. M– rbcs should be tested against the acidified serum to check for nonspecific agglutination.

Low Ionic Strength Procedures

Some blood group antibodies react preferentially in test systems using LISS solutions. LISS reagents accelerate antibody uptake (ie, the first stage of the hemagglutination reaction that involves association of antibody molecules to rbcs). Various LISS procedures have been described. Some involve the use of polycations such as protamine sulphate or Polybrene® to aggregate LISS-suspended antibody-coated rbcs and, thereby, promote the second stage of hemagglutination reactions.[5] The nonspecific aggregation caused by polycations is easily dispersed by addition of saline, phosphate buffer or sodium citrate-glucose solutions, allowing recog-

nition of agglutination due to an antigen-antibody interaction. The rbcs may subsequently be subjected to AHG testing. These methods are discussed in more detail in Chapter 7.

Polyethylene Glycol

Polyethylene glycol has also been shown to be an effective potentiator of antigen-antibody reactions. See Chapter 14 and Method 3.1.4.

Use of Thiol Reagents

Thiol reagents, such as dithiothreitol (DTT) and 2-mercaptoethanol (2-ME), cleave intersubunit disulfide bonds of IgM molecules. Intact 19S IgM molecules are cleaved into 7S subunits, which have altered serologic reactivity.[5,8] The interchain bonds of 7S IgM subunits, and IgG and IgA molecules, are relatively resistant to such cleavage (see Chapter 7 for the structure of immunoglobulin molecules). The applications of DTT and 2-ME in immunohematology include:

1. Determining the immunoglobulin class of an antibody. See Method 4.4.
2. Dissociating rbc agglutinates caused by IgM antibodies (eg, the spontaneous agglutination of rbcs caused by potent cold-reactive autoantibodies). See Method 2.13.
3. Identifying specificities in a mixture of IgM and IgG antibodies, particularly when an agglutinating IgM antibody masks the presence of IgG antibodies.
4. Dissociating IgG antibodies from rbcs using a mixture of DTT and a proteolytic enzyme (ZZAP reagent). See Method 6.4.
5. Converting nonagglutinating IgG antibodies into direct agglutinins.[9] Commercially prepared chemically modified blood grouping reagents for use in rapid saline tube, slide or

microplate tests have been manufactured in this manner. See Chapter 11.

6. Destroying selected rbc antigens (eg, those of the Kell, Dombrock, Cartwright and LW systems) for use in antibody investigations. See Method 6.4.

Inhibition Tests

Some blood group antigens exist in soluble form in such body fluids as saliva, urine or plasma. These substances are useful in antibody identification studies, either to confirm antibody specificity by inhibition or to neutralize antibodies that mask the presence of concomitant nonneutralizable antibodies. The following soluble blood group substances can be used in antibody identification tests:

1. *Lewis substances.* Le^a and Le^b substances are present in the saliva of persons with the appropriate Lewis phenotype. Le^a substance is present in the saliva of Le(a+b–) individuals, and both Le^a and Le^b substances are present in the saliva of Le(a–b+) individuals.[4,5] Saliva should be boiled immediately after collection to inactivate salivary enzymes, and should be rendered isotonic prior to use.[4] (See Method 2.5.) Commercially prepared Lewis substance is available for those laboratories that do not wish to prepare their own saliva reagents.[10]

2. *P_1 substance.* Soluble P_1 substance is present in hydatid cyst fluid. A reagent preparation derived from pigeon egg white is commercially available.[5,11]

3. *Sd^a (Sid) substance.* Sd^a blood group substance is present in soluble form in various body fluids. The most abundant source is urine.[12] If anti-Sd^a is suspected, urine from a known Sd(a+) individual can be used to inhibit the antibody. Saline or urine that does not contain Sd^a substance should be used as a negative control. Because urine may have an acidic pH and a high concentration of salts, it should be dialyzed for 48 hours against pH 7.3 phosphate-buffered saline (Method 4.9) prior to use. Once dialyzed, Sd(a+) and Sd(a–) urines can be frozen in small aliquots for future use.[13] (See Method 4.9.)

4. *Chido and Rodgers substances.* Among the antibodies most difficult to work with are those formerly known as the HTLA (high-titer, low-avidity) antibodies. Although undiluted serum gives weak to moderate reactions by the IAT, weak reactions continue to be observed in tests with progressively diluted serum. Characteristically, these antibodies produce fragile agglutinates, and the reaction scores are low.[14] (See Method 4.6.) Anti-Ch and anti-Rg can be inhibited by plasma from Ch+, Rg+ individuals.[15] (See Method 4.7.)

Ch and Rg antigens are determinants of the fourth component of human complement (C4).[16,17] Anti-Ch and anti-Rg react with trace amounts of C4 present on normal rbcs. While these antibodies react with normal rbcs only by the IAT, they may cause direct agglutination of rbcs coated in vitro with excess C4.[18] (See Method 4.6.) This is a useful test for rapid identification of anti-Ch and anti-Rg.

Confirmation of Specificity

Antibody specificity can be confirmed if the appropriate soluble substance inhibits its serologic reactivity. For example, if a serum is thought to contain anti-P_1 but insufficient reagent rbc samples are available that lack P_1 antigen to provide conclusive identification, soluble P_1 substance can be used to inhibit antibody reactivity. A volume of P_1 substance is added to the appropriate volume of serum (use volumes prescribed by the manufacturer for commercially prepared substances), and the mixture is incubated at room temperature to allow for neutralization to occur. Similarly, a control test consisting of serum plus saline, in appropriate volumes, is performed. Following incubation, P_1 rbcs are added to both mixtures. The tests are incubated at room temperature and subsequently examined for agglutination.

One of three reaction patterns will be observed:

	1	2	3
Serum + P_1 substance:	0	+	0
Serum + saline (control):	+	+	0

The interpretation is as follows:

1. If P_1 rbcs are not agglutinated by serum containing P_1 substance but the control test is reactive, it can be concluded that the serum contains anti-P_1.
2. If both tests are reactive, it is likely that: a) the antibody is not anti-P_1; b) the serum contains a potent example of anti-P_1 and only partial neutralization has occurred; or c) the serum contains anti-P_1 plus additional antibody activity.
3. If both tests are nonreactive, the antibody may be present in such a low concentration that it cannot withstand dilution.

Neutralization of Antibodies

If a serum contains multiple antibodies it may be possible to neutralize one antibody, thus facilitating recognition of other antibody specificities. For example, if a serum contains anti-P_1 and anti-S, the anti-S may not be apparent because there are no S+ rbcs that lack P_1 antigen among the available reagent rbc samples. If the anti-P_1 is neutralized with soluble P_1 substance, S+ and S– reagent rbc samples, regardless of their P system phenotype, can be used to confirm the presence or absence of anti-S. NOTE: Because of inherent dilution factors it may be necessary to increase the diluted serum-to-rbc ratio when performing inhibition tests.

Inactivation of Blood Group Antigens

Antibodies to Kell system antigens do not react with rbcs that have been treated with sulfhydryl reagents such as 2-aminoethylisothiouronium bromide (AET), DTT or 2-ME.[19,20] See Table 15-6. Thus, if an antibody is suspected of having specificity directed toward a Kell system antigen (eg, anti-Kp^b), reagent rbcs can be treated with a sulfhydryl reagent; no reactivity with treated rbcs is suggestive of Kell-related specificity. However, treatment of rbcs may denature other blood group antigens[22] so that loss of reactivity following treatment is not conclusive evidence for Kell-related specificity. A procedure for treating rbcs with DTT is described in Method 4.8. Also, a panel of DTT-treated rbcs may be used to determine the presence of other (non-Kell-related) antibodies in the

Table 15-6. Alteration of Antigens With Various Chemicals[21]

Chemical	Antigens Denatured or Altered
Proteolytic enzymes	M, N, S, Fy^a, Fy^b, Yt^a, Ch, Rg, Pr, Tn, Mg, Mi^a/V^w, Cl^a, Je^a, Ny^a, JMH
ZZAP	M, N, S, Fy^a, Fy^b, Yt^a, Ch, Rg, Pr, Tn, LW^a and all Kell blood group antigens excluding Kx
AET	JMH, Yt^a, Hy, Kn^a, McC^a, Yk^a, LW^a, Lu^b and all Kell blood group antigens excluding Kx

presence of an antibody to a high-incidence Kell system antigen (eg, anti-Fy^a + anti-Kp^b). Sulfhydryl treatment produces changes to rbcs similar to those seen in paroxysmal nocturnal hemoglobinuria such that rbcs are sensitive to the action of complement components by nonimmune mechanisms. An anti-IgG reagent should be used in tests with DTT-treated rbcs.[19]

Kell system antigens are also denatured by treatment with ZZAP reagent (see Table 15-6), a mixture of proteolytic enzyme and DTT or 2-ME, as discussed in Method 6.5.[23] Rbcs treated with ZZAP reagent can be used to exclude the presence of certain additional antibodies (eg, those to Rh and Kidd system antigens) when present in a serum containing antibody to a high-incidence Kell system antigen. However, because of the proteolytic activity of ZZAP reagent, such rbcs cannot be used to exclude the presence of antibodies to M, N, S, s, Fy^a and Fy^b antigens.[22]

Adsorption

Antibody can be removed from a serum by adsorption to rbcs carrying the corresponding antigen. The antibody forms a complex with rbc membrane-bound antigens. When the serum and rbcs are separated, the antibody remains attached to the rbcs. Subsequent elution of the bound antibody can often give additional useful information. Adsorption techniques are useful in such situations as:

1. Removing autoantibody activity to permit the detection of coexisting alloantibodies (see Chapter 16).
2. Removing unwanted antibody from a serum that contains an antibody suitable for reagent use (eg, removal of anti-A or -B from a serum containing anti-Fy^a, so that the anti-Fy^a can be used with rbcs of all ABO groups).

3. Confirming the presence of antigens on rbcs through their ability to remove a specific serum antibody.
4. Confirming the specificity of an antibody by showing that it can be adsorbed only to rbcs of a particular blood group phenotype.
5. Separating multiple antibodies present in single serum sample. Such studies require the use of combined adsorption and elution tests, and are useful in the identification of complex mixtures of antibodies (see p 661-71).

Technical Considerations

Adsorption procedures are intended for different purposes in different situations; no single procedure can be given that is satisfactory in all instances. The usual serum-to-rbc ratio used is one volume of serum to an equal volume of washed, packed rbcs. The incubation temperature should be that which is optimal for the reactivity of the antibody.

Pretreating rbcs with a proteolytic enzyme may enhance antibody uptake, reducing the number of adsorptions required for complete removal of antibody. Since some antigens such as M, N, S, Fy^a and Fy^b are destroyed by proteases, antibodies directed against these antigens may not be removed by enzyme-treated rbcs.

In separating mixtures of antibodies, selecting rbcs of the appropriate phenotype is extremely important. At least one antibody specificity should be known or suspected in order to choose rbcs that lack one antigen yet carry another. The rbcs must be available in sufficient quantity; vials of reagent rbcs will not suffice, and blood samples from staff members or donor units are the most convenient sources.

Adsorption Procedure

1. Wash the selected rbcs at least three times with saline. After the last wash, centrifuge the rbcs for at least five minutes, and remove as much of the supernatant saline as is possible. Additional saline may be removed by placing a narrow piece of filter paper into the rbcs.
2. Mix appropriate volumes of the packed rbcs and serum, and incubate at the desired temperature for 30-60 minutes. Adsorption will be more effective if the area of contact between the rbcs and serum is large; the use of a large-bore test tube (ie, 13 mm or greater) is recommended. The serum/cell mixture should be mixed periodically throughout the incubation phase.
3. Centrifuge to pack the rbcs tightly. Centrifuge at the incubation temperature if possible, to avoid antigen-antibody dissociation.
4. Transfer the supernatant fluid to a clean test tube, and label it adsorbed serum.
5. If an eluate is to be prepared, save the rbcs. Test an aliquot of the adsorbed serum to see if the procedure has removed all antibody. Preferably, test the adsorbed serum against rbcs from the original sample. Repeat the adsorption process if necessary with a fresh aliquot of washed, packed rbcs.

Elution

Elution techniques free antibody molecules from sensitized rbcs. The objective of most such procedures is to recover bound antibody in a usable form. Bound antibody may be released by changing the thermodynamics of antigen-antibody reactions, by neutralizing or reversing forces of attraction that hold antigen-antibody complexes together, or by disturbing the structural complementarity between an antigen and its corresponding binding site on an antibody molecule.

A variety of methods have been described for eluting antibody from sensitized rbcs,[24] and some procedures are given in Methods 5.1 through 5.6. While no single method is best in all clinical situations, use of heat elution should be restricted to the investigation of ABO HDN and elution with acid or an organic solvent is required for optimal elution of warm-reactive auto- and alloantibodies.

Technical Considerations

Technical factors that influence the success of elution techniques include:

1. Incorrect technique. Depending upon the elution method used, such factors as incomplete removal of organic solvents and failure to render an eluate isotonic or to a neutral pH may cause the rbcs used to test the eluate either to hemolyze or to appear "sticky." Similarly, the presence of stromal debris may interfere with the reading of tests. Careful technique and strict adherence to method protocols should eliminate such problems.
2. Incomplete washing. To prevent contamination of an eluate with serum antibody, thorough washing of the sensitized rbcs *prior to* elution is essential. Six washes with saline are usually more than adequate, but more may be needed if the rbcs have been coated in vitro with a high-titer antibody. As a means of controlling the efficacy of the washing process, it is appropriate to test the supernatant fluid from the final wash phase for antibody activity; this fluid should contain no antibody reactivity.
3. Binding of proteins to glass surfaces. If eluates are prepared from rbcs coated in vitro with purified antibody and the same test tube that was used

during the sensitization phase is also used for preparing the eluate, antibody that has become nonspecifically bound to the test tube surface may dissociate during the elution process, leading to contamination of the eluate. To avoid such contamination, it is appropriate to transfer the rbcs into a clean test tube during the washing process, before proceeding with preparation of the eluate.

4. Dissociation of antibody before elution. This is not usually a problem with IgG antibodies, unless they have a low affinity for their respective antigens. It may, however, contribute to difficulties encountered when attempting to elute predominantly cold-reactive antibodies such as anti-A or anti-M. To minimize loss of IgM antibody, cold (4 C) saline can be used for washing rbcs prior to elution when these antibodies are suspected. In the case of low-affinity IgG antibodies, substituting LISS for saline may be helpful.

5. Instability of eluates. Dilute protein solutions, such as those obtained by elution into saline, are unstable.[24] Eluates should be tested as soon after preparation as possible. Alternatively, eluates may be kept frozen following the addition of bovine albumin to a final concentration of 6% (wt/vol).

Applications

Elution techniques are useful for:

1. The investigation of a positive DAT (see Chapter 16).

2. The concentration and purification of antibodies, the detection of weakly expressed antigens and the identification of multiple antibody specificities. Such studies are used in conjunction with an appropriate adsorption technique (see p 661-71 and Method 2.4).

3. The preparation of antibody-free intact rbcs for use in phenotyping or autologous adsorption studies. Procedures used to remove cold- and warm-reactive autoantibodies from rbcs are discussed in Methods 6.1 and 6.4, and methods for autologous adsorption of warm-reactive autoantibodies are given in Chapter 16.

Combined Adsorption-Elution Tests

Combined adsorption-elution tests can often be informative when applied to detection of weakly expressed antigens on rbcs or for identification of weakly reactive antibodies. Although an antibody may not cause direct agglutination, it may be adsorbed to antigen-positive rbcs. Loss of antibody reactivity in the adsorbed serum and subsequent recovery of the antibody from the adsorbing rbcs show that an antibody-antigen interaction has occurred. Also, such procedures may be invaluable for the separation of antibody mixtures in identification studies or reagent production.

Detection of Weak Antigens or Antibodies

Adsorption of antibody, to demonstrate the presence or absence of the corresponding antigen on rbcs, is best accomplished using a low serum-to-rbc ratio (eg, 2:1 or less). Care should be taken not to dilute the serum, and hence the antibody, with residual saline from inadequately packed rbcs. Determining the protein concentrations of the serum by refractometry before or after the adsorption step is an appropriate check for such dilution. A reduction in titration score of 10 or more, using the system described in Method 4.3, is considered evidence for the presence of the relevant antigen on the adsorbing rbcs. In critical studies, control adsorptions with rbcs known to lack the antigen in question should be undertaken.

When the antibody is to be recovered from the rbcs by subsequent elution, a higher serum-to-rbc ratio (eg, 5:1 or more) should be used to sensitize the rbcs with antibody. This may permit the production of an eluate that is more potent than the original serum, if the eluate volume used is less than the volume of serum used to coat the rbcs.[18] Once prepared, the eluate should be tested against uncoated rbcs from the same sample used for adsorption, to establish that the antibody was (or was not) subject to elution.

Identification of Antibodies in Multispecific Sera

Adsorption-elution tests may be used for identification purposes with sera containing multiple antibodies of commonly encountered specificities, eg, anti-D, -K, -Fy[a], etc. Since these studies are tedious, they should be performed only when all other tests, including studies with multiple reagent rbc samples and enzyme tests, have failed to resolve the problem fully. Availability of sufficient quantities of rbcs is essential. It is useful to determine the phenotype of staff members to provide a continuing supply of rbcs, when needed.

The selection of adsorbing rbcs is crucial to the success of these studies, but often has to be an inspired choice, influenced by the phenotype of the antibody producer. Knowing which antibodies could be present should help in the selection of additional rbc samples that will prove their presence or absence. As a general rule, one or more weakly reactive rbc samples should be used, on the assumption that these will carry only one of the factors to which the serum has specificity.

The serum under investigation should be adsorbed several times, until it no longer reacts with the adsorbing rbcs. Both the adsorbed serum and an eluate, prepared from rbcs used in the first adsorption, should be examined for antibody specificity. While it is to be hoped that specific antibodies will be apparent in either or both preparations, this is not always the case. Some antibodies (eg, anti-Kn[a] and -McC[a]) are difficult to adsorb and elute. Also, the serum may be nonreactive after adsorption, yet the eluate reacts with all reagent rbc samples. Such a finding may indicate the presence of an antibody to a high-incidence antigen that has a variable expression on rbcs, or may be due to the fact that the serum antibody was subject to dilution during the adsorption process.

When the above studies are not informative, or when autoantibodies are present in the serum of a recently transfused patient such that autologous adsorption is not appropriate, adsorption with selected ZZAP-treated rbcs may be necessary. For example, if the patient's Rh and Kidd phenotypes can be determined (either from previous testing or following application of rbc separation and/or chloroquine diphosphate procedures outlined in Method 2.15), allogeneic rbcs of the same phenotype can be ZZAP-treated and used to adsorb autoantibody. (See Chapter 16.) Such rbcs should not adsorb most clinically significant alloantibodies since they will lack the same Rh and Jk antigens present on the patient's rbcs and will be devoid of all Kell system antigens as well as other antigens listed in Table 15-6.

Isolation of Specific Antibodies

Adsorption-elution procedures are effective ways of preparing antisera for use with rbcs of any ABO group, particularly antisera to high-incidence antigens, since groups A and B (or AB) rbcs lacking the relevant antigen may not be available for removing anti-A or anti-B by simple adsorption. An eluate prepared from group O rbcs that are known to react with the antibody in question should contain only the desired specific antibody, and will be devoid of anti-A and anti-B. Antibodies purified in this manner can be preserved frozen, providing the protein concentration is adjusted to 6% with bovine albumin, and may be used to phenotype rbcs from individuals whose serum appears to contain an antibody to a high-incidence rbc antigen.

A similar approach can be applied to confirm the specificity of serologic reactions, particularly when a serum reacts with a number of reagent rbc samples that do not appear to share a common antigen. The serum may contain several antibodies to low-incidence antigens, or a single antibody to an unknown determinant (for which the reagent rbcs have not been tested). In the latter instance, an eluate prepared after incubation of the serum with one of the reactive rbc samples will be seen to react with all other rbc samples with which the serum originally reacted.

Titration

The titer of an antibody is usually determined by testing serial two-fold dilutions of the serum against selected rbc samples. Results are expressed as the reciprocal of the highest serum dilution that causes macroscopic agglutination. Titration values can provide information about the relative amount of antibody present in a serum, or the relative strength of antigen expression on rbcs. Titration studies are usually performed in the following situations:

1. Prenatal studies. When the antibody is of a specificity known to cause HDN, or when the clinical signifi-

cance of the antibody is unknown, the results of titration studies, the outcome of previous pregnancies and current clinical observations are used to assess the need for amniocentesis. (See Chapter 18.)

2. Antibody identification. Some antibodies cause agglutination of virtually all reagent rbc samples, but specificity is indicated by differences in the strength of reactivity with each sample in titration studies. For example, potent autoanti-I may react in the undiluted state with both adult and cord rbcs. In titration studies, the serum may be found to react at a higher dilution with adult I+ rbcs than it does with i_{cord} rbcs.

3. HTLA-type antibodies. The obsolete term "HTLA" has been used to describe those antibodies that are weakly reactive in the undiluted state but, unlike most weakly reactive antibodies (eg, an anti-D with a titer of 4), react at a high dilution (eg, 1 in 2048). Such antibodies include anti-Ch, -Rg, - Cs^a, -Yk^a, -Kn^a, -McC^a and -JMH. When weak reactions are observed in indirect antiglobulin tests, titration studies may be used to establish whether or not the reactions are due to the presence of an HTLA-type antibody.

Details of antibody titration procedures are given in Method 4.5.[25]

References

1. Giblett ER. Blood group alloantibodies: An assessment of some laboratory practices. Transfusion 1977;17:299-308.
2. Walker RH, Lin D-T, Hartrick MB. Alloimmunization following blood transfusion. Arch Pathol Lab Med 1989;113:254-61.
3. Ellisor SS. Action and applications of enzymes in immunohematology. In: Bell, CA ed. A seminar on antigen-antibody reactions revisited. Washington, DC: American Association of Blood Banks, 1982:133-74.

4. Issitt PD. Applied blood group serology, 3rd ed. Miami: Montgomery Scientific Publications, 1985.

5. Mollison PL. Blood transfusion in clinical medicine, 9th ed. Oxford: Blackwell Scientific Publications, 1993.

6. Pierce SR. Anomalous blood bank results. In: Dawson RB, ed. Troubleshooting the crossmatch. Washington, DC: American Association of Blood Banks, 1977:85-114.

7. Beattie KM, Zuelzer WW. The frequency and properties of pH-dependent anti-M. Transfusion 1965;5:322-6.

8. Freedman J, Masters CA, Newlands M, et al. Optimal conditions for use of sulphydryl compounds in dissociating rbc antibodies. Vox Sang 1976;30:231-9.

9. Romans DG, Tilley CA, Crookston MC, et al. Conversion of incomplete antibodies to direct agglutinins by mild reduction. Evidence for segmental flexibility within the Fc fragment of immunoglobulin G. Proc Natl Acad Sci USA 1977;74:2531-5.

10. Spitalnik SL, Cowles JW, Cos MT, Blumberg N. Neutralization of Lewis blood group antibodies by synthetic immunoadsorbents. Am J Clin Pathol 1983;80:63-5.

11. Cowles JW, Blumberg N. Neutralization of P blood group antibodies by synthetic solid-phase antigens. Transfusion 1987;27:272-5.

12. Morton J, Pickles MM, Terry AM. The Sd^a blood group antigen in tissues and body fluids. Vox Sang 1970;19:472-82.

13. Judd WJ. Methods in immunohematology. Miami: Montgomery Scientific Publiations, 1988.

14. Rolih SD, ed. High-titer low-avidity antibodies and antigens: A review. Transfus Med Rev 1989;3:128-39.

15. Crookston MC. Soluble antigens and leukocyte related antibodies. Part A. Blood group antigens in plasma: An aid in the identification of antibodies. In: Dawson RD, ed. Transfusion with "crossmatch incompatible" blood. Washington, DC: American Association of Blood Banks, 1975:20-5.

16. O'Neill GJ, Yang SY, Tegoli J, et al. Chido and Rodgers blood groups are distinct antigenic components of human complement, C4. Nature 1978;273:668-70.

17. Tilley CA, Romans DG, Crookston MC. Localization of Chido and Rodgers to the C4d fragment of human C4 (abstract). Transfusion 1978;18:622.

18. Judd WJ, Kraemer K, Moulds JJ. The rapid identification of Chido and Rodgers antibodies using C4d-coated red blood cells. Transfusion 1981;21:189-92.

19. Advani H, Zamor J, Judd WJ, et al. Inactivation of Kell blood group antigens by 2-aminoethylisothiouronium bromide. Br J Haematol 1982;51:107-15.

20. Branch DR, Muensch HA, Sy Siok Hian S, Petz LD. Disulfide bonds are a requirement for Kell and Cartwright (Yt^a) blood group antigen integrity. Br J Haematol 1983;54:573-8.

21. Wilkinson SL. Serological approaches to transfusion of patients with allo- or autoantibodies. In: Nance SJ, ed. Immune destruction of red blood cells. Arlington, VA: American Association of Blood Banks, 1989: 227-61.

22. Moulds J, Moulds M. Inactivation of Kell blood group antigens by 2-amino-ethylisothiouronium bromide. Transfusion 1983;23:274-5.

23. Branch DR, Petz LD. A new reagent (ZZAP) having multiple applications in immunohematology. Am J Clin Pathol 1982;78:161-7.

24. Judd WJ. Elution of antibody from rbcs. In: Bell, CA, ed. A seminar on antigen-antibody reactions revisited. Washington, DC: American Association of Blood Banks, 1982:175-221.

25. Marsh WL. Scoring of hemagglutination reactions. Transfusion 1972;12:352-3.

16

Investigation of a Positive DAT and Immune Hemolysis

Significance of a Positive DAT

A positive direct antiglobulin test (DAT) generally means that the rbcs of the person being tested are coated in vivo with immunoglobulin and/or complement. A positive DAT, with or without an associated shortened rbc survival, may be caused by any of the following phenomena in vivo:

1. Autoantibodies to intrinsic rbc antigens that coat rbcs with immunoglobulin or complement, or both.[1-3]
2. Alloantibodies present in the recipient of a recent transfusion that react with antigens on donor rbcs.[4]
3. Antibodies present in donor plasma, plasma derivatives or blood fractions that react with antigens on a transfusion recipient's rbcs.[4]
4. Maternal alloantibodies that cross the placenta and coat fetal rbcs. These antibodies are often associated with hemolytic disease of the newborn (HDN).[4]
5. Antibodies directed against certain drugs, such as penicillin, that bind to rbc membranes.[5]
6. Rbc membrane modifications resulting from therapy with certain drugs, notably those of the cephalosporin group, leading to non-immunologic adsorption of proteins, including immunoglobulins, by rbcs.[5]
7. Drug/anti-drug complexes, formed in response to the administration of drugs such as quinidine and phenacetin,[5] that cause complement components and, rarely, IgG to be bound to rbcs.
8. Heterophile antibodies present in equine antihuman lymphocyte globulin that is used to reduce T-cell populations in organ and bone marrow transplant recipients.[6]
9. Non-antibody-mediated binding of immunoglobulins to rbcs in patients with hypergammaglobulinemia.[7-9] A positive DAT due to this phenomenon is also seen in patients treated with high-dose intravenous gammaglobulin.[7]
10. Antibodies from passenger lymphocytes in transplanted organs.[10]

A positive DAT does not necessarily mean that a person's rbcs have a shortened survival. As many as 10% of hospital patients, and between 1 in 1000 and 1 in 9000 blood donors, have a positive DAT without clinical manifestations of immune-mediated hemolysis.[11-14]

The Pretransfusion DAT or Autocontrol

Some workers routinely perform a DAT, or an autocontrol (mixing patient's serum with patient's rbcs), as part of

355

pretransfusion testing. The autocontrol serves essentially the same purpose as a DAT, [ie, to determine if rbcs are coated (or sensitized) with complement or immunoglobulins]. For the most part, the DAT detects in-vivo sensitization, whereas the autocontrol may be positive due to in-vivo or in-vitro sensitization. An autocontrol may also be positive, but the DAT negative, in rare situations involving antibodies to reagent constituents. The need to perform a DAT or autocontrol as part of routine pretransfusion testing has been the subject of considerable discussion.

It should be noted that AABB *Standards for Blood Banks and Transfusion Services*[15] (or indeed the requirements of any other accrediting agency) does not require that a DAT or autocontrol be performed as part of routine pretransfusion testing. Nonetheless, many workers advocate performing a DAT or autocontrol routinely. The purpose of such testing appears to be two-fold: 1) to screen for clinically unexpected autoimmune phenomena and 2) to detect the early manifestation of an immune response to previous recent transfusions, particularly instances in which the newly formed alloantibody has been totally adsorbed by the transfused rbcs and cannot be detected in the serum. The latter may be of concern in a multitransfused patient population.

Independent studies have shown that there is minimal risk associated with eliminating the DAT/autocontrol portion of routine pretransfusion testing.[13,16] Since performance of an antiglobulin crossmatch is also optional when unexpected antibodies are absent and there has been no history of such antibodies, streamlining of serologic testing as a means of cost-containment should also include consideration of eliminating the pretransfusion DAT/autocontrol.

The results of DATs should reflect in-vivo conditions, and should not be influenced by in-vitro phenomena associated with the collection, storage or handling of blood samples. Before further studies are undertaken on a patient with a positive DAT, causes of in-vitro rbc coating should be excluded. Causes of false-positive antiglobulin tests are discussed in Chapter 8. False-positive DAT results are most often associated with the use of refrigerated, clotted blood samples, in which complement components coat rbcs in vitro. Any positive DAT result obtained from a clotted blood sample should be confirmed using a freshly collected EDTA-anticoagulated specimen.

Evaluation of a Positive DAT

Extent of Testing

Clinical considerations should dictate the extent to which a positive DAT is evaluated. Dialogue with the attending physician is important before any additional serologic tests are undertaken. Interpreting the significance of serologic findings requires knowledge of the patient's diagnosis, recent drug and transfusion history and whether the patient has an acquired hemolytic anemia.[17] The results of serologic tests are not diagnostic; their significance can be assessed only in relationship to the patient's clinical condition and to laboratory data such as hematocrit, bilirubin, haptoglobin and reticulocyte count.

Answers to the following questions may help decide what investigations are appropriate when a positive DAT is encountered in patients other than neonates:

1. *Is there any evidence of in-vivo hemolysis?*
   Reticulocytosis, hemoglobinemia, hemoglobinuria, decreased serum haptoglobin and elevated levels of

serum unconjugated bilirubin or LDH, especially LDH1, may be associated with hemolysis.[1,18] If an anemic patient with a positive DAT manifests clinical signs and symptoms of hemolysis it is appropriate to determine if the hemolysis has an immune basis. On the other hand, IF THERE IS NO EVIDENCE OF HEMOLYSIS, NO FURTHER STUDIES ARE NECESSARY, unless unexpected antibodies are present and transfusion is necessary.

2. *Has the patient been recently transfused?*

Many workers routinely attempt to determine the cause of a positive DAT, or autocontrol, when the patient has been recently transfused (within the previous 3 months). A positive test on a recipient of a recent transfusion may be the early manifestation of an immune response to recently transfused rbcs. Alloantibodies may be present that could shorten the survival of both recently and subsequently transfused rbcs. However, as discussed earlier, antibodies to previous transfusions will usually also be detected in the serum during subsequent pretransfusion testing.

3. *Does the patient's serum contain unexpected antibodies?*

Investigation of a positive DAT may help identify unexpected serum antibodies, when present. Antibodies in the serum may coat the patient's rbcs and/or the transfused rbcs. Since the elution procedures used in the evaluation of a positive DAT may concentrate antibody activity,[19] the serologic evaluation of a positive DAT/autocontrol may facilitate the identification of weakly reactive serum antibodies.

4. *Is the patient receiving any drugs, especially α-methyldopa or intravenous penicillin?*

Approximately 3% of patients receiving intravenous penicillin and 15-20% of patients receiving α-methyldopa will develop a positive DAT,[1,5] but less than 1% of those patients who develop a positive DAT have hemolytic anemia. For patients who are receiving α-methyldopa or intravenous penicillin, the attending physician should be alerted so that appropriate surveillance for hemolysis can be maintained. If there is no hemolysis, no further studies are necessary.

5. *Has the patient received blood or components containing ABO-incompatible plasma?*

Transfusion of non-ABO group-specific plasma or intravenous immunoglobulins containing antibodies to A and/or B antigens present on the recipient's rbcs may give rise to a positive DAT and occasionally may result in accelerated destruction of those rbcs. For example, it may be necessary to give group O platelets (containing anti-A and -B) to a group A, B or AB patient because ABO group-specific platelets are not available. When signs and symptoms of immune hemolysis occur in patients who have received incompatible plasma, the investigation of the positive DAT can initially be limited to demonstrating the presence of anti-A and/or -B on the recipient's rbcs. In the absence of such antibody coating, other causes for the positive DAT should be sought.

6. *Is the patient receiving antilymphocyte globulin (ALG) or antithymocyte globulin (ATG)?*

Patients receiving ALG or ATG produced in horses develop a positive DAT within a few days after such therapy is initiated.[6] The serologic problems associated with ALG and ATG therapy appear to be related to high-titer heterophile antibodies in these products and the presence, in rabbit antihuman globulin reagents, of antibodies to equine proteins. The problems can be avoided using antihuman globulin reagents that have been partially neutralized with equine serum.[6]

Collection of Blood Samples

To verify that a positive DAT is not the result of in-vitro uptake of complement components by clotted specimens, an EDTA-anticoagulated sample must be obtained.[17] This is used for DATs and autocontrol tests, and provides a source of rbcs for adsorption and/or elution if required. A freshly collected clotted blood sample is needed for serum antibody studies. If cold agglutinin syndrome (CAS) [cold agglutinin disease (CAD), cold hemagglutinin disease (CHD)] or paroxysmal cold hemoglobinuria (PCH) is the suspected cause of the positive DAT, the clotted specimen should be maintained at 37 C until the serum has been separated.[17]

Initial Serologic Studies

If the decision has been made to evaluate a positive DAT, three areas of investigation are helpful in determining the cause of in-vivo rbc coating:

1. Tests with anti-IgG and anti-C3d antiglobulin reagents to determine the types of proteins coating the rbcs[1,17] (see Chapter 8).
2. Serum tests to detect and identify clinically significant unexpected antibodies. Such studies should be performed at 37 C and the IAT with untreated group O reagent rbcs. Tests at 37 C and the antiglobulin phase with enzyme-treated rbcs, if these are available, may also be helpful.
3. Tests with an eluate prepared from the coated rbcs to characterize the

coating protein. The eluate should be incubated at 37 C with untreated group O reagent rbcs and read at the antiglobulin phase. If the eluate is nonreactive, testing against enzyme-treated rbcs may be done. It may also be useful to prepare a more concentrated eluate for testing.[17] If the eluate is positive, further testing using panels of reagent red cells should be performed to identify the antibody. In warm autoimmune hemolytic anemia (WAIHA) the causative antibodies often show no apparent specificity. In patients having delayed-type hemolytic transfusion reactions, the most common specificities encountered are alloantibodies to Rh, Kell and Kidd blood group antigens.

Further Studies

WHEN NO UNEXPECTED ANTIBODIES ARE PRESENT IN THE SERUM, ONLY AUTOANTIBODY IS PRESENT IN THE ELUATE AND THE PATIENT HAS NOT BEEN RECENTLY TRANSFUSED, NO FURTHER SEROLOGIC TESTING IS NECESSARY. If alloantibody appears to be present in serum or eluate, or both, additional studies may be required to confirm specificity. Chapter 15 details the procedures involved in the identification of alloantibodies. If both serum and eluate are nonreactive at all test phases, and if the patient is known to have received high-dose intravenous penicillin or other drug therapy, then appropriate testing to demonstrate drug-related antibodies should be considered. Similarly, if the patient has been transfused with ABO-incompatible blood components, such as group O platelets administered to a group A recipient, tests with A and B rbcs may be done to ascertain whether passively acquired anti-A or anti-B is responsible for the positive DAT.

Some of the procedures used for differentiating between auto- and alloantibody activity are discussed in Chapter 15. The remaining sections of this chapter describe procedures used in the classification of autoimmune and drug-induced immune hemolysis, and describe tests intended to ensure safe transfusion management of the patient. Alloimmune hemolysis, resulting in HDN or associated with an immune response to recently transfused rbcs, is discussed in Chapters 18 and 19.

Immune Hemolysis

Immune hemolysis is defined as shortened rbc survival resulting from a humoral immune response. If bone marrow compensation is adequate, hemolysis may not result in anemia. Hemolysis is only one cause of anemia,[18] and many causes of hemolysis are unrelated to immune reactions.[1,2,14,18,20] The serologic investigations carried out in the blood bank do not determine whether a patient has hemolytic anemia. The diagnosis of hemolytic anemia rests on clinical findings and such laboratory data as hemoglobin or hematocrit values, reticulocyte count, rbc morphology, bilirubin, haptoglobin and LDH levels. Sometimes, rbc survival studies are informative. The serologic findings help determine whether the hemolysis has an immune basis and, if so, what type of immune hemolytic anemia is present. This is important, since the treatment for each type is different.

Immune hemolytic anemia may be classified in various ways. One classification is shown in Table 16-1. The inci-

Table 16-1. Classification of Immune Hemolytic Anemias

Autoimmune Hemolytic Anemia
1. Warm Autoimmune Hemolytic Anemia
   a. primary (idiopathic)
   b. secondary [to such conditions as lymphoma, systemic lupus erythematosus (SLE), carcinoma, or to drug therapy]
2. Cold Agglutinin Syndrome
   a. primary (idiopathic)
   b. secondary (to such conditions as lymphoma, mycoplasma pneumonia, infectious mononucleosis)
3. Mixed-Type AIHA
   a. primary (idiopathic)
   b. secondary (to such conditions as SLE, lymphoma)
4. Paroxysmal Cold Hemoglobinuria
   a. primary (idiopathic)
   b. secondary (to such conditions as syphilis, viral infections)
5. DAT-Negative AIHA
   a. primary (idiopathic)
   b. secondary (to such conditions as lymphoma, SLE)

Drug-Induced Immune Hemolytic Anemia
see Table 16-4

Alloimmune Hemolytic Anemia
1. Hemolytic disease of the newborn
2. Hemolytic transfusion reaction

Table 16-2. Serologic Findings in DAT-Positive AIHA

	WAIHA	CAS	Mixed-Type AIHA	PCH	Drug-Induced AIHA
Percent of cases	48%[23] to 70%[1]	16%[1] to 32%[23]	7%[23] to 8%[34]	Rare in adults[1] 32% in children[36]	12%[1] to 18%[23]
DAT	20%[1] to 66%[23] IgG 24%[23] to 63%[1] IgG + C3 7%[23] to 14%[1] C3	91%[23] to 98%[1] C3 only	71%[23] to 100%[34] IgG + C3	94%[23] to 100%[1] C3 only	94%[23] IgG 6%[23] IgG + C3
Immuno-globulin type	IgG (sometimes IgA or IgM, rarely alone)	IgM	IgG, IgM	IgG	IgG
Eluate	IgG antibody	Nonreactive	IgG antibody	Nonreactive	IgG antibody
Serum	57% react by IAT; 13% hemolyze enzyme-treated rbcs at 37 C; 90% agglutinate enzyme-treated rbcs at 37 C; 30% agglutinate untreated rbcs at 20 C; rarely agglutinate un-treated rbcs at 37 C[1]	IgM hemagglutinating antibody; titer usually >1000 at 4 C; usually react at 30 C in albumin; monoclonal antibody in chronic disease[1, 17]	IgG IAT-reactive antibody; IgM hemagglutinating antibody, usually react at 30–37 C in saline; titer at 4 C often <64[23, 33, 34]	IgG biphasic hemolysin (Donath-Landsteiner antibody)[1, 17]	IgG antibody similar to WAIHA[1, 17]
Specificity	80% Type I, 20% Type II[28] specificity; Rh specificity; other specificities have been reported*	Usually anti-I but can be anti-i; rarely anti-Pr[31]	Usually specificity unclear;[23, 33-35] can be anti-I, -i, or other cold agglutinin specificities	Anti-P (non-reactive with p and P[k] rbcs[1, 31]	Specificity often Rh related[1, 9]

*anti-A, -En[a], -Ge, -I[T], -Jk[a], -K1, -K4, -K5, -K13, -Lan, -LW, -N, -Sc1, -U, -Wr[b] and -Xg[a] [31]

dence of each type of autoimmune hemolytic anemia (AIHA) may vary depending on the study.[1,21-23] Estimates for frequencies of autoimmune hemolysis range as follows: 48% to 70% for WAIHA; 16% to 32% for CAS; 7% to 8% for mixed-type AIHA; 2% to 5% for PCH; and 12% to 18% for drug-induced AIHA (see Table 16-2).

The DAT, including the use of monospecific anti-IgG and anti-C3d, provides useful, although limited, information. The findings in the DAT may reduce the diagnostic possibilities; eg, the DAT in CAS is almost always positive using anti-C3d antihuman globulin serum and negative using anti-IgG. Table 16-3 summarizes the expected DAT findings in the

Table 16-3. DAT Results in AIHA Using Anti-IgG and Anti-C3 Reagents[23]

	WAIHA	CAS	Mixed-Type AIHA*	PCH	Drug-Induced
No. of patients	355	275	61	17	157
IgG only[†]	67%	1%	18%	0	94%
IgG + C3[†]	24%	1%	71%	0	6%
C3 only[†]	7%	91%	9.8%	94%	0
Poly+/Mono–[‡]	1%	0.7%	0	0	0
DAT–	1%	6.3%	1.2%	6%	0

*Patients had both cold hemagglutinating autoantibodies reactive to 30 C or higher and warm-reactive autoantibodies.
†With or without IgM and/or IgA.
‡Polyspecific antihuman globulin gives a positive result but monospecific anti-IgG and anti-C3 reagents are negative.

various autoimmune hemolytic anemias using anti-IgG and anti-C3 antisera.

Warm Autoimmune Hemolytic Anemia

The most common type of AIHA is associated with warm-reactive (37 C) antibodies.[1,22,23] Typical serologic findings are described below.

DAT

In one study,[23] when monospecific anti-IgG and anti-C3 reagents are used, one of three patterns of reactivity may be found: in 67% of cases rbcs are coated with IgG alone; in 24% of cases the rbcs are coated with both IgG and complement, in approximately 7% only with complement and in approximately 1% of cases the DAT will be negative. Further, in approximately 1% of cases the DAT will be positive when using a polyspecific antihuman globulin reagent but negative when using monospecific antiglobulin reagents. This may be related to the very rare cases where IgA or IgM was the only globulin present.[1,21,24]

Serum

The patient's serum may contain very little free autoantibody if the autoanti-body has been adsorbed by the patient's rbcs in vivo. Autoantibody usually appears in the serum when all the specific antigen sites on the rbcs have been occupied, and no more antibody can be bound in vivo. The DAT is usually strongly positive. Approximately 50% of patients with WAIHA will have sera containing autoantibody reactive in tests with untreated rbcs. The autoantibody is usually IgG and is best demonstrated by indirect antiglobulin tests (IATs). With more sensitive methods, such as tests with enzyme-treated rbcs, over 90% of sera can be shown to contain autoantibody. Autoantibodies that hemolyze or agglutinate untreated rbcs by routine techniques in vitro at 37 C are extremely rare. However, warm-reactive hemolysins can be demonstrated using enzyme-treated rbcs in approximately 15% of sera. Approximately one-third of patients with warm antibody AIHA also have cold-reactive autoagglutinins demonstrable in tests at 20 C, but cold agglutinin titers at 4 C are normal.[1] This does not necessarily mean the patient has CAS in addition to WAIHA (see mixed-type AIHA below).[1,17] Also, the serum may contain alloantibodies in addition to autoantibodies, or alloantibodies alone may be present.

Eluate

The presence of the IgG autoantibody on the rbcs can be confirmed by elution (See Methods 5.1 through 5.6). IgG may be present at such low levels that no detectable antibody is recovered by elution.[1] If only complement is found coating the rbcs, the eluate will usually be found to have no serologic activity.

Specificity of Autoantibody

The specificity of autoantibodies associated with WAIHA appears very complex.[1,25-28] However, in the most simplified description, specificity has been shown to be of two types. Type I warm-reactive autoantibodies show a preferential recognition for older rbcs, while Type II warm-reactive autoantibodies react equally well with reticulocyte-enriched or older rbcs populations.[28] It has also been suggested that specificity is often directed against the Rh antigen complex, but this can only be determined if rbcs of very rare phenotypes are available, such as –D– or Rh$_{null}$. This apparent specificity has been challenged based on the reactivity seen when using age-fractionated rbcs.[28] Apart from Rh specificity, there have been other reports of warm autoantibodies with anti-A, -En^a, -Ge, -I^T, -Jk^a, -K1, -K4, -K5, -K13, -Lan, -LW, -N, -Sc1, -U, -Wr^b, -Xg^a and other specificities.[25-27,29-31]

It is rarely, if ever, necessary to perform additional testing to ascertain autoantibody specificity in order to select antigen-negative blood for transfusion. In some patients, simple specificity will be readily apparent (eg, autoanti-e). When there is evidence of immune hemolysis and the autoantibody specificity appears to be simple, there may be some benefit in providing antigen-negative blood. However, it is important not to expose the patient to Rh antigens that their own rbcs lack, especially D. In in-stances where apparent specificity is directed to a high-incidence antigen (eg, anti-U), or when the autoantibody fails to react with rbcs of an uncommon Rh phenotype (eg, –D–, Rh$_{null}$), compatible donor blood is unlikely to be available for transfusion; thus, there is little point in determining specificity. If such blood is available, it should be reserved for alloimmunized patients of that uncommon phenotype. In rare cases where patients respond very poorly to infusion of "incompatible" rbcs, it may be appropriate to use rbcs lacking the Rh or high-incidence antigens.[17,30]

Cold Agglutinin Syndrome (Cold Agglutinin Disease)

CAS is the most common type of hemolytic anemia associated with cold-reactive autoantibodies, and accounts for approximately 16-32% of all cases of immune hemolysis.[1,2,21-23] It occurs as an acute or chronic condition. The acute form is often secondary to lymphoproliferative disorders (eg, lymphoma) or *Mycoplasma pneumoniae* infection. The chronic form is often seen in elderly patients and results in a mild to moderate degree of hemolysis; Raynaud's phenomenon and hemoglobinuria may occur in cold weather. Typical serologic findings are described below.

DAT

Complement (C3dg; see Chapter 7) is the only protein detected on the rbcs. The cold-reactive autoagglutinin is usually IgM that binds to rbcs in the peripheral circulation where the temperature may fall to 32 C. The IgM then binds complement components (C3 and C4, in particular) to the rbcs at this temperature. As the rbcs circulate to warmer areas, the IgM dissociates, leaving rbcs coated only with complement. Due to the action of Factors I and H (see Chapter 7) C3dg and C4d are the fragments of complement present on circulating rbcs, and it is the anti-C3d (-C4d) component of antiglobulin reagents that accounts for the positive DAT (see Chapter 8).

Serum

IgM cold-reactive autoagglutinins associated with immune hemolysis are usually present at titers greater than 1000 when tested at 4 C. They rarely react in vitro above 32 C in tests with saline-suspended rbcs. However, if 30% bovine albumin is included in the reaction medium, 70% of clinically significant examples will react at 37 C.[32] Hemolytic activity against untreated rbcs can sometimes be demonstrated at 20-25 C and, except in rare cases with anti-Pr specificity, enzyme-treated rbcs are hemolyzed in the presence of adequate complement. In chronic CAS the IgM autoagglutinin is usually a monoclonal protein of the kappa light-chain type. Polyclonal IgM immunoglobulin (with normal kappa and lambda light-chain distribution) is associated with the acute form of the disease. Rare examples of IgA and IgG cold-reactive autoagglutinins have also been described.

Eluate

If the rbcs have been collected properly and washed at 37 C, no antibody reactivity will be found in the eluate, as only complement components are present on the rbcs in vivo.[17]

Specificity of Autoantibody

The most common specificity associated with CAS is auto-anti-I. Less commonly, autoanti-i specificity is found, usually associated with infectious mononucleosis. On rare occasions, cold-reactive autoagglutinins with anti-Pr specificity, or other specificities, are seen (see Method 6.3).

Mixed-Type AIHA

In 1981,[23] 61 cases of an unusual AIHA were reported that serologically resembled both WAIHA and CAS. Patients having serologic features of both WAIHA and CAS had been previously reported.[1] These earlier reports indicated a WAIHA associated with a "classical" CAS (ie, titer of the cold autoagglutinin at 4 C >64). However, Sokol et al[23,33] found that the cold autoagglutinins in their patients were unusual in that they had low titers at 4 C but a high thermal amplitude (reactive at 30 C to 37 C). It was suggested that this immune hemolytic anemia may be a separate type from others and was termed mixed-type AIHA.[23] Since the original report, these observations have been confirmed and extended.[33-35]

Patients with mixed-type AIHA account for approximately 7-8% of all AIHAs.[33,34] It usually presents as an extremely acute condition primarily manifest by low hemoglobin concentrations.[34] Fortunately, these patients show a dramatic response to corticosteroid therapy and often do not need to be transfused.[34] It can be idiopathic or secondary, often associated with systemic lupus erythematosus.[33,34] Typical serologic findings are described below.

DAT

Both IgG and C3dg are usually detectable on the patients' rbcs. Presumably, the IgG is due to the warm autoantibody, while the C3dg is bound through a similar mechanism, as in CAS by IgM autoantibodies.

Serum

Both warm-reactive IgG autoantibodies and cold-reactive, hemagglutinating IgM autoantibodies are present in the patients' serum. Unlike CAS, the IgM hemagglutinating autoantibody(ies) usually have titers less than 64 at 4 C but react up to 37 C.[34]

Eluate

The eluate contains a warm-reactive IgG autoantibody.[34]

Specificity of Autoantibodies

The unusual cold-reactive IgM hemagglutinating autoantibody can have specificities typical of CAS (ie, anti-I, -i) but often has no apparent specificity.[33-35] The warm-reactive IgG autoantibody appears serologically indistinguishable from specificities encountered in typical WAIHA (see above). However, the IgG autoantibody may recognize an unusual blood group antigenic determinant distinct from that of more typical warm-reactive IgG autoantibodies.[35]

Paroxysmal Cold Hemoglobinuria

The rarest form of DAT-positive AIHA is PCH. In the past, it was characteristically associated with syphilis,[1,2] but this association is now unusual. More commonly, PCH presents as an acute transient condition secondary to viral infections, particularly in young children. It can also occur as an idiopathic chronic disease in older people. A recent, large study has shown that none of 531 adults having well-defined immune hemolytic anemias had PCH, while 22 of 68 (32%) children were shown to have PCH.[36] Typical serologic findings are described below.

DAT

The autoantibody in PCH is an IgG protein. Like IgM cold-reactive autoagglutinins, the IgG autoantibody in PCH reacts with rbcs in colder areas of the body (usually the extremities) causing complement components (C3 and C4) to be bound irreversibly to rbcs, and then elutes off the rbcs at warmer temperatures. Consequently, rbcs washed for the DAT are coated only with complement components. However, IgG may be detectable on rbcs when they are washed with cold (4 C) saline prior to the addition of cold anti-IgG AHG; this technique tends to allow antibodies of low binding affinity to remain attached to their respective epitope.

Serum

The IgG autoantibody in PCH is classically described as a biphasic hemolysin, since it binds to rbcs at low temperatures and then causes hemolysis when the coated rbcs are warmed to 37 C. This is the basis of the diagnostic test for the disease, the Donath-Landsteiner test (see Method 6.7). The autoantibody may agglutinate normal rbcs at 4 C, but rarely to titers greater than 64. Coating and complement binding are its usual properties. However, the autoantibody usually does not cause coating in vitro above 15 C.

Eluate

As in CAS, only complement components are usually present on rbcs in vivo. Consequently, eluates prepared from rbcs of patients with PCH are invariably nonreactive.

Specificity of Autoantibody

The autoantibody of PCH has most frequently been shown to have anti-P specificity; it reacts with all rbcs (including the patient's own rbcs) except those of the very rare p or P^k phenotypes. Exceptional examples with anti-I,[37] anti-i[38] and anti-Pr[39] specificity have also been described.

Investigation of Blood Samples Containing Autoantibodies

Serologic Classification of AIHAs

DATs performed with monospecific antiglobulin reagents, as well as the serum and eluate studies described earlier, can be used to classify AIHAs into one of the four major types (WAIHA, CAS, mixed-type AIHA, PCH). Three other procedures may be useful: a diagnostic cold agglutinin titer, the Donath-Landsteiner test for PCH and an eluate. These procedures are described in detail in the Methods section.

Interpretation of Results

The serologic classification of AIHA is summarized in Table 16-2. Answers to the following questions should help in the classification process:

1. *Are the patient's rbcs coated with antibody or complement, or both?*
   Most commercially prepared polyspecific antiglobulin reagents detect IgG- and C3dg-coated rbcs adequately. Complement coating may not be detected by polyspecific reagents unless negative tests are incubated at room temperature for 5-10 minutes before recentrifugation and rereading.[17] This also applies to those rare cases of WAIHA in which only IgA is present on rbcs.[24] A single nonreactive DAT obtained with a polyspecific antiglobulin reagent should not be considered conclusive evidence against AIHA in a patient with clinical signs and symptoms. Rare cases of WAIHA exist in which the

number of IgG molecules on the rbcs is below the threshold of sensitivity for the DAT, or the mechanism of immune hemolysis is unclear, and AIHA occurs in the absence of a positive DAT (termed DAT-negative AIHA).[40]

Rbcs coated with IgG alone, or with both IgG and C3dg, are encountered in the majority (87% to 91%) of cases of WAIHA.[1,23] C3dg coating alone is also seen in 7% to 13% of WAIHA cases, as well as in CAS and PCH. IgG and C3dg are usually detected using either polyspecific or monospecific antiglobulin reagents (see Chapter 8). Rarely, the DAT may be positive only when using polyspecific antihuman globulin.[23] IgA or IgM also may be present, in addition to IgG or complement, but this is not a common finding.

Care should be exercised when using monospecific antiglobulin reagents. Tests should be performed in parallel with a control, consisting of 1% bovine serum albumin in normal saline or manufacturers' diluent.[17] This control should detect any residual autoagglutination that occurs in CAS or rare cases of "spontaneous" agglutination that may occur in WAIHA. Failure to recognize this autoagglutination can lead to the incorrect conclusion that rbcs are coated with both IgG and complement (see Chapter 8). Anti-IgG, anti-C3d and the combined anti-C3b, -C3d reagents are the only licensed products available for use with human rbcs. Other antiglobulin reagents, including those prepared for use in precipitation tests such as immunodiffusion (eg, anti-IgA, -IgM, -C4), are available commercially. Their hemagglutinating reactivity should be carefully standardized by the user. Quality control must be rigid. Agglutination with antiglobulin reagents is a considerably more sensitive technique than precipitation; a serum found to be monospecific by precipitation tests may react with several different proteins in the antiglobulin test.[41]

2. *Does the serum contain antibodies? If so, are these antibodies: agglutinating or nonagglutinating? hemolytic in vitro? optimally reactive at warm (37 C) or cold (4 C) temperatures? autoantibodies? alloantibodies?*

These questions can often be answered by employing the serologic techniques usually used for the detection and identification of unexpected antibodies (see Chapters 14 and 15).

3. *Is antibody activity present in the eluate?*

If rbcs are coated only with complement, as in CAS and PCH, usually no antibody will be detected in the eluate. In some instances, autoantibody can be detected in eluates from these WAIHA cases if enzyme-treated rbcs are used, particularly if the eluate is concentrated prior to testing.

When antibody is found in the eluate, it is important to establish that it is autoantibody and not alloantibody made in response to recently transfused rbcs (see Chapter 15).

If the DAT is strongly reactive due to IgG coating and yet the eluate is nonreactive with untreated and enzyme-treated rbcs, the possibility should be considered that the immune hemolysis is secondary to transfusion with ABO-incompatible blood components or is drug-induced (eg, due to antipenicillin antibodies). See the final sections of this chapter for appropriate drug testing.

Additional Considerations

The following technical variations may be useful additions to routine tests:

1. Strict prewarmed tests.[17] The patient's serum and reagent rbcs should be warmed to 37 C separately, before mixing. The tests should be centrifuged at 37 C, and rbcs for IATs should be washed at 37 C using 37 C saline. Autoantibodies that are strongly reactive at room temperature will give the appearance of reactivity at 37 C unless temperature conditions are strictly controlled. This can confuse the classification of autoimmune hemolysis and misrepresent the clinical significance of the autoantibody.

2. Addition of complement. Patients with AIHA sometimes have low serum complement levels. Addition of complement, in the form of fresh normal serum, may yield positive tests when autoantibody activity is complement dependent.

3. Acidification of serum. Some workers[1,2] prefer to adjust the mixture of patient serum and complement to pH 6.5-6.8, as this seems to be optimal for the detection of both cold- and warm-reactive hemolysins. This can be achieved by adding one-tenth volume of 0.2 N HCl to the serum (check the final pH).

4. Enzyme tests. Both warm- and cold-reactive autoantibodies may give enhanced reactions with enzyme-treated rbcs. If these have not been used in the initial screening tests for unexpected antibodies, their use should be considered when the serological classification of autoimmune hemolysis is difficult. Enzyme-treated rbcs are usually more susceptible to hemolysis by autoantibodies than untreated rbcs.

Determining the Specificity of Warm-Reactive Autoantibodies

The specificity of warm-reactive autoantibodies is usually only of academic interest, unless the patient is actively hemolyzing and transfusion of "incompatible" blood is not adequately raising the patient's hematocrit. The undiluted serum or eluate usually reacts with all rbc samples of a common Rh phenotype, but variations in reaction strength may be observed. If rbcs of such rare phenotypes as $-D-$ or Rh_{null} are available, approximately 70% of warm-reactive autoantibodies can be shown to have an Rh-related specificity. Apparent simple Rh specificity such as anti-D, -C, -c, -E or -e is present only rarely, anti-e being the most common. If Rh-related specificity is not observed in tests with the undiluted serum or eluate, such "relative" specificity may become apparent on dilution, or may be determined from the results of adsorption and elution studies. In rare instances of WAIHA involving IgM agglutinins, determining autoantibody specificity may help differentiate such cases from CAS.[42] Examples of autoantibodies with specificities for other blood group system antigens have also been reported.[25-31]

Although warm-reactive autoantibodies, in many cases, appear to recognize some component of the Rh blood group system, this association with Rh may be a pseudophenomenon. These autoantibodies may not actually be directed to Rh antigens. Indeed, 80% of warm-reactive autoantibodies react best with older rbcs, while 20% react equally well with reticulocyte-enriched rbcs.[28] The former specificity has been termed type I and the latter termed type II.[28] Based on these findings, it has been postulated that the true specificity of most warm-reactive autoantibodies may be due to the senescence rbc antigen.[28] This hypothesis, however, requires further studies.

Determining the Specificity of Cold-Reactive Autoantibodies

The specificity of cold-reactive autoantibodies is not diagnostic for CAS.

Autoanti-I may be seen in healthy subjects and in patients with CAS.[7] The nonpathologic forms of autoanti-I rarely react to titers above 64 at 4 C, and are usually nonreactive with I$-$ (i_{cord} and i_{adult}) rbcs at room temperature. In contrast, the pathologic forms of autoanti-I that are seen in CAS may react quite strongly with I$-$ rbcs in tests at room temperature, while even stronger reactions are observed with I+ rbcs. Autoanti-i antibodies react in the opposite manner; they give much stronger reactions with I$-$ rbcs than with rbcs that are I+. Titration/thermal amplitude testing can be used to determine the specificities of cold-reactive autoantibodies. A procedure for this is given in Methods 6.2 and 6.3. In mixed-type AIHA the cold-reactive autoantibody may be weakly reactive at 4 C but usually reacts at up to 37 C.[34]

Management of Patients With Autoantibodies

In pretransfusion tests on patients with autoantibodies, the following problems may arise:

1. Cold-reactive autoantibodies can cause autoagglutination, resulting in erroneous determinations of ABO and Rh type.

2. Red cells strongly coated with globulins may undergo spontaneous agglutination when exposed to the high-protein content of some commercially prepared anti-Rh blood grouping reagents, resulting in discrepant results. Rarely, this phenomenon happens even when using low-protein reagents.[17,43]

3. The presence of free autoantibody in the serum may make it virtually impossible to obtain serologically compatible blood for transfusion. Of particular concern in this situation is

the possibility that the autoantibody may be masking the presence of a clinically significant alloantibody. Providing time permits, the presence or absence of alloantibody should be determined (see Methods 6.4 through 6.6) before blood is transfused.

Although resolving these serologic problems is important in ensuring safe transfusion management of patients with autoantibodies, delaying transfusion in the hope of finding serologically compatible blood may in some cases cause greater danger to the patient. Only clinical judgment can resolve this dilemma. Dialogue with the patient's physician is important.

Resolution of ABO Grouping Problems

There are several approaches to the resolution of ABO grouping problems associated with cold-reactive autoagglutinins. Often, it is only necessary to maintain the blood sample at 37 C immediately after collection and to wash the rbcs with warm (37-45 C) saline before testing.[1,17] In this situation, it is advisable to perform a parallel control test, using 6% bovine albumin in saline, to determine if autoagglutination still occurs.[17] If the control test is nonreactive, the results obtained with anti-A and anti-B are usually valid. When autoagglutination still occurs, interpretation of the results can be difficult, but comparing the strength of the observed reactions may be informative. If the blood sample has been kept at room temperature, or if cold-reactive autoagglutinins are particularly potent, it may be necessary to treat the rbcs with thiol reagents. Since cold-reactive autoagglutinins are invariably IgM and thiol reagents depolymerize IgM molecules (see Chapter 15), reagents such as

2-mercaptoethanol or dithiothreitol (DTT) can be used to abolish autoagglutination and permit accurate ABO and Rh typing of the rbcs (see Method 2.13). Another means of dispersing autoagglutination uses the ZZAP reagent or glycine-HCl/EDTA (see Methods 2.16 and 6.4). An alternative but less effective means of dispersing autoagglutination due to cold-reactive autoantibodies is to incubate the rbcs at 45 C for 10 minutes and wash them several times in saline at that temperature (see Method 2.14).

When the serum agglutinates group O reagent rbcs, the results of reverse typing tests may be unreliable. Repeat studies using prewarmed serum and A, B and O rbcs at 37 C will usually resolve any discrepancy. However, anti-A or -B will not always react in reverse grouping tests at 37 C. Alternatively, adsorbed serum (either autoadsorbed or adsorbed with allogeneic group O rbcs) can be used.

NOTE: Sera adsorbed with rabbit rbcs or rbc stroma may not contain anti-B since such rbcs carry a B-like antigen. Sera adsorbed in this manner should not be used for ABO reverse grouping. See later in this chapter for appropriate use and limitations of rabbit rbc adsorptions.

Resolution of Rh Typing Problems

Spontaneous agglutination of rbcs by cold- or warm-reactive autoantibodies may also cause discrepant Rh typing. These problems may be obviated by using the same procedures described for the resolution of ABO grouping problems. Rbcs strongly coated with globulins (eg, in WAIHA) may spontaneously agglutinate when mixed with antisera containing high concentrations of proteins such as bovine albumin, or other potentiators of agglutination. Most Rh typing discrepancies occur with IgG-coated rbcs when high-protein reagents designated for use by slide or rapid tube tests (sometimes referred to as modified-tube anti-Rh) are employed.[43] The use of the ZZAP reagent, with inclusion of appropriate controls, or the use of chemically modified or saline-reactive reagents may be necessary to avoid erroneous results (see Chapter 11).

Detection of Alloantibodies in the Presence of Warm-Reactive Autoantibodies

If warm-reactive autoantibodies are present in the serum, it is important to establish that alloantibodies are not also present if the patient requires blood transfusions. Alloantibodies may not be readily apparent from the results of initial studies; their presence may be masked by autoantibodies. It is helpful to know which of the common rbc antigens are lacking on the patient's rbcs. This permits prediction of the clinically significant alloantibodies a patient is capable of producing. If the patient's rbcs lack a particular blood group antigen, then the possibility exists that the serum may contain alloantibody to that antigen. When the rbcs are coated with IgG, antiglobulin-reactive reagents such as anti-Fy^a or anti-Jk^a cannot be used unless the IgG is first removed from the rbcs before testing. Procedures for this are given in the Methods section. Alternatively, blood grouping reagents can be adsorbed with the patient's rbcs, and tested by titration for a decrease in reactivity.[44] However, this is time-consuming and requires large volumes of expensive blood grouping reagents.

There are several ways to detect alloantibodies in the presence of warm-reactive autoantibodies. Some procedures involve the use of adsorption techniques, the principles of which are discussed in Chapter 15. Three widely used approaches are discussed below.

Autologous Adsorption

Autologous adsorption is the best way to detect alloantibodies in the presence of warm-reactive autoantibodies (see Method 6.4) in patients not recently transfused. Simple antibody detection tests can be done on the adsorbed serum to determine the presence or absence of unexpected alloantibodies. At 37 C, in-vivo adsorption will have occurred and all antigen sites on the patient's own rbcs may be blocked. It is necessary, therefore, to elute autoantibody from the rbcs to make the sites available for in-vitro autoantibody adsorption. In addition, treatment of the autologous rbcs with proteolytic enzymes increases their capacity to adsorb autoantibody. Once autoantibody has been removed, the adsorbed serum is examined for alloantibody activity. Autologous adsorption studies are generally used in instances where a patient has not been recently transfused (ie, there are no circulating transfused rbcs that might be capable of adsorbing an alloantibody). The word "recent" in this context is usually taken to mean within the normal rbc life span of 3-4 months. However, autologous adsorption studies may be informative even in the face of a more recent transfusion (eg, one week), although failure to detect alloantibody in "autoadsorbed" serum from a recently transfused patient should never be considered as conclusive evidence for the absence of alloantibody. It is also possible to separate the patient's own rbcs (ie, reticulocytes) from the transfused rbcs[45] and to use the harvested autologous rbcs in autoadsorption experiments. However, these techniques are highly variable, may require expensive equipment and require considerable expertise in interpretation.

Allogeneic Adsorption

Use of allogeneic rbcs for adsorption studies are appropriate when the patient has been recently transfused, or when insufficient rbcs are available for autoadsorption. When the patient's Rh phenotype is not known, group O rbc samples of three different Rh phenotypes (R_1, R_2 and r) should be selected. One should lack Jk^a and another Jk^b. These rbcs are treated with ZZAP (a mixture of papain and dithiothreitol). Such rbcs lack M, N, S, s, Fy^a, Fy^b and all Kell-system antigens.[46] A two- or threefold adsorption for each aliquot may be necessary. After adsorption the aliquots are tested against selected group O screening rbcs known either to lack or to carry common antigens of the Rh, MN, Kidd, Kell and Duffy blood group systems. Adsorbing the serum with different rbc samples provides a battery of specimens that can be used for antibody detection and identification purposes. For example, if the aliquot adsorbed with Jk(a–) rbcs subsequently reacts only with Jk(a+) rbcs, the presence of alloanti-Jk^a can be inferred.

The number of different rbc phenotypes required may be reduced if the patient's Rh and/or Kidd phenotype is known. In cases where the patient has been recently transfused, it may be possible to determine this following separation of autologous from transfused rbcs. If the patient's Rh and Kidd phenotypes are known or can be determined, it is possible to use one allogeneic rbc sample, selected to have the same Rh and Kidd phenotypes, which is ZZAP-treated, for use in a so-called one-cell ZZAP allogeneic adsorption technique (Shulman IA, personal communication; see Method 6.6).

Untreated rbcs also may be used for allogeneic adsorptions, although they may not be as efficient as ZZAP-treated rbcs in removing autoantibody. The phenotypes of the untreated rbcs should be selected to include samples lacking Fy^a, Fy^b, S and s antigens.

Autoantibodies Mimicking Alloantibodies

When interpreting the results of tests used to detect alloantibodies in the presence of autoantibodies, autoantibody reactivity may occasionally be mistaken for alloantibody.[47] For example, the serum of an r patient may have apparent anti-C and -e activity. Even though the patient's rbcs lack the C antigen, the anti-C reactivity may in fact be due to warm-reactive autoantibody. That such reactivity is due to autoantibody can be determined through the use of autologous and allogeneic adsorption studies. In the situation mentioned, the anti-e is assumed to be auto but the apparent alloanti-C will be adsorbed to both autologous and allogeneic r rbcs. This is quite unlike the behavior of a "true" alloanti-C, which will be adsorbed only by C+ rbcs.

Detection of Alloantibodies in the Presence of Cold-Reactive Autoantibodies

Usually, cold-reactive autoagglutinins will not mask clinically significant alloantibodies if serum tests are conducted at 37 C, without use of potentiating agents such as albumin, and monospecific anti-IgG reagents are used for IAT. In rare instances, it may be necessary to adsorb the serum at 4 C using the patient's own rbcs (see Method 6.1). This should reveal clinically significant alloantibodies masked by very potent cold-reactive autoantibodies. Achieving complete removal of potent cold-reactive autoagglutinins is very time-consuming. ZZAP treatment of the patient's rbcs before adsorption may facilitate removal of autoantibody.[46] If autologous adsorption studies are inappropriate because the patient has been recently transfused, or if complete removal of the autoantibody is not possible, tests for alloantibody activity may be carried out *strictly* at 37 C. The patient's serum and reagent rbcs should be warmed to 37 C prior to mixing. Since bovine albumin and other enhancement media increase the reactivity of cold-reactive autoantibodies,[17,32] their use is contraindicated in these studies. If centrifugation at 37 C is impossible, and if time permits, tests can be incubated at 37 C for 1-2 hours to allow the rbcs to settle; they can then be examined for agglutination without centrifugation. The rbcs should be washed in saline at 37 C and then tested with anti-IgG to avoid possible misleading results due to complement bound by the cold-reactive autoantibody. EDTA-anticoagulated plasma, or serum to which EDTA has been added (2 mL serum plus 0.25 mL 4.45% K_2EDTA),[48] can also be used to avoid interference by complement-binding autoantibodies.

Transfusion Considerations

Selection of Blood for Patients With WAIHA

If transfusion is essential, the smallest volume of rbcs necessary to maintain adequate oxygen transportation should be given. Serologically compatible blood is not usually obtainable, and there is substantial risk that concomitant alloantibodies could cause a severe hemolytic transfusion reaction (HTR). The clinical need must justify the risk of transfusion, but needed transfusions should not be withheld because serologically compatible blood cannot be

found.[17,18] Clinical judgment must always be the deciding factor.

It is extremely important to determine the proper ABO group of the patient and, if time permits, to determine the Rh and presence of underlying, potentially clinically significant alloantibodies present in the serum. Since autoantibodies may mask the presence of alloantibodies capable of causing a severe HTR, it is advisable to use techniques such as the autoadsorption procedures discussed in Method 6.4. If clinically significant alloantibodies are present, blood lacking the corresponding antigen(s) should be selected for transfusion.

If the autoantibody has apparent specificity for a single antigen (eg, anti-e), blood lacking that antigen (R_2) may be selected. There is evidence that such rbcs survive better than the patient's rbcs.[1,4,17,25,49,50] However, D+ blood should not be given to a D– patient with apparent anti-e autoantibody. If the autoantibody has relative Rh specificity (eg, reacts preferentially with e+ rbcs) the use of blood lacking the corresponding antigen is debatable.[17]

In many cases of WAIHA, no autoantibody specificity is apparent; the patient's serum reacts with all rbc samples tested to the same degree, or reacts with rbcs from different donors to varying degrees for reasons seemingly unrelated to their respective Rh phenotypes. In such cases, some workers test a large number of donor blood samples (eg, 12-20) and select those units that give the weakest reactions in vitro. There are no data to indicate a better in-vivo survival of these "least" incompatible rbcs, but some workers feel more comfortable issuing the least incompatible units. Other workers recommend ignoring the "specificity" of the autoantibody. After the presence of alloantibody has been excluded, they suggest giving blood of the same Rh phenotype as the patient to avoid subsequent development of Rh alloantibodies.[18,51]

While few data regarding the in-vivo significance of autoantibodies exist, a minority of these autoantibodies appear to react specifically, and there are no data to prove such specificity is insignificant. In cases of severe and progressive anemia, it may be essential to transfuse blood that does not react with the patient's autoantibody.[30] However, usually, warm-reactive autoantibodies are unlikely to cause an acute hemolytic transfusion reaction. Although rbc survival may not be normal, transfusion with incompatible blood may provide sufficient oxygen-carrying cells until other therapy can effect a more lasting benefit.[1,2,3,18,51]

In summary, transfusion of patients with WAIHA should be undertaken only if absolutely essential, with the realization that the blood is not truly compatible and its effects are likely to be brief. The volume transfused should be the least amount required to maintain adequate oxygen supply. The patient's ABO and Rh group should be determined and an attempt made to differentiate autoantibody from alloantibody in the serum. If specificity is obvious, the appropriate donor blood should, if feasible, be selected. Blood should never be withheld from a patient with severe life-threatening anemia because of incompatibility due to autoantibodies.

Selection of Blood for Patients With CAS

Patients suffering from CAS occasionally require transfusion. If the need arises, compatibility tests should be performed in ways that minimize cold-reactive autoantibody activity yet still permit detection of clinically significant alloantibodies.[17,52] Some workers perform

compatibility tests strictly at 37 C. The use of albumin and other potentiators increases the detection of these autoantibodies and, thus, should be avoided, since these enhance the complement-binding properties of the autoantibody. Further, to avoid the detection of bound complement, some workers use a monospecific anti-IgG reagent, rather than a polyspecific antiglobulin serum, for the IAT.

When these methods fail to avoid detection of cold-reactive autoantibody, it is advisable to perform autoadsorption studies (see Method 6.1). This should make it possible to detect alloantibodies masked by the cold-reactive autoantibody. This autoadsorbed serum may be used for compatibility testing, providing the patient has not been transfused within the past 3-4 months. If the patient has been recently transfused, rabbit rbcs may be used to remove autoanti-I and -IH from sera,[53] and a preparation of rabbit rbc stroma is commercially available. However, adsorption with rabbit rbc stroma may remove clinically significant alloantibodies.[54] Alternatively, allogeneic adsorption studies can be performed as for WAIHA (see above).

Selection of Blood for Patients With Mixed-Type AIHA

Patients with mixed-type AIHA, although often presenting with severe anemia, respond rapidly and dramatically to steroid therapy.[34] If blood transfusions are necessary, the considerations in the selection of blood for transfusion are identical to those described for warm antibody type AIHA (see above). In addition, the use of albumin and other potentiators of agglutination reactions should be avoided and monospecific anti-IgG, rather than a polyspecific antihuman globulin reagent, should be used for the IAT.

Selection of Blood for Patients With PCH

Sera from patients with PCH will be compatible with random donor rbcs when tested by routine crossmatch procedures. The causative antibody, demonstrated by the Donath-Landsteiner test described in Method 6.7, rarely reacts as an agglutinin above 4 C. The antibody usually has anti-P specificity; it does not react with rare p and P^k rbcs. While there is some evidence that p rbcs survive better than P+ (P_1+ or P_1−) rbcs,[55] the incidence of p blood is approximately 1 in 200,000. Moreover, PCH patients often require transfusion before rare blood can be obtained, and the transfusion of random donor blood should not be withheld from PCH patients requiring urgent transfusion.[1] Rare p blood should be considered only for those patients who do not respond to random donor blood.

Drug-Induced Immune Hemolytic Anemias

Drugs sometimes induce the formation of antibodies, either against the drug itself or against intrinsic rbc antigens.

Most drugs have a molecular weight substantially below the 5000-dalton level usually considered the threshold for effective immunogenicity. Thus, drugs may act as haptens (see Chapter 7), eliciting antibody only after they have been firmly bound to a protein carrier. Once produced, the antibody can react with the small hapten (drug) independent of any protein attachment. Drugs may cause a positive DAT, which may or may not be associated with immune hemolysis, by one of four postulated mechanisms (Table 16-4).

Mechanisms of RBC Sensitization

Drug Adsorption

Approximately 3% of patients receiving large doses of penicillin intravenously (eg, millions of units per day) will develop a positive DAT, but less than 5% of these will develop hemolytic anemia.[5] Intravascular hemolysis is rare. A possible mechanism of the positive DAT is given in Fig 16-1. The penicillin becomes covalently linked to the rbcs in vivo. If the patient has formed antibodies to penicillin, the antipenicillin will react

Table 16-4. Serologic Findings Associated With Drug-Induced Positive DATs

Mechanism	Examples	DAT	Serum and Eluate
Drug Adsorption	Penicillins, cephalosporins	IgG (sometimes C3 also)	React with drug-coated rbcs but not untreated rbcs
Immune Complex	Phenacetin, quinidine, third generation cephalosporins	C3 (sometimes IgG also)	Serum reacts with rbcs only in the presence of the drug; eluate nonreactive
Nonimmunologic Protein Adsorption	Cephalothin	IgG + C3 + albumin, etc	Serum may contain low titer anti-drug antibody; eluate nonreactive
Autoimmunity	α-methyldopa (Aldomet), procainamide	IgG (rarely C3 also)	React with normal rbcs in absence of the drug

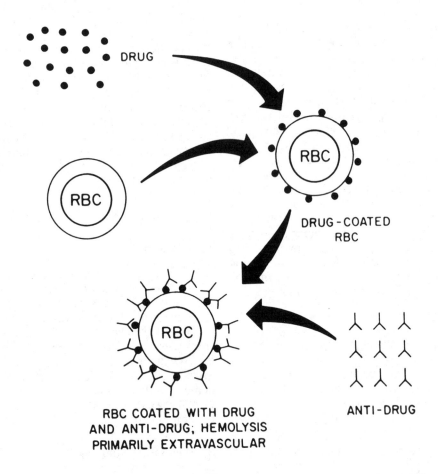

Figure 16-1. The drug-adsorption mechanism. The drug binds tightly to the rbc membrane proteins. If a patient develops a potent anti-drug antibody, it will react with the cell-bound drug. Such rbcs will yield a positive result in the DAT using anti-IgG reagents. Complement is usually not activated and lysis is primarily extravascular in nature. Penicillin-G is the prototype drug. (Reprinted with permission from Petz and Branch.[5])

with the penicillin bound to the rbcs. The result is that the penicillin-coated rbcs become coated with IgG. Complement is not usually involved. If hemolysis occurs, rbcs are usually destroyed extravascularly, probably in the same way that rbcs coated with IgG alloantibodies are destroyed. Drugs such as penicillin have several distinct haptenic groups, the most important of which is the benzyl-penicilloyl (BPO) group.[5] With sufficiently sensitive techniques, most adult human sera can be shown to contain BPO antibodies. These are usually IgM and of low titer; however, some sera contain an IgG component. The high incidence of penicillin antibodies in the normal population probably reflects the widespread exposure to this drug.[5] There is no direct correlation between the presence of IgM and IgG antibodies to penicillin and allergic reactions to the drug. These are due to IgE antibodies.

The clinical and laboratory features of drug-induced immune hemolytic anemia operating through the drug adsorption mechanism are:

1. The DAT is strongly positive due to IgG coating. Rarely, complement coating also may be present, but this is usually very weak.[1]
2. Unless rbc alloantibodies are also present, screening tests for unexpected serum antibodies will be nonreactive.
3. Antibody eluted from the rbcs will react with in-vitro drug-coated rbcs but not with uncoated rbcs.
4. At least with penicillin, a high-titer IgG antibody is always present in the serum.
5. Hemolysis typically develops only in patients receiving very large doses of intravenous drug; penicillin-induced hemolytic anemia requires millions of units daily for a week or more.
6. Hemolysis is subacute in onset, but may be life-threatening if the etiology is unrecognized and drug administration is continued.
7. Discontinuation of the causative drug is usually followed by cessation of hemolysis. However, hemolysis of decreasing severity may persist for several weeks.

Immune Complex Adsorption

Some drugs do not bind directly to rbcs but have a high affinity for their specific antibodies and form antigen-antibody complexes that circulate in the plasma. These immune complexes can attach to rbcs and initiate complement activation on the rbc surface (Fig 16-2). This may lead to intravascular or extravascular hemolysis. Rbcs that are not hemolyzed have a positive DAT because of complement coating, but immunoglobulin may also be bound. Often, only complement coating is demonstrable on the rbc surface because the immune complex binds loosely to the rbcs. The immune complexes may dissociate after activating complement and go on to react with other rbcs. This may explain why small amounts of the drug can induce acute hemolytic episodes. Although many drugs have been described as causing a positive DAT, immune hemolysis or both through this mechanism, most are reports of single cases. This mechanism is the one least often encountered when investigating drug-induced immune hemolysis. The characteristic findings are:

1. Acute intravascular hemolysis with hemoglobinemia and hemoglobinuria is the usual presentation. Renal failure occurs in approximately 50% of cases.
2. Once antibody has been formed, the patient may experience severe hemolytic episodes after taking only small quantities of the drug.
3. The antibody can be either IgM or IgG.
4. The rbcs are often coated only with complement.
5. In-vitro reactions such as agglutination, hemolysis and reactive IATs can be demonstrated only when the patient's serum and reagent rbcs are incubated in the presence of the drug.

Nonimmunologic Protein Adsorption

Drugs of the cephalosporins (primarily cephalothin) are the only drugs that are thought to react with rbc membranes in such a way that the rbcs nonimmuno-

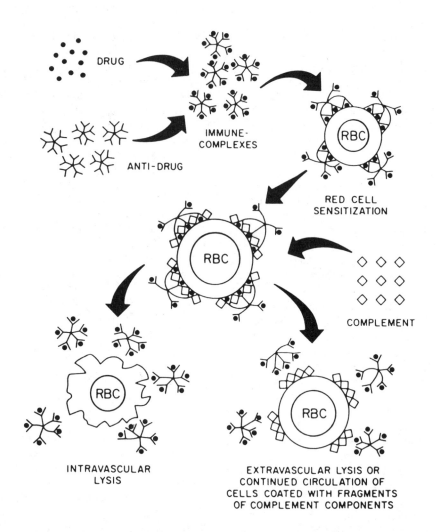

Figure 16-2. The immune-complex mechanism. Anti-drug antibody reacts with the drug to form an immune complex. The drug-antibody complex is then adsorbed onto rbcs, possibly by interaction with specific receptors. The cell-bound complexes may activate complement and result in intravascular hemolysis or may elute off the rbcs, leaving only complement components. Some of these complement-coated rbcs may be lysed by phagocytic cells of the mononuclear phagocyte system. The complement components on other erythrocytes are inactivated by complement inhibitors, leaving fragments of complement components (eg, C3dg), which are detectable by the DAT. After elution of immune complexes from rbcs in vivo, it is conceivable that they may interact with additional rbcs, thereby explaining the severity of the hemolysis even after administration of only small doses of the offending drug. Quinine and phenacetin are prototype drugs. (Reprinted with permission from Petz and Branch.[5])

logically adsorb proteins from the plasma or serum. Rbcs coated with cephalothin (Keflin) and incubated with normal plasma will adsorb albumin, IgA, IgG, IgM and β and α (ie, complement) globulins.[5,56] When this occurs in vivo, it can give rise to a positive DAT; antisera to any human serum protein, not just anti-IgG or anti-C3, will react.

Although unproven, a mechanism for this nonimmunologic adsorption of serum proteins has been proposed.[5,57] Based on experimental data indicating that cephalothin, unlike other β-lactam antibiotics, can bind firmly in vitro to rbcs at acid pH, it was hypothesized that cephalothin binds to rbcs at neutral or acid pH in a manner independent from the usual mechanism of binding to rbc membrane proteins via the alkaline pH-dependent reactive β-lactam moiety of the molecule. Once the cephalothin becomes bound to the rbc via this pH-independent mechanism, any serum protein can then become bound to the drug via an accessible, potentially reactive, β-lactam group. Figure 16-3 presents a schematic representation of this hypothetical model.

In addition to this nonimmune adsorption of proteins, the cephalosporins can also induce a positive DAT by the drug adsorption mechanism described for penicillin (see above). The drug binds firmly to rbcs, which then interact with the specific anticephalosporin antibody. These anticephalosporins cross-react with penicillin-treated rbcs.[5,58] Approximately 4% of patients receiving first- or second-generation cephalosporins develop a positive DAT.[1,5,56] There have been occasional reports of hemolysis resulting from cephalosporin therapy; these are thought to result from the effects of specific anticephalosporin antibodies, rather than from nonimmunologic adsorption of proteins following rbc membrane modifica-

tion.[1,5,58] However, the incidence and severity of cephalosporin-induced immune hemolysis appears to be increasing.[59]

Induction of Autoimmunity

The first cases of WAIHA resulting from α-methyldopa (Aldomet, Aldoclor, Aldoril, Merck Sharp and Dohme, West Point, PA) therapy were described in 1966. A closely related drug (L-dopa) has also been reported to cause a positive DAT and immune hemolysis, as have procainamide and mefenamic acid (Ponstel, Parke-Davis, Morris Plains, NJ), drugs unrelated to α-methyldopa.[1,5]

Following α-methyldopa therapy, autoantibodies are formed that react with intrinsic rbc antigens. They do not react with the drug in vitro, either directly or indirectly. The serologic findings are indistinguishable from those associated with WAIHA; often, the autoantibody can be found to have an Rh-related specificity.[1] It has been postulated that the drug alters the intrinsic rbc antigen so that this antigen is no longer recognized as self by the immune system (Fig 16-4). It has also been postulated that the drug interferes with suppressor T-cell function, allowing overproduction of autoantibody by B cells.[60] However, recent studies cannot confirm these earlier findings.[61] It has also been suggested that the autoantibody causing the hemolysis is qualitatively different from the nonhemolytic autoantibody found in the majority of DAT-positive patients receiving α-methyldopa.[62]

Therapy with α-methyldopa used to account for more cases of drug-induced positive DATs and immune hemolysis than all of the other drugs listed in Table 16-5 together. In a series of 347 patients with immune hemolytic anemia,[1] 12% were drug-induced; of these, almost 70% were due to α-methyldopa, 23% were

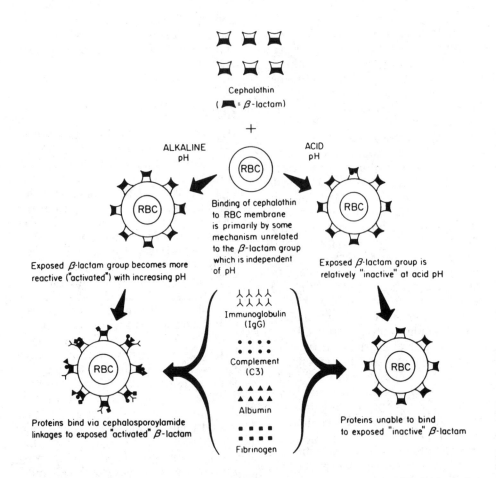

Figure 16-3. Hypothetical model for cephalothin-induced nonimmunologic protein adsorption onto rbcs. Unlike most β-lactam antibiotics, cephalothin can bind to rbc surfaces through a non β-lactam-mediated, pH-independent mechanism, possibly involving one or both side chains. Because this mechanism of cephalothin binding to rbcs does not involve the "reactive" β-lactam group, this group remains available for reaction with serum proteins under neutral or alkaline pH. This nonimmunologic mechanism results in a variety of proteins being detectable on the rbc surface when using antihuman protein reagents including anti-IgG and anti-C3. Under acid pH conditions, the cephalothin can still bind to the rbc but the β-lactam group cannot interact with other proteins. Thus, nonimmunologic protein adsorption is much less of a problem when acid conditions are used to coat rbcs with cephalothin. (See Petz and Branch,[5] Branch et al.[54])

due to penicillin and the remainder were associated with drugs that form immune complexes. The clinical and laboratory features associated with α-methyldopa-induced autoantibodies are as follows:

1. Positive DATs occur in approximately 15% of patients receiving α-methyldopa. Only 0.5-1.0% of patients taking α-methyldopa develop hemolytic anemia.[1,5]

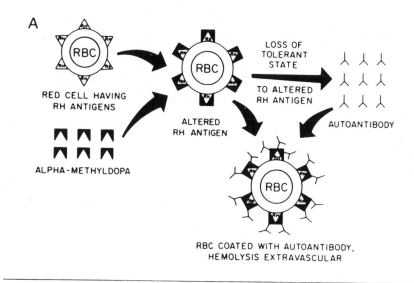

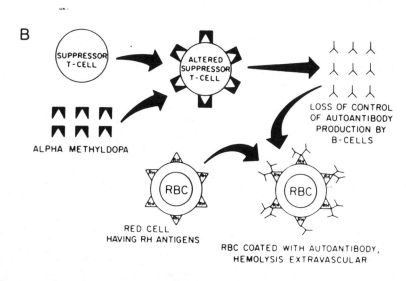

Figure 16-4. Drug-induced autoimmune hemolytic anemias, α-methyldopa is the prototype drug. (A) Altered rbc antigen hypothesis. In a susceptible host, α-methyldopa may bind tightly to the rbc membrane and alter rbc Rh-antigen protein. This alteration is such that the host loses tolerance to the altered protein antigen and forms autoantibodies. These autoantibodies will react best with the altered antigen but will also cross-react with unaltered antigen. The DAT and IAT are positive without addition of drug to the in-vitro test system. (B) Abnormal suppressor T-cell function hypothesis. In a susceptible host, α-methyldopa diminishes suppressor T-cell function. This results in unregulated autoantibody production by B cells. The DAT and IAT are positive without addition of drug to the in-vitro test system. (Reprinted with permission from Petz and Branch.[5])

Table 16-5. Compounds Reported to Cause Immune Hemolysis and/or a Positive DAT

Drug	Mechanism	Drug	Mechanism
Acetaminophen	IC	Latamoxef	?
Aminopyrine	IC	Levodopa	AI
p-Aminosalicylic acid (PAS)	IC	Mefenamic acid	AI
Antazoline	IC	Melphalan	IC
Buthizide metabolites	IC?	Methadone	?
Carbimazole	IC	Methotrexate	IC
Carbromal	DA	α-Methyldopa	AI
Cephalosporins,		Methysergide	?
first generation	DA/NA	Nomifensine	AI/IC
second generation	DA/IC	Penicillins	DA
third generation	DA/IC	Phenacetin	AI/DA/IC
Chaparral	AI?	Podophyllotoxin derivatives	?
Chlorinated hydrocarbons	IC	Probenicid	IC
Chlorproamide	IC	Procainamide	AI
Chlorpromazine	AI/IC	Pyramidon	IC
Cianidanol	AI/DA/IC	Quinidine	DA/IC
Cisplatin	NA?	Quinine	IC
Diclofenac	AI/IC	Rifampicin	IC
Diglycoaldehyde	NA	Sodium pentothal	IC
Dipyrone	DA/IC	Stibophen	IC
Erythromycin	DA	Streptomycin	AI/DA/IC
Fenfluramine	?	Sulphonamides	IC
Fluorouracil (5-FU)	IC	Sulphonylurea derivatives	IC
Furosemide	?	Suramin	NA
Glafenine	?	Teniposide (VM-26)	AI/IC
Hydralazine	IC	Tetracycline	DA/IC
Hydrochlorothiazide	IC	Thiopental	IC
9-Hydroxymethyl ellipticinium	IC	Tolbutamide	DA
Ibuprofen	AI	Tolmetin	?
Inosine dialdehyde	?	Triamterene	IC
Insulin	DA/IC	Trimellitic anhydride	?
Isoniazid	DA/IC	Zomepirac	DA/IC, ?

AI = autoimmunity; DA = drug adsorption; IC = immune complex; NA = nonimmunologic protein adsorption; ? = mechanism unclear. For most of the drugs that have been reported to cause drug-induced immune hemolysis by the IC mechanism alone, there is only a single case report.

2. Rbcs are usually coated only with IgG; rarely, weak complement coating has been reported.[1,5]

3. The DAT usually becomes positive only after 3-6 months of α-methyldopa therapy.[1,5]

4. Development of a positive DAT is dose dependent; approximately 36% of patients taking 3 g of the drug daily develop a positive DAT, compared with 11% of patients receiving 1 g per day.[1,5]

5. Antibodies in the serum and on the rbcs are indistinguishable from those found in WAIHA.[1,4,5,62]

6. The strength of the positive DAT becomes progressively weaker once α-methyldopa therapy is discontinued. This may take from 1 month to 2 years. In patients with hemolytic anemia due to α-methyldopa therapy, hematologic values usually improve within the first week or so after the drug therapy is discontinued.[62]

The above discussion of drug-induced AIHA used α-methyldopa as the prototype drug responsible for the majority of cases. However, α-methyldopa is now rarely prescribed since more effective antihypertensive drugs, having fewer side effects, have become available. Thus, the incidence of drug-induced AIHA may become lower as a result of less use of α-methyldopa. However, use of other, relatively new drugs such as nomifensine, cianidanol, diclofenac and others (see Table 16-5), which can result in AIHA as a consequence of their usage, will continue to have an impact on transfusion medicine despite the decreased usage of α-methyldopa.

Alternative Mechanisms

New insights into how drugs might induce antibodies is now accumulating that begins to raise questions regarding the previously postulated mechanisms of drug-induced immune hemolysis stated above.[63-66] Although a hapten-carrier mechanism would seem most likely as mediating drug-induced immune responses, a number of considerations raise doubt regarding this mechanism. Basic immunologic concepts indicate that the low molecular weight of drugs (haptens) allows them to be immunogenic only when bound to a carrier molecule. However, hapten-carrier-mediated immune responses require specific B-cell recognition of the hapten in conjunction with specific T helper cell recognition of a *nonself* carrier molecule. Thus, autologous proteins cannot serve a carrier function for hapten-mediated immune responses; presumably, T cells that have the potential to recognize self are deleted from the repertoire during ontogeny through the thymus (see Chapter 7). A suitable carrier molecule, however, may be provided as a constituent contained in the pharmaceutical drug preparation, by microbial proteins as a result of infection, or if an autologous protein becomes altered in some way so that it no longer appears to the host immune system as self.

However, haptens usually must bind firmly to, or are part of, the carrier molecule, while most drugs that can induce immune responses associate very weakly with cellular proteins.[63-66] Furthermore, drug-induced immune responses show extraordinary specificity to particular cellular targets such as rbcs or platelets.[66] This exquisite specificity would seem unlikely if a classical hapten-carrier-mediated mechanism was involved. Considerations such as these led investigators away from hapten-carrier-mediated mechanisms of drug-induced immune responses to alternative mechanisms, devised mainly to describe the in-vitro serologic characteristics of drug-induced immune antibodies (the immune complex, drug adsorption and autoimmune mechanisms discussed in the previous section). Recent attempts to describe the in-vivo mechanism(s) of drug-induced antibody production have led some investigators to postulate a new, unifying theory for how drugs induce antibodies.[63]

It has been proposed[63] that the production of drug-induced antibodies depends on the ability of the drug to interact with specific cell membrane components, thus altering the normal self components so that they are no longer recognized as self. This "neoantigen" that is formed appears foreign to the host immune system. This theory assumes that drugs bind with variable affinity to a particular cellular membrane component present on rbcs, granuloctyes or platelets. The degree of association would be expected to depend on numerous factors that may include the chemical structure of the drug or its metabolite(s), the concentration of the drug, the structure of cellular membrane proteins and the susceptibility of the host proteins to associate with the drug (possibly dependent on pH, temperature, ionic strength and, most probably, host genetic factors). Because conditions must be just right for this association to be of high enough affinity to provoke an immune response, instances of drug-induced immunity would be expected to be relatively rare, which is, in fact, the case.[5]

The neoantigen hypothesis allows for interesting speculations as to how drugs induce antibodies. The association of the drug with the cellular membrane may result in the formation of a previously unknown antigenic determinant, composed partly of drug and partly of membrane protein. This neoantigenic structure is not a haptenic protein and may initiate an immune response on its own, the antibody produced directly against the neoantigen itself. Alternatively, the neoantigen could serve a carrier function and thus, when processed by antigen-presenting cells and presented to a corresponding T helper cell, could result in T-cell help to those B cells that recognize that portion of the neoantigen consisting of the drug alone. (See Chapter 7.)

For efficient collaboration between T and B cells to occur, the antigenic determinant for which each cell type is specific must be on the same molecule.

Thus, the formation of a neoantigen that can induce a carrier response and that also contains the haptenic structure (in this case the drug) could in theory initiate a typical hapten-carrier humoral immune response. In this instance, it would be expected that the polyclonal antibody response would contain specificities directed at epitopes present on both the drug and the neoantigenic structure. Thus, these drug-induced antibodies may not be completely inhibited using a pure form of the drug.

For detection in vitro, these drug-related antibodies may require the simultaneous presence of both drug and antibody and, thus, would be classified as reacting by the immune complex mechanism. One can speculate that this is, at least in part, because the polyclonal antibodies produced to the neoantigen can stabilize, or crosslink, the drug (which would be in great excess in vitro) as it associates with its cellular component to form the neoantigenic structure. Thus, the increased avidity would allow for in-vitro detection.

Drugs with high binding affinities (ie, penicillins) may result in a more drug-specific immune response due to a higher degree of association with the cellular component(s). Thus, the drug may act as a true hapten, and the neoantigen formed may serve a nonself carrier function. It is also possible that these high-binding affinity drugs may be more immunogenic than drugs that bind cell membrane components with lower binding affinities. Indeed, antibodies produced to these drugs are directed predominantly to the drug (hapten) itself. Thus, these antibodies would be expected to be inhibitable using a pure form of the drug (ie, hapten inhibition), and may require that the drug bound to a solid matrix detection system (ie, rbcs; drugs previously classified as reacting by the drug adsorption mechanism) for in-vitro detection. However, with hemolytic antipenicillin, the antibody may not always be completely inhibited with pure penicillin (hapten).[5] This may simply be a quantitative effect due to the very high titers of antipenicillin found in hemolyzing patients, thus requiring higher concentrations of hapten for complete inhibition. Alternatively, this may indicate that at least a portion of the polyclonal antipenicillin antibodies recognize some shared component of the rbc membrane and drug (ie, the neoantigenic determinant). Moreover, if this occurs, the in-vitro serologic reactions may resemble both the drug adsorption and immune complex mechanisms discussed above.

Autoimmunity occurs when a drug binds to a cellular rbc component in such a way as to alter its recognition by the host immune system as self, producing an antibody that is cross-reactive with normal self antigens. This mechanism has been shown experimentally to result in the induction of autoimmunity to various protein antigens.[67] In the case of drug-induced AIHA, the resultant loss of the tolerant state to autologous cellular rbc proteins produces an antibody that is primarily directed to drug-altered antigen (ie, the neoantigen) but is cross-reactive with normal self rbcs.[62,67] In vitro, however, these antibodies may appear to react only with normal cellular components (ie, an autoantibody indistinguishable from those found in WAIHA).

The neoantigen hypothesis can explain all previously proposed mechanisms of drug-induced immune hemolytic anemias. The basic premise is that drug-induced antibody production is a result of the affinity of a given drug for a particular cellular membrane component and the degree to which that component is altered by the drug. Although current thinking has tended to dis-

miss classical hapten-carrier-mediated mechanisms,[63-66] the neoantigenic hypothesis does not preclude this mechanism (ie, the neoantigenic structure itself may serve both a hapten and carrier function).

In summary, if the drug-related neoantigenic structure formed can act as a complete antigen, the resultant antibody would be to the neoantigenic determinant(s) and the in-vitro serologic reactions would resemble the immune complex mechanism. If the neoantigen can serve as a drug hapten-carrier structure, the antibody produced would be directed against both the hapten (drug) and carrier (neoantigen). Thus, the in-vitro serologic reactions could resemble either the drug adsorption and/or the immune complex mechanisms. If the neoantigenic structure results in a particular modification of self proteins, resulting in the loss of the tolerant state with production of a cross-reactive antibody to self, the resultant in-vitro serologic reactions would resemble autoantibody. Since any one or all of the above combinations would be possible in a given individual receiving drug therapy, all types of drug-induced immune responses are explainable using only the hypothesis of neoantigen formation.

Laboratory Investigation of Drug-Induced Immune Hemolysis

The drug-related problems most commonly encountered in the blood bank are those associated with a positive DAT. Drugs of the α-methyldopa group usually cause reactive IAT in serum/rbc mixtures without added drug. The serologic evaluation of drug-induced hemolysis is carried out in essentially the same manner as that to investigate AIHA:

1. Monospecific antiglobulin reagents are useful for the DAT. Drugs that cause a positive DAT by the immune complex mechanism primarily bind complement to rbcs, in contrast to positive DATs induced by penicillin or α-methyldopa in which only IgG is usually bound. Rbcs that have adsorbed proteins nonimmunologically in association with drugs of the cephalosporin group react with some or all antiglobulin reagents (eg, anti-IgG, -IgA, -IgM, -C3) and anti-albumin reagents.

2. The patient's serum should be tested for unexpected antibodies by the routine procedures used in pretransfusion studies (see Chapter 14). If the serum does not react with untreated rbcs, the tests should be repeated against ABO-compatible rbcs in the presence of the drug(s) that the patient has been receiving. Techniques for testing may be those described in published cases, if the drug is one already reported as being immunogenic. If such information is not available, an initial screening test can be performed with a solution of the drug at a concentration of approximately 1 mg/mL in suitable phosphate-buffered saline, taking care to ensure proper pH for solubility.[5] Techniques are given in Methods 6.9 and 6.10. The physical properties of drugs, such as solubility and stability, may be found in the *Physicians' Desk Reference*,[68] in the *Merck Index*,[69] through consultation with the hospital pharmacist or by contacting the pharmaceutical company.[5]

3. If these tests are not informative, an attempt should be made to coat normal rbcs with the drug,[5] and test the patient's serum and an eluate from the patient's rbcs against the drug-coated rbcs. This is the method of choice when penicillin or the cephalosporins are the suspected cause of the positive DAT (see Method 6.8). The definitive test result for a penicillin-induced positive DAT is a positive IAT with the eluate and penicillin-coated rbcs but not with the eluate and untreated rbcs. Drugs that induce a positive DAT by the immune complex mechanism often bind only complement to rbcs, so that the eluate may be nonreactive, even when the drug is added to the test system. Drugs that have been reported to cause a positive DAT and hemolytic anemia are indicated in Table 16-5.

Resolving Problems Due to ALG/ATG Therapy

Equine preparations of ALG and ATG contain heterophile antibodies that coat recipient rbcs. Thus, patients receiving ALG/ATG develop a positive DAT within a few days. Free, unbound ALG/ATG may be found in the plasma so that IATs (antibody screen and antiglobulin crossmatch) are positive. Hemolysis is not common, but the serologic problems associated with ALG/ATG therapy can be quite difficult to resolve. Rabbit antihuman globulin reagents contain antibodies that react with equine immunoglobulin. However, this reactivity can be removed by neutralization with equine serum,[6] as shown in Method 6.11.

Other Methods

Low Ionic Polycation

Problems associated with ALG/ATG therapy are not usually encountered by the low ionic polycation (LIP) technique described in Method 3.1.5. LIP tests may, therefore, be used to screen for unexpected alloantibodies in ALG/ATG recipients.[6]

Lu(a–b–) Red Cells

ALG/ATG preparations may exhibit a Lutheran-related specificity.[70] Lu(a–b–) rbcs, if available, can be used to detect concomitant alloantibodies.

References

1. Petz LD, Garratty G. Acquired immune hemolytic anemias. New York: Churchill Livingstone, 1980.
2. Dacie JV. The haemolytic anemias. Congenital and acquired. II. The auto-immune anemias. 2nd ed. London: J & A Churchill Ltd, 1962.
3. Pirofsky B. Autoimmunization and the autoimmune hemolytic anemias. Baltimore: Williams and Wilkins, 1969.
4. Mollison PL. Blood transfusion in clinical medicine. 9th ed. Oxford: Blackwell Scientific Publications, 1993.
5. Petz LD, Branch DR. Drug-induced immune hemolytic anemia. In: Chaplin H, ed. Methods in hematology: Immune hemolytic anemias. New York: Churchill Livingstone, 1985:47-94.
6. Swanson JL, Issitt CH, Mann EW, et al. Resolution of rbc compatibility testing problems in patients receiving anti-lymphoblast or anti-thymocyte globulin. Transfusion 1984;24:141-3.
7. Heddle N, Kelton JG, Turchyn KL, Ali MAM. Hypergammaglobulinemia can be associated with a positive direct antiglobulin test, a nonreactive eluate, and no evidence of hemolysis. Transfusion 1988;28:29-33.
8. Syzmanski IO, Odgren PR, Fortier NL, Snyder LM. Red blood cell associated IgG in normal and pathologic states. Blood 1980;55:48-54.
9. Toy PT, Chin CA, Reid ME, Burns MA. Factors associated with positive direct antiglobulin tests in pretransfusion patients: A case control study. Vox Sang 1985;49:215-20.
10. Ramsey G. Red cell antibodies arising from solid organ transplants. Transfusion 1991;31:76-86.
11. Worlledge SM. The interpretation of a positive direct antiglobulin test. Br J Haematol 1978; 29:157-62.
12. Freedman J. False-positive antiglobulin tests in healthy subjects and in hospital patients. J Clin Pathol 1979;32:1014-8.
13. Judd WJ, Barnes BA, Steiner EA, et al. The evaluation of a positive direct antiglobulin test (autocontrol) in pretransfusion testing revisited. Transfusion 1986;26:220-4.
14. Garratty G. The clinical significance (and insignificance) of red-cell-bound IgG and complement. In: Wallas CE, Levitt JS, eds. Current applications and interpretations of the direct antiglobulin test. Arlington, VA: American Association of Blood Banks, 1988:1-24.
15. Widmann FK, ed. Standards for blood banks and transfusion services, 15th ed. Bethesda, MD: American Association of Blood Banks, 1993.
16. Johnson MFM, Belota MK. Determination of need for elution studies for positive direct antiglobulin tests in pretransfusion testing. Am J Clin Pathol 1988; 90:58-62.
17. Petz LD, Branch DR. Serological tests for the diagnosis of immune hemolytic anemias. In: McMillan R, ed. Methods in hematology: Immune cytopenias. New York: Churchill Livingstone, 1983:9-48.
18. Petz LD, Swisher SN, eds. Clinical practice of transfusion medicine. 2nd ed. New York: Churchill Livingstone, 1989.
19. Judd WJ. Antibody elution from red cells. In: Bell CA, ed. A seminar on antigen-antibody reactions revisited. Arlington, VA: American Association of Blood Banks, 1982:175-221.
20. Williams WJ, Beutler E, Erslev AJ, Rundles RW. Hematology. 2nd ed. New York: McGraw-Hill, 1972.
21. Dacie JV. Autoimmune hemolytic anemia. Arch Intern Med 1975;135:1293-300.
22. Worlledge SM, Blajchman MA. The autoimmune haemolytic anemias. Br J Haematol 1972;23(suppl):61-9.
23. Sokol RJ, Hewitt S, Stamps BK. Autoimmune haemolysis: An 18 year study of 865 cases referred to a regional transfusion centre. Br Med J 1981;282:2023-7.
24. Sturgeon P, Smith LE, Chum HMT, et al. Autoimmune hemolytic anemia associated exclusively with IgA of Rh specificity. Transfusion 1976;19:324-8.
25. Issitt PD. Serology and genetics of the rhesus blood group system. Cincinnati: Montgomery Scientific Publications, 1979.
26. Issitt PD, Pavone BG, Goldfinger D, et al. Anti-Wr^b and other auto-antibodies responsible for positive direct antiglobulin tests in 150 individuals. Br J Haematol 1976;34:5-18.
27. Vos GH, Petz LD, Garratty G, Fudenberg HH. Autoantibodies in acquired hemolytic anemia with special reference to the LW system. Blood 1973;42:445-53.
28. Branch DR, Shulman IA, Sy Siok Hian AL, Petz LD. Two distinct categories of warm autoantibody reactivity with age-fractionated red cells. Blood 1984;63:177-80.

29. Issitt PD. Applied blood group serology, 3rd ed. Miami: Montgomery Scientific Publications, 1986.

30. Shulman IA, Vengelen-Tyler V, Thompson JC, et al. Autoanti-Ge associated with severe autoimmune hemolytic anemia. Vox Sang 1990;59: 232-4.

31. Garratty G. Target antigens for red cell-bound autoantibodies. In: Nance SJ, ed. Clinical and basic science aspects of immunohematology. Arlington, VA: American Association of Blood Banks, 1991:33-72.

32. Garratty G, Petz LD, Hoops JK. The correlation of cold agglutinin titrations in saline and albumin with haemolytic anemia. Br J Haematol 1975;35:587-95.

33. Sokol RJ, Hewitt S, Stamps BK. Autoimmune haemolysis. Mixed warm and cold antibody type. Acta Haematol 1983;69:266-74.

34. Shulman IA, Branch DR, Nelson JM, et al. Autoimmune hemolytic anemia with both cold and warm autoantibodies. JAMA 1985; 253:1746-8.

35. Kaji E, Miura Y, Ikemoto S. Characterization of autoantibodies in mixed-type autoimmune hemolytic anemia. Vox Sang 1991;60:45-52.

36. Gottsche B, Salama A, Mueller-Eckhardt C. Donath-Landsteiner autoimmune hemolytic anemia in children. Vox Sang 1990;58:281-6.

37. Bell CA, Zwicker H, Rosenbaum DL. Paroxysmal cold hemoglobinuria (PCH) following mycoplasma infection: Anti-I specificity of the biphasic hemolysin. Transfusion 1973;13:138-41.

38. Shirey RS, Park K, Ness PM, et al. Anti-i biphasic hemolysin in chronic paroxysmal cold hemoglobinuria. Transfusion 1986;26:62-4.

39. Judd WJ, Wilkinson SL, Issitt PD, et al. Donath-Landsteiner hemolytic anemia due to an anti-Pr-like biphasic hemolysin. Transfusion 1986;26:423-5.

40. Gilliland BC, Baxter E, Evans RS. Red-cell antibodies in acquired hemolytic anemia with negative antiglobulin serum tests. N Engl J Med 1971;285:252-6.

41. Chaplin H. Clinical usefulness of specific antiglobulin reagents in autoimmune hemolytic anemias. Prog Hematol 1973;8:25-49.

42. Freedman J, Wright J, Lim FC, Garvey MB. Hemolytic warm IgM autoagglutinins in autoimmune hemolytic anemia. Transfusion 1986; 26:464-7.

43. Garratty G, Postoway N, Nance SJ, Brunt DJ. Spontaneous agglutination of red cells with a positive direct antiglobulin test in various media. Transfusion 1984;24:214-7.

44. Beattie KM. Laboratory evaluation and management of antibody specificities in warm autoimmune hemolytic anemia. In: Bell CA, ed. A seminar on the laboratory management of hemolysis. Washington, DC: American Association of Blood Banks, 1979:105-34.

45. Branch DR, Sy Siok Hian AL, Carlson F, et al. Erythrocyte age-fractionation using a Percoll-Renografin density gradient: Application to autologous red cell antigen determinations in recently transfused patients. Am J Clin Pathol 1983;80:453-8.

46. Branch DR, Petz LD. A new reagent (ZZAP) having multiple applications in immunohematology. Am J Clin Pathol 1982; 78:161-7.

47. Issitt PD, Zellner DC, Rolih SD, Duckett JB. Autoantibodies mimicking alloantibodies. Transfusion 1977;17:531-8.

48. Issitt PD, Smith TR. Evaluation of antiglobulin reagents. In: Myhre BA, ed. A seminar on performance evaluation. Washington, DC: American Association of Blood Banks, 1976.

49. von dem Borne AEG, Engelfriet CP, Beckers D, van Loghem JJ. Autoimmune haemolytic anemias: Biochemical studies of rbcs from patients with autoimmune haemolytic anemia with incomplete warm autoantibodies. Clin Exp Immunol 1971;8:377-88.

50. Salmon C. Autoimmune hemolytic anemia. In: Immunology. New York: John Wiley & Sons, 1978.

51. Pirofsky B. Immune haemolytic disease: The autoimmune haemolytic anaemias. Clin Haematol 1975;4:167-80.

52. Branch DR. Blood transfusion in autoimmune hemolytic anemias. Lab Med 1984;15:402-8.

53. Marks MR, Reid ME, Ellisor SS. Adsorption of unwanted cold autoagglutinins by formaldehyde-treated rabbit erythrocytes (abstract). Transfusion 1980;20:629.

54. Dzik W, Yang R, Blank J. Rabbit erythrocyte stroma treatment of serum interferes with recognition of delayed hemolytic transfusion reactions (letter). Transfusion 1986;26:303-4.

55. Rausen AR, Levine R, Hsu TCS, Rosenfield RE. Compatible transfusion therapy for patients with PCH. Pediatrics 1975;55:275-8.

56. Spath P, Garratty G, Petz LD. Studies on the immune response to penicillin and cephalothin in humans: 1. Optimal conditions for titration of hemagglutinating penicillin and cephalothin antibodies. J Immunol 1971;107: 845-58.

57. Branch DR, Sy Siok Hian AL, Petz LD. Mechanism of nonimmunologic adsorption of proteins using cephalothin-coated red cells (abstract). Transfusion 1984;24:415.

58. Branch DR, Berkowitz LR, Becker RL, et al. Extravascular hemolysis following the administration of cefamandole. Am J Hematol 1985; 18:213-9.

59. Garratty G, Postoway N, Schwellenbach J, McMahill PC. A fatal case of ceftriaxone (Rocephin)-induced hemolytic anemia associ-

ated with intravascular immune hemolysis. Transfusion 1991;31:176-9.

60. Kirtland HH III, Mohler DN, Horwitz DA. Methyldopa inhibition of suppressor lymphocyte function. A proposed cause of autoimmune hemolytic anemia. N Engl J Med 1980; 302:825-32.

61. Garratty G, Arndt P, Prince H, Shulman I. In vitro IgG production following preincubation of lymphocytes with methyldopa and procainamide (abstract). Blood 1986;68(Suppl 1): 108a.

62. Branch DR, Gallagher MT, Shulman IA, et al. Reticuloendothelial cell function in alpha-methyldopa-induced hemolytic anemia. Vox Sang 1983;45:278-87.

63. Mueller-Eckhardt C, Salama A. Drug-induced immune cytopenias: A unifying pathogenetic concept with special emphasis on the role of drug metabolites. Transfus Med Rev 1990;4: 69-77.

64. Garratty G. Current viewpoints on mechanisms causing drug-induced immune hemo-lytic anemia and/or positive direct antiglobulin tests. Immunohematology 1989;5:97-106.

65. Petz LD, Mueller-Eckhardt C. Drug-induced immune hemolytic anemia. Transfusion 1992; 32:202-04.

66. Salama A, Mueller-Eckhardt C. Immune-mediated blood cell dyscrasias related to drugs. Semin Hematol 1992;29:54-63.

67. Weigle WO. The antibody response in rabbits to previously tolerated antigens. Ann NY Acad Sci 1965;124:133-42.

68. Physicians' desk reference. 43rd ed. Oradell, NJ: Medical Economics, 1989.

69. Windholz M, ed. The Merck index. 15th ed. Rahway, NJ: Merck & Co, 1987.

70. Anderson HJ, Aubuchon JP, Draper EK, Ballas SK. Transfusion problems in renal allograft recipients: anti-lymphocyte globulin showing Lutheran system specificity. Transfusion 1985;25:47-50.

17

Blood Transfusion Practice

The proper use of blood components and derivatives depends on the informed assessment of the relative risks and benefits in a given clinical setting. The increased awareness of potential complications of blood transfusion has resulted in increased attention to the proper indications for transfusion. An overview of the clinical use of transfusion therapy is provided in this chapter. Readers seeking additional information are referred to several texts devoted to the topic.[1-5]

Transfusion of Red Cells

Physiologic Basis for the Transfusion of Red Cells

The primary indication for the transfusion of RBCs is to restore or maintain an adequate supply of oxygen to meet tissue demands. Since the body demand for oxygen varies greatly among different individuals in different clinical circumstances, a single laboratory measurement (the hematocrit or the hemoglobin) cannot accurately assess the need for transfusion.[6]

Normal Oxygen Supply and Demand

Tissues have a constant demand for oxygen. See Table 17-1. The oxygen content of blood (mL O_2/mL blood) is determined by the hemoglobin concentration, the binding coefficient of oxygen for normal hemoglobin, the percent saturation of hemoglobin and the quantity of oxygen dissolved in the plasma. This is described as:

$$O_2 \text{ content} = (Hb \times 1.39 \times \%sat) + (pO_2 \times 0.003)$$

Tissue oxygen consumption represents the difference between oxygen delivery in the arterial blood and oxygen return by the venous blood. This is described as:

$$O_2 \text{ consumption} = \text{Cardiac output} \times Hb \times 1.39 \times (\%sat_{arterial} - \%sat_{venous})$$

in which the units of measure are

$$(\text{mL } O_2/\text{min}) = \text{L blood/min} \times \text{g/L} \times \text{mL } O_2/\text{g} \times (\%-\%)$$

The percent saturation of arterial and venous hemoglobin with oxygen varies with the partial pressure of oxygen dissolved in the plasma. This relationship is shown in Fig 3-1 and Fig 18-1. Under normal circumstances the pO_2 falls from 100 torr in the arteries to 40 torr in the veins as the tissues extract oxygen. As a result, the saturation of hemoglobin falls from near 100% in the arteries to approximately 75% in the veins, ie, the

Table 17-1. Blood Flow and Oxygen Consumption of Body Organs at Rest[4]

	Weight (kg)	Blood Flow (mL/min/100 g)	Cardiac Output (%)	O_2 Consumption (mL/min/100 g)	Total O_2 Consumption (%)
Heart	0.32	80	5	9.00	10
Kidneys	0.30	400	22	5.00	6
Liver and gastrointestinal tract	4.00	50	23	3.00	30
Skin	2.00	10	4	0.20	2
Skeletal muscle	35.00	3	18	0.15	20
Brain	1.40	55	14	3.00	18
Remainder	27.00	3	14	0.15	14

hemoglobin "gives up" only 25% of its oxygen under normal circumstances. A primary physiologic response to increased tissue demand for oxygen or to decreased supply of oxygen is greater extraction of oxygen from the plasma and from hemoglobin, resulting in a lower pO_2 and a lower percent saturation of the venous blood. Controlled studies in primates have suggested that a critical point of limited oxygen delivery is reached when oxygen extraction approaches twice normal or 50%.[7]

Under normal resting conditions the body has a tremendous reserve of oxygen supply relative to demand:

O_2 supply
= Cardiac output × O_2 content$_{arterial}$
= 5 L blood/min × [(140 × 1.39 × 100%) + (100 × 0.003)]
= 5 L blood/min × 200 mL O_2/L blood
= 1000 mL O_2/min

O_2 consumption
= Cardiac output × (O_2 content$_{arterial}$ − O_2 content$_{venous}$)
= 5 L blood/min × (200 mL O_2/L blood − 150 mL O_2/L blood)
= 5 L blood/min × 50 mL O_2/L blood
= 250 mL O_2/min

Measuring Adequate Oxygen Supply

Measuring the hemoglobin concentration (or hematocrit) does not assess the adequacy of oxygen delivery to the tissues. This explains why a value for hemoglobin cannot serve by itself as a clinical guide for blood transfusion. The clinical assessment of adequate oxygenation is based on the patient's cardiac performance, hemoglobin mass and current oxygen demands. For patients in intensive care or in the operating room, direct measurement of the cardiac output and the systemic oxygen extraction via a pulmonary artery catheter can serve as a useful guide to the overall adequacy of oxygen supply.[8] This approach may prove to be a more physiologic measurement for determining the indication for transfusion than measurement of the hematocrit.

Although the mixed venous oxygen saturation and the extraction ratio give meaningful data on total body oxygen consumption, these values must also be interpreted in light of the clinical situation. In certain conditions, such as sepsis and adult respiratory distress syndrome, oxygen consumption is said to be supply dependent.[9] In these conditions mixed venous oxygen saturation may underestimate tissue oxygen needs.[10]

Treating Inadequate Oxygen Supply

Tissue oxygen debt results when oxygen demand exceeds supply. Deprived of adequate oxygen, tissues convert to anaerobic metabolism and produce increased quantities of lactic acid. Systemic acidemia, in turn, impairs cardiac performance, producing decreased perfusion, decreased tissue oxygen delivery and further tissue ischemia. Since the supply of oxygen depends upon blood flow, oxygenation of the blood by the lungs, hemoglobin concentration, oxygen-hemoglobin affinity and tissue demands for oxygen, each of these can be considered in treating patients who have tissue oxygen debt. Usually the oxygen-hemoglobin affinity cannot be varied greatly. Transfusion of RBCs provides an excellent means of raising the patient's hemoglobin mass. One unit of RBCs raises the average-sized adult recipient's hemoglobin concentration by 10 g/L (1 g/dL). However, increasing tissue perfusion (maximizing cardiac performance), increasing the percent hemoglobin saturation (supplemental oxygen) and decreasing tissue oxygen demands (bed rest) will all serve to improve oxygen supply vs demand independent of transfusion.

The interrelationship between oxygen delivery, cardiac output and hemoglobin mass is shown in Fig 17-1. For example, a patient with a hemoglobin of 80 g/L (8 g/dL) and a cardiac index of 4 L/min/m^2 has subnormal oxygen delivery. Assuming the need for normal oxygen delivery and assuming that oxygen extraction is constant, normal oxygen delivery could be achieved by *either* a 30 g/L (3 g/dL) increase in the hemoglobin concentration to 110 g/L (11 g/dL), *or* a 1 L/min/m^2 increase in cardiac index to 5 L/min/m^2. Increased cardiac output is an important compensation to anemia. In addition, anemia results in increased oxygen extraction, which further increases oxygen delivery to tissues.

Selection of RBCs

Fresh Whole Blood

Processing donor blood, which includes ABO and Rh grouping, antibody detection and testing for markers of transfusion-transmitted diseases, is rarely completed in less than 24 hours. Transfusing blood before necessary tests are completed carries a risk of transfusion complications that outweighs any anticipated benefit. There are no solid indications for specifically transfusing fresh Whole Blood (WB). In general, a request for fresh WB should be interpreted by the blood bank staff as a need for consultative help to establish a diagnosis and to plan specific component therapy. WB less than 5 days old is often used for exchange transfusions in newborns. Although there are no prospective, controlled trials documenting a clear benefit of WB less than 5 days old in newborns, such blood ensures plasma electrolyte concentrations within limits that are tolerable for infants, and also ensures adequate red cell content of 2,3-diphosphoglycerate (2,3-DPG). See Chapter 18.

Studies have claimed an advantage of fresh WB over component therapy for pediatric patients undergoing cardiovascular surgery.[11,12]

Stored Whole Blood

Whole Blood, which provides both oxygen-carrying capacity and blood volume expansion, is indicated for actively bleeding patients who have lost more than 30% of their blood volume. The first goal of treatment should be restoration of intravascular volume and preven-

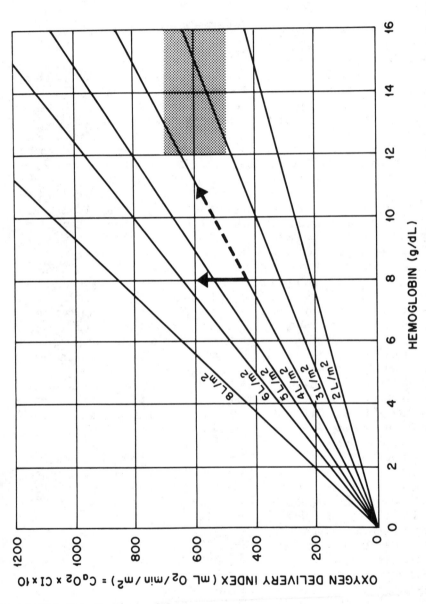

Figure 17-1. Oxygen delivery index in mL O_2/min/m^2 at various hemoglobin concentrations. Diagonal lines represent constant cardiac index (CI). C_aO_2 is the arterial content of oxygen. The shaded rectangle represents normal values at rest. An individual with a CI of 4 L/m^2 and a hemoglobin of 80 g/L (8 g/dL) has a subnormal oxygen delivery (420 mL O_2/min/m^2). Oxygen delivery could be increased to 600 mL O_2/min/m^2 by *either* an increase in hemoglobin concentration to 110 g/L (11 g/dL) (dashed arrow) *or* an increase in cardiac index to 5.5 L/min (solid arrow). (Adapted with permission from Greenburg.[4])

tion of hypovolemic shock, rather than increasing the hemoglobin concentration. Infusions of crystalloid or colloid to restore intravascular volume should be started immediately, before transfusion of blood. Because rapid blood loss of more than one blood volume replaced by a combination of RBCs without plasma can result in dilutional coagulopathy, close monitoring of clinical hemostasis and coagulation tests is important. In the setting of massive transfusion, WB is preferred because the simultaneous use of FFP with RBCs doubles the risk of transfusion-transmitted disease. WB, Modified, is prepared by returning the plasma to the RBCs after removal of PCs and/or CRYO. This component has virtually the same hemostatic properties as stored WB. Preparation of this component permits collection of PCs and/or CRYO, while ensuring a supply of WB for treating severe hemorrhage.

Red Blood Cells

RBCs are the component of choice to restore or maintain oxygen-carrying capacity. Patients who have chronic anemia or congestive heart failure, or those who are elderly or debilitated, often do not tolerate the increased volume load provided by WB. Transfusing RBCs increases oxygen-carrying capacity with minimal expansion of blood volume. For most patients with operative blood loss of only 1000-1200 mL, RBC transfusion is not required. Electrolyte and/or colloid solutions provide adequate volume replacement.[13]

Clinical Use of RBCs

Consideration of the principles of oxygen transport should emphasize that there is no single hemoglobin or hematocrit threshold that represents the proper indication for transfusion of

RBCs for all patients.[14,15] A National Institutes of Health consensus development conference on perioperative blood transfusion emphasized that preoperative transfusions should not be given simply to raise the hemoglobin concentration above 100 g/L (10 g/dL).[16] Transfusions do not improve wound healing, which depends on pO_2 rather than total oxygen content of blood.[15] Patients with chronic anemia tolerate lower hematocrit values better than those with acute anemia due to cardiovascular compensation and increased red cell 2,3-DPG. In the absence of cardiac dysfunction and critical coronary stenosis, most patients' oxygen demands are well met despite a hemoglobin concentration of 80 g/L (8 g/dL). See Appendix 17-1.

Leukocyte-Reduced Blood Components

The number of donor leukocytes present in blood components is shown in Table 17-2. Several complications of transfusion result from exposure of the recipient to donor leukocytes. These include sensitization to leukocyte antigens, febrile nonhemolytic reactions, transmission of leukotropic viruses and graft-vs-host disease (GVHD).[16] Several different methods, listed in Table 17-3, have become available for the preparation of leukocyte-reduced blood and compo-

Table 17-2. Approximate Leukocyte Content of Blood Components (per Unit)

Whole blood	10^9
RBCs	10^8
Washed RBCs	10^7
Frozen-deglycerolized	
RBCs	10^6-10^7
Apheresis platelets	10^6-10^8
Platelet concentrate	10^7

Table 17-3. Methods To Prepare Leukocyte-Reduced Blood and Components

Whole Blood
Leukocyte-adsorption filters

RBCs
Leukocyte-adsorption filters
Frozen-deglycerolized RBCs
Microaggregate-filtered RBCs
Washed RBCs
Buffy coat depleted RBCs

Platelets
Leukocyte-adsorption filters
Apheresis machines (certain models)
Centrifugation

nents.[16,17] Leukocyte-adsorption filters are highly efficient. A logarithmic scale is often used to discuss the degree of leukocyte removal. One log reduction refers to removal of 90% of the original leukocytes present. Two log reduction represents 99% removal, three log reduction is 99.9% removal and so on. See p 557. Leukocyte reduction of blood can be performed during component preparation, in the laboratory or at the bedside. However, the effectiveness of leukocyte removal varies if the methods of removal are not performed correctly. Laboratories that frequently provide leukocyte-reduced blood components should document the effectiveness of the method used. Correct use of bedside filters must be ensured. Several techniques for counting low numbers of leukocytes in blood have become available, including the use of low-cost, large volume counting chambers ideally suited for this application. See Methods 11.12 and 11.13 and Appendix 22-1. There is no single definition for a leukocyte-reduced blood component since the required degree of leukocyte removal depends on the therapeutic goal.

Prevention of HLA Sensitization

A growing body of evidence supports the concept that residual donor leukocytes bearing Class II HLA antigens provoke *primary* HLA sensitization in recipients of cellular blood components.[18-20] See Chapter 13. To prevent HLA sensitization, preliminary studies suggest that the residual donor leukocyte content should not exceed 1 to 5×10^6 leukocytes (WBCs) per bag.[21] This degree of leukocyte removal is best achieved with the use of leukocyte-adsorption filters. Since a secondary immune response occurs following exposure to a much smaller dose of donor leukocytes, use of leukocyte-reduced blood may not prevent HLA sensitization in patients with prior exposure to HLA antigens as a result of previous transfusion or pregnancy. Patients who require long-term platelet support or who may require eventual transplantation are candidates for prevention of HLA alloimmunization. Prevention of sensitization in such patients requires the use of both leukocyte-reduced RBCs and leukocyte-reduced platelets.

Other methods of preventing recipient exposure to donor HLA antigens are under investigation, including the use of ultraviolet B irradiated components.

Prevention of Febrile Nonhemolytic Transfusion Reactions

Prevention of febrile nonhemolytic (FNH) transfusion reactions can usually be achieved with a 1-2 log reduction in the leukocyte content of cellular components. (Residual leukocyte content $<5 \times 10^8$ WBCs/unit.) The use of washed cells, frozen-deglycerolized cells or microaggregate filters has been associated with successful results. Multitransfused patients receiving long-term platelet support with non-leukocyte-reduced components often develop FNH transfusion reactions. Use of leukocyte-reduced platelets to prevent febrile reactions for such patients requires individual patient evaluation. For broadly alloimmunized, refractory patients the use of leukocyte-reduced platelets may avert a febrile response, but may not improve posttransfusion increments. Febrile reactions may continue to occur despite the use of leukocyte-reduced components. For example, patients with antiplatelet antibodies may develop fever when transfused with leukocyte-reduced incompatible platelets. The use of leukocyte-reduced RBCs may allow thrombocytopenic patients to maintain a higher platelet count.[22,23]

Prevention of Transfusion-Transmitted Viruses and Bacteria

Several studies suggest that cytomegalovirus (CMV) transmission can be prevented with the use of leukocyte-reduced components regardless of the CMV serologic status of the donor. Use of leukocyte adsorption filters or use of red cells prepared by freezing and deglycerolization has been associated with success.[24,25]

The effect of leukocyte reduction on the transmission of other viruses such as human immunodeficiency virus, type 1 (HIV-1) is under investigation.[26] Preliminary studies have suggested that prestorage leukocyte reduction may decrease the incidence of bacterial overgrowth with Yersinia and other bacteria during refrigerated storage of RBCs.[27]

Prevention of Graft-vs-Host Disease

The degree of leukocyte removal necessary to prevent transfusion-associated GVHD in susceptible recipients is unknown. Although leukocyte-reduced components probably carry a lower likelihood of posttransfusion GVHD, irradiation remains the only recommended method for the prevention of transfusion-associated GVHD.[28]

Platelet Transfusion

Physiologic Principles of Platelet Transfusion

The Platelet in Hemostasis

There are four major phases to hemostasis: the vascular phase, the formation of a platelet plug, the development of fibrin clot on the platelet plug and the ultimate lysis of the clot. Platelets form a primary role in initial cessation of hemorrhage from damaged vessels. Platelets are essential to the formation of the primary hemostatic plug and provide the hemostatic surface upon which fibrin formation occurs. The clinical effects of deficiencies in platelet number and/or function are in many instances unpredictable and range from clinically insignificant prolongation of the bleeding time to major life-threatening defects in hemostasis. Platelet plug formation results from the combined processes of adhesion, activation and release, aggregation and procoagulant activity. Platelet *adhesion* to damaged endothelium is mediated in large part by von Willebrand factor, which binds to a receptor on the platelet surface termed glycoprotein Ib. Platelets also undergo a process of *activation and release*, which involves a dramatic change in the shape of the platelet with extension of long cytoplasmic pseudopod-like structures, a change in the binding properties of membrane activation proteins, the secretion of internal granule contents and the activation of several metabolic pathways. The platelet release reaction results in a number of effects, including the recruitment of additional platelets. Platelets gathering at the site of the platelet plug *aggregate* one to another, a process mediated by the binding of fibrinogen to a specific platelet surface structure termed glycoprotein IIb-IIIa. The mass of platelet plug membrane has potent *procoagul-*

ant activity, which serves to localize the formation of fibrin clot at the site of the platelet plug.

Assessing Adequate Platelet Function

Platelet function depends upon both number and function. Decreased platelet numbers result from many conditions that either decrease platelet production or increase platelet destruction. Many clinical conditions adversely affect platelet function. These include drugs, liver or kidney disease, sepsis, increased fibrin(ogen) degradation products, cardiopulmonary bypass and primary bone marrow disorders.

Adequate platelet hemostasis is best assessed by the medical history and physical exam. Patients with inadequate platelet number or function may demonstrate petechiae, easy bruising and mucous membrane bleeding. Laboratory investigation includes measurement of the platelet count and the bleeding time. The bleeding time measures the contribution of both the vascular phase and the platelet phase of hemostasis. While the bleeding time is a highly useful diagnostic test in the evaluation of patients with known abnormalities of platelet number and/or function, the bleeding time is a poor predictor of bleeding.[29,30] Thus, a prolonged bleeding time is not a sufficient indication for platelet transfusion therapy. Like the bleeding time, platelet aggregation is a useful test for investigating abnormal platelet function, but is a poor predictor of clinical bleeding.

Platelet Life Span and Kinetics

Platelets normally circulate with a life span of 9.5 days.[31] Several conditions shorten platelet life span including splenomegaly, sepsis, drugs, disseminated intravascular coagulation (DIC), alloantibodies, endothelial cell activation and platelet activation. Since a fixed number [ie, 7-10×10^9/L/day (7000-10,000/μL/day)] of platelets are required each day for routine plugging of minor defects in the vascular endothelium, the proportion of the total number of platelets required for maintenance function goes up as the total number of platelets declines.[31] As a result, platelet life span decreases with progressive thrombocytopenia. Following transfusion, platelets that have been properly collected and stored have a near normal life span when reinfused into the original donor. Platelets transfused to patients, however, frequently have a reduced survival due to the multiple factors listed above that affect circulating platelet life span.[31] In practice, the response to platelet transfusion is best assessed by observation of the cessation of clinical bleeding and by measurement of the posttransfusion platelet increment. The posttransfusion increment is generally measured between 10 minutes and 1 hour after the completion of the transfusion and expressed as a corrected count increment (CCI). The CCI corrects for the number of platelets infused and the blood volume of the recipient:

$$\text{CCI at 1 hour} = \frac{(\text{Platelet count}_{post} - \text{Platelet count}_{pre}) \times \text{BSA (m}^2)}{\text{Number of units transfused}}$$

or

$$\text{CCI at 1 hour} = \frac{(\text{Platelet count}_{post} - \text{Platelet count}_{pre}) \times \text{BSA (m}^2)}{\text{Number of platelets transfused}\ (\text{multiples of } 10^{11})}$$

where BSA is the body surface area in square meters.

A CCI of > 4000-5000 (first equation above) or > 7000-10,000 (second equation above) suggests an adequate response to allogeneic platelet transfusion. A poor CCI suggests platelet refractoriness.

Selection of Platelet Components

Pooled Platelets

Platelets prepared from individual units of whole blood are generally pooled in batches of 6-10 units prior to transfusion to adult recipients (1 unit/10 kg). Although the platelets in pooled PCs are hemostatically equal to those in apheresis PCs, pooled PCs expose the recipient to a larger number of allogeneic donors.

Random Apheresis PCs

Platelets prepared by apheresis technology are usually transfused without matching for HLA or platelet antigens. Random apheresis PCs have the advantage of representing only one donor exposure per transfusion. Some transfusion services allocate random apheresis PCs to recipients with limited allogeneic donor exposures. For example, a 56-year-old man who requires platelet therapy after cardiac surgery during which he was transfused with only two units of autologous RBCs would acquire only one additional donor exposure with the use of apheresis PCs. There is no concrete evidence that platelets prepared by apheresis technology are hemostatically better than those pooled from individual units of whole blood. Moreover, although early reports suggested that apheresis PCs were less likely than pooled PCs to result in platelet alloimmunization,[32,33] a growing body of evidence now supports the fact that the number of allogeneic donor leukocytes, not the number of donor exposures, is the major factor in the development of HLA alloimmunization and platelet refractoriness.[34]

ABO and Rh

Since ABO antigens are present on the platelet surface, recovery of group A platelets transfused into group O patients is somewhat decreased.[35] Although ABO-incompatible platelets may have slightly diminished 24-hour recovery,[36] prompt administration of available ABO-incompatible platelets is better for patient outcome than a delay to obtain ABO-compatible platelets. Higher corrected count increments have been seen when ABO-compatible platelets are transfused.[37] When many patients require PC transfusions from a limited donor pool, availability becomes the major consideration. When transfusing infants, it may be desirable to remove most of the donor plasma if the platelets contain ABO antibodies incompatible with the recipient's red cells. See Method 10.14. This is rarely necessary in adults or children.

The D antigen is not detectable on platelets and posttransfusion survival of platelets from D+ donors is normal in recipients with anti-D. Since properly prepared PCs may contain up to 0.5 mL of rbcs, D– individuals may become immunized by the small quantity of residual D+ rbcs in the component. In one study, 8% of D– patients being treated for leukemia developed anti-D after transfusion of 80-110 units of D+ pooled PCs.[38] However, another study found no anti-D alloimmunization in a similar group of patients.[39] The low rate of anti-D formation has been attributed to the immune suppression that accompanies cancer chemotherapy. The benefit of Rh Immune Globulin (RhIG) in this setting should be weighed against the risk of hemorrhage as a result of the injection. A subcutaneous injection of minidose RhIG is one alternative to traditional intramuscular therapy. For immunologically normal D– females of childbearing potential, it is desirable to avoid PCs from D+ donors. When a sufficient quantity of D– PCs are not available and platelet therapy is indicated, transfusion of PCs from D+ donors to immunologically normal D– recipients is acceptable practice. In such instances, administration of RhIG should be considered to prevent immunization. A full dose of RhIG would generally provide protection against rbcs present in 30 units of D+ PCs.

Leukocyte-Reduced Platelets

Patients who are receiving leukocyte-reduced RBCs to prevent HLA alloimmunization require leukocyte-reduced PCs as well.[40] See Section on "Leukocyte-Reduced Blood Components" in this chapter. In addition to the preparation of leukocyte-reduced PCs by leukocyte-adsorption filters, certain apheresis devices are capable of preparing leukocyte-reduced apheresis PCs. However, these techniques have not yet been shown to prevent alloimmunization in clinical trials. Whether or not apheresis PCs prepared on such devices require additional leukocyte reduction by filtration is probably best decided based on the results of WBC counting done as part of a program of quality control. Studies are evaluating whether or not ultraviolet irradiation of platelet concentrates may also have a role in the prevention of alloimmunization.[41]

HLA-Matched Apheresis Platelets

Patients who are refractory to random apheresis PCs and to random pooled PCs as a result of HLA alloimmunization may be treated with HLA-matched PCs for episodes of bleeding due to thrombocytopenia. Platelets manifest Class I HLA antigens whose expression results at least in part from adsorption of plasma antigens onto the platelet surface.[42] Because HLA antigens are not expressed on the surface of platelets as strongly as they are on the surface of leukocytes, alloimmunized recipients may sometimes respond to transfusions even if the donor has an antigen to which the recipient has an alloantibody detected by lymphocytotoxicity. The occurrence of antibodies to public antigens and/or to antigens in cross-reactive groups (Chapter 13) further complicates the proper selection of HLA-matched donors.[43] Although difficult to arrange in a reliable fashion, a limited number of HLA-compatible donors may be able to provide all of a patient's transfusion needs if PCs are obtained by repeated cytapheresis. Although many centers have large files of HLA-typed donors, a more readily available source of HLA-identical or HLA-compatible donors may be the patient's siblings. (Siblings who are potential bone marrow donors are generally not used pretransplant due to concern about sensitizing the recipient to minor transplantation antigens.) Children of the patient, who usually are two-antigen HLA mismatches, are less likely to be of benefit as platelet donors for alloimmunized, refractory recipients. Platelets collected from blood relatives of the patient should be irradiated prior to transfusion.

A grading system for HLA-based donor selection is shown in Table 17-4. Note that only grade A and BU matches lack foreign antigens. Grade BX donors have foreign antigens that are said to be "cross-reactive" with those of the recipient. See Table 13-2 for a list of cross-reactive HLA groups. In practice, the selection of "cross-reactive" donors is not always successful.[45] Patients who appear to be broadly alloimmunized to multiple private antigens may in fact be immunized to a limited number of public antigens. Thus, selecting donors based on matching for public antigens may be a more effective strategy than the use of private antigen cross-reactive groups. A scheme for donor selection that includes both public and private antigens has been proposed.[46] See Table 17-5. Studies of HLA antigens and posttransfusion in-

Table 17-4. Degree of Matching for HLA-Matched Platelets

Match Grade		Description	Examples of Donor Phenotypes for a Recipient Who Is A1,2; B13,27
A		4-antigen match	A1,2; B13,27 only
B		No mismatched antigens present	
	B1U	1 antigen unknown or blank	A1,–; B13,27
	B1X	1 cross-reactive group	A1,2; B13,7
	B2UX	1 antigen blank and 1 cross-reactive	A1,2; B40,–
C		1 mismatched antigen present	A1,25; B13,27
D		2 or more mismatched antigens present	A2,31; B8,27
R		Random	

(Adapted from Duquesnoy RJ, et al.[44])

crements indicate that: 1) the best success results with donors who are grade A or BU matches (and thus are also public antigen matches) and who are also ABO compatible with the recipient; 2) mismatching of antigens at the HLA-C locus is usually not important; 3) donor selection based on platelet cross-matching can also be used to select donors.[31,47]

Clinical Use of Platelets

The use of PCs is growing more rapidly than that of any other blood component. Nevertheless, considerable controversy

Table 17-5. Strategy for Selection of Platelet Donors Matched for Public and Private HLA Antigens

Public Epitope	Associated Private Epitopes	Approximate Frequency
1C	A1,36,10,11,19	79%
2C	A2,28,9	66%
28C	A28,33,34,26	20%
5C	B5,15,18,35,53,70	50%
7C	B7,22,27,42,40,13,47,48	51%
8C	B8,14,18,39,51	42%
12C	B12,21,13,40,41	44%
Bw4/4C	(See Table 13-1)	79%
Bw6/6C	(See Table 13-1)	87%

Example: Recipient phenotype: A1,3;B8,27
Public phenotype (see table): 1C;7C;8C;4C;6C
Potential public mismatches: 2C;5C;12C;28C
Recipient antibody screen: anti-2C (anti-A2,28,9)

If no grade A or BU match is available, select donors lacking potential public mismatches. Failing this, select any donor lacking the 2C public epitope. Otherwise, select donors based on platelet crossmatch.

(Adapted with permission from Rodey.[46])

still surrounds the proper clinical indications for platelet transfusion and studies suggest that many transfusions may not be required.[48] The decision to transfuse platelets depends on the clinical condition of the patient, the cause of bleeding and the patient's platelet count and platelet function.

Therapeutic Platelet Transfusion

Treatment of bleeding due to thrombocytopenia or abnormal platelet function is an indication for the transfusion of PCs. When the clinical and laboratory evaluation reveals that the primary hemostatic defect is thrombocytopenia, platelet transfusions are most likely to be of benefit. Platelet transfusions may also supplement other hemostatic therapies in patients with multiple defects in coagulation. Platelet transfusions will also improve hemostasis in patients who have excessive bleeding due to defects in platelet function, such as occurs following cardiopulmonary bypass or following ingestion of aspirin-containing compounds. Other acquired defects in platelet function (eg, that found in uremia) are less likely to respond to platelet transfusion since the transfused cells will acquire the same defect.

Prophylactic Platelet Transfusion

There is increasing challenge to the previously held belief that patients with chemotherapy-induced thrombocytopenia should be maintained at a platelet count of $>20 \times 10^9$/L ($>20,000/\mu$L).[48] This number is based on an outdated retrospective study that reviewed bleeding episodes in cancer patients.[49] In 1962 when the study was reported, such patients were routinely given aspirin—the antiplatelet effect of which had not yet been recognized. Intracranial bleeding occurred in eight of 92 patients with severe thrombocytopenia—seven had platelet counts $<5 \times 10^9$/L ($<5000/\mu$L) and one had a count $<10 \times 10^9$/L ($<10,000/\mu$L). Intracranial bleeding also occurred in an additional eight patients who had cerebral leukostasis and platelet counts $>20 \times 10^9$/L ($>20,000/\mu$L). It is noteworthy that one of the primary conclusions of the study was that NO distinct threshold would accurately predict major bleeding due to thrombocytopenia. However, the discussion section of the paper made the statement that the risk of bleeding was 1% for patients with platelets counts $>20 \times 10^9$/L ($>20,000/\mu$L); over time, the paper was gradually reinterpreted to mean that all patients should be maintained at a platelet count above this level. Despite the widespread use of prophylactic platelet transfusions, few studies have actually documented their clinical benefit. One study comparing patients given prophylactic transfusions with patients transfused only for clinically significant bleeding found no difference in overall survival or deaths due to bleeding between the groups[50]; however, the prophylactic group required twice as many platelet transfusions. Although one study reported that the development of alloimmunization was unrelated to the number of platelet transfusions,[51] several studies using leukocyte-reduced blood components suggest that the risk of alloimmunization increases with exposure to increasing numbers of cellular components containing an immunizing dose of donor leukocytes. Thus, the true benefit of prophylactic platelet transfusions is uncertain.[52]

Platelet transfusion therapy should be tailored to the individual patient and rigid thresholds for transfusion mistakenly assume that all patients carry the same risk of bleeding at all times. Patients with cerebral leukostasis are at high risk for fatal intracranial hemorrhage. In contrast, many stable thrombocytopenic patients can tolerate platelet counts $<5 \times 10^9$/L (<5000/µL) with evidence of minor hemorrhage (eg, petechiae, ecchymoses or epistaxis) but without serious bleeding.[52,53] Bleeding at any level of platelet count may be aggravated by fever, infection or drugs.[31,54]

Platelet Refractoriness

Platelet refractoriness, defined as a poor increment to a suitable dose of correctly prepared and stored PCs, can occur as a result of either immune or nonimmune mechanisms. Immune refractoriness is secondary to either alloantibodies or autoantibodies. Alloantibodies may be directed against either platelet alloantigens or Class I HLA antigens. Autoantibodies occur in idiopathic thrombocytopenic purpura (ITP) and may be present in some patients after bone marrow transplantation. Nonimmune causes of platelet refractoriness include splenomegaly, drugs (for example, amphotericin B) and accelerated platelet consumption. Given the multiple causes of platelet refractoriness, identifying the proper cause(s) for an individual patient can be quite difficult. Nevertheless, effective support of hemostasis often depends on identifying the dominant cause of refractoriness. See Table 17-6 and section on HLA-matched PCs.

Contraindications to Platelet Transfusion

There are several conditions for which platelet transfusions may be requested, but in which such transfusions are contraindicated. Relative contraindications include conditions in which the likelihood of benefit is remote, thus serving only to waste a valuable component that would be better used to care for another patient. An example would be the use of prophylactic PCs in a stable patient who has demonstrated platelet refractoriness and who has a condition known to cause refractoriness. Contraindications include platelet transfusions given to stable patients with thrombotic thrombocytopenic purpura or to patients with heparin-induced thrombocytopenia. These conditions are known to result in platelet thrombi and case reports have suggested major thrombotic complications immediately following platelet transfusions.[55]

Table 17-6. Etiology and Management of Platelet Refractoriness

Cause	Management
Immune	
HLA alloantibodies	HLA-matched platelets or compatible platelets
Platelet alloantibodies	Platelet-antigen matched or compatible platelets
Autoantibodies	? IV IgG, ? corticosteroids, ? splenectomy
Drug (eg, heparin)	Stop offending drug
Nonimmune	
Splenomegaly	Treat cause
Drug (eg, amphotericin)	Stop offending drug if possible
Consumption	Treat cause
Sepsis	Treat cause

Gamma Irradiation of Cellular Blood Components

Gamma irradiation of cellular blood components prevents transfusion-associated GVHD. The risk of transfusion-associated GVHD depends on the immune status of the recipient, the degree of HLA similarity between donor and recipient, and the number of viable lymphocytes transfused. Gamma irradiation is required for cellular components when the donor is a blood relative of the intended recipient. Other indications for the use of gamma-irradiated blood are evolving. See Chapter 19. The dose of gamma radiation given is 25 Gy.

Fresh Frozen Plasma

Physiologic Basis for Use of Fresh Frozen Plasma

Normal coagulation is characterized by the formation of fibrin clot on the platelet plug.[56] Coagulation results from an ordered enzyme cascade. See Fig 17-2. The central procoagulant enzyme is thrombin. The coagulation cascade is often divided into the intrinsic and extrinsic limbs, the activity of which can be measured by the activated partial thromboplastin time (aPTT) and prothrombin time (PT), respectively. In vivo, both cascades are interdependent. Fresh Frozen Plasma (FFP) contains all the clotting factors, including the labile Factors V and VIII. A minimal level of coagulation factors is required for normal formation of fibrin and normal hemostasis. These levels are shown in Table 17-7. Note that there is normally an excess of all coagulation factors. This hemostatic reserve allows patients to receive transfusions of RBCs and saline/colloid without FFP in the initial replacement of one blood volume or less. Patients with liver disease have a decrease

in this physiologic reserve and are more susceptible to dilutional coagulopathy.

Monitoring Adequate Hemostasis

The PT, aPTT and fibrinogen level are commonly used to monitor coagulation. The general relationship between the level of coagulation factors and the prolongation of the PT or aPTT is shown in Fig 17-3. Three aspects of this relationship are of note: 1) mild prolongations of the PT or aPTT occur *before* the residual factor concentration falls below the level normally needed for hemostasis; 2) significant deficiencies of coagulation factors are associated with clearly prolonged values for the PT or aPTT; and 3) an infusion of FFP that increases the concentration of factors by 20% will have a far greater impact on a greatly prolonged PT or aPTT than on a mildly prolonged PT or aPTT. As a result of the above, the infusion of two units of FFP in a patient with a PT of 14.5 seconds (normal 11-13 seconds) is unlikely to provide any clinical benefit and is also unlikely to "correct" the PT to the normal range.

Indications for Fresh Frozen Plasma

Guidelines exist for the appropriate use of FFP.[57,58] FFP is a valuable replacement component for patients with clinically significant Factor XI deficiency and for other congenital deficiencies for which no suitable clotting factor concentrate is available. FFP is most likely to be of clinical benefit in patients with deficiencies of multiple coagulation factors.[59] FFP is the replacement component of choice for plasma exchange treatment of thrombotic thrombocytopenic purpura (TTP) or hemolytic-uremic syndrome (HUS). In nonresponsive patients with TTP or HUS, cryoprecipitate-depleted FFP has been suggested as an alternative,[60] although no controlled trials document its superiority over FFP in the therapy of TTP or HUS.

Deficiencies of Multiple Coagulation Factors

Vitamin K Deficiency

The most common condition involving multiple coagulation abnormalities among hospitalized patients is deficiency of the vitamin K-dependent factors. Vitamin K deficiency results in an elevated PT with or without an associated elevated aPTT. Before patients are treated with FFP to correct a coagulopathy with an abnormal PT or aPTT, unrecognized vitamin K deficiency should be considered. See the section "Pharmacologic Alternatives to Transfusion" in this chapter.

Most patients with vitamin K deficiency do not require FFP and are better treated with parenteral vitamin K.

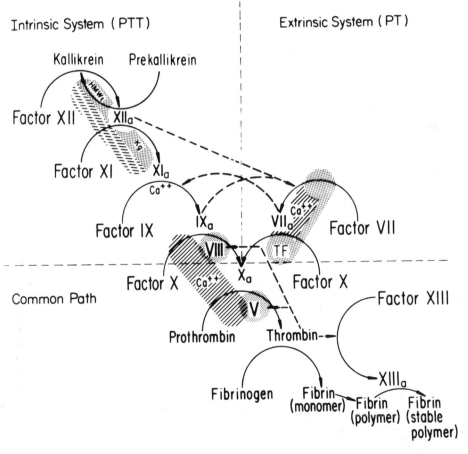

Figure 17-2. The coagulation cascade. The production of thrombin from prothrombin via the action of activated Factor X (Xa), Factor V, Ca^{++} and platelet phospholipid is the key step in the formation of a fibrin clot. Activation of Factor X can occur by either the intrinsic or extrinsic systems, but multiple areas of overlap between the two occur. (Adapted with permission from Thompson et al.[56])

Table 17-7. Biological Data of Selected Coagulation Factors[25-52]

	Approximate Plasma Concentration (mg/mL)	Biological $t_{1/2}$ (Hours)	Recommended Level for Surgery	Intravascular Fraction	Yield
Fibrinogen	2.8	99 ± 3	1 mg/mL	72%	
Prothrombin	0.13	73 ± 7	40-50%	58%	
Factor V	0.068	12-36	10-30%		83%
Factor X	0.012	33	10-40%		51%
Factor VII	0.0005	5	10-20%		100%
Factor VIII	0.00024	13 ± 3	30-100%		80-100%
Factor IX	0.005	23 ± 2	20-60%	22%	24-54%
Factor XI	0.006	61	20-30%		100%
Factor XIII	0.029	282	10%		50%
von Willebrand factor	0.006	20-40	20-50%		73%

Transfusion of plasma is occasionally needed to treat active bleeding due to vitamin K deficiency. Patients with serious hemorrhage should receive FFP or liquid plasma, since parenteral vitamin K will require several hours to completely reverse vitamin K deficiency. Since Factors II, VII, IX and X are stable during storage, plasma of any age provides effective replacement. A general guideline for plasma therapy is that 1 mL of plasma contains one unit of coagulation factor activity. Therefore, three to five units of FFP (600-1000 mL) in the averaged sized adult (3000 mL plasma volume) will generally provide sufficient coagulation factors to achieve hemostasis in coumadin overdosage. Concurrent vitamin K supplementation should also be given. The PT can provide useful information about the response to therapy. The need for additional treatment should be guided by the clinical response, however, and not the result of laboratory tests. It is rarely necessary to correct the PT or aPTT to normal to achieve adequate hemostasis.

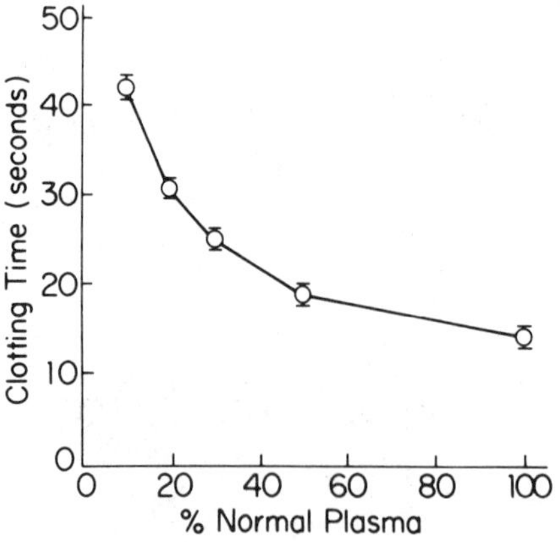

Figure 17-3. Prolongation of in-vitro clotting time as a function of the percent residual coagulation factors. (Reprinted with permission from Thompson et al.[56])

Liver Disease

Patients with liver disease exhibit a complex combination of hemostatic derangements, each of which contributes to an increased bleeding tendency. Hemostatic abnormalities include: engorged veins of the portal system and the portal-systemic collateral shunts, thrombocytopenia secondary to splenomegaly, decreased synthesis of all coagulation factors except Factor VIII, dysfibrinogenemia, decreased clearance of fibrin(ogen) degradation products, decreased clearance of fibrinolytic activators and decreased synthesis of inhibitors of the fibrinolytic system. Because Factor VII has the shortest in-vivo biologic half-life and thus requires the highest synthetic rate, decreased hepatic synthesis prolongs the PT more than the aPTT. Because hepatocellular disease results in a defect in primary protein synthesis, supplemental vitamin K will not correct the abnormality.

FFP is an appropriate replacement therapy for the multiple synthetic deficiencies found in severe liver disease. However, FFP is often used inappropriately in patients with liver disease. The most common error is to attribute bleeding to coagulation factor deficiency and thus use systemic treatment when the actual cause of bleeding is a local disruption of blood vessels best treated with local measures. For example, patients with variceal hemorrhage and a mildly elevated PT are better treated with sclerotherapy than with intravenous infusions of FFP. A second common error in the use of FFP for the treatment of coagulopathy secondary to liver disease is overdependence on the result of the PT. Stopping serious bleeding rarely, if ever, requires a normal PT. Patients who are actively bleeding with a near normal PT are very likely bleeding due to an additional hemostatic problem, such as a mucosal lesion, cut vessel, etc. Moreover, because Factor VII has such a short half-life (approximately 5 hours), the concentration of Factor VII following FFP transfusion will rapidly decline in cirrhotic patients who have little endogenous Factor VII synthesis. Thus the goal of FFP therapy in severe liver disease should *not* be to normalize the PT, but rather to remove or prevent any profound coagulation deficiency.

In addition to strict attention to local causes of bleeding and correction of profound coagulation defects, hemostatic therapy in patients with liver disease should include evaluation of platelet plug formation and the increased fibrinolysis that accompanies liver disease. The response to platelet transfusions is usually suboptimal in the presence of severe splenomegaly. Platelet function in liver disease can be enhanced by administration of 1-deamino-8-D-arginine vasopressin (DDAVP).[61] Cryoprecipitate is an appropriate supplement in the presence of severe hypofibrinogenemia; however, FFP contains sufficient concentrations of fibrinogen to treat hypofibrinogenemia in most patients with severe liver disease. Severe hepatic disease results in an increase in systemic fibrinolysis. The unregulated increase in fibrinolytic activity that accompanies terminal liver disease cannot generally be treated with FFP alone. The use of antifibrinolytic agents in combination with plasma therapy is of great practical value in these patients. See "Pharmacologic Alternatives to Transfusion."

Dilutional Coagulopathy

Loss of blood and replacement with nonplasma solutions will ultimately produce a dilutional coagulopathy. Given the significant physiologic reserve of coagulation factors, most patients can tolerate one blood volume loss and replacement without developing impaired hemostasis due to dilution. Abnormalities of platelet number and function are generally considered to develop before dilutional coagulopathy when WB or modified WB is transfused.[62,63] FFP is not likely to be of clinical benefit if the PT and aPTT are <1.5 times normal, but may be indicated to prevent dilutional coagulopathy if more transfusion support is expected. When more than one blood volume has been replaced, prolongation of the PT or aPTT to >1.8 times normal is likely to be due to either dilutional coagulopathy or hypotension with tissue ischemia.

Patients undergoing intensive daily plasmapheresis may in some cases develop significant dilutional coagulopathy. However, most patients with adequate hepatic synthetic function can tolerate daily one plasma-volume apheresis without requiring supplemental FFP.

Disseminated Intravascular Coagulation

Disseminated intravascular coagulation results from the effects of active circulating thrombin. As a consequence there is widespread fibrin formation in the microcirculation resulting in consumption of platelets and coagulation factors—particularly fibrinogen, Factor V and Factor VIII. The microcirculatory intravascular fibrin strands cause mechanical damage to rbcs and produce microangiopathic hemolysis, resulting in schistocytes. Diffuse microvascular thromboses promote tissue ischemia, release of tissue factor and further thrombin activation. Secondary fibrinolysis of microvascular fibrin results in production of increased quantities of fibrin degradation products. Numerous clinical catastrophes can initiate DIC, including shock, tissue ischemia, sepsis, disseminated cancer and obstetric complications such as abruptio placenta or amniotic fluid embolism. The common precipitating event is a procoagulant signal for thrombin production that exceeds the normal physiologic defenses against disseminated thrombin activity.

Treatment of DIC depends on treatment of the initiating event and prevention of further shock and tissue ischemia. If severe hypofibrinogenemia is present (fibrinogen <80 mg/dL), supplemental FFP or cryoprecipitate is often given. FFP plus low dose heparin (300 units/hour to inhibit thrombin activity) with or without concurrent use of antifibrinolytic agents have also been used. Infusion of concentrates of antithrombin III has also been reported.[64]

Deficiency of Protein C, Protein S or Antithrombin III

Protein C and protein S are vitamin K-dependent proteins with anticoagulant effects. Protein C is converted from an inactive to an active state via the action of protein S. Activated protein C inactivates Factor V and Factor VIII:C and increases vascular release of the fibrinolytic protein, tissue plasminogen activator. Patients with deficiencies of protein C or protein S have an increased tendency to develop thrombotic complications and are often treated with oral anticoagulants. Transfusion of plasma components can serve as an immediate source of supplemental protein C or protein S for patients with severe deficiencies.

Antithrombin III is a circulating protein with anticoagulant properties. Antithrombin III is stable in FFP and in refrigerated liquid plasma, which may be used as a source of antithrombin III. Transfusion practice for antithrombin III is discussed in the section on Plasma Derivatives and Plasma Substitutes.

Other Conditions

Hereditary angioneurotic edema (HAE) results from a congenital deficiency of C1-esterase inhibitor, an inhibitory protein regulating complement activation. Patients with HAE may experience life-threatening subglottal edema following minor triggers of complement activation. FFP or Liquid Plasma contains normal levels of C1-esterase inhibitor and can be used as replacement therapy in patients with HAE.

Misuse of Fresh Frozen Plasma

Several studies have documented that FFP is frequently used inappropriately.[65-70] Plasma should not be used to expand blood volume. Transfusing plasma for volume expansion carries a risk of transmitting disease that can be avoided by using crystalloid or colloid solutions. Plasma is also not a suitable source of immunoglobulins for patients with severe hypogammaglobulinemia, since intravenous IgG is available.

Transfusion of FFP is often given to patients with mild to moderate prolongations of the PT or aPTT prior to invasive procedures. However, there is little or no evidence that the transfusion of FFP will prevent bleeding complications in this setting. One study demonstrated that the preprocedure PT or aPTT did not correlate with the likelihood of bleeding following paracentesis or thoracentesis.[71] Two independent studies have documented that the preprocedure PT, aPTT or platelet count do not predict bleeding at the time of liver biopsy.[72,73] Since the PT and aPTT do not accurately predict the risk of bleeding,[74] there is little logic to "improving" the results of such tests by preprocedure transfusions.

Cryoprecipitate

Cryoprecipitated AHF is a concentrate of plasma high molecular weight proteins that precipitate in the cold, including von Willebrand factor (vWF), Factor VIII, fibrinogen, Factor XIII and fibronectin. The primary clinical use of CRYO is for intravenous supplementation of these factors. It has also been used topically.[75] CRYO contains donor ABO alloantibodies, and consideration should be given to ABO compatibility when large volumes are transfused.

von Willebrand Syndromes

von Willebrand syndromes are the most common major inherited coagulation abnormalities. The conditions are usually autosomal dominant and represent a collection of quantitative and qualitative abnormalities of vWF.[76,77] vWF is the major protein mediating platelet adhesion to damaged endothelium. The protein also transports Factor VIII. As a result, patients with von Willebrand syndromes have varying levels of abnormal platelet plug formation (prolonged bleeding time) and partial deficiency of Factor VIII (prolonged aPTT). Laboratory evaluation discloses a specific deficiency in the level of vWF. vWF is often measured as ristocetin cofactor activity because vWF is required for the platelet-aggregating effect of ristocetin in vitro. vWF exists in the plasma as a family of multimeric molecules with a wide range of molecular weights. The high-molecular weight species of vWF are the most hemostatically effective. The von Willebrand syndromes are subdivided based on the distribution of multimer species.

Mild cases of von Willebrand syndrome can often be treated with DDAVP, which causes a release of endogenous stores of Factor VIII and vWF. See "Pharmacologic Alternatives to Transfusion." However, DDAVP is contraindicated in the rare Type IIb von Willebrand syndrome.

The deficiency of Factor VIII and vWF seen in severe von Willebrand syndromes can be corrected with FFP or with CRYO.[78] CRYO provides a much higher concentration of high molecular vWF than is present in FFP. The quantity of CRYO required to treat bleeding episodes or to prepare for major surgery varies greatly among patients with von Willebrand syndromes. In addition to the clinical response of the patient, the template bleeding time, the level of Factor VIII or the level of ristocetin cofactor may help to guide therapy.

Commercial concentrates of Factor VIII (antihemophilic factor, AHF) will raise the patient's Factor VIII level, but usually do not provide large quantities of high-molecular weight vWF. In general, AHF is not used to treat von Willebrand syndromes. However, certain preparations of AHF do have sufficient concentrations of vWF activity to be used in the treatment of von Willebrand syndromes.[77]

Fibrinogen Abnormalities

Hypofibrinogenemia may occur as a rare isolated congenital deficiency or may be acquired as part of the DIC syndrome. CRYO is the only concentrated fibrinogen product available. On average, one unit of CRYO contains approximately 250 mg of fibrinogen.[79] The fibrinogen content of CRYO may also be of therapeutic advantage in treating dysfibrinogenemias. Dysfibrinogenemias represent conditions in which fibrinogen is immunologically present but functionally defective. A normal plasma fibrinogen level coupled with a long thrombin time in the absence of either heparin or elevated fibrin(ogen) degradation products suggests the presence of a dysfibrinogen. Dysfibrinogenemia may be congenital or acquired. Patients with severe liver disease frequently exhibit a dysfibrinogenemia.

The fibrinogen content of CRYO has also been used during surgery as a topical hemostatic preparation.[80] One to two units of CRYO are thawed and drawn into a syringe. Topical thrombin (usually of bovine origin) is drawn into a second syringe. The contents of the two syringes are simultaneously applied to the bleeding surface. The fibrinogen in the CRYO is converted to fibrin clot by the action of bovine thrombin. See Method 10.11.

Factor VIII Deficiency

Each unit of CRYO prepared from a single blood donation should contain a minimum of 80 units of Factor VIII per bag. Thus, pooled bags of CRYO can serve as replacement therapy for patients with hemophilia A. The correct number of bags of CRYO needed to deliver a therapeutic dose of Factor VIII is based on similar calculations used for AHF. See section on "Plasma Derivatives and Plasma Substitutes."

Fibronectin

Fibronectin is an opsonic glycoprotein thought to play a role in the clearance by the reticuloendothelial system of blood-borne particulate matter such as bacteria and protein aggregates.[81] Uncontrolled clinical studies suggested that infusing fibronectin might be of value in treating patients with sepsis, burns or trauma. A review of the literature on the clinical role of CRYO infusions as a means of providing supplemental fibronectin did not support the use of CRYO in this setting.[82]

Granulocyte Transfusion

There has been a great decline in the clinical use of granulocyte transfusions for adult recipients. Improved antibiotics, adverse effects attributable to granulocyte transfusions and the advent of recombinant growth factors have all contributed to this decline. Nevertheless, in selected patients transfused granulocytes may produce clinical benefits.[83,84] The preparation, storage, pretransfusion testing and quality control of granulocytes is discussed in Chapter 2. The use of granulocyte transfusions in neonates is discussed in Chapter 18.

Indications and Contraindications

Indications for granulocyte transfusions in adults are limited and the goals of therapy should be clearly defined before a course of therapy is initiated. Patients with documented granulocyte dysfunction, such as those with profound *reversible* neutropenia or those with chronic granulomatous disease, are candidates to receive granulocyte transfusions. An absolute granulocyte count below 0.5 × 10^9/L (0.5 × 10^3/µL) is a commonly used criterion, because patients with higher counts are not felt to be at increased risk of infection.[85] Granulocyte transfusions have not been proven effective in patients with localized infections or for the treatment of infections due to agents other than bacteria. Thus, granulocyte transfusions should be reserved for the treatment of bacteremia not responding to appropriate antibiotics. Septicemia should be documented by cultures to identify the infecting organism and to determine antibiotic sensitivity. Granulocyte transfusions are more commonly used to treat gram-negative septicemia than gram-positive infection since gram-negative bacteria are more often resistant to antibiotics than gram-positive organisms. Prophylactic granulocyte transfusions are not considered appropriate therapy.[86,87]

Reactions to Granulocyte Transfusions

Severe pulmonary reactions may follow granulocyte transfusions, particularly in patients with established lung infections or with alloimmunization to HLA antigens present on the donor cells. Initial symptoms may include development or acute exacerbation of cough, shortness of breath, increased respiratory rate and, usually, fever. Pulmonary reactions to granulocyte transfusions may have multiple causes including fluid overload, leukoagglutination reactions, and margination and release of granulocyte contents in the presence of pulmonary tissue infection.[88] A problem specific to granulocyte transfusion is the possibility that simultaneous use of this blood component with amphotericin B causes pulmonary infiltrates and severe respiratory distress.[89] Although controversy exists as to the cause of this clinical syndrome, many physicians prefer to avoid granulocyte transfusions in patients receiving amphotericin B. When severe respiratory distress occurs during a granulocyte transfusion, the infusion should be discontinued and supplemental oxygen given. Intravenous steroids may provide relief of symptoms. The clinical utility of granulocyte transfusions should be reconsidered in recipients who experience serious pulmonary reactions.

Febrile reactions often occur in patients receiving granulocyte concentrates. These usually mild reactions are manifested clinically as fever and chills, can usually be treated by administering non-aspirin antipyretics and slowing the rate of infusion. Meperidine injection may be useful to stop shaking chills.

Transfusion-transmitted CMV and transfusion-associated GVHD are two important complications of granulocyte transfusions.[90] See Chapters 4 and 19.

Plasma Derivatives and Plasma Substitutes

Plasma derivatives are prepared from pools of plasma and represent concentrates of specific plasma proteins. The original fractionation of plasma into albumin and other plasma proteins was developed during World War II.[91] This method, which relies on the precipitation of various plasma proteins in cold ethanol-water mixtures, is still used

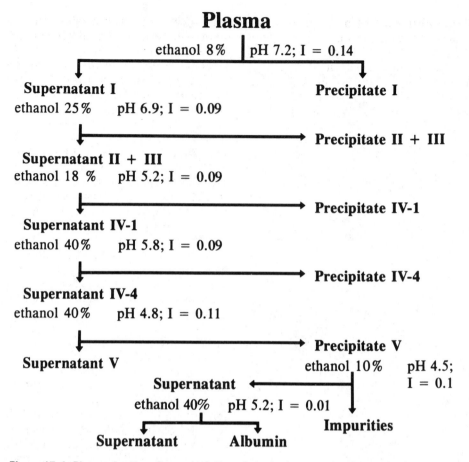

Figure 17-4. Plasma fractionation using ethanol. I = ionic strength. (Adapted with permission from Rossi et al.[1])

today with modifications. See Fig 17-4. After fractionation, derivatives undergo further processing to purify and concentrate the proteins, and inactivate any viral contaminants. Examples of virus inactivation include heat treatment, chemical solvents and detergents or affinity column purification.

Therapy for Hemophilia A

Hemophilia A is a congenital deficiency of Factor VIII resulting from an abnormality of the gene on the X chromosome and, therefore, is fully expressed in males and transmitted by female carriers. Factor VIII is critically important in the reactions leading to fibrin formation. The severity of hemophilia A depends upon the patient's level of Factor VIII. Levels of Factor VIII antigen are sometimes normal despite deficient Factor VIII coagulant activity, suggesting a functional defect of the Factor VIII molecule. Characteristic laboratory findings include prolonged aPTT, normal PT and template bleeding time, and a severe deficiency of Factor VIII activity.

As with all clotting factors, one unit of Factor VIII activity is defined as the

Factor VIII content of 1 mL of fresh, citrated, pooled, normal plasma. Thus the level of Factor VIII can be expressed as a concentration, a decimal fraction or as a percent activity. For example, a hemophiliac with one-tenth the normal activity of Factor VIII is said to have a Factor VIII level of 10 units/dL (0.1 units/mL or 10% activity). Severe hemophiliacs have Factor VIII levels below 1%. Moderate hemophiliacs typically have 1-5% activity. Mild hemophiliacs have 6-30% Factor VIII. Patients with mild to moderate hemophilia can often be managed without the use of replacement therapy. Careful attention to local hemostasis and the use of topical antifibrinolytics can often prevent the need for transfusions. Systemic levels of Factor VIII can be raised in mild hemophilia with the use of DDAVP.[92] See "Pharmacologic Alternatives to Transfusion." DDAVP stimulates the release of endogenous Factor VIII from storage sites. DDAVP is inappropriate therapy in patients with severe hemophilia A. These patients require Factor VIII replacement.

Antihemophilic Factor (AHF, Factor VIII)

AHF is prepared from large volumes of pooled normal plasma or cryoprecipitate by various separation methods. Because Factor VIII concentrates are made from pools of thousands of individual units of plasma, a high incidence of transfusion-transmitted viruses accompanied early preparations and resulted in the high incidence of hepatitis and HIV infection among hemophiliacs.[93] Within the past decade virus inactivation measures have been introduced and improved. Currently available AHF concentrates are treated either by heating in solution ("pasteurization") or by exposure to a solvent/detergent combination. The specific activity (Factor VIII units/mg pro-

tein) of current concentrates also has increased, most dramatically in concentrates prepared with affinity columns. As a result, the safety of AHF has greatly increased and the incidence of posttransfusion viral infection in hemophiliacs treated exclusively with new preparations has dramatically declined.[94] The increased complexity of manufacturing and the lower yields resulting from extensive manipulation have each contributed to the greatly increased cost of AHF. AHF is supplied in lyophilized form and the quantity of Factor VIII activity is stated on the label. After reconstitution, AHF may be administered by syringe or by an administration set.

Patients with hemophilia A may ultimately be treated with recombinant Factor VIII. Clinical studies have suggested that such material is efficacious and without serious side effects.[95]

Calculating Dosage of Factor VIII:C

The amount of transfused Factor VIII required depends upon the nature of the bleeding episode and the severity of the initial deficiency. For example, treatment for hemarthrosis ordinarily requires more Factor VIII than soft tissue hematomas. The amount of Factor VIII required for transfusion can be calculated as follows:

1. Weight (kg) × 70 mL/kg = blood volume (mL)
2. Blood volume (mL) × (1.0 − hematocrit) = plasma volume (mL)
3. Units of Factor VIII required = (Desired Factor VIII level in units/mL − initial Factor VIII level in units/mL) × Plasma volume (mL)

Example: A 70-kg severe hemophiliac with a hematocrit of 0.40 (40%) has an initial Factor VIII level of 2 units/dL (0.02 units/mL, 2% activity). How many units of Factor VIII concentrate should be given to raise his Factor VIII level to 50 units/dL?

70 kg × 70 mL/kg = 4900 mL

4900 mL × (1.0 − 0.40) = 2940 mL

2940 mL × (0.50 − 0.02) = 1411 units

This dose should produce an expected level of 50 units/dL immediately following transfusion. Although the therapy of choice for severe hemophilia A is Factor VIII concentrates, this amount of Factor VIII could be supplied by CRYO but would require at least 18 bags. Assume each bag of CRYO contains 80 IU of Factor VIII (see also Appendix 2).

During equilibration with extravascular spaces, the half-life of circulating Factor VIII is about 4 hours. The biologic half-life is about 12 hours. It is usually necessary to repeat infusions of AHF at intervals to maintain hemostatic levels.

The duration of treatment with Factor VIII transfusions depends upon the type and location of the hemorrhage and the clinical response of the patient. Following major surgery the Factor VIII level should be maintained above 40-50 units/dL for at least 10 days. When elective surgery is planned, Factor VIII assays should be made available to serve as a guide to therapy. In emergencies the aPTT can be used as a rough guide to Factor VIII activity.

Inhibitors to Factor VIII

About 10-20% of patients with hemophilia A develop a detectable inhibitor to Factor VIII. Inhibitors are antibodies that inactivate the portion of the Factor VIII molecule necessary for coagulation activity. Patients who develop inhibitors may become unresponsive to Factor VIII transfusions. The management of patients with inhibitors can be difficult. In very serious hemorrhages, an attempt is made to raise the plasma Factor VIII level in the therapeutic range. Very large doses of human Factor VIII have been tried. Porcine Factor VIII has also been tried because of low cross-reactivity with human anti-Factor VIII antibody.[96] If the inhibitor level (measured in Bethesda units) is very high and time permits, plasmapheresis may be considered prior to infusion of Factor VIII.

Factor IX complex (prothrombin complex) contains Factor II, Factor VII, Factor IX and Factor X and has been effective in treating bleeding episodes in some patients with inhibitors.[97] However, the clinical response is unpredictable.[98] It is postulated that activated factors in the preparation bypass the step in the coagulation cascade that requires Factor VIII, so that fibrin formation can occur. The exact mechanism of action, however, is uncertain. Factor IX complex is treated with heat or solvent/detergent combinations to inactivate viruses. Still, some of these products may be capable of transmitting hepatitis. They can also induce a state of DIC and have been implicated in thrombotic episodes, including myocardial infarction.

Anti-Inhibitor Coagulant Complex (AICC) is specially activated Factor IX complex concentrate intended only for treatment of patients with Factor VIII inhibitors. Brand names include Autoplex® T and FEIBA®, both of which are heat-treated to reduce the chance of virus transmission.[99,100] The risk of thrombotic complications should be kept in mind when these preparations are used.

AICCs are extremely expensive and should be used carefully in the management of hemophilia A. Clinical trials of the use of recombinant Factor VIIa in patients with inhibitors are also under way.

Therapy for Hemophilia B

Factor IX deficiency (hemophilia B, Christmas disease) is clinically indistinguishable from Factor VIII deficiency, in that both are sex-linked disorders that cause a prolonged aPTT in the presence of a normal PT and bleeding time. The disorder is confirmed by specific measurement of Factor IX activity. Defective synthesis of Factor IX is caused by an abnormal gene on the X chromosome. Factor IX complex concentrate has been used for treatment of hemophilia B for the past 2 decades. A coagulation Factor IX concentrate, containing only trace amounts of Factors II, VII or X, was licensed in December 1990. This concentrate is expected to cause fewer thrombotic complications than Factor IX complex concentrate.[101]

Formulas for calculation of Factor VIII dosage (see above) can be used to calculate Factor IX dosage if the units to be given are doubled. Upon infusion, half of Factor IX disappears immediately for unknown reasons. Factor IX equilibrates with the extravascular pool with a half-life of about 4 hours. The biologic half-life is about 24 hours.

Other Blood Derivatives

Intravenous Immunoglobulin

Intravenous IgG is prepared by modifying Cohn fraction II to render IgG safe for intravenous injection. This modification includes a combination of mild enzymatic digestion with papain or plasmin, chemical modification, treatment with polyethylene glycol or concentration at low pH. Intravenous IgG differs from blood derivatives produced for intramuscular injection, which are not suitable for intravenous administration. Intramuscular preparations contain immunoglobulin aggregates that may activate the complement and kinin systems and produce hypotensive and/or anaphylactic reactions if administered intravenously.

Table 17-8. Potential Indications and Clinical Uses for Intravenous Immunoglobulin Preparations

Congenital immune deficiencies
 Hypogammaglobulinemia and agammaglobulinemia
 Selective antibody deficiency
 IgG subclass deficiency and recurrent infection
 Premature newborns
Acquired antibody deficiency
 Malignancies with antibody deficiency and recurrent infection: multiple myeloma, chronic lymphocytic leukemia
 Protein-losing enteropathy
 Drug- or radiation-induced humoral immunodeficiency
Prophylaxis or treatment of bacterial and viral diseases
 Pediatric HIV infection for prevention of bacterial and secondary viral infections
 Cytomegalovirus infection in transplant recipients
 Neonatal sepsis
Other
 Acute immune thrombocytopenic purpura
 Kawasaki syndrome
 Guillain-Barré syndrome
 Posttransfusion purpura

The indications for the use of intravenous IgG are evolving.[102] Some conditions in which intravenous globulin is used are listed in Table 17-8. The correct dose is often a matter of speculation. A commonly used dose is 0.4 g/kg to be repeated daily for 4-5 days. This dose scheme is based on early reports of the efficacy of intravenous IgG in the treatment of childhood ITP.

Transfusion of intravenous immunoglobulin can be accompanied by reactions that include volume overload, allergic reactions and pulmonary reactions. Non-group O patients may develop a positive direct antiglobulin test due to passively transferred ABO alloantibodies. Rarely, significant hemolysis may occur.

Antiprotease Concentrates

Antithrombin III (AT III), also known as heparin cofactor,[103] is synthesized in the liver. AT III is catalytically activated by heparin. When AT III combines with heparin, an arginine site on the AT III is exposed, which neutralizes the serine site on thrombin and on other serine proteases (Factors IX, X, XI and XII), thereby inactivating potent enzyme activity. In normal plasma, AT III is present in concentrations of 230-400 mg/L. Patients who are deficient in AT III do not effectively inhibit thrombin activity and thus are prone to thromboembolic diseases. Congenital AT III deficiency can present as unexpected venous thrombosis. Acquired deficiency of AT III and venous thrombosis are occasionally seen in patients with severe nutritional deficiency. A low measured level of AT III is also seen in liver disease as a result of decreased synthesis, but the multiple other hemostatic derangements of cirrhosis result in deficient coagulation rather than thrombosis. Heparin forms a complex with AT III that results in increased clearance of the heparin-AT III complex. Thus, some patients with prolonged heparin administration can develop transient AT III deficiency and relative heparin resistance. Transfusion of additional AT III may overcome heparin resistance in such patients. A purified heat-treated concentrate of AT III is available. Liquid Plasma and FFP are alternate sources of AT III. The dosage and endpoint for plasma treatment of patients with AT III deficiency are not well defined. Other antiprotease concentrates manufactured include α_1-proteinase inhibitor (α_1-antitrypsin) and C1-esterase inhibitor.

Colloid Plasma Substitutes

Human albumin (5% and 25%) and plasma protein fraction (PPF) provide volume expansion and colloid replacement without risk of transfusion-transmitted viruses.[104] PPF is similar to 5% albumin, but PPF has a greater concentration of nonalbumin plasma proteins. Pharmacologic agents such as hydroxyethyl starch or dextran are also commonly used as plasma substitutes for volume expansion.

Physiology of Albumin

The total body albumin mass is about 300 g. Forty percent, or 120 g, is found in the plasma.[105] Daily albumin synthesis in a normal adult is about 16 g. The half-life of albumin is approximately 20 days. For each 500 mL of blood lost, a person loses only 12 g, or 4%, of the total body albumin. Thus, albumin in a four-unit hemorrhage (2000 mL) is entirely replaced by normal synthesis in 3 days.

Indications for Plasma Substitutes

Despite their widespread and frequent use, clear indications for the use of colloid plasma substitutes are few in number.[106] Albumin infusion is appropriate therapy to correct acute, large-scale loss of colloid. Examples include treatment of patients in hypovolemic shock, patients with burns, patients undergoing large volume paracentesis[107] and patients undergoing retroperitoneal surgery, in which a large volume of protein-rich fluid may pool in the atonic bowel.[108] There is long-standing debate over the necessity to use colloid solutions during large volume transfusion in surgery.

Misuse of Albumin

The use of supplemental albumin to correct hypoalbuminemia in critically ill patients is of doubtful clinical benefit.[106] In a randomized, controlled clinical trial the use of supplemental albumin in critically ill adults effectively raised the serum albumin concentration, but had no effect on clinical outcome.[109]

Although hypoalbuminemia is a reliable marker of nutritional deficiency, supplemental albumin infusions are not an appropriate source of nutrition. In cost per calorie, albumin is the most expensive nutrient supplied in the hospital. Hypoalbuminemia secondary to nutritional deficiency is better treated by enteric or parenteral alimentation.

Although severe hypoalbuminemia results in ascites and edema, not all examples of ascites and edema result from hypoalbuminemia. For example, because patients with liver disease frequently have coexistent hypoalbuminemia, their ascites is frequently misattributed to low serum albumin and low colloid oncotic pressure rather than to portal hypertension. However, patients with cirrhosis who have portal hypertension will exhibit ascites and edema even with normal serum oncotic pressure.

Complications of Transfusion With Colloid Plasma Substitutes

Problems associated with colloid therapy include:

1. Infusions of large quantities of 25% albumin may rapidly increase the intravascular oncotic pressure, drawing a significant volume of water from the interstitial and tissue spaces into the vascular space, thus risking cardiac overload and/or interstitial dehydration.

2. Hypotensive episodes were previously associated with rapid infusion of PPF and attributed to the presence of vasoactive kinins.[110] This complication is now rarely seen using present formulations of PPF. Nevertheless, caution should be exercised in the use of PPF for rapid restoration of volume, as in the treatment of hypovolemic shock.

3. Patients with anaphylactic reactions to blood due to high-titer anti-IgA antibodies may also react to plasma substitutes.

Special Situations Involving Transfusion

Autologous, Neonatal and Obstetric Transfusion Practice

See Chapters 20 and 18, respectively.

Transfusion to Patients With Autoimmune Hemolytic Anemia

Because of the serologic difficulties that accompany autoimmune hemolytic anemia and the expected short red cell survival, a conservative approach to transfusion is recommended. The presence of underlying alloantibodies should be investigated prior to beginning transfusions. It is very helpful to establish the patient's phenotype prior to transfusion to simplify subsequent investigation for the presence of possible alloantibodies.

Massive Transfusion

Massive transfusion is defined as transfusion approximating or exceeding the patient's blood volume within a 24-hour interval. The problems of massive transfusion are life-threatening and require a systematic approach outlined in several reviews.[111-113] The medical or surgical problems created by hypovolemia and hypotension pose greater risks to the patient than do the risks associated with the blood transfusions.

Emergency Issue

The transfusion service should establish in advance policies for emergency release of uncrossmatched blood. If the patient requires immediate transfusion, acceptable choices include the following: uncrossmatched, group O, D+ or D– RBCs; or uncrossmatched, group-specific, D+ or D– WB or RBCs. A combination of approaches may be best if the transfusion requirement continues to be urgent. If the pretransfusion specimen contains no unexpected antibodies, it is permissible to abbreviate the crossmatch to a saline immediate spin for confirmation of ABO compatibility. If unexpected antibodies are present, the decision whether or not to select antigen-negative units for transfusion will depend on the specific alloantibody and the clinical urgency for blood.

Following large volume transfusion over a short time, the proportion of the patient's own cells and plasma in the circulation decreases. The pretransfusion specimen ceases to represent the patient's current status and crossmatches using the initial specimen have diminished validity.

Changing Blood Groups

The transfusion service should establish guidelines for switching blood groups during massive transfusion. The age and sex of the patient are important to consider in this decision. When transfusing a young D– female, it is usually preferable to switch ABO groups before switching Rh (ie, from A– to O– RBCs, instead of a switch to A+ RBCs). The clinical situation should be evaluated and the blood bank medical director should be consulted. If the estimated transfusion requirement is likely to exceed the available supply of D– blood, the change to D+ should be done immediately in order to conserve blood for other recipients. Once the patient receives one or more units of D+ RBCs, there is little advantage to returning to D– blood until after blood loss has stopped.

Coagulation Support During Massive Transfusion

Massive transfusion is often associated with coagulation abnormalities that have been attributed to dilution, or washout, of platelets or coagulation factors.[114] During transfusion the patient's platelet count as well as a limited coagulation profile should be monitored. If abnormal bleeding occurs, support with PCs or FFP can be guided by the results of laboratory testing. Additional tests may be indicated to evaluate the possibility of DIC, acute hepatic ischemia and other complications associated with shock. As a rough guide, the patient's preoperative platelet count and fibrinogen will halve with each blood volume that is infused without supplemental platelets or plasma. Thus, platelet counts fall below $100 \times 10^9/L$ (100,000/µL) in most adult patients after infusion of 15-20 units. Supplemental FFP and PC transfusions are best administered before extreme washout and generalized bleeding occur. Although FFP transfusions are often of value in massive transfusion, mixing equal units of FFP and RBCs is rarely required. An intraoperative PT <1.5 times normal is likely to be associated with adequate hemostasis during surgery. The unpredictable occurrence of abnormal bleeding during massive transfusion indicates that simple dilution with platelet-deficient or factor-deficient blood is not the only cause of poor hemostasis.

Studies suggest that a principal cause of major hemostatic derangement during massive transfusion is shock rather than the transfusion itself.[115] Inadequate volume resuscitation and poor tissue perfusion promote not only the release of tissue procoagulant material and DIC, but also result in lactic acidosis, acidemia and poor myocardial performance.

Metabolic Side Effects of Massive Transfusion

Although the pH of stored blood is lower than normal, massive transfusion itself does not result in acidemia. Acidemia does result from lactic acidosis as a consequence of inadequate volume resuscitation and poor tissue perfusion. Although the potassium level of stored blood is elevated compared with normal, massive transfusion does not result in hyperkalemia. Rather, hypokalemia is routinely seen following massive transfusion. Hypokalemia results from the uptake of plasma potassium with glucose by the recipient's tissue cells and by the transfused donor cells. Transient impaired left ventricular performance can result from hypocalcemia induced by citrate especially when plasma components are being infused rapidly into patients who have impaired hepatic and renal function. Citrate is excreted by the kidney and metabolized in the Krebs cycle by all cells with mitochondria, par-

ticularly hepatocytes. Except in circumstances such as hepatic transplantation and neonatal exchange transfusion, treatment of citrate toxicity is rarely indicated.[115] Since calcium in bone is rapidly mobilized to blood, rules of calcium administration for each fixed number of transfusions should be discouraged. Citrate toxicity is best assessed by measuring the concentration of ionized Ca^{++}.[115] The metabolism of citrate generates a metabolic alkalosis. Hypothermia exacerbates the adverse effect of hypocalcemia on cardiac performance.

Cold Toxicity, Tissue Oxygenation and 2,3-DPG

If a large volume of refrigerated blood is rapidly transfused, there is risk of cardiac toxicity induced by hypothermia. Hypothermic conditions increase the cardiac toxicity of hypocalcemia or hyperkalemia and can result in serious ventricular arrthymias and poor left ventricular performance. The cardiac toxicity of rapid transfusion with large volumes of cold blood can be prevented by the use of blood warmers. (See below.)

In hypovolemic shock, the underlying pathophysiologic defect is inadequate tissue oxygenation. Oxygen supply to the tissues is determined by many factors, the most important of which are blood flow (perfusion) and hemoglobin concentration. Depressed levels of red cell 2,3-DPG present in stored blood have been frequently discussed as a potential cause of poor tissue oxygenation in massive transfusion. There are few clinical data to support the thesis that the low 2,3-DPG levels found in stored blood are detrimental to massively transfused patients, although in infants undergoing exchange transfusion, blood with near normal levels of DPG is frequently requested. The most important factor in supporting tissue oxygenation is maintenance of adequate blood flow and blood pressure, by transfusing enough volume to correct or prevent hypovolemic shock. Transfused RBCs regenerate 50% of normal 2,3-DPG levels in 3-8 hours.[116]

Administration of Blood and Components

Identifying Recipient and Donor Unit

Accurate identification of the donor's blood and the intended recipient may be the single most important step in ensuring transfusion safety. Most fatal hemolytic transfusion reactions occur because ABO-incompatible RBCs were inadvertently administered.[117] Plasma, platelets and blood derivatives are also capable of causing serious transfusion reactions. Accurate identification and labeling of donor blood are discussed in Chapter 1; procedures to identify the patient's specimen used for compatibility testing are discussed in Chapter 14. The final steps in safe transfusion practice occur when blood is issued for transfusion and when blood is administered.

At the Time of Issue

Both the transfusion service personnel who issue the blood and the clinical representatives who receive the unit have responsibility for identifying the blood. Before a unit of blood is released, transfusion service personnel must complete the following steps.

1. The name and identification number of the intended recipient, the ABO and Rh type of the recipient, the donation unit number, the ABO and Rh type of the donor unit and the interpretation of compatibility tests (if performed) should be recorded on a transfusion form for each unit. This form or a copy of it becomes a part of the patient's medical record.

2. The name and identification number of the intended recipient, the donation unit number and the interpretation of compatibility tests (if performed) should be securely attached to the blood bag.

3. The appearance and expiration date of the blood or component should be checked before issue and a record made of this inspection.

4. The name of the person issuing the blood, the name of the person to whom the blood is issued and the date and time of issue may be recorded.

At the Time of Infusion

The transfusionist who administers the blood is the last point at which identification errors can be detected before the patient is transfused. Some hospitals require that evidence of informed consent be checked prior to the administration of blood. The transfusionist must check all identifying information before beginning the transfusion, and record on the transfusion form that this information has been checked and found to be correct. Items to be checked are indicated below.

1. Recipient identification: The name and identification number on the patient's wristband must be identical with the name and number on the form attached to the unit.

2. Unit identification: The unit identification number must agree on the blood container and on the form attached to the unit.

3. ABO/Rh: The ABO and Rh type on the primary label on the donor unit must agree with that recorded on the transfusion form. The recipient ABO and Rh type must be recorded on the transfusion form.

4. Expiration: The expiration date of the donor unit should be verified as acceptable before infusion.

5. Compatibility: The interpretation of compatibility testing (if performed) must be recorded on the form attached to the unit. If blood was issued before compatibility tests were completed, this must be conspicuously indicated.

6. Order: The blood or component should be checked against the physician's written order, to verify that the correct component is being given.

All identification attached to the container should remain attached until the transfusion has been terminated.

Starting the Transfusion

After checking all the identifying information, the transfusionist must sign the transfusion form to indicate that the identification was correct and to document who started the transfusion. The directors of many transfusion or nursing services require that a second individual confirm the identity of the blood unit and of the patient. Notation of date and time of transfusion may also be required on the transfusion form. The date and time of transfusion, the name and volume of the component and its identification number may also be recorded.

In addition to informing the patient of the procedure and checking all identification steps, the transfusionist should observe and record the patient's vital signs before administering the blood.

Delays in Starting the Transfusion

Blood should be administered as soon as possible after issue. Blood must not be stored in unmonitored refrigerators. If the transfusion cannot be initiated within a short time, the blood should be returned to the blood bank promptly. Many blood banks set a time limit past which issued blood will not be accepted back into inventory. Often, this limit is 30 minutes, which is the time required for blood to reach 6 C when exposed to room temperature.[118] Blood remains at room temperature for several hours during transfusion; while this does not harm the red cells, prolonged periods outside the refrigerator make a unit of blood unsuitable for reissue by the blood bank. An unused unit of blood that has reached 10 C or above should not be reissued by the blood bank due to the risk of bacterial overgrowth.

Transfusion Devices

Blood Warmers

Patients receiving refrigerated blood at rates faster than 100 mL/minute for 30 minutes have an increased incidence of cardiac arrest as compared with a control group receiving blood warmed to 37 C.[119] Large volumes of rapidly infused cold blood can lower the temperature of the sino-atrial node to below 30 C, at which point ventricular arrhythmias occur. Transfusions at this rate generally occur only in the operating room or trauma room. There is no evidence that patients receiving one to three units of blood over several hours are at similar risk for arrhythmias. Routine warming of blood is unnecessary.

Several blood warmers are available.[120] AABB *Standards for Blood Banks and Transfusion Services* requires that blood warmers not allow blood to be warmed above 38 C. Electrical blood warmers should have a visible thermometer. Conventional microwave devices damage red cells[121] and should not be used for warming blood. However, an inline microwave blood warming device using a special tuned heating chamber has been developed that delivers microwave energy in a uniform and controlled manner.[122]

Electromechanical Infusion Devices

Mechanical pumps that facilitate infusion at controlled rates are useful especially for very slow rates of transfusion to pediatric or neonatal patients. When using these pumps for blood transfusion, the transfusionist must ensure that hemolysis does not occur. Some pumps use a mechanical screwdrive to advance the plunger of a syringe filled with blood; others use roller pumps or other forms of pressure applied to infusion tubing. Although some can be used with standard blood administration sets, most require plastic disposables supplied by the manufacturer. RBCs with high hematocrit and high viscosity are more likely to undergo hemolysis when infused under pressure. WB or RBCs diluted with saline have lower viscosities and are less likely to undergo hemolysis. The manufacturer should be consulted before transfusing RBCs with an infusion pump designed for use with crystalloid or colloid solutions. Studies with radiolabeled red cells and platelets administered through a pump showed no loss of in-vitro function or in-vivo recovery.[123]

Filters

Blood and components must be administered through a filter designed to retain blood clots and other debris. Standard blood filters have a pore size of 170-260 microns and can trap large blood clots. Some administration sets for PCs or CRYO have filters incorporated in tubing suitable for syringe administration. Filters are not routinely necessary for infusion of commercially prepared plasma products such as albumin, but the manufacturer's instructions should be consulted for specific recommendations.

Microaggregate filters have an effective pore size of 20-40 microns and trap microaggregates composed of degenerating platelets, white cells and fibrin strands, which form in blood after 5 or more days of refrigerated storage. Microaggregates can pass through standard blood filters and are thought to accumulate in pulmonary capillaries after transfusion. Whether or not microaggregate debris causes pulmonary dysfunction following massive transfusion has been extensively debated.[124,125] No published data support the routine use of microaggregate blood filters for low volume transfusions.[125] Some emergency room physicians, surgeons and anesthesiologists believe that the slow flow that results from use of these filters makes them inappropriate in settings requiring very rapid massive transfusion.[125] There have been reports of hemolysis induced by use of a pediatric microaggregate filter.[126] Leukocyte-adsorption blood filters are the most effective filters for removing donor leukocytes from RBCs and PCs. See "Leukocyte-Reduced Blood Components" earlier in this chapter.

Needles

Flow at high pressure through small lumen needles may damage red cells.[127,128] For infusing WB or RBCs, an 18- or 19-gauge needle gives good flow rates without excessive discomfort to the patient. For patients with small veins, much smaller needles must be used. A thin-walled, 23-gauge "scalp vein" needle is useful for pediatric transfusions and for adults whose larger veins are inaccessible. Undiluted RBCs flow very slowly through a 23-gauge needle, but diluting the cells with saline may cause unwanted volume expansion. In such cases it may be desirable to separate the unit into aliquots, keeping part of it in the blood bank while the first portion is transfused.

Either steel needles or plastic catheters can be used for transfusions. Catheters are more comfortable if infusions are to continue for a long period of time, and are less likely to become dislodged or puncture the vessel wall. The risks of infection and of thrombophlebitis increase with the length of time a catheter remains in place. Each facility should establish policy for the maximal time a catheter may remain in a vein and should outline a surveillance procedure to be sure that catheters are maintained aseptically and changed as often as specified.

Compatible Fluids

AABB *Standards* is explicit in stating that no medication may be added to blood or components. Solutions intended for intravenous use may be added to blood or components or used in an administration set if they have been approved for this use by the FDA or if documentation exists that they are safe and efficacious when added to the component. Diluting RBCs to reduce viscosity is commonly performed and intravenous solutions are sometimes used to rinse cryoprecipitate out of the bag. If fluid is to be instilled into the blood or component container, however, 0.9% saline is the only acceptable fluid.

Standards, however, is not explicit about which fluids may come in contact with blood in infusion sets, stating only that there must be adequate evidence that they are safe and approved by the FDA for admixture with blood components. Lactated Ringer's solution, 5% dextrose in water and hypotonic sodium chloride solutions should not be used. The dextrose solution causes red cells to clump in the tubing and, more important, causes red cells to swell and hemo-lyze as dextrose and associated water diffuse from the medium into the cells.[129] Lactated Ringer's solution contains enough ionized calcium (3 mEq/L) to overcome the anticoagulant effect of CPDA-1 and allow small clots to develop. When blood follows an electrolyte solution through administration tubing, 25% of the electrolyte solution remains in the tubing after 10 minutes, and 10% persists at 30 minutes.[129]

Care During Transfusion

The transfusionist should remain with the patient for the first few minutes after the start of the infusion. Catastrophic events such as anaphylactic reactions usually become apparent after a very small volume enters the patient's circulation. After the first 15 minutes, the patient should be observed and the vital signs recorded and, if there are no significant changes, the rate of infusion can be increased to that specified in the clinical order. Patient-care personnel should observe the patient frequently throughout the transfusion.

Rate of Infusion

The desirable rate of infusion varies with the patient's clinical condition. For rapid infusion, external pressure devices make it possible to administer a unit of blood within a few minutes. These should only be used with a large-bore needle. External compression devices should be equipped with a pressure gauge, and the pressure exerted should not exceed 300 torr. Blood pressure cuffs are not suitable because they do not exert uniform pressure against all parts of the bag, and irregularly applied pressure may cause the bag to leak.

While there are no experimental or clinical data to support a specific temporal restriction, the *Circular of Information* published by the AABB, the ARC and the

CCBC gives 4 hours as the maximal time permitted for an infusion. The *recommended time* for a routine transfusion should not be confused with the maximal time permitted for a transfusion.

There are also no definite rules for the length of time an administration set or filter may remain in use. A reasonable maximal time limit for use of a blood filter is 6 hours. Filters trap clumped cells, cellular debris and coagulated protein, resulting in a high protein concentration at the filter surface. If bacteria are present, the combination of room temperature incubation and high protein concentration could allow the bacteria to multiply on the filter more rapidly than they would in refrigerated blood. Accumulated material also slows the rate of flow. Standard 170-240 micron filters can ordinarily be used for two to four units of blood but filters that have remained at room temperature for prolonged periods should not be reused.

If blood flows more slowly than is desired, the filter or the needle may be obstructed, or the component may simply be too viscous for rapid flow through the administration set. Steps to investigate and correct the problem include the following:

1. Elevate the blood container to increase hydrostatic pressure.
2. Check the patency of the needle.
3. Examine the filter of the administration set for excessive debris.
4. If RBCs are flowing too slowly, and there is an order permitting addition of saline, add 50-100 mL normal saline.

Discontinuing the Transfusion

After each unit of blood has been infused, patient-care personnel should record the time, the volume and type of component given, the patient's condition and the identity of the person who stopped the transfusion and observed the patient. Many transfusion services require that a copy of the completed transfusion form be returned to the transfusion service. There is no requirement to return the empty blood bag after uncomplicated transfusions. If bags are returned, proper biohazard precautions should be used. The patient should remain under observation for at least an hour after the transfusion is completed, and posttransfusion vital signs should be recorded according to the protocol established in the institution's procedures manual.

Pharmacologic Alternatives to Transfusion

Recombinant Growth Factors

Growth factors are low molecular weight proteins that regulate hematopoiesis by specific interaction with receptors found on bone marrow progenitor cells. The use of growth factors to stimulate endogenous blood cell production is an important alternative to the use of blood.[130]

Erythropoietin

The clinical use of recombinant erythropoietin has revolutionized the transfusion support of patients with end-stage renal disease.[131] Erythropoietin is also being investigated for the treatment of patients with the anemia of chronic disease, for postsurgical or intensive care unit patients or for patients who are receiving medications that suppress the bone marrow. The use of recombinant erythropoietin in the setting of preoperative autologous blood donation is discussed in Chapter 20.

Other Blood Cell Growth Factors

Granulocyte-macrophage colony-stimulating factor (GM-CSF) and granulocyte colony-stimulating factor (G-CSF) are two recombinant growth factors that stimulate marrow production of granulocytes. G-CSF was investigated and approved in the setting of chemotherapy-induced neutropenia.[132,133] Expected clinical benefits from the use of G-CSF (or GM-CSF) include fewer days with neutropenia or fever, less mucositis and increased tolerance of cytotoxic dose schedules. These products are likely to further reduce the need for granulocyte transfusions. GM-CSF was investigated and approved for use in the setting of autologous marrow transplantation. Other potential clinical settings for the use of GM-CSF and G-CSF include the support of patients undergoing allogeneic marrow transplantation or patients receiving antiviral agents that suppress the marrow.[134]

Red Cell Substitutes

Stroma-free hemoglobin solution in which free hemoglobin has been separated from cell membranes is not suitable as a blood substitute due to several disadvantages including a low p50, short circulation time, high oncotic pressure and vasopressor/nephrotoxic properties. Chemical modifications of hemoglobin solutions may successfully overcome these disadvantages.[135] One promising modified hemoglobin adds pyridoxal-5'-phosphate to N-terminal hemoglobin chains, which are then polymerized into molecular aggregates. Pyridoxylation improves the p50 to levels similar to levels in blood, 18-22 torr. Polymerization of the hemoglobin reduces the oncotic pressure and results in a family of molecules sufficiently large to escape rapid clearance by the kidney. Clinical trials of pyridoxylated-polymerized stroma-free hemoglobin solutions suggest that with further refinement, such a product may serve as an alternative to RBCs as a short-term oxygen carrier. Another hemoglobin solution under development uses diaspirin cross-linked stroma-free hemoglobin.[136] Hemoglobin produced by recombinant DNA techniques is also being investigated.

DDAVP

DDAVP is a synthetic analog of vasopressin without significant pressor activity.[137] First used for its antidiuretic hormone effect in the treatment of diabetes insipidus, DDAVP is a useful adjunct to promote hemostasis. Although the exact mechanism of its effect is still under investigation, DDAVP appears to cause release of endogenous stores of high molecular weight vWF from Weibel-Palade bodies located in the vascular subendothelium. Because of its effect on Factor VIII and vWF, DDAVP was initially used as a hemostatic agent in patients with mild to moderate hemophilia A and in patients with von Willebrand syndromes. Because platelet adhesion and the subsequent formation of a platelet plug is dependent upon vWF, DDAVP has also been shown to be of benefit in a wide variety of platelet function disorders, including uremia,[138] cardiopulmonary bypass,[139] cirrhosis of the liver,[60] drug-induced platelet dysfunction (including aspirin), primary platelet disorders and myelodysplastic syndromes.[140]

DDAVP can be given intravenously or subcutaneously. It is usually given as a single injection to treat bleeding or as prophylactic therapy prior to a procedure. Repeated doses within a 24-48 hour period are usually not given because the drug's ability to cause release of vWF diminishes upon subsequent injections (tachyphylaxis). It causes few side effects. Some patients experience facial flushing or mild hypotension. Thrombotic complications have been reported. Repeated injections will promote water retention and hyponatremia. Its effect on vWF occurs within 30 minutes and lasts 4-6 hours. DDAVP is contraindicated in the rare Type IIb von Willebrand syndrome in which platelets have abnormally increased responsiveness to vWF.

Vitamin K

Vitamin K is a fat-soluble vitamin required for normal hemostasis. Vitamin K-dependent enzymes in the liver add a second carboxyl group to the γ-carbon of glutamyl residues found in clotting Factors II (prothrombin), VII, IX, X, protein C and protein S. These additional carboxyl groups provide a second negative charge to allow Ca^{++}-mediated binding of the factors to cell surfaces. Body stores of vitamin K last only 2 weeks. As a result, deficiency of vitamin K is one of the most common vitamin defects in nutritionally depleted, hospitalized patients. Normal gut absorption of vitamin K depends upon both bacterial metabolism of vitamin K precursors in the gut and micelle formation by bile salts. Thus, vitamin K deficiency accompanies antibiotic use as well as obstructive jaundice and fat malabsorption syndromes. Warfarin-type anticoagulants work by specifically inhibiting the action of vitamin K.

Factor VII has the shortest half-life (5 hours) of the procoagulant factors dependent on postsynthetic modification by vitamin K-dependent enzymes. Therefore, vitamin K depletion usually causes a prolongation of the PT out of proportion to the aPTT. Deficiency of vitamin K is best managed by treating the underlying condition and by providing supplemental parenteral vitamin K. If liver function is adequate, coagulation factors return to effective levels about 12 hours after intravenous or subcutaneous administration of aqueous vitamin K.

Fibrinolytic Inhibitors

Epsilon aminocaproic acid and tranexamic acid are both inhibitors of the fibrinolytic system. These drugs are synthetic analogs of lysine and competitively inhibit fibrinolysis by saturating the lysing binding sites upon which plasminogen and plasmin bind to fibrinogen and fibrin. The drugs can be used locally or systemically. When used systemically, the dose must be reduced in the presence of renal insufficiency. These drugs offer specific correction of the hemostatic defect in specialized circumstances of generalized fibrinolysis,[141] including prostatic surgery[142] and hepatic transplantation.[143] Antifibrinolytic agents are also useful adjuncts to promote hemostasis in conditions in which local fibrinolysis contributes to bleeding, eg, the local increased fibrinolysis associated with mucosal lesions of the mouth and gastrointestinal tract or following cardiopulmonary bypass surgery.[144] As a result, fibrinolytic inhibitors have been of benefit in the control of hemorrhage following dental extractions in hemophilia[145] and in the control of upper gastrointestinal bleeding.[146,147] Fibrinolytic inhibitors have also been used with success for the control of bleeding in patients with severe thrombocytopenia.[148,149]

Systemic administration of fibrinolytic inhibitors has been associated with serious thrombotic complications, including ureteral obstruction due to clot and arterial and venous large vessel thrombosis. When used in excessive doses, fibrinolytic inhibitors can *prolong* the bleeding time.[150] These drugs are best recommended by physicians with experience in their use.

Aprotinin (Trasylol®) is a proteinase inhibitor prepared from bovine lung. It inhibits plasmin, kallikrein, trypsin and, to some extent, urokinase. Randomized trials have demonstrated significantly reduced transfusion requirements when aprotinin was administered during surgery.[151,152]

Recombinant Products for Hemostasis

Recombinant gene technology is being used to develop a number of products that may serve as alternatives to plasma products in the treatment of patients with abnormalities of hemostasis. These include recombinant Factor VIII[153] and recombinant Factor VIIa.

References

1. Rossi EC, Simon TL, Moss GS, eds. Principles of transfusion medicine. 1st edition. Baltimore: Williams and Wilkins, 1991.
2. Petz LD, Swisher SN, eds. Clinical practice of transfusion medicine. 2nd edition. New York: Churchill Livingstone, 1989.
3. Hoffman R, Benz EJ, Shattil SJ, et al, eds. Hematology: Basic principles and practice. New York: Churchill Livingstone, 1991.
4. Greenburg AG. Indications for transfusion. In: Wilmore DW, Brennan MF, Harken AH, et al, eds. Care of the surgical patient. Vol. 1. Critical care. New York: Scientific American, Inc, 1989:I.6.1-19.
5. Mollison PL, Engelfriet CP, Contreras M. Blood transfusion in clinical medicine. 9th edition. Oxford: Blackwell Scientific Publications, 1993.
6. Gould SA, Rice CL, Moss GS. The physiologic basis of the use of blood and blood products. Surg Annu 1984;16:13-38.
7. Wilkerson DK, Rosen AL, Gould SA, et al. Oxygen extraction ratio: A valid indicator of myocardial metabolism in anemia. J Surg Res 1987;42:629-34.
8. Babineau TJ, Dzik WH, Borlase BC, et al. A reevaluation of current transfusion practices in surgical ICU patients. Am J Surg 1992;164: 22-5.
9. Lorente JA, Renes E, Gomez-Aguinaga MA, et al. Oxygen delivery-dependent oxygen consumption in acute respiratory failure. Crit Care Med 1991;19:770-5.
10. Kariman K, Burns SR. Regulation of tissue oxygen extraction is disturbed in adult respiratory distress syndrome. Am Rev Respir Dis 1985;132:109-14.
11. Manno CS, Hedberg KW, Kim HC, et al. Comparison of the hemostatic effects of fresh whole blood, stored whole blood, and components after open heart surgery in children. Blood 1991;77:930-6.
12. Mohr R, Martinowitz U, Lavee J, et al. The hemostatic effect of transfusing fresh whole blood versus platelet concentrates after cardiac operations. J Thorac Cardiovasc Surg 1988;96:530-4.
13. Gollub S, Svigals R, Bailey CP, et al. Electrolyte solutions in surgical patients refusing transfusion. JAMA 1971;215:2077-83.
14. Welch HG, Meehan KR, Goodnough LT. Prudent strategies for elective red blood cell transfusion. Ann Intern Med 1992;116:393-402.
15. American College of Physicians. Practice strategies for elective red blood cell transfusion. Ann Intern Med 1992;116:403-6.
16. National Institutes of Health Consensus Development Conference. Perioperative red blood cell transfusion. JAMA 1988;260:2700-3.
17. Lane TA, Anderson KC, Goodnough LT, et al. Leukocyte reduction in blood component therapy. Ann Intern Med 1992;117:151-62.
18. Claas FHJ, Smeenk RJT, Schmidt R, et al. Alloimmunization against the MHC antigens after platelet transfusion is due to contaminating leukocytes in the platelet suspension. Exp Hematol 1981;9:84-9.
19. Sniecinski I, O'Donnell MR, Nowicki B, Hill LR. Prevention of refractoriness and HLA-alloimmunization using filtered blood products. Blood 1988;71:1402-07.
20. Andreu G, Dewailly J, Leberre C, et al. Prevention of HLA immunization with leukocyte-poor packed red cells and platelet concentrates obtained by filtration. Blood 1988; 72:964-9.
21. Fisher M, Chapman JR, Ting A, Morris PJ. Alloimmunization to HLA antigens following transfusion with leukocyte-poor and purified platelet suspensions. Vox Sang 1985; 49:331-5.
22. Bareford D, Chandler ST, Hawker RJ, et al. Splenic platelet sequestration following routine blood transfusion is reduced by filtered/washed blood products. Br J Haematol 1987;67:177-80.
23. Lim S, Boughton BJ, Bareford D. Thrombocytopenia following routine blood transfusion: Microaggregate blood filters

prevent worsening thrombocytopenia in patients with low platelet counts. Vox Sang 1989;56:40-1.

24. Gilbert GL, Hayes K, Hudson IL, James J. Prevention of transfusion acquired cytomegalovirus infection in infants by blood filtration to remove leucocytes. Lancet 1989;1: 1228-31.

25. Bowden RA, Slichter SJ, Sayers MH, et al. Use of leukocyte-depleted platelets and cytomegalovirus-seronegative red blood cells for prevention of primary cytomegalovirus infection after marrow transplant. Blood 1991;78: 246-50.

26. Rawal B, Yen TSB, Vyas GN, Busch M. Leukocyte filtration removes infectious particulate debris but not free virus from experimentally lysed HIV-infected cells. Vox Sang 1991;60: 214-8.

27. Buchholz DH, AuBuchon JP, Snyder EL, et al. Removal of *Yersinia enterocolitica* from AS-1 red cells. Transfusion 1992;32:667-72.

28. Akahoshi M, Takanashi M, Masuda M, et al. A case of transfusion-associated graft-versus-host disease not prevented by white cell-reduction filters. Transfusion 1992;32:169-72.

29. Channing Rodgers RP, Levin J. A critical appraisal of the bleeding time. Semin Thromb Hemost 1990;16:1-20.

30. Lind SE. Review: The bleeding time does not predict surgical bleeding. Blood 1991;77: 2547-52.

31. Slichter SJ. Mechanisms and management of platelet refractoriness. In: Nance SJ, ed. Transfusion medicine in the 1990's. Arlington, VA: American Association of Blood Banks, 1990:95-160.

32. Gmur J, von Felten A, Osterwalder B, et al. Delayed alloimmunization using random single donor platelet transfusions: A prospective study in thrombocytopenic patients with acute leukemia. Blood 1983;62:473-9.

33. Sintnicolaas K, Sizoo W, Haije WG, et al. Delayed alloimmunization by random single donor platelet transfusions. Lancet 1981;1: 750-3.

34. Meryman HT. Transfusion-induced alloimmunization and immunosuppression and the effects of leukocyte depletion. Transfus Med Rev 1989;3:180-93.

35. Aster RH. Effect of anticoagulant and ABO incompatibility on recovery of transfused human platelets. Blood 1965;26:732-43.

36. Duquesnoy RJ, Anderson AJ, Tomasulo PA, Aster RH. ABO compatibility and platelet transfusions of alloimmunized thrombocytopenic patients. Blood 1979;54:595-9.

37. Lee EJ, Schiffer CA. ABO compatibility can influence the results of platelet transfusion. Results of a randomized trial. Transfusion 1989;29:384-9.

38. Goldfinger D, McGinniss MH. Rh-incompatible platelet transfusion—risks and consequences of sensitizing immunosuppressed patients. N Engl J Med 1971;284:942-4.

39. Lichtiger B, Surgeon J, Rhorer S. Rh-incompatible platelet transfusion therapy in cancer patients. Vox Sang 1983;45:139-43.

40. Kooy MvM, Prooijen HCv, Moes M, et al. Use of leukocyte-depleted platelet concentrates for the prevention of refractoriness and primary HLA alloimmunization: A prospective, randomized trial. Blood 1991;77:201-5.

41. Deeg HJ, Aprile J, Graham TC, et al. Ultraviolet irradiation of blood prevents transfusion induced sensitization and marrow graft rejection in dogs. Blood 1986;67:537-9.

42. Lalezari P, Driscoll AM. Ability of thrombocytes to acquire HLA specificity from plasma. Blood 1982;59:167-70.

43. Rodey GE. Class I antigens: HLA-A, -B, -C and cross-reactive groups. In: Moulds JM, Fawcett KJ, Garner RJ, eds. Scientific and technical aspects of the major histocompatibility complex. Arlington, VA: American Association of Blood Banks, 1989:23-46.

44. Duquesnoy RJ, Filip DJ, Rodey GE, et al. Successful transfusion of platelets "mismatched" for HLA antigens to alloimmunized thrombocytopenic patients. Am J Hematol 1977;2:219.

45. Dahlke MB, Weiss KL. Platelet transfusion from donors mismatched for crossreactive HLA antigens. Transfusion 1984;24:299-302.

46. Rodey GE. HLA beyond tears. Atlanta, GA: De Novo, Inc. 1991.

47. Moroff G, Farratty G, Heal JM, et al. Selection of platelets for refractory patients by HLA matching and prospective crossmatching. Transfusion 1992;32:633-40.

48. NIH Consensus Conference. Platelet transfusion therapy. JAMA 1987;257:1777-80.

49. Gaydos LA, Freireich EF, Mantel N. The quantitative relationship between platelet count and hemorrhage in patients with acute leukemia. N Engl J Med 1962;266:905-9.

50. Solomon J, Bofenkamp T, Fahey JL, et al. Platelet prophylaxis in acute non-lymphocytic leukemia (letter). Lancet 1978;1:267.

51. Dutcher JP, Schiffer CA, Aisner J, Wiernik PH. Alloimmunization following platelet transfusion: The absence of a dose-response relationship. Blood 1981;57:395-8.

52. Aderka D, Praff G, Santo M, et al. Bleeding due to thrombocytopenia in acute leukemias and reevaluation of the prophylactic platelet transfusion policy. Am J Med Sci 1986;291: 147-51.

53. Gmur J, Burger J, Schanz U, et al. Safety of stringent prophylactic platelet transfusion policy for patients with acute leukemia. Lancet 1991;338:1224-6.

54. Bishop JF, Matthews JP, McGrath K, et al. Factors influencing 20-hour increments after platelet transfusion. Transfusion 1991; 31:392-6.

55. Gordon LI, Kwaan HC, Rossi EC. Deleterious effects of platelet transfusion and recovery thrombocytosis in patients with thrombotic microangiopathy. Semin Hematol 1987;27: 194-201.

56. Thompson AR, Harker LA. Manual of hemostasis and thrombosis. 3rd edition. Philadelphia: FA Davis, 1983.

57. NIH Consensus Conference. Fresh frozen plasma: Indications and risks. JAMA 1985; 253:551-3.

58. British Committee for Standards in Hematology. Guidelines for the use of fresh frozen plasma. Transfusion Medicine 1992;2:57-63.

59. Braunstein AH, Oberman HA. Transfusion of plasma components. Transfusion 1984;24: 281-6.

60. Byrnes JJ, Moake JL, Periman P. Effectiveness of the cryosupernatant fraction of plasma in the treatment of refractory TTP. Am J Hematol 1990;34:169-74.

61. Mannucci PM, Vicente V, Vianello L, et al. Controlled trial of desmopressin in liver cirrhosis and other conditions associated with a prolonged bleeding time. Blood 1986;67: 1148-53.

62. Miller RD, Robbins TO, Tong MJ, Barton SL. Coagulation defects associated with massive blood transfusion. Ann Surg 1971;174:794-801.

63. Counts RB, Haisch C, Simon TL, et al. Hemostasis in massively transfused trauma patients. Ann Surg 1979;190:91-9.

64. Vinazzer H. Clinical use of antithrombin III concentrates. Vox Sang 1987;53:193-8.

65. Silbert JA, Bove JR, Dubin S, Bush WS. Patterns of fresh frozen plasma use. Conn Med 1981;45:507-11.

66. Solomon RR, Clifford JS, Gutman SI. The use of laboratory intervention to stem the flow of fresh-frozen plasma. Am J Clin Pathol 1988; 89:518-21.

67. Snyder AJ, Gottschall JL, Menitove JE. Why is fresh frozen plasma transfused? Transfusion 1986;26:107-12.

68. Oberman HA. Inappropriate use of fresh frozen plasma. JAMA 1985;253:556-7.

69. Blumberg N, Laczin J, McMican A, et al. A critical survey of fresh-frozen plasma use. Transfusion 1986;26:511-3.

70. Shaikh BS, Wagar D, Lau PM, Campbell EW. Transfusion pattern of fresh-frozen plasma in a medical school hospital. Vox Sang 1985; 48:366-9.

71. McVay PA, Toy P. Lack of increased bleeding after paracentesis and thoracentesis in patients with mild coagulopathy. Transfusion 1991;31:164-71.

72. Ewe K. Bleeding after liver biopsy does not correlate with indices of peripheral coagulation. Dig Dis Sci 1981;26:388-93.

73. McVay PA, Toy P. Lack of increased bleeding after liver biopsy in patients with mild hemostatic abnormalities. Am J Clin Pathol 1990; 94:747-53.

74. Suchman AL, Griner PF. Diagnostic uses of the activated partial thromboplastin time and prothrombin time. Ann Intern Med 1986; 104:810-16.

75. Gibble JW, Ness PM. Fibrin glue: The perfect operative sealant? Transfusion 1990;30:741-7.

76. Ruggeri ZM, Zimmerman TS. Von Willebrand factor and von Willebrand disease. Blood 1987;70:895-904.

77. Green D. von Willebrand's disease. In: Rossi EC, Simon TL, Moss GS, eds. Principles of transfusion medicine. 1st edition. Baltimore: Williams and Wilkins, 1991:343-53.

78. Aledort LM. Treatment of von Willebrand's disease. Mayo Clin Proc 1991;66:841-6.

79. Ness PM, Perkins HA. Cryoprecipitate as a reliable source of fibrinogen replacement. JAMA 1979;241:1690-1.

80. Rousou J, Levitsky S, Gonzalez-Lavin L, et al. Randomized clinical trial of fibrin sealant in patients undergoing resternotomy or reoperation after cardiac operations: A multicenter study. J Thorac Cardiovasc Surg 1989;97:194-203.

81. Snyder EL, Lubin NLC. Fibronectin: Applications to clinical medicine. CRC Crit Rev Clin Lab Sci 1986;23:15-34.

82. Powell FS, Doran JE. Current status of fibronectin in transfusion medicine: Focus on clinical studies. Vox Sang 1991;60:193-202.

83. Blajchman MA. Minisymposium: The role of granulocytes in transfusion medicine. Transfus Med Rev 1991;4:1-34.

84. Strauss RG. Granulocyte transfusions: uses, abuses and indications. In: Kolins J, McCarthy L, eds. Contemporary transfusion practices. Arlington, VA: American Association of Blood Banks, 1987:65-83.

85. Bodey GP, Buckley M, Sathe YS, Freireich EJ. Quantitative relationships between circulating leukocytes and infection in patients with acute leukemia. Ann Intern Med 1966;64: 328-40.

86. Rosenshein MS, Farewell VT, Price TH, et al. The cost effectiveness of therapeutic and pro-

phylactic leukocyte transfusion. N Engl J Med 1980;302:1058-62.

87. Ford JM, Cullen MH, Roberts MM, et al. Prophylactic granulocyte transfusions. Transfusion 1982;22:311-16.

88. Karp DD, Ervin TJ, Tuttle S, et al. Pulmonary complications during granulocyte transfusions: Incidence and clinical features. Vox Sang 1982;42:57-61.

89. Wright DG, Robichaud KJ, Pizzo PS, Deisseroth AB. Lethal pulmonary reactions associated with the combined use of amphotericin B and leukocyte transfusions. N Engl J Med 1981;304:1185-9.

90. Hersman J, Meyers JD, Thomas ED, et al. The effect of granulocyte transfusions on the incidence of cytomegalovirus infection after allogeneic marrow transplantation. Ann Intern Med 1982;96:149-52.

91. Cohn EJ, Gurd FRN, Surgenor DM, et al. A system for the separation of the protein components of human plasma. J Am Chem Soc 1950;72:465-74.

92. Mannucci PM. Desmopressin: A non-transfusional form of treatment for congenital and acquired bleeding disorders. Blood 1988;72:1449-55.

93. Evatt BL, Gomperts ED, McDougal JS, Ramsey RB. Coincidental appearance of LAV/HTLV III antibodies in hemophiliacs and the onset of the AIDS epidemic. N Engl J Med 1985;312:483-6.

94. Center for Disease Control. Safety of therapeutic products used for hemophilia patients. MMWR 1988;37:441-50.

95. Schwartz RS, Abildgaard CF, Aledort LM, et al. Human recombinant DNA-derived antihemophilic factor (Factor VIII) in the treatment of hemophilia A. N Engl J Med 1990;323:1800-05.

96. Hay CRM, Bolton-Maggs P. Porcine factor VIIIC in the management of patients with factor VIII inhibitors. Transfus Med Rev 1991;5:145-51.

97. Buchanan GR, Kevy SR. Use of prothrombin complex concentrates in hemophiliacs with inhibitors: Clinical and laboratory studies. Pediatrics 1978;62:767-74.

98. Lusher JM, Shapiro SS, Palascak JE, et al. Efficacy of prothrombin complex concentrates in hemophiliacs with antibodies to Factor VIII. N Engl J Med 1980;303:421-5.

99. Hilgartner MW, Knatterud GL. The use of Factor VIII inhibitor by-passing activity (FEIBA immuno) product for treatment of bleeding episodes in hemophiliacs with inhibitors. Blood 1983;61:36-40.

100. Abildgaard CF, Penner JA, Watson-Williams J. Anti-inhibitor coagulant complex (Au-toplex) for treatment of Factor VIII inhibitors in hemophilia. Blood 1980;56:978-84.

101. Smith KJ. Factor IX concentrates: The new products and their properties. Transfus Med Rev 1992;6:124-36.

102. NIH Consensus Conference. Intravenous immunoglobulin. Prevention and treatment of disease. JAMA 1990;264:3189-93.

103. Gallus AS. Replacement therapy in antithrombin III deficiency. Transfus Med Rev 1989;3:253-63.

104. Gerety RJ, Aroson DL. Plasma derivatives and viral hepatitis. Transfusion 1982;22:347-51.

105. Doweiko JP, Nompleggi DJ. The role of albumin in human physiology and pathophysiology. Part III: Albumin and disease states. JPEN J Parenter Enteral Nutr 1991;15:476-83.

106. Erstad BL, Gales BJ, Rappaport WD. The use of albumin in clinical practice. Arch Intern Med 1991;151:901-11.

107. Kellerman PS, Linas SL. Large volume paracentesis in treatment of ascites. Ann Intern Med 1990;112:889-91.

108. Snyder E. Clinical use of albumin, plasma protein fraction and isoimmune globulin products. In: Silvergleid AJ, Britten A, eds. Plasma products: Use and management. Arlington, VA: American Association of Blood Banks, 1982:87-107.

109. Foley E, Borlase B, Dzik WH, et al. Albumin supplementation in the critically ill: A prospective randomized trial. Arch Surg 1990;125:739-42.

110. Alving BM, Hojima Y, Pisano JJ, et al. Hypotension associated with prekallikrein activator (Hageman-factor fragments) in plasma protein fraction. N Engl J Med 1978;299:66-70.

111. Collins JA, Murawski K, Shafer AW. Massive transfusion in surgery and trauma. Progress in clinical and biological research. Vol. 108. New York: Alan R. Liss, 1982.

112. Dzik WH. Massive transfusion. In: Churchill H, Kurtz S, eds. Clinical blood transfusion. Oxford: Blackwell Scientific Publications, 1988:211-29.

113. Collins JA. Recent developments in the area of massive transfusion. World J Surg 1987;11:75-81.

114. Leslie SD, Toy PTCY. Laboratory hemostatic abnormalities in massively transfused patients given red blood cells and crystalloid. Am J Clin Pathol 1991;96:770-3.

115. Harke H, Rahman S. Coagulation disorders in massively injured patients. In: Collins JA, Murawski K, Shafer AW, eds. Massive transfusion in surgery and trauma. New York: Alan R. Liss, 1982:213-24.

116. Beutler E, Muel A, Wood LA. Depletion and regeneration of 2,3 diphosphoglyceric acid in stored red blood cells. Transfusion 1969;9:109-14.

117. Honig CL, Bove JR. Transfusion-associated fatalities. Transfusion 1980;20:653-61.

118. Pick P, Fabijanic J. Temperature changes in donor blood under different storage conditions. Transfusion 1971;11:213-5.

119. Boyan CP, Howland WS. Cardiac arrest and temperature of bank blood. JAMA 1963;183: 58-60.

120. Iserson KV, Huestis DW. Blood warming: Current applications and techniques. Transfusion 1991;31:558-71.

121. Linko K, Hynynen K. Erythrocyte damage caused by the Haemotherm microwave blood warmer. Acta Anaesth Scand 1979;23:320-8.

122. Holzman S, Connolly RJ, Schwaitzberg SD. The effect of in-line microwave energy on blood: A potential modality for blood warming. J Trauma 1992;33:89-94.

123. Linden JV, Snyder EL, Kalish RI, Napychank PA. In vitro and in vivo evaluation of an electromechanical blood infusion pump. Lab Med 1988;19:574-6.

124. International Forum. Does a relationship exist between massive blood transfusions and the adult respiratory distress syndrome? If so, what are the best preventative measures? Vox Sang 1977;32:311-20.

125. Snyder E, Bookbinder M. Role of microaggregate blood filtration in clinical medicine. Transfusion 1983;23:460-70.

126. Schmidt WF, Kim HC, Tomassini N, Schwartz E. Red blood cell destruction caused by a micropore blood filter. JAMA 1982;248:1629-32.

127. Wilcox GJ, Barnes A, Modanlou H. Does transfusion using a syringe infusion pump and small gauge needle cause hemolysis? Transfusion 1981;21:750-1.

128. Herrera AJ, Corless J. Blood transfusions: Effect of speed of infusion and of needle gauge on hemolysis. J Pediatr 1981;99:757-8.

129. Ryden SE, Oberman HA. Compatibility of common intravenous solutions with CPD blood. Transfusion 1975;15:250-5.

130. Klingemann HG, Shepherd JD, Eaves CJ, Eaves AC. The role of erythropoietin and other growth factors in transfusion medicine. Transfus Med Rev 1991;5:33-47.

131. Eschback JW, Kelly MR, Haley NR, et al. Treatment of the anemia of progressive renal failure with recombinant human erythropoietin. N Engl J Med 1989;321:158-63.

132. Gabrilove JL, Jakubowski A, Scher H, et al. Effect of granulocyte colony stimulating factor on neutropenia and associated morbidity due to chemotherapy for transitional cell carcinoma of the urothelium. N Engl J Med 1988;318:1414-22.

133. Crawford J, Ozer H, Stoller R, et al. Reduction by granulocyte colony-stimulating factor of fever and neutropenia induced by chemotherapy in patients with small-cell lung cancer. N Engl J Med 1991;325:164-70.

134. Lieschke GJ, Burgess AW. Drug therapy: Granulocyte colony-stimulating factor and granulocyte-macrophage colony-stimulating factor. N Engl J Med 1992;327:28-35,99-106.

135. Chang TMS. The use of modified hemoglobin as an oxygen carrying blood substitute. Transfus Med Rev 1989;3:213-18.

136. Burhop KE, Farrell L, Dunlap E, et al. Safety and efficacy evaluation of diaspirin cross-linked hemoglobin (DCLHb) in sheep and pigs (abstract). Transfusion 1991;31(Suppl): 54S.

137. Schulman S. DDAVP—the multipotent drug in patients with coagulopathies. Transfus Med Rev 1991;5:132-44.

138. Mannucci PM, Remuzzi G, Pusineri F, et al. Deamino-8-D-arginine vasopressin shortens the bleeding time in uremia. N Engl J Med 1983;308:8-12.

139. Salzman EW, Weinstein MJ, Weintraub RM, et al. Treatment with desmopressin acetate to reduce blood loss after cardiac surgery. N Engl J Med 1986;314:1402-6.

140. Kentro TB, Lottenberg R, Kitchens CS. Clinical efficacy of desmopression acetate for hemostatic control in patients with primary platelet disorders undergoing surgery. Am J Hematol 1987;24:215-9.

141. Stump DC, Taylor FB, Nesheim ME, et al. Pathological fibrinolysis as a cause of clinical bleeding. Semin Thromb Hemost 1990;16: 260-73.

142. Miller RA, May MW, Hendry WF, et al. The prevention of secondary hemorrhage after prostatectomy: The value of antifibrinolytic therapy. Br J Urol 1980;52:26-8.

143. Kang Y, Lewis JH, Navalgund A, et al. Epsilon-aminocaproic acid for treatment of fibrinolysis during liver transplantation. Anesthesiology 1987;66:766-73.

144. Lambert CJ, Marengo-Rowe AJ, Leveson JE, et al. The treatment of postperfusion bleeding using E-aminocaproic acid, cryoprecipitate, fresh frozen plasma and protamine sulfate. Ann Thorac Surg 1979;28:440-4.

145. Fobes CD, Barr RD, Reid G, et al. Tranexamic acid in control of hemorrhage after dental extraction in hemophilia and Christmas disease. Br Med J 1972;2:311-3.

146. Barer D, Ogilvie A, Henry D, et al. Cimetidine and tranexamic acid in the treatment of

acute upper gastrointestinal bleeding. N Engl J Med 1983;308:1571-5.

147. von Holstein CCSS, Eriksson SBS, Kallen R. Tranexamic acid as an aid to reducing blood transfusion requirements in gastric and duodenal bleeding. Br Med J 1987;294:7-10.

148. Gardner FH, Helmer RE. Aminocaproic acid: Use in control of hemorrhage in patients with amegakaryocytic thrombocytopenia. JAMA 1980;243:35-7.

149. Bartholomew JR, Salgia R, Bell WR. Control of bleeding in patients with immune and nonimmune thrombocytopenia with aminocaproic acid. Arch Intern Med 1989; 149:1959-61.

150. Glick R, Green D, Chung-Hsin T, et al. High dose epsilon aminocaproic acid prolongs the bleeding time and increases rebleeding and intraoperative hemorrhage in patients with subarachnoid hemorrhage. Neurosurgery 1981;9:398-401.

151. Bidstrup BP, Royston D, Sapsford RN, Taylor KM. Reduction in blood loss and blood use after cardiopulmonary bypass with high dose aprotinin (Trasylol®). J Thorac Cardiovasc Surg 1989;97:364-72.

152. Havel M, Teufelsbauer H, Knobl P, et al. Effect of intraoperative aprotinin administration on postoperative bleeding in patients undergoing cardiopulmonary bypass operation. J Thorac Cardiovasc Surg 1991;101: 968-72.

153. Growe GH, Poon MC, Scarth I. International symposium on recombinant Factor VIII: Report of the proceedings. Transfus Med Rev 1992;6:137-45.

Appendix 17-1. Clinical Guide to Blood Component Therapy

RBCs

A general clinical algorithm for the use of RBCs is shown in Fig 17-5. Decision points in the figure are numbered and discussed below:
1. Oxygen supply to tissues is dependent upon:
   a. Perfusion.
   b. Oxygen content of the blood (hemoglobin mass × % saturation).
   c. Oxygen extraction by tissues.
      Bleeding patients must first receive volume resuscitation with crystalloid or colloid volume expanders to reestablish perfusion. Due to increased oxygen extraction, most tissues that are adequately perfused will not become ischemic even in the presence of severe anemia [Hb = 70 g/L (7 g/dL)].
2. The degree of oxygen consumption should be considered before transfusions are given to stable patients with a low hematocrit. Patients at bed rest who are not febrile, who do not have congestive heart failure and who are not hypermetabolic have low oxygen requirements and, therefore, can tolerate anemia. Since the cardiac muscle has the highest O_2 extraction, a history of angina should be sought in patients with anemia. Symptomatic anemia may also present with headache, dizziness or breathlessness. Physical exam reveals pallor (not cyanosis) and tachycardia. Important laboratory data include the arterial and mixed venous oxygen saturation, and the cardiac output in addition to the hematocrit. Bleeding patients who suddenly lower their red cell mass will compensate by increasing cardiac output and by increasing oxygen extraction, resulting in a lower venous oxygen saturation. Patients with normal or elevated mixed venous oxygen saturations (75%) are unlikely to profit from additional red cells unless there is isolated critical underperfusion of a selected organ (eg, coronary stenosis). Good decisions are based on an assessment of the patient, not the hematocrit!
3. Immediate alternatives to transfusion of red cells include increasing O_2 supply (supplemental oxygen if the arterial O_2 saturation is low) and decreasing oxygen demand. Blood salvage techniques are useful adjuncts to blood transfusion in bleeding pa-

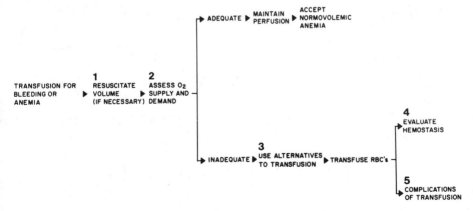

Figure 17-5. Clinical guide to the transfusion of RBCs.

tients. For stable patients with renal failure, anemia should be treated with recombinant erythropoietin rather than red cell transfusions.

4. Bleeding patients may have coexisting coagulopathies or may develop coagulopathies during resuscitation. Among the numerous complications that may accompany massive transfusion, metabolic abnormalities and coagulopathy are particularly important. Metabolic changes promoting depressed left ventricular function include hypothermia from refrigerated blood, citrate toxicity, lactic acidosis from underperfusion and hyperkalemia from tissue ischemia and acidemia. Hemostasis abnormalities include dilutional coagulopathy, DIC, shock, liver and platelet dysfunction.

Blood Components for Hemostasis

A general clinical algorithm for the use of blood components for hemostasis is shown in Fig 17-6. Decision points in the figure are numbered and discussed below.

1. Beware of inappropriate use of blood components to *prevent* bleeding in patients with abnormal laboratory coagulation values or in patients about to undergo bedside procedures. The risk of bleeding in these instances does not correlate well with the results of the PT, aPTT, bleeding time, etc. Decide whether the bleeding is local or generalized. The common error is to transfuse blood components to a patient who has mildly abnormal coagulation results and who is having local bleeding (eg, central line site) in the mistaken belief that the bleeding is due to coagulopathy. Local bleeding is best treated with local measures (stitch on central line site).

2. The four elements of normal hemostasis are:
a. Vascular integrity.
b. Platelet plugging.
c. Coagulation and fibrin formation.

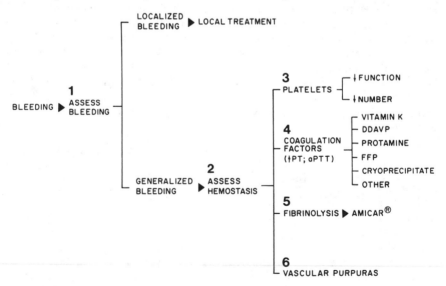

Figure 17-6. Clinical guide to the transfusion of components for hemostasis.

d. Fibrinolysis of formed clot.

Local vascular disruption remains the most common cause of bleeding. Platelet plugging is essential for the immediate hemostasis seen during surgery and with minor bedside procedures. Abnormalities of platelet function and disorders of fibrin formation are common in hospitalized patients.

3. Platelet hemostasis depends on both function and number. Although the bleeding time may be prolonged in patients with known platelet defects, the test has poor sensitivity and specificity and is a poor preoperative predictor of surgical hemostasis. Decreased platelet function resulting from drugs (especially aspirin-containing compounds and antibiotics), uremia, cardiopulmonary bypass and liver disease is common in sick, hospitalized patients. Stopping the offending drug and treating the underlying cause is the first therapy. Platelet transfusion will not correct the platelet defect in uremia. DDAVP has been shown to be an effective adjunct in most syndromes of platelet dysfunction and improves hemostasis by causing release of endogenous stores of Factor VIII:vWF, thus promoting increased platelet adhesion. Decreased platelet numbers result from decreased production, increased destruction or both. The best test to evaluate this differential is the bone marrow exam. Known platelet destructive syndromes are often clear from the history and physical examination and include splenomegaly, ITP, DIC or drug effects. Heparin-associated thrombocytopenia is a serious platelet destruction syndrome that often causes arterial thrombosis rather than bleeding. In the absence of platelet destruction, the platelet count in an average-sized adult should increase by $5\text{-}10 \times 10^9/L$ (5000-10,000/μL) for each unit transfused.

4. Abnormal PT or aPTT: Mild prolongations of the PT or aPTT (<1.5 times normal) are unlikely to reflect abnormalities that are the cause of bleeding. If prolongation of the PT is out of proportion to the aPTT, suspect vitamin K deficiency or liver disease. Vitamin K deficiency—exacerbated by poor nutrition and antibiotics—is the most common coagulation defect among hospitalized patients and should be treated with parenteral vitamin K rather than FFP. Prolongation of the aPTT out of proportion to the PT raises the possibility of von Willebrand's disease, residual heparin, a lupus-like anticoagulant or a factor deficiency. This differential can be generally resolved rapidly by repeating the test after mixing in vitro equal parts of the patient's plasma and normal plasma. DDAVP is useful in mild von Willebrand's disease and has a rapid onset of action. Protamine will neutralize residual heparin. FFP is most useful in the setting of multifactor deficiency of liver disease, but treatment should be guided chiefly by bleeding, not laboratory values. Cryoprecipitate is NOT a concentrate of all plasma coagulation factors. Cryoprecipitate is rich in fibrinogen and Factor VIII and intravenous cryoprecipitate should be reserved for patients with bleeding who have severe hypofibrinogenemia (<100 mg/dL) or for patients with hemophilia A or with severe von Willebrand's disease.

5. Pure fibrinolytic syndromes are rare. However, patients with hepatic cirrhosis exhibit chronic low grade fibrinolysis and have decreased defenses against sudden increases in blood fibrinolytic activity. Inhibitors

of fibrinolysis (such as Amicar® or tranexamic acid) may be a valuable supplement to blood components in such patients.

6. Some conditions result in excessive bleeding in the face of normal blood coagulation. Examples include systemic amyloidosis, angiodysplasia and the hemorrhagic purpuras such as cryoglobulinemia, myeloma and vasculitis.

18

Neonatal and Obstetrical Transfusion Practice

For purposes of transfusion, the neonatal period is generally considered to extend from birth to 4 months. Newborn infants present unique problems in transfusion therapy. Indications for transfusion of infants differ according to weight, gestation, circumstances of delivery and subsequent maturation.[1] Appropriate transfusion practice requires knowledge of neonatal physiology and careful clinical observation. Blood providers should be capable of furnishing components tailored to satisfy the specific requirements of these tiny recipients whose small blood volumes and impaired organ functions provide little margin for safety. The fact that ill newborn infants are more likely to receive transfusions than hospitalized patients of any other age testifies to the importance of this aspect of transfusion practice.

Fetal and Neonatal Erythropoiesis

As the embryo develops, the predominant sites of hematopoiesis change; at about the 9th week of gestation, hematopoiesis shifts from the wall of the yolk sac to the liver, and at about the 24th week from the liver to the bone marrow.[2] Hematopoiesis is regulated by gradually increasing erythropoietin levels stimulated by low oxygen tensions during intrauterine life. At 40 weeks (term), normal infants have a cord blood hemoglobin of 190 ± 22 g/L (19 ± 2.2 g/dL). Neonates of lower birth weight have lower normal hemoglobin levels following birth (Table 18-1). Fetal red cells present at birth have a life span of 45-70 days[3] and contain 53-95% hemoglobin F.[4] Red cells rich in hemoglobin F are physiologically well adapted to low intrauterine oxygen tensions; their high oxygen affinity allows fetal red cells to acquire oxygen from maternal erythrocytes throughout pregnancy. As hemoglobin A replaces hemoglobin F during extrauterine maturation, oxygen delivery to the tissues remains satisfactory despite a physiologic fall in hemoglobin concentration. The oxygen equilibrium curve shifts to the right (Fig 18-1). Premature infants have lower hematocrits and a greater percentage of hemoglobin F in their red cells than term newborns.

As tissue oxygenation in the newborn improves, levels of erythropoietin decline and erythropoiesis diminishes. This decline in red cells produces a physiologic anemia of infancy. Hemoglobin concentration at 1 week approximates that of cord blood and thereafter declines over the next 1-3 months (Table 18-1). Although some infants may be-

18

435

Table 18-1. Serial Hemoglobin Values* in Low Birth-Weight Infants

Birth Weight (Grams)	Age in Weeks				
	2	4	6	8	10
800-1000	160 (148-172)	100 (68-132)	87 (70-102)	80 (71-98)	80 (69-102)
1001-1200	164 (141-187)	128 (78-153)	105 (72-123)	91 (78-104)	85 (70-100)
1201-1400	162 (136-188)	134 (88-162)	109 (85-133)	99 (80-118)	98 (84-113)
1401-1500	156 (134-178)	117 (97-137)	105 (91-119)	98 (84-120)	99 (84-114)
1501-2000	156 (135-177)	110 (96-140)	96 (88-115)	98 (84-121)	101 (86-118)

*Values are mean figures, in g/L, with range in parentheses.
(Reproduced with permission from Stockman JA. Red cell transfusions in the newborn. Am J Pediatr Hematol/Oncol 1981;3:205–11.)

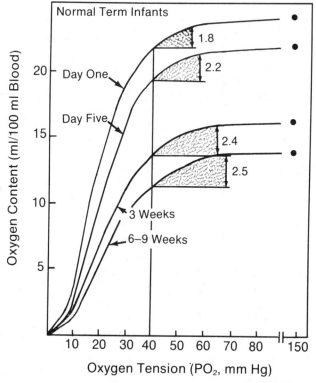

Figure 18-1. Oxygen equilibrium curves in blood from term infants at different postnatal ages. Arrows indicate the capacity to unload oxygen at given arterial and venous PO₂ levels. (Reproduced with permission from Delivoria-Papadopoulos M, et al.[5]

come quite anemic, the erythropoietin response is markedly diminished when related to the hemoglobin level. Despite hemoglobin levels that would indicate anemia in older children and adults, the normally developing infant usually maintains adequate tissue oxygenation. Arterial PO_2 rises secondary to the increase in hemoglobin A and the increase in red cell content of 2,3-diphosphoglycerate (2,3-DPG).[5] Physiologic anemia should not be confused with anemia later in infancy, which may result from dietary inadequacy. Physiologic anemia requires treatment only if the degree or timing of the anemia deviates significantly from normal, and the infant is symptomatic—a situation that occurs frequently in very low birth-weight infants who are ill and require extensive laboratory monitoring. Although transfusion is rarely indicated for the newborn who is feeding, growing and developing normally, evaluation of anemia is important in infants known to have medical or surgical problems.

Unique Aspects of Neonatal Physiology

Differences between newborns and adults may dictate differences in transfusion practice. Newborns are small and physiologically immature. Those requiring transfusion are often premature, sick and unable to tolerate even minimal stresses.

Infant Size

Full-term newborns have a blood volume of approximately 85 mL/kg; prematures have an average blood volume of 100 mL/kg. It is important to calculate transfusion needs on an individual basis. As survival rates continue to improve for infants weighing 1000 g or less at birth, blood banks are increasingly asked to provide blood components for patients whose total blood volume is less than 100 mL. The small blood volumes of neonates and the need for frequent laboratory tests make replacement of iatrogenic blood loss the most common indication for transfusion of these patients.[6]

Hypovolemia

The newborn does not compensate for hypovolemia as well as an adult. A newborn responds to a 10% volume depletion by diminishing the stroke volume ejected by the left ventricle, without increasing the heart rate. Peripheral vascular resistance increases to maintain systemic blood pressure and this, combined with the diminished cardiac output, results in poor tissue perfusion, low tissue oxygenation and metabolic acidosis.[7]

Marrow Response to Anemia

The infant's bone marrow responds more slowly than adult marrow to anemia. A hemolytic episode that would elicit a reticulocyte response within 4-6 days in adults may elicit little or no increased erythropoiesis for 2-3 weeks in the newborn.[8] This sluggish response is due primarily to low erythropoietin output.

Cold Stress

Hypothermia in the newborn causes exaggerated effects, including increased metabolic rate, hypoglycemia, metabolic acidosis and a tendency for apneic episodes that may lead to hypoxia, hypotension and cardiac arrest. Exchange transfusion using blood at room temperature may decrease the newborn's rectal temperature 0.7-2.5 C. Although an in-line blood warmer should be used for exchange transfusion, warmers are unnecessary for small volume transfusions that equilibrate to room temperature fairly rapidly. A quadruple pack or syringe placed in the isolette reaches room temperature in approximately 20 minutes. Caution should be exercised when placing blood components directly under radiant warming devices as cellular damage can occur.[9]

Immunologic Status

Infants have immature antibody-producing mechanisms, and antibodies present in their plasma originate almost entirely from the maternal circulation. IgG is the only immunoglobulin class that crosses the placenta, through mechanisms more complex than simple diffusion. Of the four IgG subclasses, IgG1 crosses the placenta first.[10] Antibody concentrations are higher in cord blood than maternal blood, suggesting an active placental transport mechanism; in addition, catabolism of IgG occurs more slowly in the fetus than in the mother.[11] Thus, passively acquired antibody is conserved during the neonatal period. Infants exposed to an infectious process in utero or shortly after birth may produce small amounts of IgM detectable by sensitive techniques, but they rarely form red cell antibodies of either IgG or IgM class during the neonatal period.[12]

The cellular immune system of neonates is similarly immature. Graft-vs-host disease (GVHD) has been reported in newborns who received intrauterine transfusion followed by postnatal exchange transfusion.[13] The lymphocytes given during intrauterine transfusion may have induced host tolerance, so that the lymphocytes given in the subsequent exchange transfusion were not rejected in the normal way. GVHD is not felt to be a significant clinical problem for immunologically normal newborns who receive multiple exchange transfusions. For exchange transfusion, irradiation of blood to prevent GVHD is probably unnecessary. However, some neonatal nursery units provide irradiated blood for low birth-weight, low gestational age or septic premature neonates based on the belief, not yet universally accepted, that such infants are immunologically more vulnerable to GVHD.[14] Blood for intrauterine transfusion is usually irradiated.

Any directed donor blood from a blood relative should also be irradiated.[15] Storage of irradiated RBCs should be avoided because of the potential problem of potassium leak.

Metabolic Problems

Because immature kidneys have reduced glomerular filtration rate and concentrating ability, the newborn may have difficulty excreting potassium, acid and/or calcium loads. Acidosis or hypocalcemia may also occur posttransfusion because the immature liver metabolizes citrate inefficiently. Although plasma potassium increases rapidly in stored red cells, small volume simple transfusions have little effect on serum potassium concentration in newborn infants. A study of sick newborns who received a total of 11 transfusions of stored red cells (10 mL/kg) revealed an insignificant posttransfusion change in mean serum potassium levels from 5.1-4.9 mEq/L.[16] On the other hand, serum potassium may rise after exchange transfusion, depending upon the plasma potassium levels in the blood used for exchange.

2,3-Diphosphoglycerate (2,3-DPG)

Tissue oxygenation is poor in sick newborns. A newborn's red cells have a high percentage of hemoglobin F, which does not deliver oxygen to the tissues with the effectiveness of adult hemoglobin. Infants with respiratory distress syndrome or septic shock have decreased levels of 2,3-DPG; alkalosis and hypothermia can further increase the oxygen affinity of hemoglobin, shifting the dissociation curve to the left and making oxygen even less available to the tissues. Respiratory distress syndrome or other pulmonary disease compromises arterial oxygenation. Mechanisms that compensate for hypoxia in adults, such as increased heart rate, are limited in newborns. If transfused blood constitutes a large proportion of the infant's blood volume, transfusion of 2,3-DPG-depleted blood may cause problems that would not affect older children or adults. Since 2,3-DPG levels decrease in stored blood, newborns should be given the freshest blood conveniently available for exchange transfusions, certainly less than 7 days old whenever possible.[17] In an attempt to ensure that the transfused red cells have adequate 2,3-DPG, many transfusion services attempt to provide similarly fresh red cells for small volume transfusions. The medical necessity to do so has never been demonstrated and arguments have been raised to suggest it is unnecessary.[1] In particular, the fact that stored adult blood will deliver more oxygen to the tissues than neonatal hemoglobin F containing blood fails to support the need for fresh blood in these situations.

Cytomegalovirus Infection

Infection by cytomegalovirus (CMV) may occur in the perinatal period, acquired either in utero or during the birth process. Newborn infants can be infected during breast feeding or by close contact with mothers or nursery personnel.[18] CMV may also be transmitted by transfusion, but evidence exists to suggest that this occurrence is very uncommon today.[19] The virus seems to be associated with leukocytes in blood and components.[20,21]

Infection in newborns is extremely variable in its manifestations, ranging from asymptomatic seroconversion to death. Symptomatic infection may produce pulmonary, hepatic, renal, hematologic and/or neurologic dysfunction.

Epidemiology and prevention of posttransfusion CMV in neonatal recipients have been under intense investigation. Some findings include:

1. The overall risk of symptomatic posttransfusion CMV infection seems to be inversely related to the incidence of seropositivity in the community. That is, where many adults are positive for CMV antibodies, there is a low rate of symptomatic CMV infection.

2. Infants born of seropositive mothers are unlikely to develop symptomatic infections during the neonatal period.

3. Premature infants weighing less than 1200 g who are born of seronegative mothers and who require multiple transfusions are at risk for symptomatic posttransfusion infections.[22]

4. The cytomegalovirus particles in the blood are associated with the leukocytes, and the cumulative number of different donor exposures incurred during transfusion correlates with the risk of acquired CMV infection.

5. The risk of transmission of CMV by blood and cellular blood components can be eliminated by transfusing blood from seronegative donors or reduced by transfusing components processed to eliminate viable CMV-containing leukocytes. Deglycerolized red cells have been used successfully.[23-25] Washed red cells may decrease the incidence of acquired CMV infection in neonates as well, but the use of washed cells for this indication remains controversial.[26] Leukocyte reduction with some blood filters may also be an effective way of reducing CMV infection.[27]

AABB *Standards for Blood Banks and Transfusion Services* states that, in geographic areas where posttransfusion CMV transmission is a problem, cellular components with minimal risk of transmitting CMV should be used for newborns weighing less than 1200 g, born to mothers who lack CMV antibodies or whose antibody status is unknown.

Hemolytic Disease of the Newborn

Pathophysiology

In hemolytic disease of the newborn (HDN), red cells of the fetus become coated with IgG alloantibody of maternal origin, directed against an antigen of paternal origin present on the fetal cells. The IgG-coated cells undergo accelerated destruction, both before and after birth. Clinical severity of the disease is extremely variable, ranging from intrauterine death to a condition that can be detected only by serologic tests on blood from an apparently healthy infant.[28]

Shortened red cell survival causes fetal hematopoietic tissue to increase production of red cells, many of which enter the circulation prematurely as nucleated cells (erythroblastosis). Organs containing hematopoietic tissue, particularly liver and spleen, increase in size. If red cell production adequately replaces lost cells, oxygen-carrying capacity is maintained. If increased hematopoiesis cannot compensate for the immune destruction, anemia becomes progressively more severe. The severely affected fetus may develop high output cardiac failure with generalized edema, a condition called hydrops fetalis, and death may occur in utero in the untreated case. If live-born, the severely affected infant exhibits heart failure and profound anemia. Less severely affected infants continue to experience accelerated red cell destruction, which generates large quantities of bilirubin.

Before birth severs the communication between maternal and fetal circulation, fetal bilirubin is processed by the mother's liver, but after birth the neonatal liver must conjugate and excrete large quantities of unconjugated bilirubin, a substance toxic to the developing central nervous system. The immature liver is deficient in uridine diphosphoglucuronyl transferase (the enzyme necessary to conjugate bilirubin for excretion) and accumulation of unconjugated bilirubin constitutes a severe threat to the infant. This threat is increased by prematurity, acidosis, hypoxia and hypoalbuminemia. For the live-born infant with HDN, rising bilirubin levels may be a greater clinical problem than the loss of oxygen-carrying capacity. The decision of when or whether to undertake exchange transfusion is based primarily on the bilirubin level, the rate of bilirubin accumulation and, to a lesser degree, on the severity of the anemia.

Mechanisms of Maternal Immunization

HDN may be classified into three categories based on serologic specificity of the causative IgG antibody. In descending order of severity these are:

1. Rh hemolytic disease, due to anti-D alone or less often in combination with anti-C or anti-E.
2. "Other" HDN, due to antibodies against other antigens in the Rh system, such as anti-c, anti-E or anti-e, or against antigens in other systems, such as anti-K, anti-Fy[a] and many others.
3. ABO HDN, due usually to anti-A,B in a group O woman, and rarely to anti-A or anti-B.

In HDN other than ABO, maternal antibodies result from immunization by previous pregnancy or transfusion. Rising titers of antibody can be documented during pregnancy, and the infant may be symptomatic at birth. In ABO HDN the immunizing stimulus is seldom known; the condition cannot be diagnosed during pregnancy and is rarely symptomatic at birth.

Pregnancy

Immunization from pregnancy results when fetal red cells possessing a paternal antigen foreign to the mother enter her circulation. The antigen that most frequently induces immunization is D, but any red cell antigen present on fetal cells and absent from the mother can, in theory, stimulate antibody production. Most immunizations result from the fetomaternal hemorrhage (FMH) that occurs during placental separation at delivery. In approximately half of all recently delivered women, small quantities of fetal cells are detectable in a post delivery blood specimen.[29] Immunization to D can occur with volumes of fetal blood less than 0.1 mL. The incidence of immunization to D correlates with the volume of Rh+ red cells entering the Rh- mother's circulation.[30] Although the usual immunizing event is delivery, small numbers of fetal cells enter the mother's circulation during the last half of pregnancy; they are usually insufficient to induce primary immunization. Immunization can also occur after amniocentesis, miscarriage, chorionic villus sampling, cordocentesis, abortion or rupture of an ectopic pregnancy.

Transfusion

In Rh- women who receive transfusions of Rh+ red cells, subsequent pregnancies with an Rh+ fetus are likely to be complicated by severe HDN. It is extremely important to avoid transfusing Rh+ WB or RBCs to Rh- females who might subsequently become pregnant. The rbcs in platelet or granulocyte concentrates can constitute an immunizing stimulus, and Rh- female recipients should be considered candidates for Rh prophylaxis if the donors are Rh+. See p 397. Further, directed donor transfusion from husband to wife should be avoided if the couple plan to have children. This form of directed donation will likely increase the risk of alloimmunization of the mother and development of alloimmune cytopenias in future children.

ABO Antibodies

The IgG antibodies that cause ABO HDN nearly always occur in the mother's circulation without a history of prior immunization by foreign transfused red cells. ABO HDN can develop in any pregnancy including the first, but it is restricted almost entirely to group A or B infants born to group O mothers. This is apparently attributable to the pathogenic antibody, anti-A,B, being present only in group O individuals.

Incidence of Immunization

Before the availability of successful prophylaxis for Rh sensitization, the incidence of anti-D formation following the first pregnancy of Rh- women who had an Rh+, ABO-compatible infant was approximately 8%.[31] An additional 8% developed detectable anti-D during their next Rh+ pregnancy. The latter group of women probably experienced primary immunization during delivery of their first Rh+ child but did not produce detectable levels of antibody. The small numbers of Rh+ fetal cells entering the maternal circulation during the next pregnancy constituted a secondary stimulus sufficient to elicit overt production of IgG anti-D. In susceptible women not immunized during their first two pregnancies, subsequent pregnancies might cause immunization, but the frequency diminishes. The overall incidence of D sensitization in multiparous D- women who deliver D+ infants is about 18%. Once immunization has occurred, successive Rh+ pregnancies often manifest HDN of increasing severity, although some families have a stable or diminishing pattern of clinical disease in subsequent pregnancies.

Rh immunization occurs in untreated Rh– women less frequently after delivery of an ABO-incompatible Rh+ infant than when the fetal cells are ABO-compatible with the mother. ABO incompatibility between mother and fetus has a substantial but not absolute protective effect against maternal immunization. With the advent of passive Rh immunoprophylaxis, both antepartum and postpartum, the incidence of Rh immunization has fallen dramatically. As a result of highly effective prevention programs, only a very small number of Rh– women continue to become immunized.[32]

Prenatal Tests

Serologic Studies

Alloimmunization that could result in HDN can be detected during pregnancy with suitable serologic tests. A recent publication recommended an appropriate battery of serologic testing for the prenatal and perinatal period.[33] Initial studies on all pregnant women should include tests for ABO and D, and a screen for unexpected antibodies. If the woman's cells are not agglutinated by

anti-D, a test for weak D (D^u) should be done. When the test for either D or weak D (D^u) is positive, the woman is classified as Rh+. Very rarely, a D+ or weak D (D^u) mother produces anti-D as a result of pregnancy, and HDN has been reported.[34]

All positive antibody screening tests require identification of the antibody.[33] The mere presence of an antibody, however, does not indicate that HDN will inevitably occur. IgM antibodies existing without known red cell stimulation, notably anti-Le^a and anti-I, are relatively common during pregnancy but do not cross the placenta. Treating the serum with 2-mercaptoethanol or dithiothreitol will aid in distinguishing the IgM antibodies from IgG. (See Method 4.4.) In addition, the fetus may be antigen negative for the mother's antibody. The results of prenatal antibody studies should be reported with sufficient additional information to indicate when a reported antibody may not be clinically significant.

When the woman has anti-D, some obstetricians test the father to estimate the likelihood of his being homozygous or heterozygous for the gene determining the presence of the D antigen. A homozygote will always transmit a gene for D to the offspring, whereas in the offspring of an Rh– woman and a heterozygous Rh+ man, half the offspring will be Rh–. See Tables 18-2 and 18-3. This

Table 18-2. Probability of Heterozygosity at D Locus in Whites for Given Rh Phenotype and *n* Previous D-Positive Offspring*

Phenotype	n=0	n=1	n=2	n=3	n=4	n=5
CcDe	0.90	0.82	0.69	0.53	0.36	0.22
CDe	0.090	0.047	0.024	0.012	0.006	0.003
cDEe	0.90	0.82	0.69	0.53	0.36	0.22
cDE	0.13	0.070	0.036	0.018	0.009	0.005
CcDEe	0.11	0.058	0.030	0.015	0.008	0.004
cDe	0.94	0.89	0.80	0.66	0.49	0.33

*If the father has had any previous D-negative children, then the probability that he is heterozygous for the D antigen is 1. (Reproduced with permission from Kanter.[35])

Table 18-3. Probability of Heterozygosity at D Locus in Blacks for Given Rh Phenotype and *n* Previous D-Positive Offspring*

Phenotype	n = 0	n = 1	n = 2	n = 3	n = 4	n = 5
CcDe	0.41	0.26	0.15	0.080	0.042	0.021
CDe	0.19	0.10	0.055	0.028	0.014	0.007
cDEe	0.37	0.23	0.13	0.068	0.035	0.018
cDE	0.01	0.005	0.003	0.001	<0.001	<0.001
CcDEe	0.10	0.053	0.027	0.014	0.007	0.003
cDe	0.54	0.37	0.23	0.13	0.068	0.035

*If the father has had any previous D-negative children, then the probability that he is heterozygous for the D antigen is 1. (Reproduced with permission from Kanter.[35])

information may be useful in counseling a couple when anti-D is known to be present.

Amniotic Fluid Analysis and Cordocentesis

During gestation, the clinical history, amniotic fluid analysis and cord hemoglobin can be used to assess the probable severity of HDN. Information about the severity of the disease in previous infants is somewhat helpful in predicting severity in subsequent infants. In a woman with anti-D, the severity of fetal HDN correlates modestly with the maternal antibody titer.[36] A better index of intrauterine hemolysis and fetal well-being is the level of bile pigment in the amniotic fluid, obtained by amniocentesis, or the hemoglobin and/or bilirubin in the infant's blood obtained by direct fetal blood sampling via the umbilical vein. Amniocentesis is usually performed in Rh– women with a history of previously affected pregnancies or with anti-D titers at or above 16.

Amniotic fluid is obtained by inserting a long needle through the mother's abdominal wall and uterus into the uterine cavity. The aspirated fluid is scanned spectrophotometrically for a change in optical density at 450 nm (the peak absorbance of bilirubin), to measure the concentration of bile pigments. This value is plotted on a semilogarithmic graph against the estimated age of gestation, because bile pigment concentration has different clinical significance at different gestational ages. (See Method 7.3.) In general, the higher the pigment concentration, the more severe the intrauterine hemolysis.

The risk of allowing a severely affected pregnancy to continue must be weighed against the risk of premature delivery and the problems of fetal lung immaturity. Respiratory distress syndrome may result when there is inadequate surfactant, lecithin and other pulmonary lipids to maintain stable pulmonary alveolar structures in the newborn. Maturity of the fetal lung is assessed by determining the ratio of lecithin to sphingomyelin (L/S ratio) and levels of phosphotidylglycerol in the amniotic fluid.[37] The L/S ratio is the current standard test for the assessment of fetal lung maturity. A ratio of >2.0:1 indicates maturity. Respiratory distress syndrome develops in about 70% of cases with a ratio of <1.5:1 and 40% of cases with a L/S of 1.5-2.0:1.[38] If the change in optical density at 450 nm indicates severe HDN but the L/S ratio indicates the lungs are not sufficiently mature to prevent respiratory distress syndrome, intrauterine transfusion may be indicated.

Amniocentesis and direct fetal blood sampling may be complicated by FMH, which can cause immunization of susceptible mothers. If amniocentesis has been performed on an Rh− woman who is not already sensitized to the D antigen, Rh immunoprophylaxis should be given. In most such cases the Rh status of the fetus will be unknown, but the likelihood is high that it is Rh+ and the bleeding induced by amniocentesis could induce anti-D in a woman not previously immunized. Due to the hazards of amniocentesis and cordocentesis, noninvasive monitoring protocols, including greater use of ultrasound evaluations of fetal well-being, are being recommended.

Intrauterine Transfusion

Intrauterine transfusion is not without risks to the fetus[39] and should be performed only after careful clinical evaluation. Intrauterine transfusion is seldom feasible before the 20th week of gestation. Once initiated, a series of transfusions is usually administered every 2 weeks until delivery. Intrauterine transfusion is performed through a needle passed with ultrasonographic monitoring through the mother's abdominal and uterine wall into the fetal abdominal cavity. The transfused red cells enter the fetal circulation by absorption from lymphatic channels draining the peritoneal cavity. Blood can also be infused directly into the umbilical vein (percutaneous umbilical blood transfusion or cordocentesis). This approach is particularly valuable for cases of severe hydrops.

For maximal survival of the transfused cells, red cells less than 5 days old should be used for intrauterine transfusion. Washed or deglycerolized red cells are preferred by many physicians because they have normal electrolyte levels, contain no anticoagulant or plasma, have very low levels of platelets and leukocytes, and have a low risk of CMV transmission. A hematocrit of 0.80 (80%) or greater is desirable to minimize the chance of volume overload in the fetus. The red cells should be group O, Rh− and negative for the antigen corresponding to the antibody in the mother's serum. The volume transfused ranges from 75-175 mL, depending on the fetal size and age. Blood for intrauterine transfusions should be irradiated because of the potential risk of GVHD.[40-42]

Newborns who have had successful intrauterine transfusions often type at birth as Rh− or very weakly positive, because at birth over 90% of their circulating red cells may be those of the donors. Similarly, the ABO grouping and a direct antiglobulin test (DAT) may give misleading results.

Intrauterine Exchange Transfusion

New medical techniques have been developed for performing intrauterine exchange transfusion. Under ultrasound guidance, the umbilical vein is cannulated and a blood sample taken for immediate hemoglobin/hematocrit measurement and verification of catheter location in the fetal circulation. The unborn fetus can then undergo an exchange transfusion.[43] Intrauterine transfusion can be performed by the intraperitoneal route or the direct approach via the umbilical vein; recent studies have shown these techniques to be effective in experienced medical centers.[44,45]

Laboratory Investigation During the Neonatal Period

A sample of cord blood, preferably collected by syringe to avoid contamination with maternal blood and debris, should be obtained on every newborn. This tube should be identified as cord blood and be labeled in the delivery suite with the mother's name, infant's identification, hospital number and date. Samples should be stored in the blood bank for at least 7 days. The cord sample is then available for testing if the mother is Rh– or if the newborn develops signs and symptoms suggestive of HDN.

Samples of both cord and maternal blood should be tested, as shown in Table 18-4. When the mother is known to have antibodies capable of causing HDN, the cord blood should be tested for hemoglobin or hematocrit and for serum bilirubin. Tests on the mother's blood present no special problems and can be done with routine techniques. Testing cord blood may present some special problems, which are described below.

ABO Testing

ABO testing on newborns relies entirely on cell grouping because alloantibodies present in cord serum are of maternal origin. If maternal alloantibodies are present, they will be IgG and, unless present at high levels, may not agglutinate reverse grouping cells on immediate spin. No useful information will be gained from routine reverse grouping tests, although in investigating possible HDN due to ABO incompatibility, tests for antiglobulin-reactive ABO antibodies may be helpful.

Rh Testing

Accurate Rh testing can be difficult if red cells are heavily coated with IgG antibodies. Either false-positive or false-negative results may occur. Blood grouping tests with anti-D reagents in a high protein diluent may be inaccurate with Rh– cells heavily coated with any antibody, or contaminated by Wharton's jelly. The discrepancy should become apparent from positive results in the tube containing reagent diluent control. If

Table 18-4. Laboratory Studies Recommended for Maternal and Cord Blood in Cases of Suspected HDN

Maternal Blood
ABO group
Rh type
Weak D (D^u), if apparently Rh –
Antibody screening test
Identification of antibody, if present

Cord Blood
ABO group
Rh type
Weak D (D^u), if apparently Rh –
Direct antiglobulin test
Eluate from red cells, if DAT is positive and clinical circumstances warrant
Identification of antibody in eluate

there is agglutination in the control system, reagents in a low protein diluent can be used to determine the Rh group.

False-negative or very weakly positive results sometimes occur when the newborn is Rh+ and the rbcs are so fully saturated with maternal anti-D that no D sites are available to react with the reagent serum, a condition sometimes called "blocked D." This should be suspected when the immunized mother is Rh– and the infant's cells give a strongly positive DAT and negative or ambiguous results with saline anti-D. Maternal anti-D can be removed from these cells by gentle heat elution (see Method 2.14) and the anti-D test repeated. Confirmation of the cause of the problem can be made by identifying the antibody contained in the eluate.

Antiglobulin Testing

The DAT usually gives strongly positive results in HDN due to anti-D or antibodies in other blood groups; reactions are much weaker or negative in HDN due to ABO. If the DAT on cord cells is positive, the antibody can be eluted from the cells and tested for specificity.

If the DAT is positive and the maternal serum has a negative antibody screening test, suspicion falls on ABO HDN or HDN due to antibody against a low-incidence antigen not present on reagent test cells. Testing the eluate from the cord cells against A and B cells, in addition to the usual O cells, confirms the diagnosis of ABO HDN.

ABO hemolytic disease may be suspected on clinical grounds even though the DAT is negative. In many cases it is possible to elute anti-A and/or anti-B from the infant's cells despite a negative DAT; if elution is performed, the eluate should be tested against A_1, B and O cells, using an antiglobulin technique. If transfusion is required, group O blood that is Rh compatible should be transfused, whether or not the diagnosis has been serologically confirmed.

If ABO hemolytic disease is ruled out, antibody against a low-incidence antigen should be suspected, and the eluate should be tested against the father's red cells, using an antiglobulin technique. The diagnosis can be confirmed by testing the mother's serum against the father's red cells, if they are ABO-compatible. If either or both of these tests are positive, it indicates that: 1) the father has transmitted an antigen to the offspring that has elicited an IgG antibody in the mother or 2) the mother may have had primary stimulation by transfusion. Since antibody to a low-incidence antigen causes no difficulty in obtaining compatible blood, these studies can be performed after initial clinical concerns have been resolved.

If the DAT is positive and all attempts to characterize the coating antibody are consistently negative, causes of a false-positive DAT should be considered. (See p 182.)

Treatment

See section on exchange transfusion later in this chapter.

Components Used for Neonatal Transfusion

Newborns may need any or all of the blood components available in other transfusion settings, but special problems exist in having to supply the small volumes needed, with adjusted hematocrits and within narrow acceptable ranges of pH and electrolyte values.

Red Cell Components

The unique small volume requirements of transfusion to neonatal recipients make it possible to provide several aliquots from a single donor unit, thus limiting donor exposure and decreasing donor-related risks such as hepatitis. Several technical approaches are available to realize this advantage and to minimize wastage.

Multiple Packs

In a multiple pack system, a single unit of blood can be apportioned into four integrally attached containers of 125 mL. Since the original seal remains intact, each container has a normal shelf life until entered. The contents of individual quad packs can be transferred to smaller containers providing two to four smaller aliquots, each with a 24-hour shelf life. Hematocrit can be adjusted at either division step. For example, most of the plasma (approximately 220 mL) can be removed as fresh frozen plasma (FFP) shortly after drawing. The remaining RBCs can be divided into each of the three attached bags without altering the shelf life of the cells. If each quad pack is apportioned, at the time of use, into four pediatric transfer packs that out-date in 24 hours, a single unit can pro-vide 12 20-mL aliquots of RBCs and a unit of FFP.[46] Alternatively, WB in the original container can be expressed into the satellite bags, which can be entered for subsequent removal of plasma or subdivision into smaller aliquots. Each aliquot must be fully labeled as it is pre-pared, including outdate time. Records must be kept of the origin and disposi-tion of each aliquot. The availability of sterile connecting devices increases the ease of preparing multiple small red cell aliquots without decreasing shelf life.

Multi-Portion System

A multi-portion system is useful in set-tings where large numbers of infants re-ceive small volume transfusions given with syringe pumps. Blood is collected either into single or multiple packs. If triple or quadruple bag sets are used, the hematocrit can be adjusted initially and FFP may be prepared from the expressed plasma if the resulting hematocrit is ac-ceptable. An alternative method of red cell concentration uses gravity sedimen-tation for 12 hours. This results in a hematocrit of approximately 0.65 (65%), which many workers consider ideal for transfusion to neonates.[47] Bags are hung in an inverted position in the refrigera-tor so that sedimented cells can be care-fully drawn through one of the access ports into a syringe.

A resealable sampling or injection site coupler inserted into the access port permits repeated entry. Once the cou-pler is inserted, the contents of the bag have a 24-hour shelf life when stored at 4 C. The precise volume of blood re-quested can be aspirated into a syringe through a large-bore needle inserted through the sampling site coupler. If de-sired, the packed or sedimented red cells can be drawn through an in-line filter when loading the syringes. If blood is not filtered during loading, a filter is re-quired in the infusion set. Aseptic tech-nique should be used and the sampling site coupler covered with sterile gauze when not in use. The sterile cap should be replaced on the filled syringe, which must be appropriately labeled for the re-cipient. The distribution of aliquots to individual recipients as filled syringes must be recorded. This flexible system can minimize wastage but, rarely, may also increase the spread of transfusion-transmitted disease.[48] A unit dose system designed to dispense precise quantities of blood components in a form ready for use by neonatal patients has been de-scribed.[49]

Deglycerolized Red Cells

After glycerolization and before freez-ing, a unit of red cells can be divided into three or four aliquots. A single unit may be designated for repeated transfusion to a single recipient, or aliquots can be as-signed to different infants. Each aliquot can be thawed as needed, with a 24-hour shelf life after thawing and deglyceroliza-tion. Aliquots may be further divided for small volume transfusions. This is an expensive system, but it provides a com-ponent with 2,3-DPG levels of freshly drawn blood and after the postthaw wash, with much reduced content of plasma proteins, electrolytes, anticoag-ulant, white cells and platelets.[50] Alter-natively, entire group O units can be thawed and deglycerolized, and aliquots removed as needed during the permitted 24-hour shelf life.

Additive Solution (AS) Red Cells

Unlike the CPDA-1 anticoagulant pre-servative, additive solutions contain additional adenine and may contain mannitol. The additional adenine, man-nitol and glucose are felt by some neonatologists to be potentially harmful to critically ill newborns. Washing or packing such units will lower the adenine levels. The amount of mannitol present (0.75 g/bag) should not present any problems, especially if the cells are washed or packed before transfusion.

A recent review suggested that red cells preserved in extended storage media present no substantive risks when used for small volume transfusions. For premature infants with hepatic or renal insufficiency, removal of the additive media is recommended based upon theoretical calculations. The authors also concluded that entire units of red cells stored with additives should be avoided in massive transfusion settings such as cardiac surgery or exchange transfusions.[51]

Half-Unit Donations

The need for small volume neonatal and pediatric transfusions provides an opportunity to use blood donors who weigh less than the 110 pounds required for donation of a 450-mL unit. It is possible to draw less than the usual volume from a small but otherwise acceptable donor. After excess anticoagulant is expressed into a satellite bag, approximately 225 mL of blood can be collected into a triple pack. Separated plasma can be expressed into the same satellite bag, which is then discarded. The remaining red cells can be apportioned between the primary container and the remaining satellite bag; this provides two units of red cells of approximately 60 mL volume. An alternative application of this approach is to draw 225 mL monthly from a group O donor of a desirable phenotype, rather than 450 mL every 8 weeks. The use of a "dedicated donor" may support the needs of an infant requiring multiple transfusions over a prolonged period.

Individual Small Units

Units containing approximately 30-60 mL of WB can be obtained by collecting blood into a container with an extra satellite bag. A unit intended for use as WB would be collected in a double bag; a unit intended for division into RBCs, platelets and FFP would be collected in a quadruple set instead of a triple set. It is permissible to draw 450 mL ± 45mL (10%) from a donor. If there is an accurate means of measuring the volume drawn, it is possible to draw 495 mL of whole blood into the primary bag. Removing 30-60 mL into the extra satellite bag leaves a satisfactory volume in the primary bag and provides an extra small volume unit with normal shelf life. The hematocrit of these small units can be adjusted by removing plasma prior to transfusion.

Walking Donor Program

This approach, a relic of less sophisticated times, is mentioned only to identify the hazards: no labeling or routine pretransfusion testing of donor blood; generally poor record-keeping; no donor sample available to work up reactions; risk of excess heparin; potential contamination through faulty technique; and risk of CMV, AIDS or hepatitis from untested blood.

Fresh Frozen Plasma

Since FFP must be frozen within 6 hours of phlebotomy, it is an excellent source of labile coagulation factors, if transfused within 24 hours after thawing. Thawed plasma stored more than 24 hours at 1-6 C provides stable coagulation factors and other plasma proteins. A thawed unit of FFP can be divided into aliquots for small volume transfusions for cases where an infant has a suspected coagulopathy; these aliquots must be used within 24 hours of entering the primary bag. Generally, unless there is a need to replace coagulation factors, the use of FFP is not necessary. Many physicians prefer to use red blood cells undiluted or diluted with albumin or a suitable crystalloid solution whenever possible since the latter do not carry a risk of transfusion-transmitted diseases. The benefit from use of any blood component must be carefully weighed against its potential risk.

Platelets

Platelet concentrate prepared from a single donation of WB contains approximately 5.5×10^{10} platelets and should raise the platelet count of an average full-term newborn 75-100 $\times$ 10^9/L (75,000-100,000/µL) if given in a dose of 5-10 mL/kg.[52] The same dose taken as an aliquot from a unit of apheresis platelets will produce a similar increment. Platelets should be group-specific if possible. Transfusion of incompatible plasma is more dangerous in neonatal recipients than adults due to their smaller blood volume. If absolutely necessary, the plasma volume of stored platelets can be reduced without adversely affecting platelet properties.[53] Incompatible plasma should be removed to the maximum extent possible (see Method 10.14), and the platelets resuspended in saline or albumin. FFP can also be used if clotting factors are required by the patient, but a safer approach would be the use of a platelet-rich plasma.

Granulocyte Concentrates

Optimal use of granulocyte transfusion for neonatal recipients is under investigation.[54] Granulocytes may be harvested by standard apheresis techniques or, for newborns, smaller quantities of granulocytes can be harvested from the buffy coat of units of freshly donated blood by gravity sedimentation or by an automated process. Several reports,[55,56] however, have cast doubt on the efficacy of buffy coat transfusions. The dose currently recommended is 1×10^9 neutrophils/kg body weight. Because granulocyte concentrates contain large numbers of lymphocytes, many feel it is desirable to irradiate granulocyte concentrates for neonatal transfusion to prevent GVHD. Granulocyte transfusions to neonates are usually collected from CMV seronegative donors.

Compatibility Testing

Because the immunologic system of the newborn is immature and relatively unresponsive to antigenic stimulation during the first 4 months of life, standards for compatibility testing for neonates are different from those for adults. In a report of 65 neonates who received 572 transfusions from different donors, even with very sensitive detection techniques, no patients were shown to form red cell alloantibodies.[57]

The most common indication for transfusion of sick neonates is to replace blood drawn for laboratory studies.[58] Samples drawn for repeated compatibility testing contribute to this iatrogenic blood loss. Since infants seem not to produce antibodies despite multiple transfusions and since repeated blood bank testing causes demonstrable harm through blood loss, AABB *Standards* permits a reduction in pretransfusion serologic testing for neonates. Initial testing must include ABO and Rh typing of a neonatal recipient's red cells and an antibody screening test, which may be done on the newborn's or the mother's serum or plasma. If, during any one hospitalization, the antibody screen is negative and if all red cells transfused during the neonatal period are group O or

ABO identical or compatible with both mother and child, and are either Rh– or the same Rh type as the neonate, compatibility testing and further grouping may be omitted during the first 4 months of life. If unexpected antibody is detected in the initial sample from the infant, or the mother's serum contains clinically significant antibody, then antigen-negative units are necessary, for as long as maternal antibody persists in the infant's blood. If transfusions are to continue for several days or longer, the antibody screening test should be repeated on each sample of the infant's blood received with a request for transfusion. Once a negative result is obtained, subsequent crossmatches are unnecessary.

AABB *Standards* states that if the cells selected for transfusion are not group O, the infant's serum or plasma shall be tested, as appropriate, for anti-A or anti-B by methods that include the antiglobulin phase, using either reagent or donor red cells. Tests for anti-A shall use A_1 cells. If no anti-A or anti-B is detected, no subsequent crossmatching is necessary during the remainder of the infant's hospital admission. If anti-A or anti-B is detected, ABO-compatible RBCs shall be transfused. These units need not be crossmatched. If a non-group-O infant has received blood components containing alloagglutinins directed against his/her own A and/or B antigens, and if subsequent donor RBCs selected for transfusion are not group O, then the infant's serum or plasma shall be tested for anti-A and/or anti-B.[59(p 26)]

A special group of infant recipients will inevitably receive regular or frequent transfusions (eg, those with thalassemia, sickle cell disease or aplastic anemia). It is desirable to group their red cell antigens as completely as possible before beginning transfusion therapy because transfusions will result in a mixed population of red cells unsuitable for antigen grouping. These patients are liable to develop complex combinations of antibodies, and knowing their true phenotype can be helpful in selecting compatible blood. Records of this testing should be retained indefinitely. Since approximately 30% of these patients may become alloimmunized, some experts advocate providing blood that has been extensively phenotyped.[60]

Transfusion Administration

Vascular access is often difficult in the tiny newborn and in any infant requiring long-term or repeated intravenous infusions. The umbilical artery may be cannulated in newborns. Thereafter, a vein large enough to accommodate a 23- or 25-gauge needle or a 22- or 24-gauge vascular catheter should be chosen for blood administration. It is not usually necessary to warm small volume transfusions that are given slowly.

Constant rate syringe delivery pumps are satisfactory for transfusion of red cells through small-gauge needles.[61] Hemolysis increases with cells stored longer than 7 days and with slow rates of infusion.

The length of the plastic tubing used can add significantly to the amount of blood required for a transfusion. Platelet or component infusion sets have much less dead space than standard transfusion sets because they have short tubing and a small 170-micron blood filter. All blood components must be infused through filters. Microaggregate filters (20- or 40-micron) are superfluous, since microaggregates do not accumulate significantly in blood stored less than 1 week,[62] and blood transfused to infants is usually less than 7 days old. There have been reports[63,64] of hemolysis occurring when stored blood was infused through a 20-micron stainless steel mesh filter.

Indications for Red Cell Transfusion

Because the tissue need for oxygen cannot be measured directly, and so many variables determine oxygen availability, no universally accepted criteria exist for transfusion of premature or term infants.[1] The decision to transfuse a newborn for anemia should include evaluation of expected hemoglobin levels ascertained from the literature (Table 18-1) and an evaluation of the infant's clinical status. Other potentially useful considerations include the presence or absence of reticulocytes as an index of bone marrow erythroid function, and development of adaptive mechanisms, such as the increased intracellular 2,3-DPG occurring in physiologic anemia of infancy. Table 18-5 lists representative criteria for replacement transfusion in a high-risk newborn.[65] Because the neonate in respiratory distress is hypoxic and more vulnerable to cerebral hemor-

rhage, RBC transfusions are given more aggressively.

Iatrogenic Blood Loss

Although specialized care in neonatal intensive care units requires close laboratory monitoring, unnecessary laboratory testing should be avoided. Repeated blood sampling to measure blood gases, pH and electrolytes often results in anemia. The volume of blood removed from infants must be carefully recorded. When blood loss equals 10% of the infant's calculated blood volume, it is usual practice to replace with RBCs on a volume-for-volume basis. If an anemic infant develops congestive heart failure, it may be better to remove aliquots of dilute blood from the infant and replace with concentrated red cells. This is sometimes called a "partial exchange" transfusion.

Causes of Blood Loss

A variety of acute or chronic problems occurring prenatally, during delivery or postnatally may lead to anemia. Causes of prenatal blood loss include spontaneous fetomaternal or fetoplacental hem-

Table 18-5. Guidelines for Red Cell Transfusions in the Neonate*

1. To restore the hematocrit to >0.40 (40%) at birth.

2. To maintain a hematocrit of >0.40 (40%) in infants requiring ventilators and/or oxygen support or in the presence of cyanotic heart disease.

3. To maintain a hematocrit of >0.30 (30%) during the neonatal period to treat significant problems such as tachycardia, tachypnea, apnea, poor weight gain and diminished vigor (ie, poor cry, eating, etc).

4. To correct for iatrogenic blood loss when >10% of the blood volume is removed for laboratory tests (over 10 days):
     if the initial hematocrit is >0.50 (50%) within 72 hours of birth, or
     if the hematocrit is <0.40 (40%).
         Otherwise
   Correct for iatrogenic blood loss when >5% of the blood volume is removed for laboratory tests.

*Modified from Sacher et al.[65]

orrhage, traumatic amniocentesis, complications of intrauterine transfusion or twin-twin transfusion (when monozygotic twins share a monochorionic placenta). Clinically significant twin-twin transfusion causes a hemoglobin difference of at least 50 g/L (5 g/dL); if twin-twin transfusion continues chronically, the infants will differ markedly in birth weight and organ size. The smaller, anemic twin is at risk of congestive heart failure; the larger, plethoric twin is at risk for hyperbilirubinemia or hyperviscosity. The condition of the smaller twin, however, is nearly always more critical.

The fetus may lose blood into the placenta if the cord is wrapped tightly around the neck, or if the infant is placed above the placenta before the cord is clamped. Obstetric accidents, umbilical cord rupture, abruptio placentae, placenta previa and other cord and placenta abnormalities can also result in hemorrhage and an anemic, hypovolemic newborn.

Postnatal anemia may result from internal hemorrhage, usually the result of traumatic delivery. This deficit may not become apparent until 24-72 hours of age. Common bleeding sites include the brain, liver, lungs, spleen, adrenal glands and scalp. However, the major source of chronic blood loss is iatrogenic anemia resulting from laboratory testing.

Failure To Thrive

An indication for transfusion unique to this age group is lack of expected weight gain in the absence of other known causes of failure to thrive. Anemia in newborns increases oxygen consumption, probably because anemia increases cardiac workload. Increased oxygen consumption at a fixed caloric intake causes diminished rate of weight gain. A group of premature infants[66] with no other medical problems had an average weight gain of only 21 g/day, compared with normal average gain of 28 g/day. Of these 13 infants, 11 gained weight when transfused from a mean hemoglobin of 85 to 114 g/L (8.5 to 11.4 g/dL). There was an associated 11% decrease in oxygen consumption. In contrast, others have shown little overall benefit from transfusions simply given for failure to thrive in the absence of obvious clinical causes.

Indications for Exchange Transfusion

Exchange transfusion, originally used almost exclusively as treatment for hemolytic disease of the newborn, has recently been advocated as adjunctive therapy for a variety of life-threatening diseases affecting newborns including respiratory distress, disseminated intravascular coagulation (DIC) and sepsis. The potential risks of exchange transfusion are listed in Table 18-6. The procedure carries a mortality rate of approximately 1% and there may be substantial morbidity.[67] Exchange transfusion is often quantified (eg, two-volume, single-volume) to reflect the effect on the infant's total blood volume.

Hemolytic Disease of the Newborn

Exchange transfusion is the indicated treatment for severe HDN. Removing the infant's plasma reduces the load of accumulated bilirubin and the number of unbound antibody molecules. Replacement with donor plasma restores albumin and any deficient coagulation factors. Antibody-coated cells, whose destruction would further raise the bilirubin load, are removed and replaced with red cells compatible with the maternal antibody. For a discussion of hematologic and mechanical considerations of exchange transfusion, see p 458.

Table 18-6. Possible Complications of Exchange Transfusion

Cardiac
Arrhythmias and/or arrest due to hyperkalemia, hypocalcemia and citrate toxicity
Myocardial infarct

Vascular-Mechanical
Volume overload or depletion
Perforation of vessels
Thrombosis of hepatic or portal veins
Embolization with air or thrombi
Injury to donor cells—mechanical, thermal or osmotic
Perforation of bowel with or without necrotizing enterocolitis

Infectious
Bacterial (eg, sepsis, omphalitis, septic thrombophlebitis, hepatic abscess)
Viral (eg, hepatitis, cytomegalovirus, human immunodeficiency virus)

Hematologic-Coagulation
Over-heparinization (if heparinized blood is used)
Aggravation of thrombocytopenia in severe disease
Sickling of donor blood

Immunologic
Incompatible erythrocytes or plasma
Graft-vs-host disease

Other
Hypoglycemia
Hypothermia
Retrolental fibroplasia
Intracranial hemorrhage

Selection of Blood

In most cases the mother's serum is used for crossmatching and the transfused cells are compatible with her ABO antibodies as well as with whatever antibody or antibodies have caused the hemolytic process. Since the mother and the infant may be of different ABO groups, group O cells are commonly used. In ABO hemolytic disease, the cells used for exchange must be group O. If the antibody is anti-D the cells must, of course, be Rh–. Not every exchange transfusion, however, requires group O, Rh– blood. If the mother and the infant have the same ABO group, group-specific cells can be used. If the pathogenic antibody is not anti-D, the cells given to an Rh+ infant may be Rh+.

To crossmatch blood for exchange transfusion, the serum or plasma of either the mother or the infant may be used. The mother's serum is available in large quantity, has the antibody present in high concentration and is capable of being accurately and completely analyzed before birth. If the infant is to be transferred to another facility from the place where delivery occurred, a specimen of maternal blood should accompany the infant.

Problems With Crossmatching

If maternal blood is not available, or if it is unsuitable for immediate use in cross-matching, the infant's serum, an eluate from the infant's cells or both can be used for crossmatching.

Maternal serum may contain antibodies directed against antigens other than those on the infant's cells, or IgM antibodies that have not crossed the placenta. The eluate provides a concentrated preparation of the antibodies responsible for red cell destruction, but will not contain antibodies against antigens absent from the infant's cells. The infant's serum, on the other hand, may not contain a high concentration of antibody if most of the molecules are bound to the red cells. Use of either or both may, however, be preferable to delaying transfusion while a maternal specimen is obtained.

Subsequent Transfusion

In severe HDN, bilirubin may reaccumulate rapidly after an initial successful exchange, partly because a large quantity of extravascular bilirubin will reenter the intravascular space, (see p 456) and partly because hemolysis characteristically continues at a reduced but nonetheless significant rate. If rising bilirubin levels make a second or third exchange transfusion necessary, the same considerations of cell selection and crossmatching apply.

Transfusion When Antibody Reacts With a High-Incidence Antigen

Rarely, the mother's serum may contain an antibody to a high-incidence antigen and no compatible blood is available. If this problem is recognized and identified in the prenatal period, there will be time to test the siblings of the mother for compatibility and suitability, and to work with the rare donor file to locate compatible donors. If this problem is not recognized until after delivery, three choices are open:

1. Collect a unit of blood from the mother, if the obstetrician agrees that this is safe. Centrifuge the WB and remove as much plasma as possible. Alternatively, the unit can be washed. Resuspend the red cells to the desired hematocrit in group AB plasma. The unit should be irradiated due to the genetic relationship of the infant and mother.

2. Test the mother's siblings for compatibility and suitability, if they are available.

3. Use available donor blood that possesses the antigen and is incompatible. If no compatible blood is available and the clinical situation is urgent, exchange transfusion with incompatible blood may be required. The procedure does remove antibody and bilirubin, but it will likely have to be followed with several additional incompatible exchanges, since the transfused cells will be destroyed and will generate additional bilirubin.

Hyperbilirubinemia

The most common indication for neonatal exchange transfusion is excessive unconjugated bilirubin. Whenever unconjugated bilirubin in serum exceeds the level at which free bilirubin crosses the blood-brain barrier, bilirubin may concentrate in the basal ganglia and cerebellum, causing central nervous system (CNS) damage called kernicterus. The fetal liver has limited capacity to conjugate bilirubin. During intrauterine existence, unconjugated bilirubin crosses the placenta for excretion through the mother's hepatobiliary system; after delivery, the fetal liver is incapable of handling the increased bilirubin load arising from HDN.

Several mechanisms may cause unconjugated bilirubin to accumulate in the newborn. Normal newborns rarely develop dangerous hyperbilirubinemia, but there are several processes that lead to rising bilirubin levels. These include:

1. Poor hepatic uptake of bilirubin, due in part to low levels of albumin, which functions as a bilirubin carrier protein.

2. Transient deficiency of the hepatic microsomal enzyme, uridine diphosphoglucuronyl transferase, responsible for converting bilirubin from an indirect-unconjugated lipid-soluble form to the direct water-soluble glucuronide conjugate that is excreted without damage to the CNS.

3. Rapid bilirubin production caused by the shortened life span of fetal red cells.

4. Efficient enterohepatic resorption of bilirubin.

Prematurity amplifies all of the processes listed above. Neonatal patients who require exchange transfusion are usually premature and also have one or more of the following pathologic processes:

1. Hemolysis secondary to maternal alloantibody, most commonly those of the ABO system and anti-D, but occasionally other antibodies in the Rh system or in systems such as Kidd, Duffy or Kell.

2. Hemolysis secondary to:
   a. inherited deficiencies of red cell enzymes, most commonly glucose-6-phosphate dehydrogenase or, less often, pyruvate kinase
   b. congenital red blood cell membrane defects, such as hereditary spherocytosis
   c. hemoglobinopathies, associated with shortened red cell survival

3. Hemorrhage into an enclosed space, especially likely in prolonged labor or difficult delivery.

4. Increased enterohepatic circulation due to any form of intestinal obstruction or delay in bowel transit time, allowing deconjugation and reabsorption.

5. Displacement of bound bilirubin from albumin by competing substances, usually drugs given to the mother or infant, such as sulfonamides, vitamin K or salicylates.

6. Sepsis.

Phototherapy with fluorescent blue lights sometimes prevents the need for exchange transfusion. When bilirubin near the surface of the skin is exposed to light it undergoes photoisomerization to form "photobilirubin." These isomers of bilirubin are transported in the plasma to the liver where they are rapidly excreted in bile without being conjugated.[68]

Effects of Exchange

Exchange transfusion removes unconjugated bilirubin and provides additional albumin to bind residual bilirubin. If there is antibody-mediated hemolysis, exchange transfusion is additionally beneficial in removing free antibody and antibody-coated red cells and providing red cells that will survive normally.

Exchange transfusion should be done before bilirubin rises to levels at which CNS damage occurs. Several factors affect the threshold for toxicity. CNS damage occurs at lower levels if there is prematurity, decreased albumin binding capacity or the presence of such complicating conditions as sepsis, hypoxia, acidosis, hypothermia or hypoglycemia. In infants with very low birth-weights, kernicterus may occur at levels of unconjugated bilirubin as low as 103-154 μmol/L (6-9 mg/dL).[69] The level of hyperbilirubinemia, not the cause, influences the decision to perform exchange transfusion; representative danger levels are listed in Table 18-7.

The rate at which bilirubin rises is a better predictor of the need for exchange transfusion than any single value. Infants with an accumulation rate greater than 8.6 μmol/L/hour and/or significant anemia usually require exchange transfusion.[70] A two-volume exchange transfusion decreases the serum bilirubin to 45-50% of its preexchange value.[70] This observed efficiency is less than the predicted theoretical efficiency (see p 36) because exchange transfusion permits reequilibration between bilirubin in plasma and in extravascular tissues. Within the subsequent few hours, more extravascular bilirubin enters the circulation to equilibrate with lowered serum levels. This rebound rise in bilirubin, combined with continued bilirubin production, may restore serum concentration to a level requiring a repeat exchange transfusion. The indications for repeat exchange are similar to those for the initial exchange.

Respiratory Distress

Exchange transfusion has been shown to improve survival in low birth-weight infants with respiratory distress,[5] possibly because substitution of hemoglobin A for hemoglobin F results in a shift of the oxyhemoglobin curve to the right and increases tissue oxygenation. However, the clinical utility of this approach is debatable and exchange transfusion is not employed widely as treatment of respiratory disease. Infants who are hypoxic due to respiratory distress are also more susceptible to intracerebral hemorrhage. Other effects, including improvement in coagulation status, removal of toxic substances and repletion of serum proteins, have been suggested to explain the beneficial effects of exchange transfusion.

Disseminated Intravascular Coagulation

In the neonatal period DIC occurs secondary to many conditions, particularly sepsis and necrotizing enterocolitis. In spite of demonstrated severe shortening of both platelet and fibrinogen survival times in these patients, the tests for fibrin degradation products and the routine coagulation screening tests (PT, PTT, TT) may remain normal.[71] Thrombocytopenia and a low fibrinogen are the most important indices of DIC in low birth-weight infants in whom DIC is not infrequent.

The most important therapy for neonatal DIC is to treat the underlying disease. Exchange transfusion has produced variable results, perhaps due to

Table 18-7. Bilirubin Values (in μmol/L) Indicating the Need for Exchange Transfusion in the Newborn Patient[69]

Birthweight (g)	<1250	1250–1499	1500–1999	2000–2500	>2500
Uncomplicated	222	257	291	308	342
Complicated*	171	222	257	291	308

*Complicated includes the presence of any of the following: 5-minute Apgar less than 3; PaO$_2$ less than 40 torr for 1 hour; pH less than 7.15 for 1 hour; rectal temperature 35 C or less; serum albumin 25 g/L or less; signs of CNS deterioration; proven sepsis or meningitis; hemolytic anemia; birth weight less than 1000 g.

the fact that only the sickest infants have been selected to receive this therapy. Exchange transfusion appears to be effective therapy for infants who suffer severe, symptomatic DIC following birth asphyxia.

Sepsis

Newborn infants experience exceedingly high morbidity and mortality from bacterial infections, particularly from group B streptococcus. Treatments including exchange transfusion and transfusion of WB or granulocytes have been shown to improve survival.[72,73] There may be a potential role for intravenous immunoglobin to prevent late onset sepsis in very low birth-weight infants.

Other Toxins

Exchange transfusion is occasionally used to remove other toxins, such as drugs or chemicals given to the mother near the time of delivery, drugs given in toxic doses to the infant or substances such as ammonia that accumulate in the newborn because of prematurity or inherited metabolic diseases.

Partial Exchange Transfusion for Polycythemia

A venous hematocrit greater than 0.65 (65%) or hemoglobin in excess of 220 g/L (22 g/dL) any time in the first week of life defines polycythemia. As hematocrit rises above 0.50 (50%) the viscosity of blood increases exponentially and oxygen transport decreases.[74] The infant has limited ability to increase cardiac output to compensate for hyperviscosity and may develop congestive heart failure.

Polycythemia in the newborn generally requires treatment whether or not it produces symptoms. If untreated, the re-

sulting hyperviscosity can produce sludging of blood flow, hyperbilirubinemia, reduced tissue oxygenation and increased incidence of microthrombi. Many organs may be affected, resulting in CNS abnormalities, pulmonary or renal failure or necrotizing enterocolitis. Newborn polycythemia may be due to maternal-to-fetal transfusion, placental-to-fetal transfusion, twin-to-twin transfusion or intrauterine hypoxia. Males, infants small for gestational age and infants of diabetic mothers are at increased risk.[75]

The goal of partial exchange with plasma is to lower the hematocrit to 0.55-0.60 (55-60%). Whole blood is removed and replaced with an equal volume of 5% albumin or crystalloid, the choice being based on the infant's clinical condition and the volume to be replaced. Plasma is usually not recommended because the volume given is insufficient to correct significant clotting abnormalities. This procedure lowers the hematocrit while maintaining blood volume. A formula for the volume of replacement fluid required for the exchange is:

Volume of replacement fluid =

$$\frac{\text{blood volume} \times (\text{observed hemoglobin} - \text{desired hemoglobin})}{\text{observed hemoglobin}}$$

Example: Calculations for volume of replacement fluid needed for a partial exchange to achieve a hemoglobin of 200 g/L (20 g/dL) in a 2-kg infant who has a hemoglobin of 240 g/L (24 g/dL). The blood volume of a full-term newborn is approximately 85 mL/kg.

Blood volume = $2 \times 85 = 170$ mL
Volume of fluid needed =

$$\frac{170 \, \text{mL} \times (24 - 20 \, \text{g/dL})}{24 \, \text{g/dL}} = 28 \, \text{mL}$$

Technique of Exchange Transfusion

Vascular Access

Exchange transfusions in the newborn period are usually accomplished via catheters in the umbilical vessels. Catheterization is easiest within hours of birth, but it may be possible to achieve vascular access at this site for several days. The catheters should be radiopaque to facilitate radiographic monitoring during and after placement. Once placed, they should be secured with sutures. Holes should be at the end, and the catheter should be kept filled with solution at all times. If umbilical catheters are not available for exchange transfusion, small central venous or saphenous catheters may be used.

Choice of Components for Exchange Transfusion

Many different combinations of blood components have provided safe and effective exchange transfusion; no single component or combination is unequivocally best. Most frequently used are fresh (<1 week old) RBCs in CPDA-1. These can be used alone, with 5% albumin or with FFP if clotting factors are required. Heparinized blood is no longer recommended due to the risk of bleeding associated with its use. WB collected in CPDA-1 appears satisfactory for exchange transfusion in term infants.[76] Blood components of the infant's ABO and Rh types are generally used, except in hemolytic disease due to maternal alloantibodies (see p 453). For infants who are hypoxic or acidotic, some pediatricians request that blood for exchange transfusion lack hemoglobin S.[77]

Traditionally, calcium has been administered to infants receiving blood anticoagulated with citrate, to offset the calcium-binding effects of citrate. There is little documentation to support this practice. In one study, posttransfusion levels of ionized calcium did not differ significantly between infants given 100 mg of calcium gluconate after each 100 mL of blood exchanged and a similar group receiving no supplemental calcium.[78] If used, it is recommended that calcium not be infused through the same IV line with transfused blood because it will cause clots to form.

Albumin binds unconjugated bilirubin. Increased intravascular binding is thought to enhance diffusion of bilirubin from the extravascular compartment into the circulation, thereby increasing the total quantity of bilirubin removed during the exchange and protecting the infant's brain from bilirubin toxicity. Some physicians give 25% serum albumin, either 1 hour prior to the exchange (1 g/kg) or at 100-mL intervals during exchanges intended to reduce hyperbilirubinemia. However, in a study comparing 15 hyperbilirubinemic infants given albumin with 27 who received none, the efficiency of bilirubin removal was the same in both groups.[79] Because infusing albumin raises the colloid osmotic pressure and increases intravascular volume, it should be given cautiously, if at all, to severely anemic infants, infants in renal or congestive heart failure or infants with increased central venous pressure.

Volume and Hematocrit

An exchange transfusion equal to twice the patient's blood volume is typically recommended for newborns. Rarely is more than one full unit of donor blood needed during an exchange transfusion, since bilirubin, antibody, sensitized cells and/or toxins are removed with progressively less efficiency in the late stages of an exchange. In practice, the calculated volume for exchange is used as an estimate, with the actual volume exchanged being one unit of fresh WB or one unit of RBCs reconstituted with one unit of compatible FFP. Thus, the final hematocrit of the unit selected for exchange will be approximately 40-50% and sufficient plasma will be present to offer an optimal efficiency of exchange and to provide clotting factors. In the unusual event that the infant's condition warrants a high postexchange hematocrit, a small volume transfusion of red blood cells can also be given. It is important to mix the donor blood during the exchange. If WB is allowed to settle in the container, the final aliquots will not have the intended hematocrit. Samples should be obtained from the last aliquot removed in the exchange for determination of the infant's hematocrit and bilirubin.

Methods Used

Two methods of exchange transfusion are in common use. The isovolumetric method requires vascular access through two catheters of identical size. Withdrawal and infusion occur simultaneously, regulated by a single peristaltic pump. The umbilical artery is usually used for withdrawal, and the umbilical vein is used for infusion. The push-pull technique can be accomplished through a single vascular access if necessary. A three-way stopcock joins the unit of blood, the infant and an extension tube that leads to the graduated discard container. A maximum of 5 mL/kg is used for each withdrawal and infusion.

An in-line blood warmer and a standard blood filter should be incorporated in the administration set.

The following additional considerations may apply to exchange transfusion in newborns:

1. The infant's oxygenation, ventilation and acid-base balance should be monitored frequently; it is often necessary to increase the inspired oxygen concentration during the procedure.

2. If the postexchange platelet count is less than 25×10^9/L (25,000/µL) many physicians administer platelets.

3. Hypoglycemia may occur as a rebound phenomenon after the sudden glucose increase from the exchange or secondary to the hyperinsulinism that may accompany severe hemolytic disease. Infusion of 10% dextrose solution after the exchange is completed may be desirable.

4. If the initial exchange transfusion was performed for hyperbilirubinemia, phototherapy using fluorescent blue light bulbs should be instituted when the exchange is completed.

Platelet Transfusion

The normal range of the platelet count in newborns is similar to that in adults. A platelet count less than 100×10^9/L (100,000/µL) in a full-term or premature infant is abnormal and requires evaluation. In the absence of other coagulopathy, however, the thrombocytopenic term infant who is in stable clinical condition rarely bleeds unless the platelet count is less than 10×10^9/L (10,000/µL). Small premature infants, or those with other complicating illnesses, may bleed at higher platelet counts and should be considered for platelet transfusion. Due to platelet dysfunction, clinically significant bleeding may occur in such infants at platelet counts of $75-150 \times 10^9$ (75-150,000/µL).[80] When platelet transfusions are given, a 1-hour posttransfusion platelet count should be obtained to evaluate efficacy.

Neonatal thrombocytopenia may result from decreased platelet production, increased platelet destruction or both.[81] Decreased production occurs in congenital megakaryocytic hypoplasia, an entity usually associated with skeletal deformities, in congenital leukemia or systemic histiocytosis, and in rare, genetically determined thrombocytopenias. Increased platelet destruction occurs in conditions such as infection, immune thrombocytopenia, large cavernous hemangioma or DIC. Platelet transfusion is indicated if bleeding occurs with these forms of thrombocytopenia.

Neonatal Immune Thrombocytopenia

Maternal IgG antibodies can cross the placenta and damage fetal platelets, causing severe antenatal thrombocytopenia. Although the stress of labor and delivery can cause petechiae to develop in the first few hours postpartum, caesarean section in pregnant women with immune thrombocytopenia is generally only performed for appropriate maternal indications. Two categories of immune thrombocytopenia are recognized, and the distinction between them is therapeutically important.

Secondary to Maternal ITP

Of infants born to mothers with active idiopathic (autoimmune) thrombocytopenic purpura (ITP), many are not profoundly thrombocytopenic and the risk of hemorrhage is relatively small when compared to alloimmune thrombocytopenia. The circulating platelet antibody is usually IgG, which readily crosses the placenta. Some women with systemic lupus erythematosus have similar circulating platelet antibodies. If maternal ITP is in remission throughout gestation and delivery, fetal risk may persist, since any platelet antibodies that remain in the mother's circulation may affect the infant. Occasionally, delivery of a severely thrombocytopenic infant has led to the diagnosis of previously unsuspected ITP in a moderately affected mother [platelet count 75-100 × 10^9/L (75-100,000/μL) postpartum]. In cases of mild gestational thrombocytopenia, defined as a maternal platelet count usually between 100-150 × 10^9/L (100-150,000/μL) with no history of autoimmune disorder, little to no risk to either the mother or fetus/neonate occurs.

The platelet antibody of ITP has broad reactivity against all platelets. When the quantity of antibody is high in the infant, transfusions of platelets from random donors, the mother or other family members have uniformly short survival. However, responses sometimes will occur, and platelet transfusions can be used as emergency therapy for hemorrhage. Exchange transfusion may be used to remove circulating antibodies and to provide platelets. Heparinized blood should be avoided, since it may increase the risk of hemorrhage. Intravenous immunoglobulin therapy has become an effective therapy and should be used for severe thrombocytopenia.[82]

Neonatal Alloimmune Thrombocytopenia

A fetus whose platelets possess a paternal antigen absent from maternal platelets may immunize the mother during gestation or delivery, in a pathologic process similar to HDN. The result is formation of maternal IgG alloantibody that crosses the placenta, usually in a subsequent pregnancy, and causes neonatal thrombocytopenia.[83] However, first-born children are frequently affected as well, and the severity in successive pregnancies is unpredictable. The maternal platelet count remains normal. Most important, the fetus can be seriously affected and antenatal care is mandatory when high risk pregnancies are recognized. IVIG administration to the mother is frequently employed and fetal intrauterine platelet transfusions may also be used. Although the infant's thrombocytopenia is self-limited (usually persisting less than 3 weeks after delivery), transfusion therapy is indicated if there is birth trauma, progressive purpura or hemorrhage.

Several dominantly inherited platelet antigens have been implicated in alloimmune neonatal thrombocytopenia. The most commonly involved antigen is HPA-1a (Pl^{A1}), present in 98% of unselected individuals. Platelets from random donors are usually positive for HPA-1a (Pl^{A1}) and are ineffective because of rapid destruction by the alloantibody. Often the most readily available source of compatible platelets is the mother. It is usually safe to collect platelets from the mother by plateletpheresis (see p 32), even in the postpartum period. Before the platelets are transfused, the mother's antibody-containing plasma must be removed and the platelets must be irradiated.

Granulocyte Transfusion

The role of granulocyte transfusion for neonates remains controversial.[84-86] Neonates are more susceptible to severe bacterial infection than are older children. Mortality for infants with fulminant group B streptococcal sepsis approaches 100% when treated with antibiotics alone. Neutrophils found in the neonate have been shown to be deficient both quantitatively and qualitatively. Areas of controversy regarding the use of granulocyte transfusions in neonates include such fundamental areas as dose, neutrophil level at which to transfuse and type of product to use. In addition, encouraging data are emerging to suggest that IVIG may be equal in efficacy to granulocyte transfusions.

Strauss[86] has analyzed the data from seven reports of granulocyte transfusions used to treat infected neonates. His recommendations are summarized below:

1. The precise role of granulocyte transfusion for neonatal sepsis is unclear. Although mortality is high, some infants respond to antibiotics alone.

2. Infants with an absolute neutropenia of $<3 \times 10^9$ PMN/L during the first week of life, or $<1 \times 10^9$ PMN/L thereafter with strong evidence of bacterial septicemia, should be considered candidates for granulocyte transfusions.

3. Septic infants without neutropenia should be considered for treatment with antibiotics alone.

4. The efficacy of exchange transfusion vs use of granulocyte concentrates collected by mechanical apheresis is unproven at this time.

Current recommendations are that if a decision is made to use granulocyte transfusions for a septic neonatal patient, mechanical leukapheresis should be used to provide the child with a dose of $>1 \times 10^9$ PMN/kg in a volume of 15 mL/kg. Fresh blood buffy coats have recently been criticized as being ineffective and as currently of unproven value. Irradiation of the granulocyte concentrates before transfusion is recommended because of the large quantity of lymphocytes contained in the product. Donors should be ABO and Rh compatible.

Other Blood Components

Hemorrhagic disease of the newborn, caused by deficiency of vitamin K-dependent coagulation factors (Factors II, VII, IX and X), may result in significant cutaneous, gastrointestinal or CNS hemorrhage at 2-4 days of age. This disease is now rare because intramuscular vitamin K is routinely given at birth. If vitamin

K therapy is omitted, and especially if the infant is breast fed, hemorrhagic disease may occur. If there is life-threatening hemorrhage, the treatment is FFP.

Because maternal clotting factors do not cross the placenta, hereditary deficiencies of coagulation factors may be apparent in the newborn. Significant bleeding, however, is rare. If hemorrhage occurs, therapy includes local thrombin for small superficial bleeds, virus-inactivated factor concentrates for hemophilia A, cryoprecipitate for von Willebrand's disease and FFP for other congenital disorders.[87]

Obstetrical Considerations

Rh Immune Globulin

Rh Immune Globulin (RhIG) is a concentrated solution of IgG anti-D derived from human plasma. A 1-mL full dose vial, containing 300 μg of anti-D, is sufficient to counteract the immunizing effects of 15 mL of Rh+ red cells; this corresponds to 30 mL of fetal whole blood. RhIG, like other immunoglobulin preparations, does not transmit hepatitis or HIV infection.[88,89] The protective effect of RhIG on Rh− individuals exposed to Rh+ cells probably results from interference with antigen recognition in the induction phase of primary immunization.

Antepartum Administration

The Rh− mother of an Rh+, ABO-compatible infant, who receives no protection, has a 7-8% chance of developing anti-D. When a full dose vial of RhIG is administered postpartum, the risk of immunization decreases to about 1%. A further decrease in risk, to 0.1%, is achieved if RhIG is given antepartum at 28 weeks of gestation, in addition to the postpartum dose.[90] No adverse effects

have been observed in infants of mothers who have received up to two antepartum doses of RhIG.[91] The American College of Obstetricians and Gynecologists (ACOG) has recommended RhIG antepartum prophylaxis.[92] When antepartum RhIG is given, good communication must exist between the patient's physician and the blood bank staff of the hospital where the patient will give birth, so that laboratory tests made at the time of delivery will be correctly interpreted.

Testing at Delivery

Standards does not require that blood from Rh− women be tested at the time of delivery for the presence of unexpected antibodies. It does recommend Rh testing of all women admitted for delivery, abortion or any invasive obstetric procedure. Neither the pre- nor postdelivery specimen need be tested for antibodies, provided there is not a request for red cell transfusion. The Rh test on the mother should include a test for weak D (D^u) if there is not direct agglutination with anti-D.

Cord blood from infants born to Rh− mothers should be tested for D; ABO testing is not required but is desirable. The mother's antibody status and the infant's clinical condition dictate whether or not a DAT should be done. In some hospitals it is routine to perform ABO testing and a DAT on cord blood from all infants born to group O mothers, but in other centers these tests are performed only if symptoms develop.

The following women are not candidates for RhIG:

1. Rh− women who have Rh− infants.
2. Rh+ women. Although cases of HDN have been reported involving infants whose mothers were of the weak D (D^u) phenotype, this rare event does not justify routine RhIG prophylaxis

in women of the weak D (D^u) pheno-type.[93]

3. Rh– women known to be immunized to D. Since the presence of anti-D in the postpartum specimen may actually be due to prenatal passive immunization, postpartum RhIG may be indicated. An accurate history is essential in such cases.

Anti-D in a Postpartum Specimen

The woman who has received antepartum RhIG often has anti-D present in an antibody screening test done at delivery. Such a woman should receive postpartum RhIG. Only if the anti-D present at delivery is known to be the result of active immunization can administration of RhIG be omitted. There are some laboratory clues that may help distinguish the origin of the antibody. Passively administered RhIG is IgG. If a woman's anti-D is saline-reactive or can be inactivated by treating the serum with 2-mercaptoethanol or dithiothreitol, it probably represents active immunization. Passively acquired anti-D is usually weakly reactive, rarely achieving a titer above 4. High-titered anti-D is likely to be of maternal origin. However, confirmation should always be sought from the physician's records. RhIG should be given whenever there is doubt that cannot be resolved.

Administration of RhIG

The antepartum dose of RhIG is given between 28 and 30 weeks of gestation, a recommendation based on the fact that, of women who develop anti-D during pregnancy, 92% do so at 28 weeks or later.[94] A sample for laboratory testing should be obtained before injection of RhIG. Tests on the specimen drawn at 28-30 weeks should include[33]:

1. ABO group.

2. Rh type and a test for weak D (D^u) if reagent anti-D does not cause immediate agglutination.

3. Antibody screen.

4. Identification of antibody, if present.

The presence, in an Rh– woman, of antibodies other than anti-D must not preclude giving RhIG.

The anti-D from an injected dose of RhIG may remain detectible for as long as 6 months. The half-life of an injected dose is approximately 23 days; of 300 μg of antibody given at 28 weeks, 20-30 μg should remain at the time of delivery 12 weeks later. Postpartum RhIG should be injected within 72 hours of delivery, in addition to the antepartum dose given at 28 weeks of gestation. Some data suggest that the presence of antibody at levels around 20 μg may enhance the likelihood of immunization if FMH has occurred.[95] It is extremely important that RhIG administration not be omitted or delayed because of uncertainty in interpreting an antibody screening test. If for some reason RhIG was not given within 72 hours, later administration should not be withheld.

The "Utilization Gap"

Administration of RhIG is indicated, but sometimes inadvertently omitted, after several common events: abortion, ectopic pregnancy, amniocentesis, chorionic villus sampling, antepartum hemorrhage or fetal death. If pregnancy in an Rh– woman terminates before 13 weeks of gestation, a low dose vial of 50 μg is adequate to cover the small fetal blood volume during the first trimester. From 13 weeks until term, the standard full dose vial (300 μg) should be given.

Amniocentesis

Since FMH may accompany amniocentesis, the procedure can cause Rh immunization.[96] The Rh– woman who has amniocentesis at 16-18 weeks for genetic analysis should receive a 300-µg dose of RhIG. A second dose should be given 12 weeks later or at 28 weeks of gestation and a third dose given after delivery if the infant is Rh+. Amniocentesis performed in the second or third trimester of pregnancy on the nonimmunized Rh– woman should be followed by the injection of 300 µg RhIG. If a subsequent amniocentesis is done more than 21 days later, an additional injection of 300 µg RhIG should be given. A mother who gives birth within 21 days of receiving a 300-µg dose of RhIG may not need a postpartum injection unless there is evidence of a massive FMH.

If amniocentesis is performed to assess fetal maturity, and if delivery occurs within 48 hours of the amniocentesis, the 300 µg RhIG can be withheld until after the infant is confirmed to be Rh+. If amniocentesis precedes delivery by more than 48 hours, the patient should receive 300 µg RhIG following amniocentesis. Although additional RhIG may not need to be given if delivery occurs within 21 days and there is no evidence of a massive FMH,[92] prudent management would suggest an additional dose at delivery.

Detection and Quantitation of FMH Screening Procedures

Postpartum Rh immunization can occur despite RhIG administration if the quantity of Rh+ fetal red cells entering the mother's circulation exceeds the 30 mL of whole blood covered by a single 300 µg dose of RhIG. The incidence of transplacental hemorrhage greater than 30 mL has been estimated as only about 0.3%, but large FMH is an important and preventable cause of failure of immunoprophylaxis.[97] *Standards* requires that a postpartum specimen be examined from all Rh– women at risk of immunization to detect the presence of

FMH larger than that for which one dose of RhIG provides protection. In the past, a microscopic examination of the weak D (D^u) test was used to screen for Rh+ red cells in the maternal circulation, but it is not sufficiently sensitive. In a survey of laboratories, 12% failed to detect Rh+ cells in a specimen simulating hemorrhage of approximately 30 mL.[98]

Although the Kleihauer-Betke acid elution technique is used for detecting and quantitating small volumes of fetal cells in the maternal circulation, the difficulty of performance and interpretation makes it less desirable than other procedures as a screening test.[98]

The Rosette Test

The rosette test is a very practical method to use as a screening test for the detection of a large FMH.[99,100] The rosette test uses D+ indicator red cells to form easily identified rosettes around individual D+ fetal cells that may be present in the maternal circulation. (See Method 7.1.) This method will detect FMHs of approximately 10 mL. Such sensitivity provides a margin of safety that is desirable for a screening test. The rosette test gives only qualitative results, and positive results must be followed by the quantitative Kleihauer-Betke acid elution test or an enzyme-linked antiglobulin test (ELAT) to quantify the hemorrhage.[101] Weak D (D^u) positive cells from the infant do not react as strongly in the rosette procedure as normal D+ cells. If the mother or the newborn types as weak D (D^u) positive, then a Kleihauer-Betke acid elution test should be done routinely.

Acid Elution

Results of the Kleihauer-Betke acid elution test are reported as percentage of fetal cells, but the precision and accuracy of the procedure may be poor. To calculate the volume of FMH, this percentage of fetal cells is multiplied by

50.[101] Since one 300-µg dose of RhIG will protect against a transplacental hemorrhage of 30 mL of Rh+ fetal blood, the volume of fetal blood should be divided by 30 to determine the number of doses of RhIG required.

For example:

1. Kleihauer-Betke reported as 1.3%
2. 1.3 × 50* = 65 mL of fetal blood
3. 65/30 = 2.2 doses of RhIG required
   * 5000 mL (mother's arbitrarily assigned blood volume) × 1/100 = 50.

Because quantification by this procedure is inherently imprecise and because the consequences of undertreatment can be serious, it is important to provide a safety margin in calculating RhIG dosage. One approach is as follows:

1. When the number to the right of the decimal point is less than 5, round down and add one dose of RhIG (Example: 2.2 doses—give 3 doses).
2. When the number to the right of the decimal point is 5 or greater, round up to the next number and add one dose of RhIG (Example: 2.8 doses—give 4 doses).

Not more than five doses of RhIG should be injected at one time into each buttock. If more than five doses are required, the injections may be spaced over a 72-hour period; the optimal time sequence for these injections has not been established. A more conservative approach uses the dose schedule shown in Table 18-8. When the Kleihauer-Betke technique was compared to flow cytometry, the Kleihauer-Betke test was found to be useful and precise for hemorrhages of 25 mL or greater, but flow cytometric determinations appeared to be more accurate and precise.[102]

Enzyme-Linked Antiglobulin Test

An ELAT has been described that has excellent sensitivity and can be used as a screening test for FMH as well as a procedure to quantitate the occasional case of large FMH that occurs.[103]

Indications for FMH Screening

The American College of Obstetrics and Gynecology recommends that testing for large FMH should be performed only for high risk pregnancies. However, a recent study demonstrated that ACOG criteria would miss 50% of mothers at risk for large FMH.[104] For this reason, AABB *Standards* continues to mandate FMH screening for all postpartum RhIG candidates.[105]

Table 18-8. RhIG Dosage for Massive Fetomaternal Hemorrhage, Based on the Acid Elution Test[101]

% Fetal Cells	Fetomaternal Hemorrhage Volume (mL Whole Blood)		Vials of RhIG To Inject
	Average	Range*	
0.3–0.5	20	<50	2
0.6–0.8	35	15– 80	3
0.9–1.1	50	22–110	4
1.2–1.4	65	30–140	5
1.5–2.0	88	37–200	6
2.1–2.5	115	52–250	6

*The range provides for the poor accuracy and precision of the acid elution test. These recommendations are based upon 1 vial needed for each 15 mL rbcs or 30 mL whole blood.

References

1. Strauss RG. Transfusion therapy in neonates. Am J Dis Child. 1991;145:904-91.
2. DePalma L, Ness PM, Luban NLC. Red blood cell transfusion. In: Luban NLC, ed. Transfusion therapy in infants and children. Baltimore, MD: The Johns Hopkins University Press, 1991:1-30.
3. Batteby L, Garby L, Wadman B. Studies on erythro-kinetics in infancy. XII. Survival in adult recipients of cord blood cells labeled in vitro with di-isopropyl fluoro-phosphate (DF^{32}P). Acta Paediatr Scand 1968;57:305-10.
4. Oski FA, Naiman JL. Hematologic problems in the newborn. 3rd ed. Philadelphia: WB Saunders, 1982.
5. Delivoria-Papadopoulos M, Roncevic NP, Oski FA. Postnatal changes in oxygen transport of term, premature and sick infants: The role of red cell 2,3-diphospho-glycerate and adult hemoglobin. Pediatr Res 1971;5:235-45.
6. Smoller BR, Kruskall MS. Phlebotomy for diagnostic laboratory tests in adults: Pattern of use and effect on transfusion requirements. N Engl J Med 1986;314:1233-5.
7. Wallgren G, Hanson JS, Lind J. Quantitative studies of the human neonatal circulation. Acta Paediatr Scand 1967;179(suppl):43-54.
8. Oski FA. The erythrocyte and its disorders. In: Nathan OG, Oski FA, eds. Hematology of infancy and childhood. 3rd ed. Philadelphia: WB Saunders, 1987:16-43.
9. Luban NLC, Mikesell G, Sacher RA. Techniques for warming red blood cells packaged in different containers for neonatal use. Clin Pediatr. 1985;24:642-5.
10. Parinaud J, Blanc M, Grandjean H, et al. IgG subclasses and Gm allotypes of anti-D antibodies during pregnancy: Correlation with the gravity of the fetal disease. Am J Obstet Gynecol 1985;151:1111-5.
11. Pollock JM, Bowman JM. Placental transfer of Rh antibody (anti-D IgG) during pregnancy. Vox Sang 1982;43:327-34.
12. Floss AM, Strauss RG, Goeken N, Knox L. Multiple transfusions fail to provide antibodies against blood cell antigens in human infants. Transfusion 1986;26:419-22.
13. Parkman R, Mosier D, Umansky I, et al. Graft-versus-host disease after intrauterine and exchange transfusions for hemolytic disease of the newborn. N Engl J Med 1974;290:359-63.
14. Sanders MR, Graeber JE. Posttransfusion graft-versus-host disease in infancy. J Pediatr 1990;117:159-63.
15. Anderson KC, Weinstein HJ. Transfusion-associated graft-versus-host disease. N Engl J Med 1990;322:315-21.
16. Batton DG, Maisels MJ, Shulman G. Serum potassium changes following packed red cell transfusions in newborn infants. Transfusion 1983;23:163-4.
17. Delivoria-Papadopoulos M, Martens RJ, Anday EK, Kumar SP. Neonatal oxygen transport: The role of exchange transfusion. In: Sherwood WS, Cohen A, eds. Transfusion therapy: The fetus, infant, and child. New York: Masson, 1980:63-74.
18. Stagno S, Pass RF, Dworsky ME, et al. Congenital cytomegalovirus infection: The relative importance of primary and recurrent maternal infection. N Engl J Med 1982;306:945-9.
19. Skinnider L, Wrobel H, McSheffrey B. The nature of leukocyte contamination in platelet concentrates. Vox Sang 1985;49:309-14.
20. Tegtmeier GE. The use of cytomegalovirus-screened blood in neonates. Transfusion 1988;28:201-3.
21. Hersman J, Meyers JD, Thomas D, et al. The effect of granulocyte transfusion on the incidence of cytomegalovirus infection after allogeneic marrow transplantation. Ann Intern Med 1982;96:149-52.
22. Yeager AS, Grumet FC, Hafleigh EB, et al. Prevention of transfusion-acquired cytomegalovirus infections in newborn infants. J Pediatr 1981;98:281-7.
23. Land DJ, Ebert PA, Rodgers BM, et al. Reduction of postperfusion cytomegalovirus infections following the use of leukocyte depleted blood. Transfusion 1977;17:391-5.
24. Brady M, Anderson D, Milam J, Hawkins E, et al. Prevention of posttransfusion cytomegalovirus infection in neonates by the use of frozen-washed red blood cells. Clin Res 1982;30:895A.
25. Simon T, Johnson J, Koffler H, et al. Impact of previously frozen deglycerolized red blood cells on cytomegalovirus transmission to newborn infants (abstract). Blood 1983;62(Suppl):238a.
26. Luban NLC, Williams AE, MacDonald MG, et al. Low incidence of acquired cytomegalovirus infection in neonates transfused with washed red blood cells. Am J Dis Child 1987;141:406-19.
27. Gilbert GL, Hayes K, Hudson IL, James J. Prevention of transfusion-acquired cytomegalovirus infection in infants by blood filtered to remove leucocytes. Lancet 1989;1:1228-31.
28. Polesky HP. Diagnosis, prevention, and therapy in hemolytic disease of the newborn. In: Myhre BA, ed. Clinics in laboratory medicine. Philadelphia: WB Saunders, 1982:107-22.
29. Cohen F, Zuelzer WW. Mechanisms of isoimmunization. II. Transplacental passage and postnatal survival of fetal erythrocytes in

heterospecific pregnancies. Blood 1967;30: 796-804.

30. Ascari WO, Levine P, Pollack W. Incidence of maternal immunization by ABO compatible and incompatible pregnancies. Br Med J 1969; 1:399-401.

31. Woodrow JC, Donohue WTA. Rh-immunization by pregnancy: Results of a survey and their relevance to prophylactic therapy. Br Med J 1968;4:139-44.

32. Bowman JM. The prevention of Rh immunization. Transfus Med Rev 1988;2:129.

33. Judd WJ, Luban NLC, Ness PM, et al. Prenatal and perinatal immunohematology: Recommendations for serologic management of the fetus, newborn infant, and obstetric patient. Transfusion 1990;30:175-83.

34. Lacey PA, Caskey CR, Werner DJ, Moulds JJ. Fatal hemolytic disease of a newborn due to anti-D in an Rh+ D^u variant mother. Transfusion 1983;23:91-4.

35. Kanter MH. Derivation of new mathematic formulas for determining whether a D-positive father is heterozygous or homozygous for the D antigen. Am J Obstet Gynecol 1992;166:61-3.

36. Goldsmith KLG, Mourant AE, Banghan DR. The international standard for anti-Rh$_0$(D) incomplete blood typing serum. Bull WHO 1967; 36:435-45.

37. Gluck L. Fetal maturity and amniotic fluid surfactant determinations. In: Spellecy WN, ed. Management of the high risk pregnancy. Baltimore: University Park Press, 1976:189-207.

38. Wennberg RP, Goetzman BW. Neonatal intensive care manual. Chicago: Yearbook Publishers, 1985:6-7.

39. Bowman JM. Treatment options for the fetus with alloimmune hemolytic disease. Transfus Med Rev 1990;4:191-207.

40. Naiman JL, Punnett HH, Lischner HW, et al. Possible graft-versus-host reaction after intrauterine transfusion in Rh erythroblastosis fetalis. N Engl J Med 1969;281:697-701.

41. Leitman SF, Holland PV. Irradiation of blood products. Transfusion 1985;25:293-300.

42. McMican A, Luban NLC, Sacher RA. Practical aspects of blood irradiation. Lab Med 1987;18:299-303.

43. Grannum PA, Copel JA, Plaxe SC, et al. In utero exchange transfusion by direct intravascular injection in severe erythroblastosis fetalis. N Engl J Med 1986;314:1431-4.

44. Gravenhorst JB, Kanhaii HHH, Meerman RH, et al. Twenty-one years of intra-uterine intraperitoneal transfusions. Eur J Obstet Gynecol Reprod Biol 1989;33:71-7.

45. Poissonnier MH, Brossard Y, Demedeiros N, et al. Two hundred intrauterine exchange trans-

fusions in severe blood incompatibilities. Am J Obstet Gynecol 1989;161:709-13.

46. Konugres AA. Transfusion therapy for the neonate. In: Bell CA, ed. A seminar on perinatal blood banking. Washington, DC: American Association of Blood Banks, 1981:93-107.

47. White KJ, Wilson JK, Barnes A. Sedimented red cells. Transfusion 1980;20:476.

48. Noble RC, Kane MA, Reeves SA, Roeckel I. Posttransfusion hepatitis A in a neonatal intensive care unit. JAMA 1984;252:2711-5.

49. Strauss RG, Crawford GF, Elbert C, et al. Sterility and quality of blood dispensed in syringes for infants. Transfusion 1986;26:163-6.

50. Valeri CR, Valeri DA, Gray A, et al. Cryopreserved red blood cells for pediatric transfusion: Frozen storage of small aliquots in polyvinyl chloride (PVC) plastic bags. Transfusion 1981;21:517-36.

51. Luban NLC, Strauss RG, Hume HA. Commentary on the safety of red cells preserved in extended-storage media for neonatal transfusions. Transfusion 1991;31:229-35.

52. Hathaway WE. The bleeding newborn. Semin Hematol 1975;12:175-88.

53. Moroff G, Friedman A, Robkin-Kline L, et al. Reduction of the volume of stored platelet concentrates for use in neonatal patients. Transfusion 1984;24:144-52.

54. Strauss RG. Current status of granulocyte transfusions to treat neonatal sepsis. J Clin Apheresis 1989;5:25-9.

55. Baley JE, Stork EK, Warkentin PI, Shurin SB. Buffy coat transfusion in neutropenic neonates with presumed sepsis: A prospective randomized trial. Pediatrics 1987;80:712-20.

56. Wheeler JC, Chauvenet AR, Johnson CA, et al. Buffy coat transfusion in neonates with sepsis and neutrophil storage pool depletion. Pediatrics 1987;79:422-5.

57. Ludvigsen C, Swanson JL, Thompson TR, McCullough J. The failure of neonates to form red cell alloantibodies in response to multiple transfusions. Am J Clin Pathol 1987: 87:250-1.

58. Cohen AR, Schwartz E. Transfusion in the newborn period. In: Sherwood WS, Cohen A, eds. Transfusion therapy: The fetus, infant and child. New York: Masson, 1980:37-50.

59. Widmann FK, ed. Standards for blood banks and transfusion services, 15th ed. Bethesda, MD: American Association of Blood Banks, 1993.

60. Vichinsky EP, Earles A, Johnson RA, et al. Alloimmunization in sickle cell anemia and transfusion of racially unmatched blood. N Engl J Med 1990;322:1617-21.

61. Wilcox GJ, Barnes A, Modanlou H. Does transfusion using a syringe infusion pump and small-gauge needle cause hemolysis? Transfusion 1981;21:750-1.

62. Solis RT, Goldfinger D, Gibbs MB, Zeller JA. Physical characteristics of microaggregates in stored blood. Transfusion 1974;14:538-50.

63. Schmidt WF, Kim HC, Tomassini N, Schwartz E. RBC destruction caused by a micropore blood filter. JAMA 1982;248:1629-32.

64. Longhurst DM, Gooch W, Castillo RA. In vitro evaluation of a pediatric microaggregate blood filter. Transfusion 1983;23:170-2.

65. Sacher RA, Luban NLC, Strauss RG. Current practice and guidelines for the transfusion of cellular blood components in the newborn. Transfus Med Rev 1989;3:39-54.

66. Stockman JA III, Clark DA, Levin EA. Weight gain, a response to transfusion in preterm infants. Pediatr Res 1980;14:612.

67. Bowman JM. Rh erythroblastosis fetalis. Semin Hematol 1975;12:189-207.

68. Tan K. Comparison of the effectiveness of phototherapy and exchange transfusion in the management of non-hemolytic hyperbilirubinemia. J Pediatr 1975;87:605.

69. Lee K, Gartner LM, Eidelman AI, Ezhuthachan S. Unconjugated hyperbilirubinemia in very low birth weight infants. Clin Perinatol 1977;4:305-20.

70. Maisels MJ. Jaundice in the newborn. Pediatr Rev 1982;3:305-19.

71. Feusner JH, Slichter SJ, Harker LA. Acquired hemostatic defects in the ill newborn. Br J Haematol 1983;53:73-84.

72. Tollner U, Pohlandt F, Heinze F, Henrichs I. Treatment of septicemia in the newborn infant: Choice of initial antimicrobial drugs and role of exchange transfusion. Acta Paediatr Scand 1977;66:605-10.

73. Shigeoka AO, Hall RT, Hill HR. Blood transfusion in group B streptococcal sepsis. Lancet 1978;1:636-8.

74. Erslev AJ. Clinical manifestations and classification of erythrocyte disorders. In: Williams WJ, Beutler E, Erslev AJ, Lichtman ML, eds. Hematology. New York: McGraw-Hill, 1990:423-9.

75. Ramamurthy RS, Brans YW. Neonatal polycythemia: criteria for diagnosis and treatment. Pediatrics 1981;68:168-74.

76. Kreuger A. Adenine metabolism during and after exchange transfusions in newborn infants with CPD-adenine blood. Transfusion 1976;16:249-52.

77. Murphy RJC, Malhorta C, Sweet AY. Death following an exchange transfusion with hemoglobin SC blood. J Pediatr 1980;96:110-20.

78. Gershanik JJ, Levkoff AH, Duncan R. Serum ionized calcium values in relation to exchange transfusion. J Pediatr 1973;82:589-93.

79. Chan G, Schoff D. Variance in albumin loading in exchange transfusions. J Pediatr 1976;88:609-13.

80. Andrew M, Castle V, Saigel S, et al. Clinical impact of neonatal thrombocytopenia. J Pediatr 1987;110:457-64.

81. Deaver JE, Leppert PC, Zaroulis CG. Neonatal alloimmune thrombocytopenic purpura. Am J Perinatol 1986;3:127-31.

82. Bussell JB, McFarland JG, Berkowitz RL. Antenatal management of fetal alloimmune and autoimmune thrombocytopenia. Transfus Med Rev 1990;4:149-62.

83. Blanchette VS, Chen L, Salomon de Friedberg Z, et al. Alloimmunization to the Pl^{A1} platelet antigen: Results of a prospective study. Br J Haematol 1990;74:209-15.

84. Cairo MS. The use of granulocyte transfusions in neonatal sepsis. Transfus Med Rev 1990;4:14-22.

85. Christensen RD, Rothstein G, Anstall HB, Bybee B. Granulocyte transfusions in neonates with bacterial infection, neutropenia, and depletion of mature marrow neutrophils. Pediatrics 1982;70:1-6.

86. Strauss RG. Current issues in neonatal transfusions. Vox Sang 1986;51:1-9.

87. Centers for Disease Control. Safety of therapeutic products used for hemophilia patients. MMWR 1988;37:441-50.

88. Centers for Disease Control. Lack of transmission of human immunodeficiency virus through Rh₀(D) immune globulin (human). MMWR 1987;36:728-30.

89. Wood C, Williams A, McNamara JG. Antibody against the human immunodeficiency virus in commercial intravenous gammaglobulin preparations. Ann Intern Med 1986;105:536-8.

90. Bowman JM, Chown B, Lewis M, Pollock JM. Rh isoimmunization during pregnancy: Antenatal prophylaxis. Can Med Assn J 1978;118:623-7.

91. Jennings ER, Dibbern HH, Hodell FH, et al. Prevention of Rh hemolytic disease of the newborn. Calif Med 1969;10:130-3.

92. American College of Obstetrics and Gynecology. Prevention of D isoimmunization. ACOG Technical Bulletin. Number 147. Washington DC: ACOG, 1990.

93. Konugres A, Polesky H, Walker R. Rh Immune globulin and the Rh positive, D^u variant mother. Transfusion 1982;22:76-7.

94. Frigoletto FD Jr. Risk perspectives of Rh sensitization. In: Frigoletto FD Jr, Jewett JF, Konugres AA, eds. Rh hemolytic disease: New strategy for eradication. Boston: GK Hall, 1982:103-10.

95. Contreras M, Mollison PL. Rh immunization facilitated by passively-administered anti-Rh? Br J Haematol 1983;53:153-9.

96. Lele AS, Carmody PJ, Hurd ME, O'Leary JA. Fetomaternal bleeding following diagnostic amniocentesis. Obstet Gynecol 1982;60:60-4.

97. Zipursky A, Israels LG. The pathogenesis and prevention of Rh immunization. Can Med Assn J 1967;97:1245-57.

98. Polesky HF, Sebring ES. Evaluation of methods for detection and quantitation of fetal cells and their effect on Rh IgG usage. Am J Clin Pathol 1981;76:525-9.

99. Sebring ES, Polesky HF. Detection of fetal maternal hemorrhage in Rh immune globulin candidates. Transfusion 1982;22:468-71.

100. Taswell HF, Reisner RK. Prevention of Rh_0 hemolytic disease of the newborn: The rosette method—a rapid, sensitive screening test. Mayo Clin Proc 1983;58:342-3.

101. Walker RH. Relevancy in the selection of serologic tests for the obstetric patient. In: Garratty G, ed. Hemolytic disease of the newborn. Arlington, VA: American Association of Blood Banks, 1984:173-203.

102. Corsetti JP, Cox MT, Leary JF, et al. Comparison of quantitative acid-elution technique and flow cytometry for detecting fetomaternal hemorrhage. Ann Clin Lab Sci 1987;17:197-206.

103. Riley JZ, Ness PM, Taddie SJ, et al. The detection and quantitation of fetal-maternal hemorrhage using an enzyme-linked antiglobulin test (ELAT). Transfusion 1982; 22:472-4.

104. Ness PM, Baldwin ML, Niebyl JR. Clinical high risk designation does not predict excess fetal maternal hemorrhage. Am J Obstet Gynecol 1987;156:154-8.

105. Sebring ES, Polesky HF. Fetomaternal hemorrhage: Incidence, risk factors, time of occurrence, and clinical effects. Transfusion 1990;30:344-57.

19

Adverse Effects of Blood Transfusion

Transfusion of blood and components is ordinarily a safe and effective way to correct hematologic deficits, but untoward results may occur. These adverse effects are commonly called "transfusion reactions," but the deleterious results include a range of events and problems broader than this limited term implies (Table 19-1). Some adverse effects can be prevented; others cannot. Health-care providers should know the risks of blood transfusion and evaluate them against potential therapeutic benefits.

Evaluation of Suspected Hemolytic Transfusion Reactions

The time between suspicion of a hemolytic transfusion reaction (HTR) and the investigation and initiation of appropriate therapy should be as short as possible. Responsibility for recognizing a reaction rests with the transfusionist, who may be a nurse, physician or other member of the clinical team. The presenting events of fever and chills may be the same for life-threatening HTRs and less serious febrile reactions. Any adverse symptom or physical sign occurring during transfusion of blood or its components should be initially considered as a potentially life-threatening reaction;

the following actions must be taken by the clinical personnel:

1. Stop the transfusion immediately to limit the amount of blood infused. Notify a responsible physician.
2. Keep the intravenous line open with infusion of normal saline (0.9% sodium chloride).
3. At the patient's bedside, check all labels, forms and patient identification to determine if the transfused component was intended for the recipient.
4. Report the suspected reaction to blood bank personnel immediately.
5. Send required blood samples, carefully drawn to avoid mechanical hemolysis, to the blood bank as soon as possible, together with the discontinued bag of blood, the administration set without the needle, attached intravenous solutions and all related forms and labels. Smaller volumes of posttransfusion samples are appropriate for pediatric patients.
6. Send other blood or urine samples for evaluation of acute hemolysis as directed by the blood bank director or the patient's physician.

If clinical events suggest the possibility of an HTR, the following steps must be taken.

1. Check identification of patient samples and of the donor blood component. If there is a discrepancy, imme-

Table 19-1. Immediate and Delayed Adverse Effects of Transfusion

Immediate Effects	
Immunologic Effects	**Usual Etiology**
Hemolysis with symptoms	Red cell incompatibility
Febrile nonhemolytic reaction	Donor's granulocytes
Anaphylaxis	Antibody to IgA
Urticaria	Antibody to plasma proteins
Noncardiac pulmonary edema	Antibody to leukocytes or complement activation
Nonimmunologic Effects	
Marked fever with shock	Bacterial contamination
Congestive heart failure	Volume overload
Hemolysis with symptoms	Physical destruction of blood, eg, freezing or overheating
	Mixing nonisotonic solutions with red blood cells
Delayed Effects	
Immunologic Effects	**Usual Etiology**
Hemolysis	Anamnestic antibody to red cell antigens
Graft-vs-host disease	Engraftment of transfused functional lymphocytes
Posttransfusion purpura	Development of antiplatelet antibody (usually anti-HPA-1a)
Alloimmunization to RBC or WBC antigens, platelets or plasma proteins	Exposure to antigens of donor origin
Nonimmunologic Effects	
Iron overload	Multiple transfusions (100 +)
Hepatitis	HCV (and undetermined incidence of non-A, non-B, non-C), occasionally B (rarely A)
Acquired immune deficiency syndrome	HIV-1
Protozoal infection	Malaria parasites, Babesia, trypanosomes

diately notify the patient's physician or other responsible health-care professional and search appropriate records to determine whether other patient samples or donor units have been misidentified or incorrectly issued. After eliminating the possibility of risk to other patients, and after appropriate diagnostic procedures, trace each step of the transfusion process to find the error.

2. Compare the color of serum or plasma in the patient's pretransfusion specimen to the posttransfusion specimen. Pink or red discoloration specimen. Pink or red discoloration in the posttransfusion specimen but not in the pretransfusion specimen may indicate free hemoglobin from destruction of donor red cells. Intravascular hemolysis of as little as 5 mL of red cells can produce visible hemoglobinemia. Mechanical hemolysis occurring during sample collection or other medical interventions can also produce pink or red-tinged serum or plasma. If faulty sampling is suspected, a second specimen should be requested. A slightly hemolyzed sample is acceptable for the direct antiglobulin test (DAT). Yellow

or brown discoloration from hemoglobin breakdown products such as bilirubin may indicate recent hemolysis in samples drawn 5-7 hours after transfusion.

3. Perform a DAT on the posttransfusion specimen. If incompatible transfused cells had not been immediately destroyed, the DAT from the posttransfusion specimen will be positive, with a mixed-field appearance. Since circulating antibody- or complement-coated cells may be rapidly destroyed, the DAT may be negative if the specimen was drawn several hours after the suspected reaction. Nonimmune hemolysis (eg, from thermal damage or mechanical trauma, as from extracorporeal systems) can produce hemoglobinemia without a positive DAT. Other causes of nonimmune hemolysis should be considered whenever hemoglobinemia occurs without an obvious immune etiology (see below).

Interpretation of Laboratory Observations

The absence of hemoglobinemia and a negative DAT in an immediate posttransfusion specimen strongly suggest that an acute immune hemolytic reaction has not occurred. Positive results in any of these procedures require additional investigation. If any findings are positive or doubtful, some or all of the tests described below should be performed and the results and interpretations recorded. If the patient's clinical condition suggests a hemolytic reaction, further investigation is warranted despite negative results from preliminary testing.

Investigation for Possible Alloantibodies

To determine if an antibody has caused the reaction and to identify the antibody:

1. Repeat ABO and Rh tests on the patient's pretransfusion sample and on blood from the unit or an attached segment. Test the posttransfusion sample for ABO and Rh; a mixed-field pattern with microscopic reading suggests the presence of incompatible donor cells.

   If ABO and Rh typing on the patient's two samples do not agree, there has been an error in patient or sample identification, or in the testing. If so, another patient's blood may have been drawn and incorrectly labeled, making it important to check records of all specimens received at approximately the same time.

   If the donor blood is not of the ABO group on the bag label, there has been an error in labeling, processing and, almost certainly, an error in the crossmatch as well.

2. Repeat the crossmatch, including an antiglobulin phase, testing both the pretransfusion and posttransfusion serum sample against a sample of red blood cells from the bag or from a segment still attached to the unit.

   If results are incompatible with both specimens, an error was almost surely made during pretransfusion testing. The donor specimen used for the crossmatch may have been taken from a different unit or the patient's antibody screen was incorrectly read as negative. Whenever possible the crossmatch should be repeated with cells from the segment that was actually used in the initial crossmatch. Both pretransfusion and posttransfusion samples should be used. If the crossmatch is incompatible with the posttransfusion specimen but compatible with the pretransfusion specimen, a delayed HTR is possible. This is most likely if the reaction has occurred, or if the posttransfusion sample was drawn, several days after transfusion. If only a short time has elapsed since transfusion, check the patient's previous transfusion history. It is possible that an antibody has developed to red cells transfused in the preceding few days. Less likely, antibody might have been present in a transfused blood component.

If both crossmatches are compatible and there is strong reason to believe that an acute immune hemolytic reaction has occurred, further testing is necessary. Check the records and performance of the original crossmatch. For other investigations, see section on special testing on p 475.

3. Repeat the antibody detection tests on the pretransfusion and posttransfusion samples and on the donor blood. If any tests are positive, identify the antibody specificity (see Chapter 15). Test donor units for the corresponding antigen. If the patient's pretransfusion sample or the donor blood has an antibody not previously reported, check records to see how the discrepancy occurred. If the donor blood has a previously undetected antibody, perform a minor crossmatch using the patient's pretransfusion sample or type the patient's cells for the suspected antigen. If the posttransfusion specimen has an antibody not present before transfusion, suspect an anamnestic antibody reaction or passive transfusion of antibody in a recently transfused component.

If an antibody is identified, phenotype the patient's red cells using the pretransfusion sample to verify that the patient lacks the corresponding antigen. Check transfusion records to determine whether there may be transfused cells in the pretransfusion specimen. Such cells would give a mixed-field or weak reaction with typing reagents, and could confuse the interpretation of results. Such cells could also be the stimulus for an anamnestic antibody response.

Investigation for Nonimmune Hemolysis

1. Consider bacterial contamination of the donor unit if 1) the cells or plasma have brownish or purple discoloration, 2) there are clots or abnormal masses in the liquid blood, 3) the plasma is opaque or muddy or 4) there is gas or a peculiar odor.
   a. Before manipulating the bag excessively, take specimens from the bag for cultures at various temperatures as bacterial contaminants may grow preferentially at different temperatures.
   b. Examine a blood smear stained with Gram's stain or acridine orange, which stains bacterial DNA.[1]

2. Examine supernatant plasma from the donor blood container for free hemoglobin. If present, the unit may have been damaged by improper temperatures in shipping or storage, mishandling at the time of administration, by the injection of drugs or hypotonic solutions, or by bacterial contamination.

3. Examine the blood remaining in the administration tubing for free hemoglobin. If the administration set had previously been used for hypotonic solutions or dextrose solutions, there could be hemolysis in the tubing but not in the bag.

Excessive heat from a faulty in-line blood warmer can also damage transfused blood without causing abnormalities in the blood container. The possibility should be pursued if the patient has posttransfusion hemoglobinemia with no other apparent cause.

4. Consider the possibility that either the patient or donor has an intrinsic red cell defect. Patients with glucose-6-phosphate dehydrogenase deficiency or with sickle cell anemia may experience intravascular hemolysis because of medical problems not related to the transfusion. Paroxysmal nocturnal hemoglobinuria is a rare disease that may produce severe hemoglobinemia and hemoglobinuria.

5. Consider the possibility of mechanical hemolysis. Mechanical hemolysis may be caused by roller pumps such as those used in cardiac bypass surgery, pressure infusion pumps, pressure cuffs or small bore needles (see Chapter 17).

6. Consider osmotic hemolysis due to inadequate deglycerolization of frozen-thawed RBCs or inadvertent entry into the circulation of hypotonic fluids, such as distilled water used for postprostatectomy bladder irrigation.

7. Exclude myoglobinemia by the use of ammonium sulfate precipitation or electrophoretic studies.[2]

Clinical Evaluation

To follow the patient's clinical condition when hemolysis is proven or strongly suspected:

1. Examine posttransfusion urine and plasma specimens for the presence of free hemoglobin. Intact red cells in the urine (hematuria) are a sign of hemorrhage in the urinary tract; HTRs do not cause red cells to enter the urine. Following hemolysis, hemoglobin from damaged cells can enter the urine, but the cells do not. The test for hemoglobin should be done on the supernatant of a centrifuged specimen of freshly collected urine. If the urine does contain red cells that hemolyze in vitro, however, the results will be misleading.

If there has been a delay of several days before diagnosing hemolysis or before obtaining a urine sample, it may be appropriate to test for hemosiderin in the urine.

2. Test posttransfusion serum samples for bilirubin, carefully recording the timing of sample collection. The rate and magnitude of bilirubin rise are variable. Rising bilirubin may be detectable as early as 1 hour posttransfusion. Peak levels occur at 5-7 hours and disappear within 24 hours if liver function is normal.

Special Tests To Diagnose Red Cell Incompatibility

If routine tests are uninformative and if immune hemolysis continues to be suspected:

1. Perform antibody detection tests and compatibility tests with additional techniques. (See Chapter 14.) Previously undetected antibody in the pretransfusion specimen may become apparent by using low ionic strength salt solution, Polybrene® or enzyme techniques, or by increasing the ratio of serum to cells.

2. Perform direct antiglobulin and antibody detection tests on posttransfusion specimens at daily or other frequent intervals. The immediate posttransfusion specimen may have a negative DAT if all the antibody-coated cells had been removed from the circulation. Similarly, the serum may contain no free antibody because all of it had reacted with the transfused cells. Under these circumstances antibody concentration usually rises rapidly, so detection and identification become possible within a few days.

3. Measure hematocrit or hemoglobin values at frequent intervals post-transfusion to document whether the transfused cells have or have not produced the expected therapeutic rise, or to demonstrate that a decrease in hematocrit has occurred after an initial increase.

   A unit of RBCs is expected to increase the hemoglobin level by approximately 10 g/L (1g/dL) (see p 391) and the hematocrit by about 0.03-0.04 (3-4%) when administered to a hemodynamically stable 70-kg recipient.

4. Type the cells of the recipient and of the implicated donor unit to find antigens present in the donor and absent in the recipient, and examine the patient's posttransfusion blood for the presence of cells bearing these antigens. The recipient's specimen must be a pretransfusion sample that contains only the patient's cells. This may be difficult if the patient has received transfusions within the previous several weeks. For a technique to obtain autologous cells (reticulocytes) from a patient who has been transfused, see Method 2.17.

   If an antigen can be found that is present on the donor cells and absent from the patient's cells, its presence or absence in posttransfusion samples indicates whether the transfused cells have survived and remain in the circulation. Special techniques can be used to estimate the quantity of remaining donor cells.

5. In patients with sickle cell anemia, hemoglobin electrophoresis can be used to determine if transfused cells containing hemoglobin A have survived.

6. In rare cases, transfusion reactions have occurred in the absence of detectable alloantibody. In these situations, red cell survival studies may be useful to demonstrate rapid destruction of transfused cells and/or to identify the incompatible antigen.[3]

7. Haptoglobin measurements are rarely useful except to evaluate minimal degrees of hemolysis. It is important to compare prereaction and postreaction values to evaluate haptoglobin kinetics.[4]

Acute Adverse Effects of Transfusion

Acute Hemolytic Transfusion Reactions

An acute HTR is triggered by an antigen-antibody reaction that activates the complement and coagulation systems and prompts endocrine responses. Catastrophic clinical events that may occur include shock, disseminated intravascular coagulation (DIC) and acute renal failure. Life-threatening HTRs are almost always due to ABO incompatibility attributable to an identification error that results in the recipient receiving the wrong blood. Incompatibility in other blood groups may also cause acute hemolysis in a recipient with alloantibodies stimulated by previous transfusions or pregnancies. These reactions, however, are rarely as severe as those involving ABO incompatibility.

Diagnosis

Initial signs and symptoms that may occur with an acute HTR are listed in Table 19-2. The most common initial sign is fever, frequently accompanied by symptomatic chills.[5] Reactions may occur after as little as 10-15 mL of incompatible blood has been infused. The onset of symptoms may be misleadingly mild, such as vague uneasiness or an aching back. The first sign may be red urine, which may be accompanied by

Table 19-2. Signs and Symptoms That May Accompany Hemolytic Transfusion Reactions

Fever	Hemoglobinuria
Chills	Shock
Chest pain	Generalized bleeding
Hypotension	Oliguria or anuria
Nausea	Back pain
Flushing	Pain at infusion site
Dyspnea	

back pain or may be completely painless. The severity of initial symptoms is often related to the amount of blood transfused and may presage the severity of the ensuing clinical problems. In anesthetized recipients the only manifestations of an acute HTR may be diffuse bleeding at the surgical site (due to DIC), hypotension or hemoglobinuria. Whenever an HTR is suspected, the transfusion must be stopped immediately. However, the intravenous line should be maintained for therapeutic interventions that may be required.

The posttransfusion blood samples should be used for diagnostic testing as a baseline against which evolving clinical findings can be compared. Laboratory tests that may be useful in evaluating acute hemolysis have been outlined above and are listed in Table 19-3.

Pathophysiology of Acute Hemolytic Transfusion Reactions

Interaction of antibody with antigen initiates the pathophysiologic events of immunologically mediated acute HTRs, through activation of the following three interrelated mechanisms.[6]

The Neuroendocrine Response. Antigen-antibody complexes activate Hageman factor (Factor XIIa), which, in turn, acts on the kinin system to produce bradykinin. Bradykinin increases capillary permeability and dilates arterioles. Be-

cause of resulting hypotension, and/or as a direct effect of immune complexes, the sympathetic nervous system is stimulated and norepinephrine and other catecholamine levels rise. These catecholamines produce vasoconstriction in organs with a vascular bed in which adrenergic receptors are highly concentrated—renal, splanchnic, pulmonary and cutaneous capillaries. Coronary and cerebral vessels have few α-adrenergic receptors and these vascular beds partic-

Table 19-3. Tests for Red Cell Destruction in Hemolytic Transfusion Reactions

Immediate

Visual or photometric comparison of free hemoglobin (pink) or bilirubin (yellow-brown) in serum of prereaction and postreaction specimens

Direct antiglobulin test on postreaction sample

As Indicated

Repeat ABO and Rh determinations on pre- and postreaction samples and unit of blood

Crossmatch prereaction and postreaction samples with red blood cells from unit or stored, sealed segment

Measure unconjugated bilirubin, preferably on specimen drawn 5 to 7 hours after transfusion

Look for free hemoglobin in urine (rule out intact red blood cells)

Look for hemosiderin in urine (delayed)

Perform routine and/or specially sensitive tests for unexpected antibody in donor and patient

Evaluate response to transfusion with hemoglobin and hematocrit results [in a 70-kg recipient, an increment of 10 g/L (1 g/dL) hemoglobin or 0.03 (3%) hematocrit per unit of blood or packed cells transfused]

Make Gram's stain of blood smear from unit

Culture unit at 4 C, 22 C and 35-37 C

Look for free hemoglobin in plasma or donor unit

Measure serum haptoglobin on both prereaction and postreaction samples

ipate minimally in the reaction. In addition, antigen-antibody complexes activate the complement system, resulting in stimulation of mast cells, which release histamine and serotonin. Serotonin and histamine are also released from platelets, stimulated by antigen-antibody complexes or through initiation of clotting (DIC). These vasoactive amines mediate many of the clinical signs and symptoms of the reaction.

The Complement System. Antigen-antibody complexes fixed to red cell membrane can activate complement. When complement is activated and the enzymatic cascade proceeds to completion, intravascular hemolysis results. If complement activation does not proceed to completion, red cells coated with C3b are removed by interaction with phagocytes that have receptors for C3b. In some instances C3b inactivator converts C3b to C3dg. Cells coated with C3dg survive normally, since macrophages do not have C3dg receptors. In an ABO mismatch, complement activation usually proceeds to completion with activation of C9. With the C5-C9 membrane attack complex bound to the red cell, osmotic red cell lysis occurs within the vascular system, releasing both free hemoglobin and red cell stroma into the plasma. Free hemoglobin was formerly thought to play a major role in renal ischemia, but current thought attributes renal vasoconstriction, acute tubular necrosis and renal failure largely to the presence of antibody-coated cell stroma. With most other (non-ABO) blood group antibodies, complement activation is, at most, incomplete. For a more complete discussion of the actions of complement, see Chapter 7.

The Coagulation System. The intrinsic clotting cascade may be activated by antigen-antibody complexes through Hageman factor activation or directly by the presence of incompatible red cell stroma. DIC, thus initiated, may cause: 1) formation of thrombi within the microvasculature; 2) consumption of fibrinogen, platelets and Factors V and VIII; 3) activation of the fibrinolytic system with generation of plasmin; 4) generation of fibrin degradation products; and, possibly, 5) uncontrolled bleeding.[7]

The cumulative effect of systemic hypotension, renal vasoconstriction and formation of intravascular thrombi compromises the blood supply to the kidney. This renal ischemia may be transient or may progress to acute tubular necrosis.

Therapy

Vigorous treatment of hypotension and promotion of adequate renal blood flow are the cornerstones of therapy for HTRs. If shock can be prevented or adequately treated, renal failure can usually be avoided. Adequacy of renal perfusion can be monitored by measuring urine output. Fluid therapy should be directed at maintaining urine flow rates above 100 mL/hour in adults for at least 18-24 hours. Underlying cardiac and/or renal disease may complicate therapy. To improve blood flow to the kidneys and increase urine output, diuretic agents can also be administered. Intravenous furosemide improves renal blood flow and produces diuresis. Mannitol is an osmotic diuretic that increases blood volume and thereby may also increase renal blood flow.

Vasopressor agents that decrease renal blood flow are contraindicated, but dopamine, which in low doses dilates the renal vasculature while increasing cardiac output, may be useful in treating the hypotension that occurs in the acute phase of HTRs.[8]

DIC with resultant bleeding is a predominant clinical finding in some HTRs and may be the initial presentation in anesthetized patients. It is largely due to hypotension and shock. Heparin treatment is controversial because heparin, an anticoagulant that can cause bleeding, may be hazardous in patients who have recently undergone surgical procedures. In the majority of cases, treatment of the primary disease process causing DIC is the therapy of choice and heparin is not indicated. Since DIC from an HTR is rare, consultation with a hematologist is recommended before administering heparin.

In summary, an acute HTR is a rare event that requires vigorous therapy to prevent serious morbidity or mortality. Since the medical management may become complicated and include aggressive interventions such as hemodialysis, a physician experienced in intensive care medicine should be involved in the treatment of patients with renal failure or shock.

Prevention

Prevention of all HTRs is impossible because hemolysis may occur even when the crossmatch is compatible.[5] Errors in labeling samples or donor units, or in identifying recipients, are the most common causes of severe, acute HTRs.[9] Human errors are difficult to prevent, but opportunities for error can be minimized through careful delineation of every step in the transfusion procedure in a readily available procedures manual, and careful adherence to detail by every member of the transfusion service and clinical team, from phlebotomist to medical technologist to transfusionist.

Starting a transfusion is a critical step because the transfusionist has the last opportunity to prevent misidentification and the first opportunity to detect a transfusion reaction.

Febrile Nonhemolytic Reactions

A febrile nonhemolytic (FNH) reaction is usually defined by a temperature increase of 1 C or more occurring in association with transfusion and without any other explanation. Some FNH reactions are caused by antibodies in recipient's plasma reacting against antigens present on the cell membranes of transfused lymphocytes, granulocytes or platelets.[10] Since these antibodies can be difficult to demonstrate in vitro, it is unrewarding to pursue a search for leukocyte antibodies. Transfusion of leukocyte-reduced components may minimize the occurrence of fevers.[11] (See Chapter 17.) The temperature rise may be mild to severe and may begin any time, from early in the transfusion to the time when most of the unit has been transfused or even an hour or two after the transfusion has finished. The fever usually responds to antipyretics. FNH reactions tend to occur in recipients who have been repeatedly transfused or who have had multiple pregnancies.

Fever may be the initial manifestation of several types of transfusion reactions, some of which are potentially fatal. Although true FNH reactions are seldom dangerous, it is important to establish the cause of fever occurring during transfusion. For example, fever may be the first sign of an acute HTR, or of a response to transfusion of a unit of blood contaminated with bacteria. FNH reactions are often more uncomfortable and frightening than life-threatening; signs and symptoms are usually self-limiting.

True rigors may be a sign of bacteremia, especially when associated with cardiovascular collapse or fever more than 40 C. The diagnosis of a FNH reaction is one of exclusion; other causes of fever must first be ruled out. These usually benign reactions are common and usually can be prevented or ameliorated by giving antipyretics or leukocyte-reduced blood components. Experience has shown that the patient who experiences a FNH reaction for the first time does not always have a similar reaction to the next blood transfusion.[12] Thus, it seems reasonable to recommend leukocyte-reduced preparations only after a patient has had two or more FNH reactions.[13] Antipyretics such as aspirin or acetaminophen can be given before the transfusion to patients with a history of previous FNH reactions. Aspirin, however, alters platelet function and should not be given to thrombocytopenic patients or those with qualitative platelet disorders (thrombocytopathy).

Bacterial Contamination

Bacteria may enter the blood during phlebotomy or contaminate the port of the bag during preparation of the component for infusion.[14] Bacteria are more likely to multiply in components stored at room temperature but growth and release of endotoxin may also occur in refrigerated components. The relatively long storage time permissible with platelet concentrates in containers that have enhanced gas permeability has been associated with an increased number of reports of bacterial contamination of platelets.[15] With sterile disposable equipment, bacterial contamination of refrigerated blood and components is rare, especially when there is strict adherence to appropriate protocols during donor phlebotomy, scrupulous attention to sterile techniques during component preparation and storage, and careful screening of donors to exclude transient bacteremia.

Although a rare occurrence, bacteria in blood, platelet concentrates or other components can cause a devastating septic transfusion reaction. Such reactions are usually due to endotoxin produced by psychrophilic (cold-growing), gram-negative bacteria, which include *Pseudomonas* species, *Citrobacter freundii*, *Escherichia coli* and *Yersinia entero-*colitica. *Yersinia enterocolitica* contamination has occurred when blood is collected from healthy donors with asymptomatic gastrointestinal disease.[16] *Bartonella* and *Brucella* species have also been the causes of septic transfusion reactions. Severe reactions are characterized by high fever, shock, hemoglobinuria, DIC and renal failure. Clinically, this type of shock is the "warm" type with flushing and dryness of skin. Abdominal cramps, diarrhea, vomiting and generalized muscle pain also may occur.

If bacterial contamination is suspected, the transfusion should be stopped immediately and the unit examined for the presence of bacterial growth. A purple color, clots in the bag or hemolysis suggest contamination, but the appearance of the blood in the bag is often unremarkable. A Gram's stain of the component revealing bacteria is confirmatory, but the absence of visible organisms does not exclude this possibility. The patient's blood, the suspect component, and all intravenous solutions used should be cultured for aerobic and anaerobic organisms at various temperatures.

Bacterial contamination is rare but such reactions may be fatal. Treatment includes immediate intravenous administration of antibiotics combined with therapy for shock, including steroids or vasopressor drugs such as dopamine. Prevention depends upon careful preparation of the phlebotomy site when blood is drawn, maintenance of sterility during component preparation, attention to prescribed storage conditions and inspection of blood components prior to issue.

Anaphylactic Reactions

Features that distinguish anaphylactic reactions from other immediate reactions are: 1) occurrence after infusion of only a few milliliters of blood or plasma and 2) absence of fever. The onset may be characterized by coughing, bronchospasm, respiratory distress, vascular instability, nausea, abdominal cramps, vomiting, diarrhea, shock and loss of consciousness.

Some of these reactions occur in IgA-deficient patients who have developed anti-IgA antibodies after immunization by previous transfusion or pregnancy,[12,17] although the immunizing event cannot always be identified. Although IgA deficiency occurs in about 1 out of 700 persons, anaphylactic reactions due to anti-IgA are very rare since the reaction depends on the presence of antibody. IgA-deficient individuals occasionally may have antibodies against the IgA alpha heavy chain, called class-specific antibodies, or type-specific antibodies directed against heavy chain subclass specificities. Individuals with normal IgA levels can have type-specific antibodies but do not make class-specific antibody.

Most authorities recommend that IgA-deficient blood components be given only if anti-IgA has been detected and prior anaphylactic reactions have occurred. Indeed, unless there has been large-scale population screening or there is a family history of IgA deficiency, individuals with IgA deficiency and anti-IgA will be detected only if they have an anaphylactic transfusion reaction and the investigation reveals anti-IgA.

ously. Steroid therapy may also be useful. Under no circumstances should the transfusion be restarted. Treatment is initiated on the basis of clinical impression of anaphylaxis; diagnosis is made retrospectively. Demonstration of anti-IgA remains primarily a research procedure, not readily available in most laboratories, but suggestive evidence can be obtained by documenting the absence of serum IgA by immunodiffusion or immunoelectrophoresis.

IgA-deficient patients with anti-IgA and a prior reaction should be transfused with blood components that lack IgA.[17] Files of IgA-negative donors are maintained by the AABB Rare Donor File, the American Red Cross National Reference Laboratory in Rockville, MD, and the Canadian Red Cross in Toronto, Ontario. The immediate need for red cells only may be met by using deglycerolized red cells or extensively washed red blood cells.[18] For components that contain plasma, IgA-deficient donors will be needed. It may be possible to collect and store frozen autologous red cells or plasma from patients known to have experienced anaphylactic reactions.

There are other causes of anaphylactic reactions such as antibodies to soluble plasma antigens or to drugs such as penicillin contained in transfused blood components.[19] Immediate treatment is the same as for reactions due to anti-IgA; prevention requires identifying the antibody and avoiding exposure to the antigen.

Treatment and Prevention

Immediate treatment of any anaphylactic transfusion reaction in an adult should include measures to: 1) stop the transfusion; 2) keep the IV line open with normal saline and treat hypotension; and 3) give epinephrine subcutane-

Cutaneous Hypersensitivity Reactions

Urticarial reactions are commonly encountered, second in frequency only to febrile nonhemolytic reactions. The typical urticarial reaction is characterized by local erythema, hives and itching, usually without fever or other adverse findings. If localized urticaria is the only manifestation, it is usually not necessary to discontinue transfusion. Indeed, the risk of transfusion-transmitted viral infection from a replacement unit of blood may pose a greater threat to the patient than does continuation of the original unit once the urticaria has resolved following treatment with an antihistamine. The infusion can be interrupted while an antihistamine such as diphenhydramine is administered orally or parenterally. After relief of symptoms, the transfusion is continued slowly. Recipients who have frequent urticarial reactions may be pretreated with an antihistamine.

The etiology of these limited cutaneous reactions is unknown, but allergy to some soluble substance in donor plasma is suspected. Transfusion of washed or deglycerolized red cells prevents urticarial reactions but is rarely necessary unless the patient has repeated and/or severe reactions. If a patient develops extensive urticaria or a confluent total body rash during transfusion, it would be prudent to discontinue the transfusion and not restart the same unit even after symptoms have responded to treatment.

Circulatory Overload

Rapid increases in blood volume are poorly tolerated by patients with compromised cardiac or pulmonary status and/or chronic anemia with expanded plasma volume. Even transfusion of small amounts of blood may cause circulatory overload in infants. Infusion of 25% albumin, which shifts large volumes of interstitial fluid into the vascular space, may also cause circulatory overload.

Hypervolemia must be considered if dyspnea, severe headache, peripheral edema or other signs of congestive heart failure occur during or soon after trans-

fusion. Symptoms of circulatory overload include coughing, cyanosis, orthopnea and difficulty in breathing. A rapid increase in systolic blood pressure supports the diagnosis. Symptoms usually improve when the infusion is stopped and the patient is placed in a sitting position and given diuretics and oxygen. If symptoms are not relieved, more aggressive therapy including phlebotomy may be necessary.

Prevention

Patients susceptible to circulatory overload should receive RBCs, not whole blood, in small volume increments, slowly infused. When necessary, the donor unit can be divided into aliquots, so that part of the unit can be stored at 1-6 C while the remainder is slowly administered. Subsequent aliquots can be issued as needed so that the rate of infusion does not exceed 1 mL/kg of body weight/hour.[20] Giving diuretics before the transfusion may be helpful. For some patients with hematocrits in the 0.10-0.20 (10-20%) range, phlebotomy followed by transfusion may be useful in increasing oxygen-carrying capacity without expanding blood volume. The blood removed may be discarded and replaced with allogeneic RBCs with a higher hematocrit, or the blood removed can be centrifuged and the autologous cells reinfused after removal of supernatant plasma. Caution must be exercised before phlebotomy, however, to ensure that the patient's cardiovascular system can tolerate an acute volume loss of up to 450 mL of blood if a full unit is to be removed.

The blood bank director and members of the medical staff must agree on protocols for these situations, and the blood bank procedures manual should have detailed instructions for the approved procedures. Among the concerns to be addressed are: the ratio of blood to anticoagulant if the cells are to be reinfused, proper labeling of the blood bag, sterile phlebotomy technique and proper patient identification.

Noncardiogenic Pulmonary Reactions

Transfusion recipients rarely experience clinically apparent pulmonary edema without concurrent changes in cardiac pressures. A series of 36 cases of transfusion-related acute lung injury (TRALI), however, suggests that these cases may be more common than previously appreciated.[21] The chest x-ray is typical of acute pulmonary edema. There is acute respiratory insufficiency, but no evidence of heart failure. Symptoms of respiratory distress, at times severe, occur after infusion of volumes too small to produce hypervolemia and may be accompanied by chills, fever, cyanosis and hypotension.

At least two mechanisms for noncardiogenic pulmonary reactions have been postulated. One is a reaction between the donor's leukocyte antibodies and recipient's leukocytes; this mechanism produces white cell aggregates that are trapped in the pulmonary microcirculation, producing transient changes in vascular permeability.[22] Fluid enters the alveolar air spaces, causing problems with adequate gas exchange. During transfusion of granulocyte concentrates, the reverse is also possible, ie, leukocyte antibodies in the recipient aggregate the transfused granulocytes.[23] An alternative pathogenic mechanism may be activation of complement to generate the anaphylatoxins C3a and C5a, which release histamine and serotonin from tissue basophils and platelets, and directly aggregate granulocytes to produce leukoemboli that lodge in the microvasculature of the lungs.[24]

As with all acute transfusion reactions, the transfusion should be stopped immediately. Treatment includes intravenous steroids and respiratory support as required. If subsequent transfusions are needed, leukocyte-reduced red cells may prevent such reactions. If the reaction was due to an antibody in the donor unit, future transfusions can be administered by routine techniques. Donors whose blood has been found to contain leukocyte antibodies because specific testing was initiated after a suspected transfusion reaction should have any future donations restricted to use as washed RBCs.

Delayed Adverse Effects of Transfusion

Delayed Hemolytic Transfusion Reactions

Primary Immunization

There are two different types of delayed HTRs—primary immunization and anamnestic response. The first is mild, occurs several weeks after transfusion and is the result of primary alloimmunization.[25] The overall risk of immunizing a recipient to a red cell antigen other than the D antigen has been estimated as 1-1.6% for each unit of blood transfused.[26] Antibodies are detectable no earlier than 7-10 days after transfusion and usually several weeks or months later. As the antibody increases in titer and avidity, it may react with transfused cells that are still circulating. The degree of hemolysis depends on the quantity of antibody produced and the quantity of transfused cells remaining. Primary immunization rarely causes significant hemolysis of transfused red cells, and such delayed hemolysis is usually unsuspected. The diagnosis may be suggested by an unexplained fall in hemoglobin concentration coupled with a positive DAT and/or the detection of a new red cell alloantibody.

Anamnestic Responses

The second type of delayed HTR occurs in a previously immunized recipient who experiences an anamnestic, or secondary, response to transfused red cell antigens. Some alloantibodies formed after primary immunization may diminish to levels undetectable in serum. Antibodies in the Kidd system (anti-Jk[a] and anti-Jk[b]) often disappear. Pretransfusion testing reveals no unexpected antibody and no serologic incompatibility, but within 3-7 days after transfusion, an anamnestic response leads to high levels of IgG antibodies that react with the transfused cells. The combination of high antibody levels and large numbers of transfused cells in the circulation may produce readily apparent manifestations. The most common presenting signs are fever, an unexplained fall in the patient's hemoglobin and mild jaundice, but associated clinical problems are infrequent. Hemoglobinuria may occur; acute renal failure is uncommon.[27] Treatment is rarely necessary, but the patient's urine output and renal function should be monitored.

The blood bank may detect a delayed hemolytic reaction, through serologic findings in patients without symptoms. In fact, the majority of cases once considered to be delayed HTRs are asymptomatic and more appropriately considered to be delayed serologic transfusion reactions.[28] If additional transfusions are required, the new blood specimen may have a positive DAT. In addition, positive antibody detection tests and crossmatch incompatibilities might be noted. The specimen used for compatibility testing must be no more than 72 hours old at the time of transfusion if the patient has been transfused or pregnant within the past 3 months. This is to detect rapidly developing antibodies that, if undetected, might cause an acute HTR upon subsequent transfusion. If a DAT is performed at this time, or is part of a routinely performed autologous control, antibody-coated transfused cells may be detected even though serum antibody is not yet detectable.

Elution and identification of the antibody is critical when the DAT becomes positive in a patient who has been transfused within the previous 2-3 weeks.[29] In cases where the DAT is positive but results on testing the patient's serum are negative or equivocal, crossmatching with the red cell eluate may be useful.

Infectious Complications of Transfusions

The most common and feared infectious complications of blood transfusions are diseases transmitted by viruses. These transfusion complications (hepatitis, cytomegalovirus infection and AIDS) are considered in Chapter 4. Although the following diseases are much less prevalent and are not a major concern for patients and their physicians in the United States, they can cause serious medical illness and may become issues in blood transfusion practice in the United States. If a case of transfusion-transmitted disease is confirmed, the blood collecting facility must be notified of the units involved in a written report.[30(p 34)]

Malaria

There are no practical laboratory screening tests for malaria. Although still rare in the United States, the number of cases of transfusion-associated malaria increased to the highest level in the past 25 years in the 1980's; the rate is now lower.[31] Travel and immigration are among the primary factors responsible for this persistent problem. Exclusion of donors at high risk of harboring parasites is the only effective preventive measure. This requires careful questioning of donors for a history of immigration from or travel in areas where malaria is endemic. See p 768.

Babesia

Another parasitic disease, babesiosis, can be mistaken for malaria. This disease can be transmitted by an asymptomatic blood donor who had been bitten by a tick in the past. Babesiosis is a more serious infection in immunocompromised or asplenic patients.[32,33]

Syphilis

Transmission of syphilis by transfusion is possible, but requires that blood be drawn during the rather brief period of spirochetemia, and that the organisms remain viable at the time of transfusion. The treponemal spirochete does not ordinarily survive more than 72 hours at 4 C, so only components stored at room temperature (platelet concentrate) or transfused very promptly after donation can transmit syphilis.[34,35] Performing a serologic test for syphilis (STS) on donor blood does not prevent transmission of syphilis because a positive test does not occur until well after the brief period of potential infectivity. The test is characteristically negative in primary syphilis and most positive STS results occur in donors whose reactions are unrelated to syphilitic infection, so-called biologic false-positive reactions. AABB *Standards* requires syphilis testing of donor blood since a positive test result may reflect a life-style of high risk activities.

Chagas' Disease

Chagas' disease is an infectious disease that may become a greater problem for the United States blood supply as more individuals migrate from endemic areas.[36] This infection is caused by the parasite *Trypanosoma cruzi*, endemic to most areas of Mexico, Central America and South America. Many persons in these endemic areas have chronic infection and can transmit the disease via blood. A few cases have been reported in the United States.[37,38] Approaches to prevention under investigation include eliminating donors with exposure in endemic areas, serologic testing and the addition of the medication Gentian violet to donor blood.

Toxoplasmosis

Toxoplasmosis has been reported as an unusual complication of transfusions, particularly in patients who are immunosuppressed.[39] Although clinical illness has been reported in granulocyte recipients, the disease is not a problem in routine transfusion practice.

Lyme Disease

Lyme disease may be a potential problem in transfusion. Although transfusion-related cases have not been reported, the disease is associated with chronic subclinical infections and has other features suggesting the potential for transfusion as a vector. Lyme disease is associated with the bite of the eastern deer tick and a spirochete, *Borrelia burgdorferi*, has been isolated from these ticks and from patient specimens.[40] An antibody response has been detected in patients as well.[41] Donors with a history of Lyme disease should be asymptomatic and a full course of antibiotic therapy must have been completed before donating blood.[42]

Graft-vs-Host Disease

Graft-vs-host disease (GVHD) is a rare complication following transfusion to patients who are severely immuno-suppressed, such as those being inten-sively treated with chemotherapy and ir-radiation.[43] Patients at risk include those with lymphopenia (absolute lym-phocyte count less than 500/μL) and bone marrow suppression. GVHD has oc-curred in infants who received intrauter-ine transfusions followed by exchange transfusion for hemolytic disease of the newborn.[44]

GVHD occurs if immunocompetent donor lymphocytes engraft and multiply in the recipient, who is usually im-munocompromised. These engrafted donor cells react against the "foreign" tissues of the host-recipient. The clinical syndrome of GVHD may include fever, skin rash, hepatitis, diarrhea, bone mar-row suppression and infection, usually progressing to a fatal outcome.[45] Pre-transfusion irradiation with a dose of 25 Gy of all blood components containing lymphocytes should reduce the risk of GVHD.[30(p 30)] A radiation dose of 15-50 Gy renders 85-95% of the lymphocytes in a unit of blood, granulocyte or platelet concentrate incapable of replication. The function of red cells, granulocytes and platelets is not affected by such irra-diation.[46]

Several cases have recently been de-scribed where immunocompetent pa-tients developed GVHD after transfu-sions when the patient was found to share an HLA haplotype with an HLA homozygous blood donor.[47] This situa-tion is most likely to occur in genetically homogeneous populations or among first-degree family members. Based upon these cases, the AABB requires that directed donations from all blood rela-tives be irradiated.

The indications for irradiated blood components for other conditions con-tinue to evolve. It is well accepted that patients with congenital immuno-deficiencies or those who undergo bone marrow transplantation should rou-tinely receive only irradiated blood com-ponents. Blood components for intra-uterine transfusion and for patients with Hodgkin's disease should also be irradi-ated. Many centers have extended blood irradiation to include cellular compo-nents intended for transfusion to prema-ture newborn recipients, recipients of HLA-matched components and compo-nents for patients receiving high dose chemoradiotherapy in preparation for an autologous marrow transplant, but these indications remain controver-sial.[48]

Posttransfusion Purpura

Posttransfusion purpura is a rare event, occurring almost exclusively in multip-arous women. A precipitous fall in plate-let count produces generalized purpura about a week after a blood transfusion. Some patients have been shown to have developed a platelet-specific alloanti-body, anti-HPA-1a (anti-Pl^{A1}, in Europe, anti-Zw^a). This antigen has a prevalence of 98.3% in the population, so only 1.7% of recipients are at risk of developing the alloantibody. The antibody destroys not only the transfused HPA-1a-positive platelets, but also the patient's own HPA-1a-negative platelets. The mechanism for the destruction of autologous plate-lets remains the subject of intense inves-tigation.[49] The thrombocytopenia is usu-ally severe, and if treatment is needed exchange plasmapheresis has been sug-gested as possible therapy.[50] The thrombocytopenia is usually self-limit-ing and platelet transfusions are usually not beneficial.

Iron Overload

Every unit of red cells contains approxi-mately 200 mg of iron. For chronically transfused patients, such as those with thalassemia, progressive and continual accumulation of iron in the mitochondria of cells can be hazardous. When patients have received more than 100 transfusions, iron deposition may interfere with function of the heart, liver or endocrine glands. Treatment is indicated and is directed at removing iron without reducing the patient's circulating hemoglobin.[51] Metered subcutaneous infusion of desferrioxamine, an iron-chelating agent, is valuable for reducing body iron stores in such patients.[52]

Immunomodulation by Transfusion

Transfusion has been known to modulate immune system responses since the reports of improved renal allograft survival in transfused patients in the 1970's.[53] Transfusion-modulated immune responses have been implicated in other clinical settings, including increased rates of solid tumor recurrence[54] and increased rates of postoperative bacterial infection.[55] These effects are somewhat controversial and have not been confirmed in prospective controlled trials, but suggest that the relationship between transfusion and the immune system is more complex than previously considered.

Records of Transfusion Complications

The blood bank or transfusion service must keep reports of transfusion complications. Cases of transfusion-associated disease (including but not confined to hepatitis B, hepatitis C and transfusion-associated AIDS) must be reported to the center that drew the blood. Fatalities resulting directly from transfusion complications, eg, hemolytic reactions or viral hepatitis, must be reported to the FDA, Director, Office of Compliance, Center for Biologics Evaluation and Research by telephone (301-295-8191) within 24 hours and by written report within 7 days (21 *CFR* 606.170). See also p 550.

References

1. McCarthy LR, Senne JE. Evaluation of acridine orange stain for detection of microorganisms in blood cultures. J Clin Microbiol 1980;11:281-5.
2. Henry JB. Clinical diagnosis and management by laboratory methods. 18th ed. Philadelphia: WB Saunders Co, 1991.
3. Baldwin ML, Barrasso C, Ness PM, Garratty G. A clinically significant erythrocyte antibody detectable only by ^{51}Cr survival studies. Transfusion 1983;23:40-4.
4. Fink DJ, Petz LD, Black MD. Serum haptoglobin: A valuable diagnostic aid in suspected hemolytic transfusion reactions. JAMA 1967;199:615-8.
5. Pineda AA, Brzica SM Jr, Taswell HF. Hemolytic transfusion reaction: Recent experience in a large blood bank. Mayo Clin Proc 1978;53:378-90.
6. Goldfinger D. Acute hemolytic transfusion reactions—a fresh look at pathogenesis and considerations regarding therapy. Transfusion 1977;17:85-98.
7. Bick RL. The clinical significance of fibrinogen degradation products. Semin Thromb Hemost 1984;8:302-30.
8. Goldberg LI. Cardiovascular and renal actions of dopamine: Potential clinical application. Pharmacol Rev 1972;24:1-29.
9. Honig CL, Bove JR. Transfusion-associated fatalities: A review of Bureau of Biologics reports 1976-1978. Transfusion 1980;20:653-61.
10. Brittingham TE, Chaplin H. Febrile transfusion reactions caused by sensitivity to donor leukocytes and platelets. JAMA 1957;165:819-25.
11. Meryman HT, Hornblower M. The preparation of red cells depleted of leukocytes: Review and evaluation. Transfusion 1986;26:101-6.
12. Kevy SV, Schmidt PJ, McGinniss MH, Workman WG. Febrile, non-hemolytic transfusion reactions and the limited role of leukoagglutinin in their etiology. Transfusion 1962;2:7-16.
13. Menitove JE, McElligott MC, Aster RH. Febrile transfusion reaction: What blood component should be given next? Vox Sang 1982;42:318-21.
14. Goldman M, Blajchman MA. Blood product-associated bacterial sepsis. Transfus Med Rev 1991;5:73-83.

15. Morrow JW, Braine HG, Kickler TS, et al. Septic reactions to platelets, a persistent problem. JAMA 1991;266:555-8.

16. Tipple MA, Bland JJ, Murphy MJ, et al. Sepsis associated with transfusion of red cells contaminated with *Yersinia enterocolitica*. Transfusion 1990;30:207-13.

17. Vyas GN, Holmdahl L, Perkins HA, Fudenberg HH. Serologic specificity of human anti-IgA and its significance in transfusion. Blood 1969;34:573-81.

18. Yap PL, Pryde EAD, McClelland DBL. IgA content of frozen-thawed-washed red blood cells and blood products measured by radioimmunoassay. Transfusion 1982;22:36-8.

19. Wells JV, King MA. Adverse reactions to human plasma proteins. Anaesth Intensive Care 1980;8:139-44.

20. Marriott HL, Kekwick A. Volume and rate in blood transfusion for relief of anemia. Br Med J 1940;1:1043-6.

21. Popovsky MA, Moore SB. Diagnostic and pathogenetic considerations in transfusion-related acute lung injury. Transfusion 1985;25:573-7.

22. Latson TW, Kickler TS, Baumgartner WA. Pulmonary hypertension and noncardiogenic pulmonary edema following cardiopulmonary bypass associated with an antigranulocyte antibody. Anesthesiology 1986;64:106-11.

23. Higby DJ, Burnett D. Granulocyte transfusions: Current status. Blood 1980;55:2-8.

24. Hammerschmidt DE, Weaver J, Hudson LD, et al. Association of complement activation and elevated plasma-C5a with adult respiratory distress syndrome. Lancet 1980;1:947-9.

25. Taddie SJ, Barrasso C, Ness PM. A delayed transfusion reaction caused by anti-K6. Transfusion 1982;22:68-9.

26. Lostumbo MM, Holland PV, Schmidt PJ. Isoimmunization after multiple transfusions. N Engl J Med 1966;275:141-4.

27. Holland PV, Wallerstein RO. Delayed hemolytic transfusion reaction with acute renal failure. JAMA 1968;204:1007-8.

28. Ness PM, Shirey RS, Thoman SK, Buck SA. The differentiation of delayed serologic and delayed hemolytic transfusion reactions: Incidence, long-term serologic findings, and clinical significance. Transfusion 1990;30:688-93.

29. Judd WJ, Butch SH, Oberman HA, et al. The evaluation of a positive DAT in pretransfusion testing. Transfusion 1980:20;17-23.

30. Widmann FK, ed. Standards for blood banks and transfusion services. 15th ed. Bethesda, MD: American Association of Blood Banks, 1993.

31. Nahlen BL, Lobel HO, Cannon SE, Campbell CC. Reassessment of blood donor selection criteria for United States travelers to malarious areas. Transfusion 1991;31:798-804.

32. Rosner F, Zarrabi MH, Benach J, et al. Babesiosis in splenectomized adults: Review of 22 reported cases. Am J Med 1984;76:696-701.

33. Mintz ED, Anderson JF, Cable RG, Hadler JL. Transfusion-transmitted babesiosis: A case report from a new endemic area. Transfusion 1991;31:365-8.

34. Chambers RW, Foley HT, Schmidt PJ. Transmission of syphilis by fresh blood components. Transfusion 1969;9:32-4.

35. Van der Sluis JJ, Tenkate FJW, Vuzevski VD, et al. Transfusion syphilis, survival of *Treponema pallidum* in stored donor blood. Vox Sang 1985;49:390-9.

36. Schmunis GA. *Trypanosoma cruzi*, the etiologic agent of Chagas' disease: Status in the blood supply in endemic and nonendemic countries. Transfusion 1991;31:547-57.

37. Grant IH, Gold JWM, Wittner M, et al. Transfusion-associated Chagas' disease acquired in the United States. Ann Intern Med 1989;111:849-51.

38. Nickerson P, Orr P, Schroeder ML, et al. Transfusion-associated *Trypanosoma cruzi* infection in a non-endemic area. Ann Intern Med 1989;111:851-3.

39. Siegel SE, Lunde MN, Gelderman AH, et al. Transfusion of toxoplasmosis by leukocyte transfusions. Blood 1971;37:388-94.

40. Burgdorfer W, Barbour AG, Hayes SF, et al. Lyme disease—a tick-borne spirochetosis? Science 1982;216:1317-9.

41. Benach JL, Bosler EM, Hanrahan JP, et al. Spirochetes isolated from the blood of two patients with Lyme disease. N Engl J Med 1983;308:740-2.

42. Aoki SY, Holland PV. Lyme disease—another transfusion risk? Transfusion 1989;29:646-50.

43. Greenbaum BH. Transfusion-associated graft-versus-host disease: Historical perspectives, incidence, and current use of irradiated blood products. J Clin Oncol 1991;9:1889-1902.

44. Parkman R, Mosier D, Umansky I, et al. Graft-versus-host disease after intrauterine and exchange transfusion for hemolytic disease of the newborn. N Engl J Med 1974;290:359-63.

45. Anderson KC, Weinstein HJ. Transfusion-associated graft versus host disease. N Engl J Med 1990;323:315-21.

46. Leitman SF, Holland PV. Irradiation of blood products. Transfusion 1985;25:293-300.

47. Juji T, Takahashi K, Shibata Y, et al. Posttransfusion graft-vs-host disease in immunocompetent patients after cardiac surgery in Japan. N Engl J Med 1989;321:56.

48. Anderson KC, Goodnough LT, Sayers M, et al. Variation in blood component irradiation practice: Implications for prevention of transfusion-associated graft-versus-host disease. Blood 1991;77:2096-102.

49. Kickler TS, Ness PM, Herman JH, Bell WR. Studies on the pathophysiology of post-transfusion purpura. Blood 1986;68:347-50.

50. Vogelsang G, Kickler TS, Bell WR. Post-transfusion purpura: A report of five patients and a review of the pathogenesis and management. Am J Hematol 1986;21:259-67.

51. Jacobs A. Iron chelation therapy for iron loaded patients. Br J Haematol 1979;43:1-5.

52. Cohen A, Mizanin J, Shwartz E. Treatment of iron overload in Cooley's anemia. Ann NY Acad Sci 1985;445:274-81.

53. Opelz G, Sengar DPS, Mickey MR, et al. Effect of blood transfusions on subsequent kidney transplants. Transplant Proc 1973;5:253-9.

54. Blumberg N, Heal JM. Transfusion and host defenses against cancer recurrence and infection. Transfusion 1989;29:236-45.

55. Triulzi DJ, Blumberg N. Association of transfusion with postoperative bacterial infection. CRC Crit Rev Clin Lab Sci 1990;28:95-107.

20

Autologous Transfusion

Autologous transfusion indicates that the blood donor and transfusion recipient are identical. Although autologous transfusion practice has existed for over 100 years, the last decade has seen explosive growth in the use of autologous blood. This growth has occurred in large part as a result of concern over the risk of transfusion-transmitted diseases. Despite the growth in autologous services, studies have suggested that autologous blood is still being underutilized.[1] Numerous national professional organizations and federal agencies have endorsed the use of autologous blood services and The National Blood Resource Education Program has published a statement specifically focused on autologous services.[2] Frequently cited advantages and disadvantages of autologous blood are listed in Table 20-1.

Autologous blood services are best used as part of a comprehensive strategy of blood conservation that includes careful attention to the proper indications for transfusion, acceptance of normovolemic anemia and avoidance of excessive blood sampling for diagnostic testing. Four categories of autologous blood services exist: 1) preoperative donation, in which blood is drawn prior to anticipated need; 2) intraoperative hemodilution, in which blood is collected at the start of surgery and then reinfused during or at the end of surgery; 3) intraoperative blood collection, in which blood is recovered from the surgical field and

then reinfused; and 4) postoperative collection, in which blood shed from surgical drains is collected for reinfusion to the patient. When these are used in a coordinated approach, their advantages to the patient are additive.[3-5] Each hospital must analyze its own transfusion practices to determine the optimal autologous technique or combination of techniques to be used.

Preoperative Autologous Blood Donation

Numerous studies have documented that the use of preoperative autologous blood in selected patient subgroups can significantly reduce or completely avoid allogeneic blood exposures. In principle, stable patients scheduled for most surgical procedures in which blood transfusion is likely are candidates for preoperative autologous donation. In practice the technique has found widest application for orthopedic,[6] vascular, urologic and cardiac surgery.[4,7] For procedures in which the likelihood of transfusion is remote, the use of preoperative donation is not cost-effective. A hospital's surgical blood order schedule can serve as an objective guide for those procedures in which preoperative donation is most likely to benefit the patient.[8] For such patients, autologous blood services have become a necessary medical service available in all states. AABB *Standards*

491

Table 20-1. Advantages and Disadvantages of Autologous Blood Services

Advantages
- Prevent transfusion-transmitted disease
- Prevent alloimmunization
- Prevent certain transfusion reactions (allergic, febrile, hemolytic, graft-vs-host)
- Supplement blood supply
- Reassure donor-patient
- Source of blood for patients with multiple alloantibodies
- Stimulate erythropoiesis

Disadvantages
- Donation reactions
- Increased cost and complexity of services
- Outdating of units if surgery is postponed

for Blood Banks and Transfusion Services must be followed in the selection of the donor, collection of the unit and subsequent testing, labeling and pretransfusion testing requirements.[9(p 35-36)] Several unanswered questions remain concerning the proper design of autologous programs.[10-13] A fundamental issue in program design is whether or not unused autologous blood will be released to the general supply, a practice termed "crossover."[11] Some of the differences between programs without crossover and with crossover are discussed below.

Preoperative Autologous Donation Without Crossover

Each blood center or hospital must establish its own procedures, documents and supporting information for the proper conduct of an autologous blood collection program. Guidelines exist that aid in establishing a new program or in improving an existing one.[14-18] A visit to a larger program is very useful for programs that anticipate growth in preoperative collections. Education of the medical staff and of eligible patients is important so that all suitable patients are considered candidates for autologous blood donation. Table 20-2 lists the issues of medical staff education that are important in order to set up and maintain an effective preoperative autologous program. Requests for autologous blood collection are made in writing by the patient's physician and the request (which may simply be a prescription) is kept by the collecting facility. Requests should include the patient's name, the number of units and kind of component requested, the anticipated surgical date and surgical procedure, and the physician's signature. Although the donation process for autologous blood follows the same general outline as that used for regular volunteer donors (Chapter 1), there are numerous special issues for the autologous donor.

Information for the Donor

In addition to general information about blood donation, autologous donors need information about any special fees for autologous services.

Medical Interview

The medical interview should be restructured to the special needs of autologous donors. For example, more attention should be given to the donor's medications, associated medical illnesses and cardiovascular fitness.[19]

Questions should address the possibility of intermittent bacteremia in the donor. In programs that do not intend crossover, many of the interview questions that probe for transfusion-transmittable diseases need not be asked.

Physician Responsibility

There should be a transfusion medicine physician available to help assess the suitability of autologous donors who appear to be at higher risk for complications of blood donation by virtue of their medical history or physical exam. Although the donor's attending physician initiates the request for autologous services, the responsibility for the health and safety of the donor while giving blood rests with the medical director in charge of the blood collecting facility.

Informed Consent and Testing for Transfusion-Transmitted Diseases

If the blood is to remain within the collecting facility and if crossover is not practiced, there is no requirement to test for transfusion-transmitted diseases. However, if testing is not done, then special precautions are required by the FDA for the collection and distribution of untested components. If units are to be shipped from the collecting facility, then it is required that the first unit from a given donor during a 30-day period must be tested for the same markers of transfusion-transmitted diseases that are used for routine allogeneic units. Some programs that do not practice crossover will test autologous donations in the same manner as allogeneic donations to simplify the logistics of testing.[11] Depending on the level of testing to be done, the informed consent provided by the autologous donor may need to be different from that provided by regular volunteer donors. Informed consent for donation may also need to include the possibility of unexpected outcomes, including loss or destruction of the autologous unit.

Supplemental Iron

Provision should be made for advising the donor about the use of supplemental iron. Supplemental iron is ideally prescribed by the requesting physician even before the first donation to allow maximum time for iron intake. Insufficient storage of iron is frequently the limiting factor for individuals seeking to donate multiple units of blood. Oral iron is commonly given to autologous blood donors but may be insufficient to maintain iron stores.[20] Oral iron is usually taken with meals and the dose should be adjusted to the individual's tolerance of iron's gastrointestinal side effects.

Table 20-2. Issues in the Education of Medical Staff

- Medical advantages of autologous services to the patient
- Range of autologous services provided
- Importance of a comprehensive program
- Appropriate patient selection
- Contraindications to use of autologous services
- Recommended intervals for preoperative collections
- Oral iron supplementation
- Details of logistic arrangements
- Policy regarding crossover
- Charges
- Sources for additional information

Donation Schedule

A schedule for donations should be established with the donor. A weekly schedule is often used. Usually, the last donation occurs at least 72 hours before the scheduled surgery. This is intended to allow time for adequate volume repletion prior to the general anesthesia.[21] Under ideal circumstances, the donor's final donation is more than 2 weeks before the intended surgery to allow sufficient time to rebuild red cell mass. According to AABB *Standards*, autologous blood is generally not collected when the patient's hematocrit is less than 0.33 (33%). This level may be adjusted to higher or lower values by the medical director depending on the clinical circumstances of the donor. Many programs notify the requesting physician when each unit is successfully collected.

Each program should establish a policy regarding action to be taken in the event of postponement of surgery beyond the expiration date of the autologous units. Options include: 1) discarding the unit; 2) reinfusing it back into the donor-patient prior to its expiration and then drawing a new autologous unit; and 3) freezing the unit either with or without prior rejuvenation.

Volume Collected

For patients weighing >50 kg, standard units are collected. If a low volume unit (300-405 mL) is inadvertently collected, it is still suitable for storage and subsequent autologous transfusion. Undercollected units (<300 mL) may still be suitable for autologous use with approval of the medical director. For patients weighing <50 kg there should be a proportional reduction in the volume of blood collected (not to exceed 15% of the donor's blood volume), and a proportional reduction in the volume of antico-

agulant/preservative solution used. See Chapter 1. By using a double pack, the unwanted anticoagulant/preservative solution can be easily transferred to the satellite bag prior to phlebotomy without opening the system.

Serologic Testing

ABO and Rh testing must be done on all units. Transfusing facilities must retest units drawn at other facilities. Testing for unexpected antibodies is optional if the blood is for autologous use only.

Labeling

Labeling requirements for autologous units are detailed in the AABB *Standards*. Units should be clearly labeled with the autologous donor's name, identifying number and expiration date. The unit should be clearly marked "For Autologous Use Only." In addition, the unit should be labeled as Autologous Donor Blood. Although many programs store all autologous blood as whole blood, components may also be prepared, but are for autologous transfusion use only. A biohazard label must be applied if the donor tests positive for hepatitis C virus antibodies, hepatitis B core antibodies, hepatitis B surface antigen (HBsAg), human immunodeficiency virus antibodies (anti-HIV-1/2) or a serologic test for syphilis.

Storage and Shipment

Long liquid shelf life has obvious advantages for autologous programs including flexibility and the opportunity for the donor to rebuild red cell mass after donation and before surgery. Some programs collect autologous units more than 6 weeks prior to scheduled surgery and freeze the blood. Although this provides greater time for the donor to recover lost red cell mass, glycerolization and freezing add to the cost of the program and complicate blood availability during the perioperative period. If the unit is to be shipped to another institution and if the donor has a positive confirmatory test for anti-HIV or HBsAg, the ordering physician should provide written agreement to accept the unit.

Transfusion of Autologous Units Before Allogeneic Units

A system must be established that identifies the availability of autologous blood for the recipient. The system should ensure the use of autologous components before nonautologous components. Transfusing anesthesiologists, surgeons and physicians need education about the importance of selecting autologous components first.

Pretransfusion Testing and Component Modification

In general, requirements for pretransfusion testing are similar for patients about to receive autologous units or allogeneic units. See Chapter 14. Except in the circumstance of autologous units collected prior to allogeneic marrow transplantation, autologous units do not require gamma irradiation prior to transfusion to the donor-recipient. It is presumed that there is little clinical benefit to leukocyte reduction of autologous components prior to autologous transfusion.

Issue and Return of Unused Components; Records; Reactions

AABB *Standards* regarding the proper issue and return of unused autologous units follow the same outline as for regular volunteer units. Records must be maintained that connect the original donation and all components made from it to their eventual disposition. The initial investigation of suspected transfusion reactions should be the same for autologous and allogeneic units.

Preoperative Autologous Donation With Crossover

Crossover refers to use of autologous units for the general blood supply if not used by the original intended recipient. Approval from the appropriate hospital governing committee should be obtained and the details of the policy explained to the medical staff. Hospitals that adopt a crossover policy need to take special precautions to comply with standards of the AABB and the FDA.

Information for the Donor-Patient

The policy governing release of the donor's unit to the general supply should be clearly explained to the donor-patient.

Medical Interview

In addition to questions designed particularly for autologous donation, the medical interview must include all questions that are routinely used to assess the suitability of regular volunteer donors. In crossover programs it is important that donors understand that their answers to certain questions during the medical interview must be given in light of the possibility of crossover. Autologous donors have special motivation to avoid exclusion as donors. It may be helpful to segregate the questions into two groups: a first set to decide donor suitability for autologous collection and a second set to determine donor suitability for crossover should the donor not need his/her blood.

Physician Responsibility

Clear, written criteria for decisions about the suitability of crossover are the responsibility of the medical director. Crossover is ill-advised in situations in which the collecting facility and the transfusing facility are different. In addition to meeting acceptable criteria for allogeneic use based on the donor interview, physical examination, exclusion form, required serologic testing and testing for transfusion-transmitted diseases, autologous units considered suitable for crossover should meet equivalent criteria as regular volunteer units for red cell mass (hematocrit × volume). Plasma from autologous donations may not be salvaged for manufacturing purposes unless the donor meets all the criteria for acceptance applied to a routine allogeneic donor.

Informed Consent and Testing for Transfusion-Transmitted Diseases

Testing for all required markers of transfusion-transmitted diseases should be done on samples obtained at the time of collection of the unit. If the donor fails to meet any of the donor suitability criteria applied to allogeneic donors, then the unit should be stored separately from allogeneic units and must be restricted for autologous use only. Informed consent should carefully explain the policy by which the donor's blood will not be available once it has been crossed over to the general supply. Donor consent to testing for markers of transfusion-transmitted diseases is required. The donor should be informed about which persons will be notified if such tests are positive.

Notification of Crossover to the Clinical Team

Programs that use crossover frequently choose to notify the clinical team when the time reserved for autologous use is about to expire.

Labeling

There must be a system that clearly differentiates those units suitable for crossover from those units that must be restricted for autologous use only. When a unit is crossed over, the label that identified the original donor is obliterated, but the label that identifies the unit as autologous blood remains.

Records

Records must be able to trace the original source of the blood as well as its final disposition. A record of the date/time of crossover is desirable.

Special Patient Categories

Special considerations apply for autologous donations by several patient groups. Pediatric donors will require more preparation, attention and parental participation.[22] Consultation with programs that regularly collect autologous units from pediatric patients may be very useful. Autologous blood donations by pregnant women remain controversial.[23,24] Antepartum autologous donations by pregnant women are likely to be of benefit only in selected circumstances: in women with alloantibodies to multiple or high-incidence antigens, in women with placenta previa or high risk pregnancy and in women with bleeding disorders. Autologous blood is not generally collected prior to routine pregnancy and delivery.[11] Patients with sickle cell disease may present special difficulties because their red cells (if glycerolized) cannot be deglycerolized easily by standard techniques.[25] The successful use of autologous blood in sickle cell disease has been reported.[26] However, allogeneic red cell transfusions offer the advantage of providing hemoglobin A, which may prevent sickling complications during and after surgery.

Patients with valvular heart disease or with disease of the left main coronary (or left main equivalent) have been traditionally considered at too high a risk for autologous donation.[11] However, some programs having experience with such patients and having ready access to advanced medical support do not exclude such patients from autologous blood services.[7,27,28] A similar situation exists with patients facing major organ transplantation. Each program must establish general criteria for donor acceptability in the context of the medical support available in the donation area.[29]

Unresolved Issues in Preoperative Autologous Services

Several issues in the management of preoperative autologous services remain unresolved. These issues include the use of erythropoietin, the appropriate "transfusion trigger" for autologous blood, the role of autologous collections in the absence of identified need and the preoperative collection of special autologous blood components.

Use of Erythropoietin

Measurements of the endogenous release of erythropoietin in response to the mild anemia associated with blood donations [Hct generally >0.33 (>33%)] have shown little elevation in erythropoietin levels.[30] However, pharmacologic doses of supplemental erythropoietin can stimulate erythrocyte production within a week. Adequate reticulocyte response is dependent on sufficient iron stores. Several studies have claimed that administration of erythropoietin to autologous donors allows a greater number of participants to complete their prescribed course of donations.[31,32] In one study, erythropoietin-treated donors were able to donate 5.4 units in 3 weeks vs 4.1 units for placebo controls.[33] How-

ever, given the high cost of erythropoietin and its marginal benefit for donors who will give three units or less, the exact role of erythropoietin in autologous services remains uncertain.

Transfusion Trigger

There is disagreement about the proper "transfusion trigger" for autologous blood.[11] Some claim that one set of criteria should be used to decide if a given patient needs a transfusion and that the decision to transfuse should be made independent of whether or not autologous blood is available. Others observe that some physicians will elect to transfuse autologous blood under circumstances in which allogeneic blood would not be used. Transfusion of autologous blood is not without some risks to the recipient, including clerical errors that result in giving an unintended unit, bacterial contamination of the unit and volume overload. However, autologous blood carries less risk to the recipient than allogeneic blood. The theory of risk/benefit analysis would favor the use of two separate criteria for judging the transfusion trigger of autologous vs allogeneic blood and would support the reinfusion of autologous units under circumstances in which allogeneic blood would not be used. However, there are no clinical studies supporting or refuting such a dual standard.

Autologous Services in the Absence of Anticipated Need

Public concern over the risk of transfusion-transmitted diseases has resulted in the development of facilities that provide long-term storage of autologous frozen blood.[34] Donors pay these services to maintain a supply of autologous blood should it become needed for an unanticipated illness. The cost of such services and the unproven availability for emergency transfusion are generally felt to outweigh the benefit. Long-term frozen storage is, however, suitable and recommended for individuals with rare phenotypes and alloantibodies to clinically significant high-incidence antigens.[11]

Preoperative Collection of Components

Some studies have suggested that preoperative collection of platelet-rich plasma may improve hemostasis following cardiopulmonary bypass.[35] Such collections may be done preoperatively or intraoperatively. One randomized study suggested decreased allogeneic exposures resulted from the use of this technique.[36] However, an independent randomized, blinded trial found no benefit.[37] The preoperative preparation of autologous Cryoprecipitated AHF for topical use during surgery has also been described.[38]

Intraoperative Hemodilution

Intraoperative hemodilution (IH) refers to the removal of one or more units of blood at the beginning of surgery for reinfusion during or at the end of the operation. There is increasing interest in IH and proponents of the technique attest to its value.[11,39,40] One randomized trial of IH vs preoperative autologous blood donation in 50 patients undergoing retropubic prostatectomy suggested the two autologous blood techniques were of equal efficacy.[41] The magnitude of the contribution of IH to blood conservation has been difficult to measure precisely.

Theoretical Considerations

The expected benefit of IH rests on three principles: 1) improved oxygenation in the microcirculation is expected to occur when blood viscosity is reduced by hemodilution; 2) less red cell mass is

expected to be lost if the patient's blood is diluted at the start of surgery; and 3) removal of blood at the beginning of surgery would conserve a small supply of normal platelets and coagulation factors for the end of surgery.

Improved Oxygenation

Studies in animals using tissue oxygen probes suggested improved oxygen delivery to tissues during acute normovolemic hemodilution. However, in humans changes in regional blood flow in the microcirculation resulting from IH have not been measured. Studies in humans have measured total systemic oxygen delivery and have provided conflicting results. One study used dextran-60 or hydroxyethyl starch as the replacement solution and noted a 5-7% increase in total oxygen delivery following hemodilution to hematocrits in the 0.28-0.33 (28-33%) range. When 5% albumin was used as a replacement solution in a different study, total oxygen delivery declined by 17% as the hematocrit decreased to 0.33 (33%). The difference in results between studies using dextran/starch vs albumin has been attributed to the hyperoncotic effect of dextran/starch resulting in a hypervolemic state and improved total blood flow relative to controls.[42,43] The bulk of evidence supports the idea that if the heart is able to increase cardiac output in compensation for acute normovolemic anemia, overall tissue oxygen delivery at hematocrits of 0.25-0.30 (25-30%) is as good as (but no better than) delivery at hematocrits of 0.35-0.45 (35-45%).

Conserved Red Cell Mass

Surgical bleeding at a low hematocrit results in less loss of red cell mass than bleeding at a normal hematocrit. In practice, the actual red cell mass saved by IH depends on the patient's predilution hematocrit, the quantity of blood removed during IH, the blood volume of the recipient, the total blood loss for the operation and the "transfusion trigger" for administering blood during surgery. Although the final hematocrit may be slightly higher with IH, the use of IH usually results in a lower hematocrit than that found in a control patient during surgery.

Preservation of Hemostasis

Because blood collected by IH is usually stored at room temperature in the operating room and is returned to the patient within 8 hours of collection, there is little deterioration of platelets or coagulation factors. Although the hemostatic value of blood collected by IH is as yet unproven, interest remains in the hemostatic potential of fresh whole blood.[44,45]

Clinical Studies

The safety and efficacy of intraoperative hemodilution as a method of reducing allogeneic blood exposure has been investigated in several clinical studies.[40,46] The technique has been applied in patients undergoing cardiac surgery,[47,48] vascular surgery,[49] orthopedic surgery[50] and major general surgery.[51] Reductions in allogeneic blood use between 18% and 90% have been reported. Given the limited theoretical savings in red cell mass resulting from the technique, the reduction in allogeneic blood use seems unexpected. One possible explanation for these results may be that the autologous units collected by IH are used as a replacement fluid for the volume losses that occur during surgery. This may have implications for the reported results of clinical studies using other autologous blood techniques as well. More studies are needed to clarify the role and value of hemodilution in blood conservation.

Practical Considerations

Hospitals offering IH must identify key individuals from anesthesia, surgery and transfusion medicine to establish a local knowledge base upon which others can depend. Criteria for patient selection have been published. See Table 20-3. The

Table 20-3. Selection of Patients for Intraoperative Hemodilution

General Surgery[39]

- Expected total blood loss approximately 1–2 liters
- Hemoglobin >120 g/L (>12 g/dL)
- Absence of coronary heart disease
- Absence of restrictive or obstructive lung disease
- Absence of renal disease
- Absence of severe hypertension or cirrhosis
- Absence of clotting deficiencies

Cardiac Surgery[47]

- Hemoglobin >140 g/L (>14 g/dL)
- Absence of all of the following:
  —Unstable angina
  —Abnormal left ventricular function, ejection fraction <0.5 or cardiac index <2.5 L/min/m^2
  —Left main coronary stenosis
  —Ischemic electrocardiogram changes at rest
  —Impaired lung function

procedure is generally performed by an anesthesiologist and the amount of blood removed is determined by published nomograms or simple calculations.[11,40,52] Simultaneous crystalloid or colloid replacement is given while monitoring cardiac performance.[42,53]

The following transfusion medicine issues are of practical importance in establishing a program in IH:

1. The local indications for IH should be established based on the patient's preoperative blood volume and hematocrit, the target hemodilution hematocrit, the surgical procedure and other physiologic criteria.
2. Written policy, procedure and mechanisms for education of staff should be established and periodically reviewed.
3. Careful monitoring of the volume and perfusion of the patient during the procedure is required.
4. Blood should be collected in an aseptic fashion into standard blood collection bags with citrate anticoagulant. Blood should not be collected and stored in empty saline bags or other crystalloid solution bags.
5. The unit must be properly labeled and stored. The bag label must contain at a minimum the patient's full name, medical record number and the statement "For Autologous Use Only." In addition, the date/time of collection is recommended. The suggested upper limit of storage at room temperature is 8 hours.

Intraoperative Blood Collection

Intraoperative blood collection (IBC) refers to the collection and return of blood recovered from the operative site or from associated extracorporeal blood circuits. The use of IBC has ex-perienced widespread growth. Several publications provide useful information for hospitals or blood centers contemplating IBC services as well as for those with established programs.[14,54-56] The technique has been widely used in cardiac, vascular and orthopedic surgery. In addition to decreasing allogeneic donor exposures, IBC may provide an important source of red cells during massive transfusion. The use of IBC is most suitable in operations in which the surgical field is sterile and free of tumor cells, in which blood may be aspirated without excessive hemolysis and in which the anticipated blood loss is 20% or more of the patient's estimated blood volume.

Most IBC programs use machines in which shed blood is collected and the red cells concentrated and washed prior to reinfusion. This process typically results in a final transfusate consisting of 225 mL of saline-suspended red cells with a hematocrit of 0.50-0.60 (50-60%). Red cell survival of blood collected by IBC is no less than that of transfused allogeneic red cells. The concentration of plasma-free hemoglobin varies widely and is often higher than that found in allogeneic packed cells. Sodium and chloride concentrations are those of the saline wash and potassium concentrations are low. Washed recovered blood contains no clinically useful concentrations of coagulation factors or platelets.

Clinical Studies

IBC has proved to be an effective component of an overall blood conservation program for a number of surgical procedures including cardiac,[57,58] vascular,[59,60] orthopedic,[5,61] urologic,[62,63] trauma,[64,65] gynecologic[66,67] and transplantation surgery.[68] The precise contribution of IBC to preventing patient exposure to allogeneic blood varies widely among different studies. The overall decline in blood use, the use of comparisons to historical controls and the influence of other autologous techniques undoubtedly contribute to the variable effectiveness seen in clinical studies. IBC has been used for Jehovah's Witnesses and a publication by the church indicates that the use of IBC techniques in which the blood does not leave the operating room will be acceptable to many Jehovah's Witness patients.[69]

Relative contraindications to IBC include malignancy, infection and contaminants in the operative field. In general, IBC is not used for the resection of a nonmetastatic tumor because of concern over reinfusion of tumor cells. However, IBC has been used in some centers during resection of malignant tumors.[70] Because studies document that washing does not remove bacterial contamination from recovered blood, it is generally recommended that IBC not be used if the operative field has gross bacterial soilage. A variety of contaminants (Table 20-4) may also be present in the operative field and caution should be used prior to reinfusion of these contaminants to the patient.[14]

Medical Controversies

Several medical controversies listed in Table 20-4 surround the use of IBC. With the development of devices that neither concentrate nor wash shed blood prior to reinfusion, there is interest in the relative risks of reinfusing unwashed shed blood collected by IBC.[11,14] Blood collected during IBC has undergone varying degrees of both hemolysis and coagulation/fibrinolysis. Some degree of hemolysis occurs in blood collected by IBS as a result of the high suction pressure used for aspiration of blood, turbulence of blood during collection or mechanical compression in roller pumps and plastic tubing. Surface skimming during collection and high negative pressure during collection are the major causes of hemolysis.

Washing recovered blood prior to reinfusion decreases the concentration of free hemoglobin. Concern has been expressed that reinfusion of high concentrations of free hemoglobin may be nephrotoxic if given to patients with impaired renal function. Although there has not been direct proof that nephrotoxicity occurs more frequently without washing recovered blood,[71] many programs establish limits to the quantity of unwashed recovered blood that may be reinfused without processing.

Several factors contribute to the degree of coagulation and clot lysis present in recovered blood. These include: 1) whether or not the patient is systemically anticoagulated at the time of IBC; 2) the degree of contact of the blood with serosal body cavities prior to aspiration; 3) the degree of contact of the blood with artificial surfaces during collection; 4)

Table 20-4. Controversies in Intraoperative Blood Collection

- Use in patients with malignancy
- Use in presence of wounds contaminated with bacteria
- Reinfusion of unwashed blood collected by IBC
    - —Reinfusion of free hemoglobin
    - —Reinfusion of procoagulants and fibrin degradation products
    - —Reinfusion of debris, fat particles, amniotic fluid, ascitic fluid, urine, methacrylate, topical antiseptics and topical hemostatic agents

the degree of turbulence induced during collection; and 5) the amount and kind of anticoagulant used. In general, blood collected from patients who are not systemically anticoagulated has already undergone coagulation followed by fibrinolysis prior to recovery and will not contribute to hemostasis upon reinfusion. Concern has existed that such blood, which is rich in fibrin degradation products, may adversely affect coagulation in the patient if reinfused in large volumes over a short period of time. Patients with advanced liver disease and impaired ability to clear procoagulant material and fibrin degradation products may be at greatest risk for developing a coagulopathy resulting from reinfusion of unwashed recovered blood.

Practical Considerations

IBC services require the coordinated effort of surgeons, anesthesiologists, transfusion medicine specialists and specific personnel trained in the use of special equipment. Some hospitals develop "in-house" IBC services, whereas others employ outside contract services for IBC. Each hospital's own needs should dictate the kind of IBC services that are selected for use. Options may include: 1) devices that collect recovered blood for direct reinfusion; 2) devices that collect recovered blood, which is then concentrated and washed in a separate cell washer; 3) high speed machines that automatically concentrate and wash recovered red cells.

IBC With Processing Prior to Reinfusion

Several devices are available that automatically process recovered blood prior to reinfusion. Blood is collected by vacuum suction while being mixed with anticoagulant. It is suggested that the vacuum level not exceed 100 mmHg in order to minimize hemolysis, although higher levels of suction occasionally may be needed during periods of rapid bleeding. Either citrate (ACD) or heparin may be used as an anticoagulant. When ACD is used, the ratio of ACD to blood is generally adjusted to a 1:5 to 1:10 ratio.[14] When heparin is used, 30,000 units of heparin are typically added to a liter of saline and the flow adjusted to achieve a 1:5 to 1:10 ratio with shed blood.[14] The blood collects in a holding reservoir prior to centrifugation and washing. The volume of saline used for washing varies between 500 and 1500 mL, depending on the clinical circumstances. The washed concentrated red cells are then pumped to a transfer pack, labeled and made available for reinfusion through a filter. An alternative approach is to collect blood in a canister system designed for direct reinfusion and then concentrate and wash the recovered red cells in a blood bank cell washer.

IBC With Direct Reinfusion

Commercially available systems have been developed for collection and direct return of recovered blood. These systems generally consist of a suction catheter attached to a disposable collection bag or rigid plastic canister to which anticoagulant (usually citrate or heparin) may have been added. Blood is suctioned into the holding canister prior to direct reinfusion through a microaggregate filter. Low vacuum suction and minimal hemolysis are preferred in nonwashed systems. Low cost and simple design are the major advantages of these devices. An important disadvantage is the concern about the adverse consequences of direct reinfusion of unprocessed recovered blood. See Table 20-4.

Standards

If collected under aseptic conditions with a device that washes with normal saline and if properly labeled, blood collected by IBC may be stored. Storage may be at room temperature for up to 6 hours or at 1-6 C for up to 24 hours, provided that storage at 1-6 C is begun within 6 hours of initiating the collection.[9(p 37)] Proper labeling should include at a minimum the name and identifying number of the patient, the component name, the statement "For Autologous Use Only" and the expiration date and time. If the blood leaves the patient for cell washing in a remote location, appropriate procedures must be undertaken to ensure proper identification of the blood for the intended recipient.

Hospitals with IBC programs should establish written policies and procedures that are regularly reviewed by a physician who has been assigned responsibility for the conduct of the program. Transfusion medicine specialists should play an active role in design, implementation and activity of an IBC program. There must be written policy for the proper collection, labeling and storage of blood collected by IBC. Collection equipment and technique must ensure that the blood is aseptic. Periodic quality control testing of recovered blood is recommended. Such testing may include measurements of the sterility, the red cell mass recovered and the degree of hemolysis present. In addition, some programs may choose to monitor the amount of vacuum suction and the concentration of residual heparin (if used). Quality assurance for IBC focuses on the appropriate use of IBC services and adequate training of personnel.

Administrative Aspects

In addition to a responsible head for the IBC program, an adequate number of personnel should be specifically trained in the proper use of the collection equipment and handling of the collected blood. Most programs establish some system of coverage for off hours, weekends and holidays. Written protocols, procedure logs, machine maintenance procedures, procedures for handling adverse events and documentation are recommended.[14]

Postoperative Blood Collection

Postoperative blood collection (PBC) refers to the collection of blood from surgical drains and reinfusion with or without processing. PBC has been used after cardiac[72] and orthopedic surgery.[73] The contribution of PBC to overall blood conservation is generally less than that of preoperative blood donation or IBC techniques.[74-76] In some programs, postoperative shed blood is collected into sterile canisters and directly reinfused through a microaggregate filter without further processing. Blood collected by PBC is dilute, partially hemolyzed and has undergone clotting and lysis prior to collection. The concentration of fibrin degradation products is elevated in shed mediastinal blood and can cause measurable levels in the patient postinfusion.[77] Most programs choose to set upper limits on the quantity of PBC blood that can be reinfused without processing. Because of the possibility of bacterial contamination, PBC blood should be either reinfused or discarded within 6 hours of collection. Hospitals with PBC programs need to establish written policies, procedures, labeling requirements, quality assurance and review consistent with AABB *Standards*.

References

1. Toy P, Strauss RG, Stehling LC, et al. Predeposited autologous blood for elective surgery: A national multicenter study. N Engl J Med 1987;316:517-20.
2. The National Blood Resource Education Program Expert Panel. The use of autologous blood. JAMA 1990;263:414-7.
3. Breyer RH, Engelman RM, Rousou JA, Lemeshow S. Blood conservation for myocardial revascularization: Is it cost effective? J Thorac Cardiovasc Surg 1987;93:512-22.
4. Dietrich W, Barankay A, Dilthey G, et al. Reduction of blood utilization during myocardial revascularization. J Thorac Cardiovasc Surg 1989;97:213-9.
5. Goulet JA, Bray TJ, Timmerman LA, et al. Intraoperative autologous transfusion in orthopedic patients. J Bone Joint Surg [Am] 1989;71:3-8.
6. Turner RH, Capozzi JD, Kim A, et al. Blood conservation in major orthopedic surgery. Clin Orthop 1990;256:299-305.
7. Owings DV, Kruskall MS, Thurer RL, Donovan LM. Autologous blood donations prior to elective cardiac surgery - Safety and effect on subsequent blood use. JAMA 1989;262:1963-8.
8. Axelrod FB, Pepkowitz SH, Goldfinger D. Establishment of a schedule of optimal preoperative collection of autologous blood. Transfusion 1989;29:677-80.
9. Widmann FK, ed. Standards for blood banks and transfusion services. 15th ed. Bethesda, MD: American Association of Blood Banks, 1993.
10. Anderson BV, Tomasulo PA. Current autologous transfusion practices: Implications for the future. Transfusion 1988;28:394-6.
11. Maffei LM, Thurer RL, eds. Autologous blood transfusion: Current issues. Arlington, VA: American Association of Blood Banks, 1988.
12. Simon TL, Smith KJ. The issues in autologous transfusion. Hum Pathol 1989;20:3-6.
13. Chambers LA, Kruskall MS. Preoperative autologous blood donation. Transfus Med Rev 1990;4:35-46.
14. Autologous Transfusion Committee. Guidelines for blood salvage and reinfusion in surgery and trauma. Arlington, VA: American Association of Blood Banks, 1990.
15. Sandler SG, Silvergleid AJ, eds. Autologous transfusion. Arlington, VA: American Association of Blood Banks, 1983.
16. Toy P. Preoperative autologous blood donation. In: Rossi EC, Simon TL, Moss GS, eds. Principles of transfusion medicine. Baltimore, MD: Williams and Wilkins, 1991:401-4.
17. Silvergleid AJ. Autologous, directed and home transfusion programs. In: Petz LD, Swisher SN, eds. Clinical practice of transfusion medicine, 2nd ed. New York: Churchill Livingstone, 1989:327-44.
18. Kruskall M. Autologous blood collection and transfusion in a tertiary care center. In: Taswell HF, Pineda AA, eds. Autologous transfusion and hemotherapy. Boston: Blackwell Scientific, 1991:53-77.
19. McVay PA, Andrews A, Kaplan EB, et al. Donation reactions among autologous donors. Transfusion 1990;30:249-52.
20. Biesma DH, Kraaijenhagen RJ, Poortman J, et al. The effect of oral iron supplementation on erythropoiesis in autologous blood donors. Transfusion 1992;32:162-5.
21. Adamson J, Hillman RS. Blood volume and plasma protein replacement following acute blood loss in normal men. JAMA 1968;205:609-12.
22. Silvergleid AJ. Safety and effectiveness of predeposit autologous transfusions in preteen and adolescent children. JAMA 1987;257:3403-4.
23. Sayers MH. Controversies in transfusion medicine. Autologous blood donation in pregnancy: Con. Transfusion 1990;30:172-4.
24. Kruskall MS. Controversies in transfusion medicine. The safety and utility of autologous donations by pregnant patients: Pro. Transfusion 1990;30:168-71.
25. Meryman HT, Hornblower M. Freezing and deglycerolizing sickle-trait red blood cells. Transfusion 1976;16:627-32.
26. Chaplin H, Mischeaux JR, Inkster MD, Sherman LA. Frozen storage of 11 units of sickle cell red cells for autologous transfusion of a single patient. Transfusion 1986;26:341-5.
27. Mann M, Sacks HJ, Goldfinger D. Safety of autologous blood donation prior to elective surgery for a variety of potentially "high risk" patients. Transfusion 1983;23:229-32.
28. Dzik WH, Fleisher AG, Ciavarella D, et al. Safety and efficacy of autologous blood donation prior to elective aortic valve replacement. Ann Thorac Surg 1992;54:1177-81.
29. Sandler SG, Sacher RA. Preoperative autologous blood donations by high-risk patients. Transfusion 1992;32:1-2.
30. Goodnough LT, Brittenham GM. Limitations of the erythropoietic response to serial phlebotomy: Implications for autologous blood donor programs. J Lab Clin Med 1990;115:28-35.
31. Goodnough LT, Wasman J, Corlucci K, Chernosky A. Limitations to donating adequate autologous blood prior to elective orthopedic surgery. Arch Surg 1989;124:494-6.
32. Graf H, Watzinger U, Ludvik B, et al. Recombinant human erythropoietin as adjuvant

treatment for autologous blood donation. BMJ 1990;300:1627-8.

33. Goodnough LT, Rudnick S, Price TH, et al. Increased preoperative collection of autologous blood with recombinant human erythropoietin therapy. N Engl J Med 1989;321:1163-8.

34. Avoy DR. Private enterprise, nontraditional blood banking. In: Garner RJ, Silvergleid AJ, eds. Autologous and directed blood programs. Arlington, VA: American Association of Blood Banks, 1987:65-76.

35. Giordano GF, Giordano GF Jr, Rivers SL, et al. Determinants of homologous blood usage utilizing autologous platelet-rich plasma in cardiac operations. Ann Thorac Surg 1989;47:897-902.

36. Jones JW, McCoy TA, Rawitscher RE, et al. Effects of intraoperative plasmapheresis on blood loss in cardiac surgery. Ann Thorac Surg 1990;49:585-90.

37. Klapper E, Capon S, Jacobs A, et al. Postoperative infusion of autologous platelets in cardiac surgery (abstract). Transfusion 1991;31(Suppl):59S.

38. Silberstein LE, Williams LJ, Hughlett MA, et al. An autologous fibrinogen-based adhesive for use in otologic surgery. Transfusion 1988;28:319-21.

39. Messmer K. Preoperative hemodilution. In: Rossi EC, Simon TL, Moss GS, eds. Principles of transfusion medicine. Baltimore, MD: Williams and Wilkins, 1991:405-9.

40. Stehling L, Zauder HL. Acute normovolemic hemodilution. Transfusion 1991;31:857-68.

41. Ness PM, Bourke DL, Walsh PC. A randomized trial of perioperative hemodilution vs transfusion of preoperatively deposited autologous blood in elective surgery. Transfusion 1992;32:226-30.

42. Martin E, Hansen E, Peter K. Acute limited normovolemic hemodilution: A method for avoiding homologous transfusion. World J Surg 1987;11:53-9.

43. Lundsgaard-Hansen P. Hemodilution: New clothes for an anemic emperor. Vox Sang 1979;36:321-36.

44. Manno CS, Hedberg KW, Kim HC, et al. Comparison of hemostatic effects of fresh whole blood, stored whole blood, and components after open heart surgery in children. Blood 1991;77:930-6.

45. Mohr R, Martinowitz U, Lavee J, et al. The hemostatic effect of transfusing fresh whole blood versus platelet concentrates after cardiac operations. J Thorac Cardiovasc Surg 1988;96:530-4.

46. Tuma RF, White JV, Messmer K. The role of hemodilution in optimal patient care. Munich: Zuckschwerdt Verlag, 1989.

47. Klovekorn WP, Richter J, Sebening F. Hemodilution in coronary bypass operations. Bibl Haematol 1981;47:297-302.

48. Baron JF, Vicaut E, Duvelleroy M. Limits of hemodilution in patients with coronary artery disease. In: Vincent JL, ed. Update in intensive care and emergency medicine. Eighth International Symposium on Intensive Care and Emergency Medicine. Berlin: Springer-Verlag, 1988:32-9.

49. Cutler BS. Avoidance of homologous transfusion in aortic operations. The role of autotransfusion, hemodilution, and surgical technique. Surgery 1984;6:717-23.

50. Vara-Thorbeck R, Guerrero-Fernandez Marcote JA. Hemodynamic response of elderly patients undergoing major surgery under moderate normovolemic hemodilution. Eur Surg Res 1985;17:372-6.

51. Rose D, Coutsoftides T. Intraoperative normovolemic hemodilution. J Surg Res 1981;31:375-81.

52. Zetterstrom H, Wiklund L. A new nomogram facilitating adequate haemodilution. Acta Anaesthesiol Scand 1986;30:300-4.

53. Messmer K, Kreimeier U, Intaglietta M. Present state of intentional hemodilution. Eur Surg Res 1986;18:254-63.

54. Stehling L, ed. Perioperative autologous transfusion. Arlington, VA: American Association of Blood Banks, 1991.

55. Dzik WH, Sherburne B. Intraoperative blood salvage: Medical controversies. Transfus Med Rev 1990;4:208-35.

56. Williamson KR, Taswell HF. Intraoperative blood salvage: A review. Transfusion 1991;31:662-75.

57. McCarthy PM, Popovsky MA, Schaff HV, et al. Effect of blood conservation efforts in cardiac operations at the Mayo Clinic. Mayo Clin Proc 1988;63:225-9.

58. Thurer RL. Blood conservation in cardiac operations. Mayo Clin Proc 1988;63:292-3.

59. Hallett JW, Popovsky M, Ilstrup D. Minimizing blood transfusion during abdominal aortic surgery: Recent advances in rapid autotransfusion. J Vasc Surg 1987;5:601-6.

60. Clifford PC, Kruger AR, Smith A, et al. Salvage autotransfusion in aortic surgery: Initial studies using a disposable reservoir. Br J Surg 1987;74:755-7.

61. Bovill DF, Moulton CW, Jackson WST, et al. The efficacy of intraoperative autologous transfusion in major orthopedic surgery: A regression analysis. Orthopedics 1986;9:1403-7.

62. Klimberg I, Sirois R, Wajsman Z, Baker J. Intraoperative autotransfusion in urologic oncology. Arch Surg 1986;121:1326-9.

63. Hart OJ, Klimberg IW, Wajsman Z, Baker J. Intraoperative autotransfusion in radical cystectomy for carcinoma of the bladder. Surg Gynecol Obstet 1989;168:302-6.

64. Jurkovich GJ, Moore EE, Medina G. Autotransfusion in trauma: A pragmatic analysis. Am J Surg 1984;184:782-5.

65. Timberlake GA, McSwain NE. Autotransfusion of blood contaminated by enteric contents: A potentially life-saving measure in the massively hemorrhaging trauma patient? J Trauma 1988;28:855-7.

66. Merrill BS, Mitts DL, Rogers W, Weinberg PC. Autotransfusion: Intraoperative use in ruptured ectopic pregnancy. J Reprod Med 1980;24:14-6.

67. Silva PD, Beguin EA. Intraoperative rapid autologous blood transfusion. Am J Obstet Gynecol 1989;160:1226-7.

68. Williamson KR, Taswell HF, Rettke SR, Krom RA. Intraoperative autologous transfusion: Its role in orthotopic liver transplantation. Mayo Clin Proc 1989;64:340-5.

69. The Watchtower Bible and Tract Society. Questions from readers. The Watchtower 1989;110:30-1.

70. Hart OJ, Klimberg IW, Wajsman Z, Baker J. Intraoperative autotransfusion in radical cystectomy for carcinoma of the bladder. Surg Gynecol Obstet 1989;165:302-6.

71. Stanton PE, Shannon J, Rosenthal D, et al. Intraoperative autologous transfusion during major aortic reconstructive procedures. South Med J 1987;80:315-9.

72. Lane TA. Blood salvage in cardiovascular surgery. In: Stehling L, ed. Perioperative autologous transfusion. Arlington, VA: American Association of Blood Banks, 1991:67-83.

73. Semkiw LB, Schurman DJ, Goodman SB, Woolson ST. Postoperative blood salvage using the Cell Saver after total joint arthroplasty. J Bone Joint Surg 1988;71:823-7.

74. Johnson RG. Postoperative salvage. In: Maffei LM, Thurer RL, eds. Autologous blood transfusion: Current issues. Arlington, VA: American Association of Blood Banks, 1988:57-67.

75. Lepore V, Radegram K. Autotransfusion of mediastinal blood in cardiac surgery. Scand J Thorac Cardiovasc Surg 1989;23:47-9.

76. Page R, Russell GN, Fox MA, et al. Hard shell cardiotomy reservoir for reinfusion of shed mediastinal blood. Ann Thorac Surg 1989;48:514-7.

77. Griffith LD, Billman GF, Daily PO, Lane TA. Apparent coagulopathy caused by infusion of shed mediastinal blood and its prevention by washing of the infusate. Ann Thorac Surg 1989;47:400-6.

21

Safety

Introduction

Preventing disability and death is the objective of all safety programs and must become a primary goal of every employer/employee team. Unfortunately, prevention is a complex process involving the timely completion of several tasks. Significant among them is the successful identification and removal of hazardous conditions or the nullification of the risks they pose through effective communication, proper training and the provision and use of protective equipment. Also of importance is the need to identify and change habitual behaviors in individuals who, due to the nature of their responsibilities, are at increased risk for injury or death.

Such tasks are difficult to accomplish especially when the risks or dangerous elements inherent in a given object or action are not easily perceived or, as is often the case with biohazardous material, cannot be seen. These essential tasks are almost impossible to accomplish in an environment that resists change.

A prevention mind set must become a part of the corporate attitude. There often persists a certain stubborn adherence to old ways—the very sort of arrogance that yields only to fiscal disasters or governmental intervention. These attitudes must change.

This chapter does not address all of the safety concerns present in blood centers and transfusion services. An alarm-

ing number of hazards that may be even more significant than biosafety, radiation or chemical exposure may threaten laboratory staff. For example, in an informal survey of 29 blood banking institutions conducted by the AABB Safety Committee, a total of 600 injury incidents reported during 1989 and 1990 could be grouped into the following specific categories: 1) puncture wounds; 2) cuts and abrasions; 3) injuries involving twisting, bending, lifting, pushing and pulling; 4) slips, trips and falls; 5) nonpuncture exposures; 6) impact injuries; 7) strains, sprains and bruises; 8) burns; 9) electric shock; 10) eye injuries and 11) vehicle collisions. It is clear that much consideration needs to be given to such "unexciting" safety issues as training employees in the proper use of tools and electrical equipment, lifting techniques, use of stairs, defensive driving and facility maintenance.

An awareness of biosafety issues has significantly increased since it became known that AIDS could be transmitted through exposure to blood or body fluids. However, the principles discussed in this chapter have their foundation in good laboratory practices that have been applied to varying degrees throughout health-related settings ever since Koch's postulates concerning infection were described. For nearly 25 years, there has been concern about hepatitis B virus (HBV) and, more recently, hepatitis C virus (HCV) transmission due to occupational exposure. Recent interest in and emphasis on biosafety have made hospitals and institutions employing healthcare workers more conscious of providing the necessary information and tools to staff for maintaining a safe work environment. These concerns, along with recent regulatory requirements of the Occupational Safety and Health Administration (OSHA),[1] have led to an increased need for documentation of safety program requirements and compliance with those requirements.

In this chapter the recommended measures described to minimize the potential risks of infection that are inherent in working with blood are outlined with the following assumptions in mind:

1. The ultimate responsibility for safety rests with both the employer and the employee; neither can be effective alone.

2. Biosafety technology will continue to evolve with increased knowledge about infectious agents and their control. Specific procedures frequently must be reevaluated as new information becomes available.

3. All blood should be handled as if potentially infectious; however, the general precautions described here are not proposed for handling very high risk materials such as virus cultures or blood known to be infected with HBV, human immunodeficiency virus (HIV-1/2) or other human retroviruses. Although patient samples will generally be considered more likely to be infectious than the blood from normal, healthy, prescreened donors who have denied having risk factors for hepatitis B and AIDS, the concept of "universal precautions" to prevent transmission of blood-borne infections as recommended by the Centers for Disease Control and Prevention (CDC) should be applied.[2] In

areas such as blood collection, however, where exposure to blood is unlikely if no open containers are handled, Biosafety Level 2 (see p 511) has not been rigidly enforced.

4. In addition to blood, other tissues and body fluids are known to be potentially infectious. Precautions similar to those outlined for blood are applicable. Solid organs and tissues used for transplantation may require additional procedures due to their complex structure and biology.

5. Likewise, equipment contaminated with blood may present special challenges beyond the scope of this general information. Whenever there is any doubt, it would be reasonable to apply the more stringent criteria.

6. Every workplace has unique features. The biosafety precautions described here must be tailored to meet the individual needs of each establishment. This chapter is intended to serve as background to assist in developing standard operating procedures (SOPs); it should not be construed as an SOP manual itself.

7. In blood banks or transfusion services there are many safety concerns besides biosafety. Chemical hazards and radiation safety are also briefly discussed. A comprehensive safety program will consider all of the occupational hazards, including those discussed in this chapter.

8. Many of the principles abstracted here assume an understanding of laboratory operation and infection control objectives. It is highly recommended that the key references be read in their entirety to ensure a more thorough and accurate background for proper design and implementation of a safety program.

9. Federal requirements in place, and proposed rules published before July 1992, were considered in developing

these recommendations. However, the CDC, OSHA, the Food and Drug Administration (FDA) and the Environmental Protection Agency (EPA) all have an interest in biosafety and many policies continue to evolve. It will be necessary for each laboratory to stay abreast of current federal requirements as well as any state or local regulations that may apply. The references and Table 21-1 may be helpful in identifying information sources and applicable regulations.

10. Throughout this chapter, the general term "blood" is defined to include any part of human blood or blood components. Not all blood-derived products and reagents prepared from human blood require the same precautions if virus inactivation procedures have eliminated their potential infectivity. This is particularly pertinent to shipping requirements for FDA-regulated products that are exempt from the general requirements for shipping clinical specimens.[3]

The term "staff" is interpreted here to include all persons performing tasks at a work site, whether or not they are paid workers or volunteers.

4. A surveillance program that addresses confidentiality issues and includes reporting, investigating, documenting laboratory incidents and counseling of exposed persons. Programs for periodic routine collection or testing of serum specimens from staff (serum banks), if deemed appropriate as part of surveillance programs, require careful planning and appropriate employee consent.

The safety program development should take into account the procedures that will be used to monitor compliance and the corrective action plan, as well as any punitive consequences for staff who fail to comply. Periodic surveys of all areas where work is conducted should be performed by designated safety professionals to update procedures and document safe practice. A designated person should have specific responsibility for the occupational safety and health program within each institution. The flow of information and data should be defined in detail and management review specified. The findings and recommendations of surveys and reviews should be part of the records maintained.[4]

Overview of Safety Program Development

Every institution should develop a comprehensive safety program that includes special consideration of infection control, chemical hazards and radiation safety. The goals of this part of the safety program should provide for:

1. Appropriate facilities and equipment, and the proper maintenance of both.
2. Safe practices and procedures.
3. Identification of staff at risk and development of programs to educate and train these persons prior to exposure.

Terminology

Biosafety terminology can be confusing. Early publications referred to OSHA Categories I, II and III as a classification of risk levels of tasks performed by employees. Public Health Service (PHS) Biosafety Levels 1, 2 and 3 describe the relative risk that may be encountered in a work area. These definitions must be kept separate because an OSHA "Category I" task is the *most* dangerous, but a PHS "Biosafety Level 1" area is the *least* threatening. The references should be consulted for a complete understanding of these subjects, but the brief descrip-

Table 21-1. Safety Resources*

Centers for Disease Control and Prevention
Health and Biosafety Branch
1600 Clifton Road NE, MS F05
Atlanta, GA 30333
(404) 639-3238
FAX: (404) 639-2294

Department of Agriculture
APHIS
Federal Bldg. Rm 754
6505 Bellcrest Road
Hyattsville, MD 20782
(301) 436-7815

Department of Transportation
Office of Hazardous Materials Standards
Research and Special Programs
Administration
400 7th Street, SW
Washington, DC 20590
(202) 366-4488

Environmental Protection Agency
Office of Solid Waste
Special Programs Section
Mail Code OS 332
401 M Street, SW
Washington, DC 20460
(800) 424-9346
(703) 920-9810

Division of Blood Collection and Processing
  HFM-350
Center for Biologics Evaluation and Research
Food and Drug Administration
1401 Rockville Pike, Suite 200N
Rockville, MD 20852-1448
(301) 227-6700

International Air Transportation Association
2000 Peel Street
Montreal, Quebec
Canada H3A 2R4
(514) 844-6311

International Civil Aviation Organization
1000 Sherbrook Street W
Montreal, Quebec
Canada H3A 2R2
(514) 285-8219

National Committee for Clinical Laboratory
  Standards
771 East Lancaster Avenue
Villanova, PA 19085
(215) 525-2435

National Institutes of Health
Division of Safety
Safety Operations Section
Bld. 13, Rm. 3K04
Bethesda, MD 20892
(301) 496-2346
(301) 496-3353 (import/export)

National Institute for Occupational Safety and
  Health
Robert A. Taft Laboratory
4676 Columbia Parkway
C14
Cincinnati, OH 45226
(800) 356-4674

Nuclear Regulatory Commission
Region 1
475 Allandale Road
King of Prussia, PA 19406
(215) 337-5000

Occupational Safety and Health Administration
Office of Information Consumer Affairs
US Department of Labor
Room N-3647
200 Constitution Avenue, NW
Washington, DC 20210
(202) 523-8151
(202) 523-8061 (Standards)
(202) 523-7725 (Inspections)

US Postal Service
Office of Safety and Health
475 L'Enfant Plaza
Rm. 9301
Washington, DC 20260
(202) 268-3692

*Information current as of March 1993.

tions below will help in recalling the terminology.[3-7(p11-21)]

OSHA Categories

Although now obsolete, OSHA categories for risk levels of tasks performed by employees provide useful classification when planning training programs for staff:

Category I:
Tasks that involve exposure to blood, body fluids or tissues.
Category II:
Tasks that involve no exposure to blood, body fluids or tissues, but employment may require performing unplanned Category I tasks.
Category III:
Tasks that involve no exposure to blood, body fluids or tissues.

PHS Biosafety Levels

PHS biosafety levels of risk that may be encountered in a work area are:

Level 1:
Work that involves agents of no known or of minimal potential hazard to laboratory personnel and the environment.
Level 2:
Work that involves agents of moderate potential hazard to personnel and the environment. Note: Most work with blood requires Biosafety Level 2 precautions. Exceptions may be appropriate if no open specimens will be encountered.
Level 3:
Work that involves indigenous or exotic agents that may cause serious or potentially lethal disease as a result of exposure by inhalation.

Protection of Personnel

Safety programs should include consideration of the needs of all persons who may be affected by the work environment. Although the most obvious consideration is usually the safety of technical staff, the potential risks for ancillary personnel, volunteers, visitors, housekeeping, maintenance and repair staff must also be evaluated and appropriate provisions applied if they cannot be protected by exclusion from the risk area.[1]

The CDC has made recommendations for "universal precautions for prevention of transmission of HIV, HBV, and other blood-borne pathogens in healthcare settings."[2] These recommendations apply to the handling of blood and body fluids from *all* patients regardless of their blood-borne infection status. Since no distinction is made in these CDC recommendations between patients known to be infected and others, the precautions included are intended to be adequate for all routine practices. Blood units from persons with negative test results for HBsAg and anti-HIV-1/2 may transmit infection through transfusion or accidental inoculation of personnel. The "universal precautions" are believed to be a safe approach to infection prevention because employees can follow a single standard, and errors in correctly assessing patient status will not adversely affect employee safety. The "universal precautions" do acknowledge the difference between hospital patients and healthy donors, however, because the prevalence of infectious disease markers is significantly lower in the latter group. Some blood banks, therefore, have modified the precautions for low risk tasks where blood exposure is not expected, eg, in performing donor phlebotomies.

Training

It is essential that programs be tailored to the target group, both in level and content. General background knowledge of biohazards, work experience or understanding of control procedures is never assumed to fulfill the requirement for specific training, although an assessment of such knowledge is a first step in planning program content. The frequency of training updates will depend on many factors but must reflect at a minimum any changes in work environment and any important new knowledge of hazards.

The mandate for employee training programs not only is based on good practice, but also reflects OSHA requirements.[1,6,8] Every employer must evaluate the work conditions and tasks that workers are expected to encounter and identify the exposure category of each employee's tasks. Persons who may encounter blood, tissue or body fluids in their work must have prior training that enables them to appropriately protect themselves.

The OSHA training and education recommendations state that the employer should establish an initial and periodic training program for all employees who perform tasks with infectious exposure risk.[6] Workers should not engage in any task that places them at risk before receiving training pertaining to the SOPs, work practices and protective equipment for that task. The training program should ensure that all workers:

1. Understand the modes and rates of transmission of HBV and HIV, and the consequences of HIV and HBV infection.

2. Can recognize and differentiate tasks that pose infectious risk from other duties.

3. Know the types of protective clothing and equipment generally appropriate for procedures that may expose the employee to the risk of infection and understand the basis for selection of clothing and equipment.

4. Know the appropriate actions to take and persons to contact if unplanned

exposure to blood or other potentially infectious materials occurs.

5. Are familiar with and understand the requirements for work practice and protective equipment specified in SOPs covering the tasks they perform.

6. Know where protective clothing and equipment are kept, how to use them properly and how to remove, handle, decontaminate and dispose of contaminated clothing or equipment.

7. Know and understand the limitation of protective clothing and equipment. For example, ordinary gloves offer no protection against needlestick injuries. Employers and workers should be forewarned against sense of security that is not warranted by the use of protective equipment.

8. Know the corrective actions to take in the event of spills or personal exposure to fluids or tissues, the appropriate reporting procedures and the medical monitoring recommended in cases of suspected parenteral exposure.

Restricted Work Areas

Concerns for safety as well as requirements for maintaining an environment where errors are minimized dictate that casual visitors be eliminated from areas where blood may be encountered.[7(p11-21),9] In addition, Biosafety Level 2, which applies wherever open blood specimens are handled, requires that visitors be excluded from the work area at all times.

Volunteers are considered "staff" and require at least as much safety training as paid staff performing similar functions. More frequent training may be necessary because volunteers may be less aware of hazards if infrequently involved. Children must be closely supervised whenever they are present. Even the blood of a parent may be potentially infectious, and children should not be allowed in areas where they could be exposed to blood or other hazards.

Staff on the premises where blood is handled who are not normally assigned to tasks that include potential exposure to blood should receive enough training to avoid placing themselves at risk in case of an error or accident involving blood or by entering a restricted work area.[4(p72-4),5] Whenever possible, functions not requiring special precautions should be clearly separated from those that require a restricted area. For example, all nonessential clerical work should be removed from the laboratory area.

Specific training programs should be designed for housekeeping personnel. They should understand when to refuse assignments or to raise questions concerning hazards they may occasionally encounter if errors occur in their work situation. Biosafety Level 2 areas should be cleaned only by fully trained, technically competent personnel or by persons under the direct supervision of technically competent staff.

Equipment to be repaired or scheduled for preventive maintenance, if potentially exposed to blood, must be decontaminated before release to a repair technician. Maintenance personnel should have appropriate training in recognition and control of hazards as well as authority to refuse hazardous work.

Employee Performance

Applicable safety procedures should be reviewed with every new employee at the time of orientation and training prior to workplace exposure. The employee's understanding and application of all necessary precautions should be documented in writing by a supervisor before independent work is permitted. Any temporary work assignments must also include prior safety training if any significant differences exist in potential hazards. Periodic performance evaluations should include rating the employee's adherence to standard safety procedures.

Supervisory personnel must monitor safety practices in their areas of responsibility. Continuing attention to safety issues should be reflected in routine staff meetings and training sessions. Periodic audits performed by a safety professional are recommended.

Written warnings should be issued and recorded when the rules are broken. The corporate discipline policy should be explained to all staff and applied consistently to each infraction.

Specific Prophylaxis

All employees routinely exposed to blood should be offered hepatitis B vaccine if they do not already have HBV antibodies. Pretesting for antibody cannot be required of the employee. The CDC has published recommendations for both pre- and postexposure prophylaxis.[10] Hepatitis B immune globulin (HBIG) is usually given concurrently with hepatitis B vaccine postexposure to penetrating injuries. When administered in accordance with the manufacturer's directions, both products are very safe and have been proven free of any risk for infection with HBV and HIV.[11] OSHA requires that persons at risk be offered hepatitis B vaccine at no cost to the employee.

Medical Follow-up and Records of Accidental Exposure

When requested by the worker, monitoring for HBV and HIV antibodies following known or suspected parenteral exposure must be provided free of charge along with appropriate counseling. The usual schedule would include immediate tests on the source of the potentially infectious material and the worker, and follow-up on the worker at intervals after exposure.[10,12] Informed consent is required for this voluntary testing.

All aspects of accident follow-up should be appropriately documented, including the employee's rejection of testing, if applicable.

Personal Injury Investigations

When investigating cases of personal injury, investigators should not give the impression that they are attempting to fix blame. Otherwise, an attitude of "covering up" may develop, which would make it difficult or impossible to get all the facts. Whenever possible, the first report of injury should include[13]:

- Name and address of the injured person.
- Time of the accident (hour, day, month, year).
- Specific place where the accident occurred.
- Details of the injured person's activities at the time of injury.
- Nature of injury (bruise, laceration, burn, etc).
- Part of the body injured (head, arm, leg, etc).
- Date the injured person stopped work.
- Date the injured person returned to work.
- Estimated cost of damage to property or to equipment.
- Injured person's statement of the events leading to the accident.
- Statement from witnesses.
- Cause of the accident.
- Corrective action taken or recommendations for corrective action.

In addition, the supervisor should complete the insurance company's accident report and investigation form.

OSHA requires that health services employers with 11 or more workers keep records of occupational injuries and illnesses. Logs, summaries and supplemental records (within 6 days of injury) are all required; they must be maintained for at least 5 years beyond the calendar year of occurrence.[14] Reports to OSHA of fatalities and of hospitalization of five or more employees are required.

Restrictions for Staff

HIV- or HBV-infected employees may safely perform many tasks provided they have no open lesions; each individual case should be considered on its own merits including concern for the potential risk to immunocompromised persons.[2] It is not considered necessary to exclude pregnant women from routine blood bank tasks unless hazardous chemicals or radiation exposure pose risks to the fetus.

General Considerations in Safety Programs

OSHA regulations protecting workers from blood-borne diseases were published December 6, 1991 and require employers to[1]:

- Provide a hazard-free workplace.
- Educate and train staff.
- Evaluate infectious exposure potential for all procedures.
- Determine worker potential for exposure.
- Implement labeling and post signs.
- Apply universal precautions for blood and body fluids.
- Provide personal protective equipment such as gloves or other barriers.
- Make available hepatitis B vaccine prophylaxis to all staff who have occupational exposure unless previously vaccinated or immune, and HBIG treatment for percutaneous injury.

Whenever possible the potential hazards should be eliminated by proper facility design, work organization and choice of procedures. This may not be completely possible in every situation, especially in mobile blood collection operations, and workable alternatives must be sought. An advance visit to the site by someone trained in safety considerations is necessary to ensure that threats are minimized.

Ready access to hand washing is essential at all blood collection sites. Any carpeted or difficult-to-clean surfaces will require an absorbent overlay with waterproof backing in any area where blood spills may occur.[7(p11-21)] Traffic flow may require restriction with portable screens or roping to maintain safe work areas. Food service areas should be clearly separated from blood collection and storage. All blood-contaminated trash must be returned to the central location or be packaged and incinerated by trained staff. Particular attention should be paid to postcollection cleanup of mobile sites. The training of personnel must include recognition of unsafe conditions and understanding of the objectives of infection control procedures. Site safety responsibility should be an assigned function of a senior level employee.

Housekeeping methods, schedule and responsibility should be clearly defined for every area. Good housekeeping reduces all potential hazards and is essential to minimizing biosafety concerns. Written procedures, personnel training and continuous monitoring of housekeeping effectiveness are all essential to safe operations.

Protective Clothing and Devices

It is the employer's obligation to ensure that appropriate protection is available at no cost to the employee.[1] In addition, the employer may be considered negligent if breaches of good laboratory practice are ignored when staff fail to follow prescribed procedures.

Uniforms and Laboratory Coats

Closed laboratory coats or full aprons over long-sleeved uniforms should be worn by all personnel routinely exposed to blood. The type of material required will vary depending upon whether tasks may result in large fluid spills that would be expected to soak the garment. Any obviously contaminated clothing should be removed immediately. Protective clothing should be removed before leaving the work area. Place soiled garments in appropriate bag and launder as potentially infectious. Home laundry of garments worn in a Biosafety Level 2 area is not permitted because of the added risk in unpredictable methods of transportation, handling and laundry options.[1] OSHA requires that the employer furnish personal protective equipment (PPE) and clothing, and clean, launder or dispose of PPE at no cost to the employee.

Masks, Safety Glasses or Face Shields

Whenever splashes of blood are likely, the eyes and the mucous membranes of the mouth and nose should be protected. If shields are worn for long periods of time, they should be changed periodically. Permanent shields fixed in place are preferable when equipment use permits this, eg, splash barrier above dielectric tubing sealer or centrifuge cabinets. Such shields should be cleaned and disinfected on a regular schedule by technical staff.

Biological Safety Cabinets (BSC)

Biological safety cabinets are containment devices that facilitate safe manipulation of infectious materials and reduce the risk to personnel and the laboratory environment.[15] A vertical laminar flow cabinet is an example of a BSC that protects both the worker and the material handled.[7(p94-95)] Blood bank procedures that would appropriately be done in a BSC include centrifugation of open blood samples or manipulation of units known to be positive for HBsAg or anti-HIV, although BSCs are not a required part of universal precautions.

The National Institutes of Health recommends the following for effective use of biological safety cabinets.[15]

General Suggestions

1. Keep the laboratory meticulously clean. Minimize storage of boxes and supplies, particularly near the BSC.
2. Wash hands thoroughly before and after working in a BSC. Wear a clean lab coat and gloves while working in a BSC to increase safety and help reduce contamination of research materials.
3. The effectiveness of the BSC is a function of directional airflow (inward and downward, through a high efficiency filter). Anything that disrupts the airflow pattern reduces cabinet effectiveness, such as: rapidly moving arms in and out of the BSC; people walking rapidly behind the employee using the BSC; downdrafts from ventilation systems; open laboratory doors.
4. Understand how the cabinet works. Plan the work to be done in the BSC to provide maximal protection for the worker, the material and any coworkers.

BSC Operational Suggestions

1. Turn on the BSC. Wipe work surface with 70% EtOH. Wipe off each item needed for the procedures and place in the cabinet. Allow the cabinet to run at least 5 minutes before beginning work.
   a. *DO NOT* place anything over the front air intake grill; *DO NOT* block the rear exhaust grill.
   b. Arrange materials to segregate contaminated and clean items. Minimize movement of contaminated items over clean ones. Remember, "work from clean to dirty."
   c. Perform work at least six inches back from the front air intake grill.
2. Put on clean lab coat (wrap-around style with elastic wrists may be useful). Thoroughly wash hands and put on gloves, as appropriate.
3. Continue to follow good microbiological techniques, such as holding open tubes and bottles as horizontal as possible.
   a. Use convenient pipetting aids. Do not pipet by mouth.
   b. Use horizontal discard pans containing appropriate disinfectant inside the BSC. Do not use vertical pipet discard canisters on floor outside cabinet.
   c. It is not necessary to flame items. The flame creates turbulence in airflow and will compromise sterility; heat buildup may damage the filters.
4. If it is necessary to remove items from the BSC or introduce new items, move arms slowly in and out of the cabinet to minimize disruption of the airflow.
5. If a piece of equipment is used that creates air turbulence in the BSC (such as a centrifuge, blender, sonicator), place the equipment in the back 1/3 of the cabinet; stop other work while equipment is operating.
6. Protect the building vacuum system from biohazards by placing a cartridge filter between the vacuum

trap and the source valve in the cabinet (eg, Pall Ultipor® DFA 3001 AXPK5 or equivalent).

7. Clean up all spills in the cabinet immediately. Wait 3-5 minutes before resuming work if procedures allow.

8. Remove all materials and wipe all interior surfaces with 70% alcohol when work is finished. Let cabinet run 10 minutes, turn off. Examine the tray under the work surface, and disinfect and clean as necessary.

9. Discard waste materials appropriately (eg, autoclave or incinerate).

10. Remove lab coat and wash hands thoroughly before leaving laboratory.

Hand Washing

Frequent effective handwashing is the first line of defense in infection control. The blood-borne pathogens of concern generally do not penetrate intact skin; thus, immediate removal helps prevent spread to others or transfer to a mucous membrane or broken skin area.

Hands should always be washed before leaving a restricted work area, before using the BSC, between medical examinations, immediately after soiling with blood, after removing gloves or finger cots, and after using the toilet. Routine donor phlebotomy does not require gloves, or changing of unsoiled gloves between donors if gloves are worn. The effectiveness of hand wipe disinfectants or sanitizing pledges has not been demonstrated as a safe alternative to hand washing.

Eye Wash

Laboratory areas that contain chemicals toxic to the eye must be equipped with eye wash devices. Procedures for use in case of accidents must be posted and routine maintenance checks should ensure safe operation. Employees should be trained in the proper use of eye wash

devices; however, protection through use of safety glasses or shields is preventive. Solutions other than water should be used only upon a physician's direction. The effectiveness of eye washing in preventing infection has not been demonstrated but is assumed to be desirable when accidents occur.

Gloves

Examination gloves or equivalent barriers should be used when tasks are likely to involve exposure to blood.[1,2] Staff should be aware of the potentially serious hazard resulting from latex hypersensitivities, and other potential allergic responses to glove materials. According to OSHA standards, phlebotomists working with healthy prescreened donors do not routinely require gloves, because experience has demonstrated that donors have low rates of infectious disease markers, exposure to blood during most phlebotomies is very rare and other effective barrier alternatives suited to the task are available.[1] For example, when removing a needle from a donor's arm, the minimal blood flow expected can be controlled effectively with a suitable gauze pad.

The CDC recommendations for prevention of transmission of blood-borne pathogens include the following general guidelines for determining when gloves are necessary[2]:

1. Use gloves for performing phlebotomy when the health-care worker has cuts, scratches or other breaks in his/her skin.

2. Use gloves in situations where the health-care worker judges that hand contamination with blood may occur (eg, when performing phlebotomy on an uncooperative patient).

3. Use gloves for performing finger and/or heel sticks on infants and children.

4. Use gloves when persons are receiving training in phlebotomy.
5. Use gloves when handling any "open" blood container or specimen.
6. Use gloves when collecting or handling blood or samples from all patients, or from donors known to be infected with a blood-borne pathogen.
7. Use gloves when cleaning up spills or handling waste materials.
8. Use gloves when potential exposure cannot be assessed because of lack of experience with a procedure or situation.
9. Use gloves when examining mucous membranes or open lesions.

Institutions with policies and procedures that do not require routine gloving for all phlebotomies should periodically reevaluate the potential need for gloves. Employees should never be discouraged from using gloves, and gloves should always be available. Guidelines for the safe use of gloves include[1,4(p72-4)]:

1. Change gloves immediately if they are torn, punctured or contaminated, and after handling high risk samples or performing a physical examination (eg, on an apheresis donor).
2. Remove gloves by keeping outside surfaces in contact only with outside, and by turning the glove inside out as it is being removed from the hand.
3. Use gloves only where needed and avoid touching clean surfaces such as telephones, door knobs or computer terminals with gloves. It may be useful to designate "clean" telephones where no gloves are allowed. Work area phones can be equipped with speakers to eliminate the need to pick up the receiver.
4. Wash hands with soap after removing gloves.
5. Use sterile gloves for procedures involving contact with normally sterile areas of the body.
6. Use examination gloves for procedures involving contact with mucous membranes, unless otherwise indicated, and for other patient care or diagnostic procedures that do not require the use of sterile gloves.
7. Change gloves between patient contacts. Unsoiled gloves do not have to be changed between donors.
8. Do not wash or disinfect surgical or examination gloves for reuse. Washing with surfactants may cause "wicking" (ie, the enhanced penetration of liquids through undetected holes in the glove). Disinfecting agents may cause deterioration of gloves.
9. Use general purpose utility gloves (eg, rubber household gloves) for housekeeping chores involving potential blood contact and for instrument cleaning and decontamination procedures. Utility gloves may be decontaminated and reused but should be discarded if they are peeling, cracked or discolored, or if they have punctures, tears or other evidence of deterioration.

Procedures

All existing and new procedures should be evaluated with the objective of minimizing any potential infectious risks for donors, staff or the general public. This review should include identifying those tasks that require Biosafety Level 2 safeguards.

Biosafety Level 2 Summary

All blood should be handled as if it were infectious. All areas where blood is handled in open containers should conform to the following Biosafety Level 2 criteria.[7(p11-21)] Staff should have training in handling pathogenic agents, access to work areas should be restricted and procedures that create aerosols should be conducted in biological safety cabinets. The SOP manual should describe biosafety precautions, and biosafety SOP review by all staff should be documented.

Biosafety Level 2 Precautions[7(p11-21)]

Biosafety Level 2 precautions as applied in the blood establishment setting include at least the following:

1. Bench tops are constructed of non-absorbent material and work surfaces are decontaminated daily with an EPA-approved hospital disinfectant. [Although a freshly prepared dilution of household bleach (eg, 1:10 dilution of 5% sodium hypochlorite) is effective it may damage surfaces.] See section on Choice of Disinfectant, p 521.

2. Laboratory rooms have closable doors. A "one pass, in flow" air system with no recirculation is preferred, but not required. Sinks and waste decontamination facilities are available within the area. Procedures that may create aerosols (eg, opening evacuated tubes, centrifuging, mixing, sonicating) are contained within a BSC or equivalent, or workers wear masks and goggles in addition to gloves and gowns during such procedures. (See section on Protective Clothing and Devices p 515.) Open tubes of blood should not be centrifuged. Closed overwraps are recommended to contain leaks when centrifuging whole units of blood or plasma.

3. Gowns and gloves are used routinely. Staff with actively exudative skin lesions on the hands and arms are excluded unless lesions are securely bandaged. All staff wash their hands every time gloves are removed and after completing activities; protective clothing must be re-moved before leaving the work area for any reason.

4. No mouth pipetting is permitted.

5. All blood specimens must be placed in well-constructed containers with secure lids to prevent leaking during transport. All blood samples are packaged for shipment to others in accordance with CDC requirements for etiologic agents or clinical specimens, as appropriate.

6. Infectious waste is not compacted and is decontaminated before disposal in leakproof containers. Proper packaging includes double, seamless, tear-resistant, orange or red bags and protective cartons. The carton, as well as the bag inside, is labeled with the biohazard symbol and is handled only by trained personnel throughout delivery to an incinerator or autoclave. If a waste management contractor is used, the agreement should clearly define responsibilities of the staff and the contractor.

7. No eating, drinking, smoking or application of cosmetics or contact lenses occurs in the work area. All food and drink are stored separately outside the restricted area. Laboratory glassware is never used for food or drink. Personnel are instructed to avoid touching faces, ears, mouth, eyes or noses with hands or other objects such as pencils and telephones.

8. High risk activities are appropriately segregated from lower risk activities and the boundaries are clearly defined.

9. Extreme caution is used in handling and disposing of needles and syringes. Needles are never bent, broken, sheared, replaced in sheath or detached from syringe before being placed in puncture-proof, leakproof containers for controlled disposal.

Procedures are designed to minimize exposure to sharp objects.

10. Any accidental exposure to suspicious or actual hazardous material is reported to the laboratory director immediately.

Special Precautions

Some procedures are known to result in more frequent injury. Special attention should be given to finding alternatives, if possible, or providing extra training and protective devices to the staff performing functions such as using lancets for finger puncture, handling capillary tubes, crushing vials for arm disinfection, handling any unsheathed needle (including filling of pilot tubes or disposing of collection sets), cleaning scissors and giving mouth-to-mouth resuscitation.

Direct Patient Care

Blood bank staff may at times be involved in dealing with patients. These situations include autologous blood collection from persons who do not meet donor suitability criteria, therapeutic hemapheresis, therapeutic plasma exchange, therapeutic phlebotomy and intraoperative or postoperative red cell collection. The CDC recommends that gloves be worn routinely whenever exposure to a patient's blood or body fluids is possible. Avoid direct contact with blood as much as is feasible and follow the recommendations above for the safe use of gloves.

Known Infectious Donors

It is necessary in special circumstances (eg, autologous donors or vaccine production) to collect blood from donors known to be at high risk because of their behavior history or test results. FDA recommendations for collection of blood from high risk donors include[16]:

1. The informed consent acknowledges that blood collection and processing staff will be informed of any positive test results and that special biohazard labeling of the component will be required.

2. The procedure is performed away from normal, healthy donors by timing, or by use of a separate area.

3. Complete cleaning and disinfection of the area and all equipment used are performed after each procedure on a donor known to have positive hepatitis B surface antigen (HBsAg) or anti-HIV-1/2 test results.

4. Personnel wear protective gowns, gloves, masks and eye shields throughout all aspects of the donor processing.

5. Only closed, disposable systems with integrally attached satellite containers are used.

6. These components are stored separately from other blood components in double overwraps, which are sealed at all times.

7. Labeling, packaging and shipping complies with applicable CDC and Department of Transportation regulations for biohazardous materials.[17,18]

8. All disposable materials used are autoclaved or incinerated without undue delay under the supervision of trained staff.

9. Employees working with HBsAg-reactive donors are not permitted to waive HBV vaccination if they are not HBV antibody-positive.

10. The most recent FDA regulations and guidelines should be consulted for any changes or additions to these procedures. Additional donor protection precautions such as examination by the personal physician apply to serial apheresis programs.

Organ, Sperm and Tissue Banks

The Public Health Service has recommended that selection and testing procedures for organ, sperm and tissue donors be similar to those applied to blood donors. At a minimum, donors with risk factors should be excluded and tests for HBsAg, anti-HIV, anti-HCV, anti-HTLV-I and syphilis should be negative. In addition, whenever possible, the donated material should be stored frozen for at least 6 months (preferably 12) and the donor retested before the initial donated tissue is used. In critical situations, however, transplants may be performed in spite of positive results or without a waiting period when the relative risk justifies this medical decision.

If cadaveric donors are used, this retesting obviously cannot be done; however, any autopsy report available should be consulted. Whenever possible, processing should be delayed until test results and history are known. Workers should take special precautions to prevent cuts, especially when collecting or cleaning bones; heavy protective gloves may be appropriate.

Decontamination

All reusable equipment and surfaces that are contaminated with blood require daily cleaning and decontamination. Obvious spills should be cleaned up immediately and routine wipe-downs performed at the end of each shift or on some other regular basis that provides equivalent safety.

Choice of Disinfectants

In general, an EPA-approved hospital disinfectant is recommended. Consult EPA list for acceptable solutions.[19,20] Whenever there is organic material present, the effectiveness of the disinfectant is diminished; therefore, all surfaces should be superficially clean before disinfectant is applied. The length of contact time necessary for effective kill varies with the solution chosen.[21] Most solutions must be freshly diluted on a daily basis.

Spill Cleanup

Every facility handling blood should prepare in advance for the inevitable spills. This preparation includes at least the following elements:

1. Design work areas to permit easy cleanup.
2. Prepare a spill cart with instructions and all necessary supplies and equipment. Place such a cart near any areas where spills are anticipated.
3. Train all personnel who may be involved in cleanup and reporting of significant incidents.
4. Assign responsibility for cart maintenance, spill handling, record-keeping and review of significant incidents.

When blood spills occur, the following steps should be taken in the order listed[4]:

1. Leave the area for 30 minutes if an aerosol has been created. Remove clothing if it is contaminated. Post warnings to keep area clear. If spill occurs in the centrifuge, turn off power immediately and leave cover closed for 30 minutes. The use of overwraps helps prevent aerosols in the event of breakage.
2. Wear appropriate protective clothing and gloves; if sharp objects are involved, gloves must be puncture-resistant. [Note: OSHA may require use of instruments (eg, broom) to avoid cutting hands.[1]]
3. Totally cover the spill with absorbent paper. Remove the paper and any broken glass with brush and pan.

4. Clean with detergent.
5. Flood the area with 1:10 dilution of freshly made sodium hypochlorite (bleach) solution or other appropriate disinfectant, and let it stand for 15 minutes.
6. Wipe up the disinfectant.
7. Dispose all materials safely in accordance with biohazard guidelines. All blood-contaminated items require autoclaving or incineration.

Waste Management

It is essential that biosafety programs include appropriate training and procedures for handling waste that may be contaminated with blood or body fluids. Laboratory staff or other technically trained personnel must have the responsibility for identifying wastes that require special handling and disposal.

It will be necessary for the safety manager to design a waste management program that both adequately protects staff and meets federal, state and local regulatory requirements.[22] The principles described here will provide a basis for procedure development but will not provide enough detail to be used independently of a thorough understanding of safety objectives. Consult Table 21-1 for further resources in designing programs and resolving problems.

The first goal of any waste management program is to reduce the volume of hazardous material to be handled to an absolute minimum. Sometimes substitutions in techniques or materials give a less hazardous waste or reduce the volume of infectious waste. Consider all such options carefully and seek employee support in identifying safer alternatives wherever possible. Separate completely all noninfectious waste from infectious waste to reduce the volume of the latter. Employee training is absolutely essential; even packaged waste should not be left to chance with untrained personnel.

Hazardous waste, which may or may not be infectious, is defined as "a solid waste or a combination of solid wastes which because of its quantity, concentration, physical or chemical or infectious characteristics may pose a substantial or potential threat to human health or the environment when improperly treated, stored, transported or disposed of, or otherwise managed."[23] Infectious waste includes disposable equipment, utensils and articles or substances that may harbor or transmit pathogenic organisms from individuals who are suspected to have or have been diagnosed as having a communicable disease.[24,25]

Medical waste as defined by the EPA includes, but is not limited to, infectious waste.[22] Medical waste is any solid waste (including semisolids and liquids) generated in the diagnosis, treatment or immunization of human beings or animals in related research or production or testing of biologics.[26]

The EPA interprets infectious waste to include wastes that probably contain pathogenic organisms. Thirteen types of infectious waste appear in the EPA list:

1. Isolation wastes.
2. Cultures and stocks of etiologic agents.
3. Blood and blood products.
4. Pathologic wastes.
5. Other wastes from surgery and autopsy.
6. Contaminated laboratory wastes.
7. Sharps.
8. Dialysis unit wastes.
9. Animal carcasses and body parts.
10. Animal bedding and other waste from animal rooms.
11. Discarded biologics.
12. Contaminated food and other products.
13. Contaminated equipment.

Waste management program design should include attention to all applicable regulations, the types of waste and quantity of each, the availability of treatment equipment and alternatives (eg, autoclaves, incinerators), physical constraints, and capital and operational costs for necessary personnel, equipment and supplies.

Essential Precautions for Packaging Waste

The following basic precautions must be observed in whatever system is chosen to meet the needs of the institution:

1. Identify hazardous waste consistently; red or orange seamless plastic bags are recommended; always use the biohazard symbol.
2. Double bag or place in a protective container to preserve integrity when storing or transporting.
3. Discard sharps only in rigid, puncture-proof, leakproof containers.
4. Put liquids only in leakproof unbreakable containers.
5. Do not compact.
6. Use appropriate materials.

Treating Infectious or Medical Waste

At the present time, incineration or decontamination by autoclaving are the recommended disposal methods for blood samples and blood products. The following elements should be considered in any procedure:

1. Size of load being autoclaved.
2. Type of container/packaging of item(s) being autoclaved.
3. Density of item(s) being autoclaved.
4. Number of items in single load being autoclaved.
5. Placement of items(s) in the autoclave allowing for steam penetration.

Verification of the procedure can be addressed by placing a biological indicator in the center of loads varying in size and contents and evaluating the procedure for optimal steam penetration times.

Consult the EPA requirements for detailed information on equipment choice and operation.[24]

Any infectious material storage area must be secured to prevent accidents in handling. Generally, public trash collection is not a suitable means for disposal of raw infectious waste. Contracts with private carriers should include disclosure of the risks and specify the carrier's acknowledgment of an understanding of safety requirements.

Blood Storage

Concern for reducing infectious risk by maintaining a clean and orderly facility at all times extends to the blood storage area as well. Segregation of hazardous materials and clear demarcation of areas for different types of storage are required. Although blood itself is considered hazardous, it must also be protected from unnecessary exposure to other hazardous materials. Products for transfusion should be separated from reagents and pilot tubes as well as all unrelated materials. If a separate refrigerator is not available for blood component storage, extra care must be taken to reduce the likelihood of spills or other accidents and the areas within the refrigerator must be clearly segregated. No food or drink should be allowed anywhere in the area. No open containers should be permitted during storage or transportation. The type of container closure should be adequate to protect against spilling under the conditions that can reasonably be anticipated. Construction should be adequate for safely storing the maximum anticipated volumes and should facilitate easy and thorough cleaning. Surfaces should be kept clean and dry at all times. Any items that could result in punctures of containers should be removed from the area.

Transportation, Shipping and Labeling of Blood

All specimens, products and components should be superficially clean and should be placed in secure containers to prevent leakage during transport. Accompanying paperwork should be sealed in watertight pouches to prevent contamination if leaks occur.

Blood that is being transported from one location of an establishment to another by trained staff is considered to be under the control of the establishment. It does not require the same packaging and labeling as shipments made on common carriers. Deliveries of fully tested and labeled blood components without full protective packaging may also be made by trained staff. The following recommendations for shipping procedures apply to shipments handled by common carriers or personnel not under the direct authority of the shipper.[17,27,28]

Both tested and untested blood are potentially infectious materials. Current interpretation of the requirements for packaging and labeling shipments has permitted untested blood to be shipped without the special precautions applied to known etiologic agents.

Procedures for Shipment of Clinical Specimens

Clinical specimens and biological products that are reasonably believed not to contain an etiologic agent may be shipped with minimum packaging requirements.[28] Untested blood from healthy donors meeting all of the FDA donor suitability criteria are generally considered in this category and are

shipped without the extra packaging precautions mandated for known hazards.

The packaging of clinical specimens is the same as that for etiologic agents except that the special labeling and tertiary containers are unnecessary, and the 50 mL volume limit for etiologic agents does not apply. Primary and secondary containers must not contain more than 1 liter and the outer shipping container must not exceed 4 L. The contents (eg, clinical blood sample) should be noted on the shipping carton. See Method 1.1.

Suggested Self-Audit Biosafety Assessment

The following questions may serve as a first step in reviewing the compliance of a facility with currently accepted biosafety objectives:

1. Is there documentation of an appropriately leveled biosafety training program for all staff potentially exposed to blood-borne pathogens?
2. Is there appropriate segregation of potentially hazardous activity (eg, clearly designated Biosafety Level 2 for handling all open blood samples)?
3. Do written policies exist for reporting and follow-up of accidental exposure to blood if the skin barrier is breached, including:
   a. Serologic evaluation of source?
   b. HBIG prophylaxis if appropriate?
   c. Counseling and testing postexposure?
   d. Storage of employee sample?
4. Is there documentation of hepatitis B immunization (or written refusals) for all staff who will potentially be exposed to blood?
5. Do waste handling, labeling and disposal procedures ensure appropriate segregation and safe disposition of contaminated wastes?

6. Is PPE (eg, gloves) readily available to staff and does training program provide knowledge of appropriate use?
7. Is facility design, organization and housekeeping consistent with good biosafety procedure?
8. Is responsibility for biosafety programs clearly defined and are effective mechanisms for problem resolution available?
9. Are known infectious donors drawn? If yes, are procedures that meet FDA recommendations applied?

Chemical Hazards

The addition of several new tests for infectious disease markers has challenged the blood bank laboratory to provide appropriate training and procedures for the chemical hazards involved in performing these tests. Therefore, some of the basic elements of a chemical safety program are outlined here. As with biosafety, however, the reader is urged to consult the applicable state and federal regulations for a more complete description of requirements.[29]

Laboratory supervisors must monitor employee exposure and the procurement and storage of new chemicals, maintain a composite list of all hazardous chemicals in the laboratory [material safety data sheet, (MSDS)], conduct annual verification and updating and ensure that all staff are appropriately trained in the use of personal protective equipment and in applying the procedures pertinent to storage, handling, use and disposal of hazardous substances. Do not overlook as a resource the MSDS, which supplies critical information. The more specific instructions in the MSDS take precedence if there is any conflict with the generic information included here. See Appendix 21-1.

Operational Principles

1. Adequate physical facilities (especially ventilation) must be ensured relative to the work conducted and its scale.
2. Excess quantities of chemicals should be kept outside work areas and fume hoods. Observe volume limits for flammable solvents.
3. Lists of materials requiring higher level approval must be reviewed before beginning any new project.
4. Technical personnel must review written procedures and related safety precautions before beginning new tasks.

Chemical Labeling and Signs

Any solution containing a hazardous chemical must be prominently labeled with hazard identification at the time of preparation. Acids and alkalis should be labeled as caustic or corrosive. Skin absorption hazards must be identified.

Signs meeting OSHA requirements must be posted in any area where hazardous chemicals are used. Both alcohol and sodium hypochlorite (bleach) meet OSHA's definition of a hazard and require a sign.

Personal Protective Equipment

1. Appropriate, chemical-resistant neoprene gloves are recommended for handling concentrated acids and organic solvents.
2. Latex or vinyl gloves are adequate for handling most other chemicals and for specimens.
3. Goggles or face shields are necessary when pouring concentrated acids, alkalis or organic solvents; handling irritants, unstable or explosive materials; or when there is a risk of spraying (eg, reagent lines under pressure).

4. Masks should be worn whenever there is danger of inhalation. A simple, disposable dust mask is adequate for dry chemical transfers. A respirator with organic vapor filters is preferred for cleaning up spills of noxious materials.
5. Fume hoods must be available for use with organic solvents, volatile liquids and dry chemicals with significant inhalation hazard.
6. Showers and eyewashes must be available if caustic, corrosive, flammable or combustible liquids are used.
7. Protective gowns or lab coats should be worn at all times within the laboratory, but should not leave the laboratory.
8. Fire blankets and extinguishers should be readily available and all staff should be trained in their use.
9. Appropriate tongs and insulated gloves must be available for handling hot or frozen materials.
10. Spill cleanup kits tailored to the hazards present must be available in each area.
11. All safety equipment requires regular maintenance at documented intervals.

Disposal

Unless local regulations are in conflict, the following guidelines are to be followed for chemical disposal:

1. Nonmiscible organic liquids (not soluble in water), whether flammable or not, must *not* be poured down the drain. (Refer to the Flammable Solvents section for specific details.) Water-soluble organic liquids such as alcohol may be poured down the drain.
2. Water-reactive chemicals (eg, concentrated sodium hydroxide) must not be poured down the drain. Contact the manufacturer for disposal recommendations.
3. Radioactive reagents must not be poured down the drain except as approved by the facility's Nuclear Regulatory Commission (NRC) license. Refer to the CDC *Radiation Safety Manual* for specific details.
4. Carcinogens, corrosives, oxidizers, irritants, sensitizers and toxic chemicals may be generally discarded into the sanitary sewer system if they are water-soluble. Check local regulations, which vary widely, before disposing of any questionable material.

   Dilute and flush with copious amounts of water after dumping. If large volumes (eg, multiple jugs of concentrated acids) are involved, spread the disposal over several days. Wear goggles and gloves as appropriate if caustic solutions are involved. Pour slowly with water running so as to minimize splashing.
5. Water-soluble dry chemicals may be poured down the drain unless they are potentially toxic (eg, salts of heavy metals such as mercury, lead or cadmium). In such cases, commercial disposal may be needed. Consult with a chemist or the manufacturer.
6. Toxic dry chemicals may require commercial disposal. Consult with a chemist or the manufacturer.
7. Reagents containing sodium azide may be flushed down the drain with excess running water. Allow water to run for 2-3 minutes after disposal to clear the trap and lines of any chemical. Refer to p 527 for specific details.
8. Mercury should be collected in a plastic bottle for commercial disposal. Store in a fume hood if possible. Keep bottle tightly closed. Broken thermometers should have as much mercury removed as possible without creating increased risk due to handling. They should be placed in unbreakable containers, such as a plas-

tic bottle, and disposed of in the solid trash.

Acids, Alkalis and Corrosive Compounds

Strong acids and alkalis and certain other corrosive compounds can produce irritation, severe burns and tissue damage. During transport, large containers should be protected by plastic or rubber bucket carriers and small containers secured with both hands.

Pour with great care; eye protection is essential and gloves and gowns are recommended. Always add acid to water when diluting. Hold large jugs with one hand each on neck and base and position well away from face. Filling small-necked vessels requires a funnel or stirring rod, and intermediate transfer to a beaker is recommended if the stock bottle is large. Always wipe up spills immediately and wash hands promptly.

Concentrated acids should be stored in floor cabinets and local use volumes should be limited to 1 liter. Specific cautions for materials in the area should be posted. For example, perchloric acid may be explosive if yellowish or brown; notify a supervisor if liquid is not clear.

Acrylamide

Acrylamide is on the list of "cancer-causing agents," can be absorbed through the skin and is neurotoxic. Avoid contaminating hands, wear gloves and wash hands immediately after any exposure. Small amounts of acrylamide may be disposed of in a sink with running water. More than a few milligrams requires professional disposal.

Liquid Laboratory Wastes Containing Sodium Azide

Sodium azide is used in in-vitro diagnostic products as a preservative or as an active ingredient. The amounts involved are generally very small. Waste products containing sodium azide are commonly discarded into a laboratory's drain system. However, in view of the significant problems that azide can create, many laboratories will want to consider putting azide in the chemical waste instead of the drain system. See Method 1.11 for a procedure for decontamination of metallic azides.

Compressed Gases

All tanks must be labeled as to content and concentration and must be secured by an approved restraint system. Valves should be closed and regulator pressure relieved between uses. Regulators must be properly fitted and clean. Tanks generally should not be drained below 50 psi and acetylene should not be used below 60 psi. Empty tanks should be labeled as such. Stored tanks should have protective valve caps and safety chains. Oxygen should not be stored close to combustible gas or solvents. A properly designed hand truck should be used for transport and hand rolling eliminated as much as possible.

Liquid Nitrogen

Due to the extremely cold temperature of liquid nitrogen, there is a risk of freeze injury or severe burn to areas of the skin or eyes. Heavy insulated gloves and goggles should be worn when liquid nitrogen is poured from the Dewar bottle. Pour a more than adequate amount from the Dewar into an appropriate transfer container to make transfer to a final container easier. Some liquid will be lost due to evaporation. Pour from the transfer vessel into the final container. Be certain the final container is securely supported to eliminate any risk of spill.

Flammable Solvents

Liquids are categorized as flammable or combustible depending on whether their flash point is below or above 100 F (38 C). Flammable liquids are further subclassified according to their volatility by the National Fire Protection Association (NFPA), the Joint Commission on Accreditation of Healthcare Organizations (JCAHO) as well as OSHA. See Tables 21-2 and 21-3.

Any area in which flammable solvents will be used must have NO SMOKING signs posted. A fire extinguisher, fire blanket and solvent cleanup kit must be readily available in the area. Containers larger than 1 gallon must be kept in the flammable solvent storage room or in a local fire safety cabinet. Local storage under a hood is acceptable for 1 gallon, or smaller, glass or plastic containers depending on the class of the liquid as indicated in the list for flammable liquids. Glass or plastic bottles kept at the bench for routine use should not exceed 1 pint in capacity.

Ethyl ether must be stored either in the flammable storage room or in an explosion-proof refrigerator, which is so labeled on the door. It should be stored only in safety cans no larger than 1 gallon in size. Organic extracts of specimens that must be stored should be stored only in an explosion-proof refrigerator or freezer.

Unless drawing from a large drum or can in the solvent storage room, volatile solvents (flammable or nonflammable) should be poured in a suitable hood. Eye protection (goggles, face shield, etc) must be worn when pouring or working with flammable solvents. Chemical-resistant neoprene gloves should be worn while pouring solvents.

When flammable liquids are poured from a metal container, it is possible for an electrostatic charge to build up on the container, which might cause a spark and ignite the solvent vapors. The best way to prevent this is to ground the container by connecting it to a water pipe or other ground connection. If the recipient container is also metal, it should be kept electrically connected to the delivery container during pouring to prevent any discharge between the two containers. For proper connection, the clips on the cans must contact bare metal. If glass or plastic containers are involved, no such precautions are necessary. No flame or other source of possible ignition should be in the vicinity where flammable solvents are being poured or used.

Centrifugation of organic solvents or specimen extracts should be done only in screwcap tubes. Reagents containing

Table 21-2. Maximum Allowable Container Size—Flammable Liquids

| Container | Class of Liquid* | | |
	IA	IB	IC
Glass or approved plastic	1 pt or 500 mL	1 qt or L	1 gal
Safety cans: NFPA, JCAHO	1 gal	2 gal	2 gal
OSHA	2 gal	5 gal	5 gal

*Class IA = FP < 73 F, BP < 100 F
Class IB = FP < 73 F, BP ≥ 100 F
Class IC = FP 73–100 F, BP > 100 F

FP = Flash Point (temperature at which the vapors will support a flash fire across the liquid surface)
BP = Boiling Point

Table 21-3. Maximum Allowable Container Size—Combustible Liquids

Container	Class of Liquid*	
	II	III
Glass or approved plastic	1 gal	1 gal
Safety cans: NFPA, JCAHO	2 gal	2 gal
OSHA	2 gal	5 gal

*Class II = FP 100–140 F
Class III = FP ≥ 140 F
FP = Flash Point (temperature at which the vapors will support a flash fire across the liquid surface)

flammable solvents must be labeled "FLAMMABLE."

Disposal

After use, solvents or other non-water-soluble organic liquids should be discarded into a self-closing metal safety can designated for this purpose. Halogenated solvents should be discarded into separate, designated cans because disposal procedures are different for these solvents. Under no circumstances should waste solvents be poured down the drain.

Chemical Spill Cleanup

Acids and Alkalis

Wear eye protection and rubber gloves; use breathing protection if indicated. Ventilate the area if fumes are present. Neutralize acids with sodium carbonate (Na_2CO_3) or soda ash/sand. Neutralize alkalis with boric acid (H_3BO_3). Stir to ensure neutralization and check results with pH paper. Mop up and discard down the drain. If sand was used, discard with solid trash.

Flammable Solvents

Recruit help and prepare for possible fire by notifying facility personnel and readying an extinguisher at the site. Extinguish all source of flames and venti-late area. Wear eye protection, gloves and a respirator mask and leave area every few minutes if it is poorly ventilated. Soak up spill with absorbent material and place in plastic bag. Seal and dispose with solid trash.

Water-Reactive Chemicals

Sweep up dry chemicals, place in plastic bag and discard as solid trash. Soak up liquids with absorbent material, place in plastic bag and discard as solid trash. Clean area with detergent solution.

Carcinogenic Agents

Contact a designated supervisor. Wear gloves, gown and, if dry powder is spilled, a dust mask. Mop up as ordinary spill and discard down the drain, unless prohibited by local regulations.

Radiation Hazards

Overview of Radiation Hazards

Radiation may be defined as energy in the form of waves or particles emitted and propagated through space or a material medium. Gamma rays are electromagnetic radiation while alpha rays and beta rays are examples of particulate radiation. Although blood banks may have only small quantities of radioactive materials, the presence of these hazards requires unique precautions and training in addition to general laboratory safety rules. In addition to training in safe handling, monitoring procedures, emergency procedures and safety rules concerning radioactivity, the employee needs an understanding of the biological effect of and standards for exposure to radiation.

Biological Effects of Radiation

All the effects of radiation on tissue begin with the absorption of radiation energy and the resulting disruption of chemical bonds. Molecules and atoms become ionized and/or excited with the absorption of this energy. The "direct action" path leads to radiolysis or formation of free radicals that in turn alter the structure and function of molecules in the cell.

The molecular alterations may cause chromosomal or cellular changes that are dependent upon the amount and type of radiation energy. The cellular changes can be expressed as somatic effects such as erythema. Chromosomal changes can be expressed within the individual as leukemia or other cancers, or within the germ cells for transmission to future generations.

Two factors affecting biological damage are the total absorbed dose and the dose rate. The total absorbed dose refers to the actual amount of radiation absorbed in the tissue. The greater the dose the greater the biological damage. The dose rate can be acute or chronic in nature.

Demonstrated radiation effects can have acute or latent (delayed) effects. Acute effects include radiation sickness, hematopoietic syndrome, gastrointestinal syndrome and central nervous system syndrome. Latent or delayed effects include carcinogenesis, developmental effects and genetic effects.

Standards for Radiation Exposure

The NRC sets regulatory standards for protection against radiation hazards arising out of licensed activities.[30] Some of these standards are for dose limits, waste disposal, instructions to employees, individual monitoring, warning signs and labels, and shipping and handling.

Dose limits are a measure of the radiation risk over time. They are also named maximum permissible dose equivalents and serve as standards for exposure. Whole body occupational dose limits are 1250 mrem/quarter or 5000 mrem/year. In general, the employer is required not only to maintain certain standards of radiation exposure that cannot be exceeded but also to keep exposure levels as far below these limits as reasonably achievable.

License To Perform Tests and Employee Training

The NRC controls the usage of radioactive materials by establishing requirements of licensure. There may also be requirements for state inspection and/or licensure. The type of license under which radioisotopes or irradiators are obtained depends on the scope and size of the use of radioactivity. Under a specific NRC license, each hospital or blood establishment must have a radiation safety officer who is responsible for meeting the legal safety requirements for personnel surveillance and monitoring, and proper disposal and handling of shipments of radioactive materials. Training sessions for all personnel handling radioactive materials should be held annually. Training courses should include health protection problems, emergency procedures, proper storage, transfer and use of radioactive materials, and explanation of the presence and potential hazards of radioactive materials found in the employees' work area.

Notices and Instructions to Workers

These regulations explaining notifications, instructions and reports to employees are found in the *CFR*.[31] Notices and instructions to workers should include:
1. Precautions to minimize exposure.
2. NRC regulations and license conditions.
3. How to observe license conditions and regulations and how to report any violations or conditions of unnecessary exposure.
4. How to interpret results of monitoring devices.
5. Specific instruction to pregnant workers.
6. Rights during inspections.
7. Maintenance of records, reports and notices.
8. Storage, transfer or use of radioactive materials in restricted areas.

In addition, emergency procedures should be clearly defined and made available to staff.

Radiation Monitoring

Radiation monitoring is a valuable tool for early detection and prevention of problems due to radiation exposure. Radiation monitoring is used to evaluate the radiation environment, radiation work practices and procedures and to comply with regulations, including the NRC license conditions. Two types of monitoring devices are 1) the film badge and 2) the survey meter.

The film badge provides a permanent record of a measure of the exposure received by an individual over a fixed period of time. The film badge is sensitive for X and gamma rays. It must be changed monthly and protected from high temperature and humidity. The film badge should be stored at work and away from sources of radiation. It is important that the worker wear the film badge in accordance with NRC license conditions. Minors are not permitted in areas requiring radiation monitors.

The survey meter is used to detect the presence of radiation and to provide a quantitative assessment of radiation hazards. It is sensitive to low levels of gamma radiation. The survey meter must be calibrated annually by an authorized NRC licensee.

All laboratory work surfaces and irradiator surfaces should be checked for surface contamination with a wipe test (also called leak test) regularly. The wipe test consists of wiping the surface with a moistened absorbent material (the wipe) and counting the radiation contained in each wipe. Kits are available for this purpose.

Radiation Safety Practices

In addition to general laboratory safety practices, there are four basic principles of radiation safety.
1. Minimize time of exposure by working in the most efficient manner.
2. Maximize distance from the source of the radiation. This may be achieved by stepping back from the source.
3. Maximize shielding by wearing lead aprons, if needed, or using a self-shielded irradiator. These requirements are usually stipulated in the license conditions.
4. Use good housekeeping practices, which will minimize the spread of radioactivity to uncontrolled areas.
   a. Gloves and lab coats should be worn when handling radioactive materials.
   b. Radioisotope work should be performed in a tray or pan lined with absorbent paper to prevent contamination of lab surfaces.

c. Dispose of liquid and solid waste such as glassware, vials, paper towels, etc, in clearly labeled containers.
d. Notify the supervisor and radiation safety officer when spills are detected. Begin cleanup immediately.
e. Decontamination procedures should be written and accessible to employees.

7. Any clothing or apparatus that becomes contaminated is to be removed and placed in a plastic bag if possible, labeled properly and stored in the hot locker.
8. If the skin becomes contaminated, wash the area several times and take readings. If the reading is not less than 0.02 mR/hr, seek advice from the radiation safety officer.

Radioactive Spills

A spill can be construed as a dispersal of radioactive substance in a manner that in the judgment of the user or the radiation safety officer may constitute a serious health hazard or be in noncompliance with the NRC regulation.

1. When a radioactive substance is spilled on the floor, clear the area, tape it off and monitor it.
2. If the spill is confined to an area less than 1 sq ft and the reading at 1 ft is less than 5 mR/hr and the half-life of the radionuclide is 5 days or less, a technician wearing gloves may proceed to clean the area.
3. Soap and water or a solution approved for cleaning up radioactive spills may be used to wash up the area after blotting the spill with paper towel.
4. It may be necessary to wash the area several times, taking a reading after each wash to make sure background level is achieved.
5. Discard the gloves and paper towels in a plastic bag and label the bag properly before it is put into the "hot locker." Label with date and name of radioactive material.
6. If a spill is registering over 5 mR/hr and the half-life is over 5 days, notify supervisory personnel at once to direct the cleanup procedure.

References

1. Occupational Safety and Health Administration. OSHA Standard on bloodborne pathogens. Final rule. Federal Register, December 6, 1991. FR 64175-64182.
2. Centers for Disease Control. Update: Universal precautions for prevention of transmission of human immunodeficiency virus, hepatitis B virus, and other blood-borne pathogens in health-care settings. MMWR 1988;37:377-86.
3. Code of federal regulations. Title 42, Part 72. Interstate shipment of biological material that contains or may contain etiologic agents. Washington, DC: US Government Printing Office, 1993. (Revised annually.)
4. National Committee for Clinical Laboratory Standards. Protection of laboratory workers from infectious disease transmitted by blood, body fluids and tissue. Second edition; Tentative Guideline. NCCLS document M29-T2 (ISBN 1-56238-123-7). Villanova, PA: NCCLS, 1991.
5. Department of Labor/Department of Health and Human Services. Joint Advisory Notice. HBV/HIV. Fed Regist, 1987; 52(210):41818-24.
6. Occupational Safety and Health Administration. OSHA, Instruction CPL 2-2.44b. Enforcement procedures for occupational exposure to hepatitis B virus (HBV) and human immunodeficiency virus (HIV). Washington, DC: US Government Printing Office, 1990.
7. Centers for Disease Control and National Institutes of Health. Department of Health and Human Services. Biosafety in microbiological and biomedical laboratories. DHHS Publication No. (CDC) 88-8395. 2nd edition. Washington, DC: US Government Printing Office, 1988.
8. Occupational Safety and Health Act of 1970, Section 5(a)(1). Washington, DC: US Government Printing Office, 1970.
9. Code of federal regulations. Title 21, Part 600.10 (c). Washington, DC: US Government Printing Office, 1993. (Revised annually.)

10. Centers for Disease Control. Recommendations of the Immunization Practices Advisory Committee. ACIP. MMWR 1990;39:1-26.
11. Centers for Disease Control. Recommendations for preventing transmission of infection with human T-lymphotropic virus type III/lymphadenopathy-associated virus during invasive procedures. MMWR 1986;35(14):221-3.
12. Occupational Safety and Health Administration. OSHA, Instruction CPL 2-2.44C. Enforcement procedures for the occupational exposure to bloodborne pathogens standards, 29 CFR 1910.1030. Washington, DC: US Government Printing Office, 1992.
13. American Red Cross. Loss control manual. Washington, DC: American Red Cross, 1988.
14. Code of federal regulations. Title 29, Part 1904.2. Washington, DC: US Government Printing Office, 1992. (Revised annually.)
15. Richmond JY. Safe practices and procedures for working with human specimens in biomedical research laboratories. J Clin Immunoassay 1988;11(3):115-9.
16. FDA Memorandum. Revision to 26 October 1989 guideline for collection of blood products from donors with positive tests for infectious disease markers ("High Risk" Donors). Bethesda, MD: Food and Drug Administration, 17 April 1991.
17. Code of federal regulations, Title 42, Part 72. Washington, DC: US Government Printing Office, 1992. (Revised annually.)
18. Code of federal regulations. Title 49, Parts 173. 386-388. Washington, DC: US Government Printing Office, 1992. (Revised annually.)
19. Environmental Protection Agency. Registered hospital disinfectants and sterilants. (TS767C). Washington, DC: Antimicrobial Program Branch, 1992. (Continually updated and available from Antimicrobial Program Branch, 401 M Street SW, Washington, DC 20460).
20. Vastly D, Lauer J. Decontamination, sterilization, disinfection and antisepsis in the microbiology laboratory. In: Miller BM, ed. Laboratory safety: Principles and practice. Washington, DC: American Society for Microbiology, 1986:182-98.
21. Resnick L, Veren K, Salahuddin Z, et al. Stability and inactivation of HTLV-III/LAV under clinical and laboratory environments. JAMA 1986;255:1887-91.
22. Environmental Protection Agency. Standards for the tracking and management of medical waste. Interim final rule and request for comments. Fed Regist 1989;54(56):12326-95.
23. Resource Conservation and Recovery Act of 1976. Public Law 94-580, Section 1004. Washington, DC: US Government Printing Office, 1976.
24. Environmental Protection Agency. EPA guide for infectious waste management. EPA/530-SW-86-014. (NTIS #PB86-199130). Washington, DC: National Technical Information Service, 1986.
25. National Committee for Clinical Laboratory Standards. Clinical laboratory hazardous waste. Proposed Standard Doc. 6P5-P. Villanova, PA: NCCLS, 1986.
26. Code of federal regulations, Title 40, Part 259. Washington, DC: US Government Printing Office, 1992. (Revised annually.)
27. Code of federal regulations. Title 49, Parts 171-173. Washington, DC: US Government Printing Office, 1992. (Revised annually.)
28. United States Postal Service. Mailability of etiologic agents. Fed Regist 1989;54(156):33823-5.
29. Occupational Safety and Health Administration. OSHA, 29 CFR Part 1910. Occupational exposures to hazardous chemicals in laboratories; final rule. Washington, DC: US Government Printing Office, January 31, 1990.
30. Code of federal regulations. Title 10, Part 20. Washington, DC: US Government Printing Office, 1992. (Revised annually.)
31. Code of federal regulations. Title 10, Part 19. Washington, DC: US Government Printing Office, 1992. (Revised annually.)

Suggested Reading

1988 Agent summary statement for human immunodeficiency virus and report on laboratory acquired infection with human immunodeficiency virus. MMWR (Supplement) 1988;37:1S-22S.

ABRA HIV infection control guidelines. Annapolis, MD: American Blood Resources Association, 1987.

AuBuchon JP. A review: Occupational safety in blood banking—concepts and conundrums. Immunohematology 1988;4:23-30.

CAP Environment, Safety and Health Committee. Guidelines for laboratory safety. Chicago, IL: College of American Pathologists, 1989.

Centers for Disease Control. Recommendations for prevention of HIV transmission in health-care settings. MMWR (Supplement) 1987;36(2S):1S-18S.

Code of federal regulations. Title 21, Part 600-699. Washington, DC: US Government Printing Office, 1992. (Revised annually.)

Gerberding JL, Bryant-LeBlanc CE, Nelson K, et al. Risk of transmitting the human immunodeficiency virus, cytomegalovirus and hepatitis B virus to health care workers exposed to patients with

AIDS and AIDS-related conditions. J Infect Dis 1987;156:1-8.

Gerberding JL, Henderson DK. Design of rational infection control policies for human immunodeficiency virus infection. J Infect Dis 1987;156(6):861-4.

Gibbs FL, Kasprisin CA, eds. Environmental safety in the blood bank. Arlington, VA: American Association of Blood Banks, 1987.

International Air Transportation Association. Dangerous goods regulations. Montreal, Quebec: IATA, 1988.

International Civil Aviation Organization. Technical instruction for the safe transport of dangerous goods by air. Montreal, Quebec: ICAO, 1989-1990. (Available from American Label Mark, 5724 N. Pulaski Road, Chicago, IL 60646.)

Kuhls TL, Cherry JD. The management of health care workers' accidental parenteral exposures to biological specimens of HIV seropositive individuals. Infect Control 1987;8(5):211-13.

McEvoy M, Porter K, Mortimer P, et al. Prospective study of clinical, laboratory, and ancillary staff with accidental exposures to blood or body fluids from patients infected with HIV. Br Med J 1987;294:1595-7.

National Committee for Clinical Laboratory Standards. Procedures for the domestic handling and transport of diagnostic specimens and etiologic agents. Approved Standard. Villanova, PA: NCCLS, 1985.

Radiation safety manual. Atlanta, GA: Office of Biosafety, Centers for Disease Control, 1992.

United States Postal Service. Acceptance of hazardous, restricted or perishable matter and domestic mail manual. Section 124.38. Nonmailable matter—articles and substances; special mailing rules; disease germs and biological products. January 1989. (Available from USPS Eastern Area Supply Center, Route 206 VA Supply Center, Sommerville, NJ 08877.)

Appendix 21-1. Sample Hazardous Chemical Data Sheet

The following information should be a part of the procedures for use of hazardous chemicals:

FACILITY
IDENTIFICATION   : _____

LAB NAME: : _____

ROOM NUMBER   : _____

NAME OF CHEMICAL : _____

SYNONYMS   : _____

CHEMICAL ABSTRACT
NO. (CAS#)   : _____

COMMON NAME   : _____

PRIMARY HAZARD   : Carcinogen: _____ Reproductive toxin: _____
                    High acute toxicity: _____
                    Other health hazard: _____
                    Safety hazard: _____
                    MSDS or other reference available: _____
                    Is prior approval required for use of the chemical; if so,
                    by whom? _____

GENERAL AND SPECIAL PRECAUTIONS:

SIGNS REQUIRED (Warning signs indicating presence of hazardous chemicals/
operations): _____

STORAGE (Secondary containment, temperature-sensitive, incompatibilities, water-reactive,
etc): _____

SPECIAL CONTROLS AND LOCATION (Fume hood, glove box, etc): _____

SPECIAL EQUIPMENT AND LOCATION (Vacuum line filter, liquid or other traps, special
shielding): _____

PERSONAL PROTECTIVE EQUIPMENT (Glove type, eye protection, special clothing, etc): _____

EMERGENCY PROCEDURES:

Spill or release: _____
Fire: _____
Decontamination procedures: _____

DISPOSAL PROCEDURES:

Appendix 21-2. Example of an Emergency Instructions Checklist

1. Phone numbers and instructions posted for fire, police, medical assistance, chemical and biological hazards; supervisor to be notified and report requirements.

2. Designated assistance for handicapped persons; alert responsibility assigned for hearing impaired, visually handicapped and others as appropriate.

Fire:

Designated responsibility to ensure alarm sounded, area is evacuated completely, gas and electric appliances shut off, hazardous materials confined in cabinets and fire doors shut.

Bomb Threats:

Obtain maximum information from caller; notify emergency response authorities immediately; avoid all suspicious items but turn off all radios or transceiver equipment; evacuate calmly.

Radiation Incident:

Confine contamination with absorbent material if possible; remove shoes and clothing before entering a clean area; wash body if contact possible; notify emergency response authorities; report to medical service, quarantine area until safe reentry is determined by authorities.

Chemical or Biological Hazards:

Leave room (do not open windows; close doors); call emergency response authorities; wash body if contact occurred; report to medical service; quarantine area until safe reentry is determined by authorities.

Appendix 21-3. Hazardous Chemicals in the Blood Bank

Chemical	Hazard
Ammonium chloride	Irritant
Bromelain	Irritant, sensitizer
Calcium chloride	Irritant
Carbon dioxide, frozen (dry ice)	Corrosive
Carbonyl iron powder	Oxidizer
Chloroform	Toxic, suspected carcinogen
Chloroquine	Irritant, corrosive
Chromium (III) chloride hexahydrate	Toxic, irritant, sensitizer
Citric acid	Irritant
Copper sulfate (cupric sulfate)	Toxic, irritant
Dichloromethane	Toxic, irritant
Digitonin	Toxic
Dry ice (carbon dioxide, frozen)	Corrosive
Ethidium bromide	Carcinogen, irritant
Ethylenediaminetetraacetic acid (EDTA)	Irritant
Ethyl ether	Highly flammable and explosive, toxic, irritant
Ficin (powder)	Irritant, sensitizer
34.9% Formaldehyde solution	Suspected carcinogen, combustible, toxic
Glycerol	Irritant
Hydrochloric acid	Highly toxic, corrosive
Imidazole	Irritant
Isopropyl (rubbing) alcohol	Flammable, irritant
Liquid nitrogen	Corrosive
Lyphogel	Corrosive
2-Mercaptoethanol	Toxic, stench
Mineral oil	Irritant, carcinogen, combustible
Papain	Irritant, sensitizer
Polybrene	Toxic
Potassium hydroxide	Corrosive, toxic
Saponin	Irritant
Sodium azide	Toxic, irritant, explosive when heated
Sodium ethylmercurithiosalicylate (thimerosal)	Highly toxic, irritant
Sodium hydrosulfite	Toxic, irritant
Sodium hydroxide	Corrosive, toxic
Sodium hypochlorite (bleach)	Corrosive
Sodium phosphate	Irritant, hygroscopic
Sulfosalicylic acid	Toxic, corrosive
Trichloroacetic acid (TCA)	Corrosive, toxic
Trypsin	Irritant, sensitizer
Xylene	Highly flammable, toxic, irritant

22

Quality Management

The pursuit of quality requires a comprehensive and coordinated management program that is prospectively designed to promote desired outcomes. This program is used in blood centers and hospital transfusion services to: 1) protect donors and patients from harm, 2) maximize progress in reaching defined objectives and 3) meet the needs of users of the services offered. This does not just happen, but rather is the result of a conscious effort by staff, supervisors and directors to achieve excellence in daily practice. Quality Control (QC) is concerned with the *process* while Quality Assessment (QA) is concerned with the *outcome*. Prevention of problems and Continuous Improvement (CI) are additional elements in this activity, which is also called a Total Quality Management (TQM) program.

The Joint Commission on Accreditation of Healthcare Organizations (JCAHO) has stimulated new interest in the monitoring and evaluation of hospital and blood center activities through a process that involves the following[1]:

1. Identification of the most important aspects of the care (for example, procedures or treatments) that the organization (or department or service) provides.
2. Use of measurable indicators to systematically monitor these aspects of care in an ongoing way.
3. Evaluation of the care when thresholds are reached in the monitoring process to identify opportunities for improvement or problems in the quality and appropriateness of care.
4. Taking actions to improve care or solve problems, and evaluation of the effectiveness of those actions.

The JCAHO has suggested 10 steps to accomplish this activity (see Table 22-1).

A Quality Assessment and Continuous Improvement (QACI) Plan

Each blood center and transfusion service must have a written QACI plan and designate an individual who will be responsible for the QACI program of the facility.[2] The director and supervisors should develop the facets of the QACI program *after* examining the entire activity of the facility.

The primary goal of QACI in transfusion medicine is a safe transfusion. The best guarantee of meeting the objectives of QACI is careful adherence to standard operating procedures (SOPs) by trained staff.[3] The importance of QACI to blood banking can be seen by the development of comprehensive QACI guidelines by the FDA,[4] JCAHO,[1] AABB[2,5] and CAP.[6] Most serious transfusion errors, as well as regulatory compliance problems, result from carelessness; specifically, from inaccurate identification of the donor, donor specimen, donor unit, patient, patient's blood specimen, test results or requisition forms.[7] Meticulous accuracy is essential in all aspects of donor and

539

Table 22-1. Steps Suggested by the JCAHO for the Monitoring and Evaluation Process[1]

1. Assign responsibility for monitoring and evaluation activities.
2. Delineate the scope of care provided by the organization.
3. Identify the most important aspects of care provided by the organization.
4. Identify indicators (and appropriate clinical criteria) for monitoring the important aspects of care.
5. Establish thresholds (levels, patterns, trends) for the indicators that trigger evaluation of the care.
6. Monitor the important aspects of care by collecting and organizing the data for each indicator.
7. Evaluate care when thresholds are reached in order to identify either opportunities to improve care or problems.
8. Take actions to improve care or to correct identified problems.
9. Assess the effectiveness of the actions and document the improvement in care.
10. Communicate the results of the monitoring and evaluation process to relevant individuals, departments or services and to the organization's quality assurance program.

patient contact, laboratory technique and record-keeping. QC programs monitor whether equipment and procedures fulfill their expected functions, and whether personnel perform these procedures in an approved, reproducible fashion. QACI programs must be practical and realistic. Testing should not be excessively time-consuming nor should it result in the accumulation of unnecessary data. All QACI efforts must be legibly documented to allow proper verification and to provide a historical record with which to analyze deviant trends and to allow prompt correction.

Quality Indicators and Performance Thresholds

After examining the entire activity of the facility and determining desired outcomes, the director and supervisors can establish indicators to monitor results and progress in reaching objectives. Each indicator should be developed with specific thresholds or criteria of performance set. Performance thresholds are derived by reviewing the historical data of the facility and the scientific literature or other sources. After input from the staff of the facility, a consensus of the indicators chosen and the thresholds used should be developed by management. Threshold target values for the indicators should be defined in numerical terms in order to assess the degree to which desired goals are reached. Below are listed some examples of appropriate indicators:

1. Blood Collection and Processing
   a. Success in meeting blood donor recruitment goals.
   b. Length of time (mean and range) that blood donors wait from registration to phlebotomy.
   c. Number of incompletely filled blood component requests that have been received from hospitals.
   d. Satisfaction of donors (first time, repeat, apheresis, etc).
   e. Completeness of donor history/physical exam record.
   f. Number of labeling errors.
2. Hospital Transfusion Service
   a. Percent of all red cell transfusions that are autologous.
   b. Frequency of gaps in records or unreported transfusion reactions.
   c. Availability and appropriate use of blood components and RhIG.

d. Frequency of patients without wristbands or samples inappropriately labeled.

Once the indicators have been selected and thresholds of performance defined, the method, frequency and responsibility for review should be determined. For example, will the review include all observations or rather a sample of the total? If a sample, what fraction will be included and how should the sample be selected? These choices will vary according to local needs and situations.

Quality assessment indicators should be reported on an established, regular basis. Plans for corrective action should be documented and program results evaluated by management. The collected data are critically evaluated to determine the degree of success in meeting the established target values and/or not exceeding thresholds of defined criteria. Appropriate corrective action should follow the review. Documentation of the effectiveness of action taken should be included in the evaluation by management. The personnel involved in the process of monitoring should receive feedback, not only when there have been failures, but also praise when the indicators show compliance with target values. The specific indicators should periodically be reviewed for appropriateness, as improvement and success are achieved, in order to substitute new indicators when applicable for monitoring. Previous indicators may occasionally be reinstituted on a rotating basis in order to make comparisons and to determine if the desired objectives have been sustained over time. Consideration should be given in the ongoing evaluation process to making the thresholds more stringent.

Personnel

Qualified, trained and highly motivated personnel constitute the key to success- ful performance. Every effort should be made to employ staff with the necessary educational background and appropriate experience. Job descriptions should define the essential prerequisite requirements and the competencies expected for the position. References and recommendations should be sought. An orientation should be planned in order to acquaint new staff members with the institutional policies and procedures, safety matters and personal expectations. Special attention by the supervisors or designated senior staff will facilitate the adjustment of new staff members. A probationary period is desirable in order for the employer and employee to develop confidence and respect for each other. New staff members must be checked by the supervisor or an experienced staff person to ensure that they can perform required tasks. Additional competencies should be added as the employee gains confidence and demonstrates ability and motivation. Periodic performance evaluations by the supervisor afford opportunities for critical review and positive and negative feedback to the employee. These evaluations should be based upon written performance standards rather than subjective opinions.[8,9] Continuing education on relevant laboratory topics, including the practical and theoretical aspects of procedures, as well as safety, clerical and computer skills, should be required of each staff member.

Procedures Manual

Each facility must have documents that constitute the standard operating procedures. The SOP manual should contain a complete description of the QACI program as well as all policies and directions for all technical procedures performed. It should be readily available for reference and written in a consistent format such as the guidelines given in Table 23-1. SOP manuals must properly incorporate the directions supplied by the manufacturers of the reagents and equipment that are currently being used. If a manufacturer's guidance is not followed, data that fully support any deviation from that guidance must be on file. These data must substantiate the efficacy of the altered method and meet regulatory requirements. The AABB *Accreditation Requirements Manual*[5] (*ARM*) states that SOPs must include examples of forms used to record test results and interpretations. Procedures for the maintenance and disposition of these records must also be available. The SOP manual must contain written and/or pictorial descriptions of how to read, score and record all test results and interpretations, when applicable. Regulatory agencies require a system to document that the laboratory director has approved SOPs and that all personnel are aware of and will comply with changes in the SOP manual.

AABB *Standards for Blood Banks and Transfusion Services* requires a review of the SOP manual each year.[2(p 1)] When procedures are added to or replaced in the manual, the new instructions must be marked with the date they went into effect. Material removed from the manual must be retained at least 5 years, with the date of removal recorded.[5] Electronic media such as magnetic tapes, optical disks or on-line computer data storage are widely used for archiving records. Blood bank record storage on optical disks requires special consideration of the limitations because FDA policy has not been clearly defined. Microfiched records can be stored for years. The potential also exists for the increasing use of optical character reading devices to archive written records onto electronic media.

Commitment to Excellence

Quality and improvement require a positive attitude on the part of every individual in the facility. This attitude is a desire to achieve excellence in the performance of all tasks in order to ensure the desired outcomes.

Good Records and Checking Results

Careful documentation of critical activities protects both patient and donor, as well as the staff of the facility. The laboratory information system (computer) must be monitored continuously for validation, modification, errors, backup and security. See Chapter 23.

When the consequences of erroneous testing or interpretations are potentially catastrophic, it may be desirable to have two different people perform the tasks independently and then compare the results and interpretations. For example, this is effectively done when two individuals are involved in the manual labeling of blood donor units. Unfortunately, even repeated checking does not guarantee that discrepancies will be detected. Once an error is undetected on the initial check, it tends to be perpetuated. All personnel should be instructed on the importance of confirming independently all data. Computer controls are used to reduce errors. For instance, bar code labels may be used to identify donor and patient samples, to prepare expiration date labels, product description, and to identify and track test trays in automated testing instruments.

Checking results previously obtained on the same individual helps monitor accurate sample identification and also allows observation of significant changes in serologic status. AABB *Standards*[2] requires (H1.100) that, for potential transfusion recipients, current findings be checked against records of ABO and Rh tests done in the preceding 12 months and records of difficulty in blood typing, clinically significant unexpected antibodies and severe adverse reactions to transfusion within at least the preceding 5 years. Checking previous ABO and Rh test results on donors is not required, but is a desirable form of QA. The *ARM* requires that there be a written system to prevent collection of blood from previously deferred or otherwise unsuitable donors as well as prohibiting the release of unacceptable blood components.[5] It also requires that there be a system for the receiving facility to notify the blood collecting facility of any unsuitable units.

The Food and Drug Administration (FDA) requires that all manufacturing records be retained for 5 years or "6 months after the latest expiration date for the individual product, whichever is later."[4] Each blood center and transfusion service must design a system to ensure that records (especially those associated with frozen components) are retained for the required length of time. Record retention has assumed greater importance due to the recent intensity of "look-backs" on donations made prior to positive tests in blood donors.

Quality Control

Various QC activities must be established to check specific elements of procedures in order to determine whether or not certain critical steps in processing are being performed within established limits of acceptability. In addition, all equipment must be tested to determine that optimal operating conditions are being met and that there is periodic maintenance of critical functions. This information should be documented. Some of the QC procedures and instrument function checks are listed below.

Selection of materials and equipment should be tailored to optimize results for each facility based upon local needs. Survey data of the College of American Pathologists provide comparative results that may be of value in this regard.

Reagents

Since commercial antisera and reagent rbc products are licensed by the FDA, Center for Biologics Evaluation and Research, the manufacturers must demonstrate that their products meet minimum standards for specificity and potency before they are licensed. It is neither necessary nor meaningful for individual users to test reagent antisera for titer or avidity. Each laboratory must confirm that each reagent on each day of use reacts as expected when used as described in the facility's SOP manual. If the local procedure differs from that recommended by the manufacturer, there must be documentation that the modification gives satisfactory results. For unlicensed reagents that are locally produced, there must be records of reactivity and specificity that document that FDA requirements are met. IgG-coated rbcs and A and B cells for serum (reverse) grouping may be prepared locally, with records documenting their reactivity and specificity. Reagents for all other required tests must be shown to meet or exceed FDA criteria, as outlined in 21 CFR 660,[4] a requirement that precludes local preparation of most reagents except at very well-equipped centers.

Records of testing must include results and interpretation of the results, identification of the personnel involved, the source and identification numbers of all reagents tested, the date of testing and the source and nature of controls, when used.

Antisera

The manufacturer's directions should be reviewed for changes with each new lot number and the package inserts should be saved from every lot in use. Procedural modifications used in individual blood banks or transfusion services must not conflict with the directions of the manufacturer. Antisera may lose potency or specificity or both, due to poor storage or shipping conditions. Contamination during preparation or use can also impair reactivity. Reagents should be observed at each use for abnormal appearance, cloudiness or turbidity and should be stored in accordance with label instructions when not in use.

Frozen Storage

Freezing is not recommended for storing most commercially prepared reagents, which often contain additives adversely affected by freezing. Antibody-containing sera and other materials prepared locally without preservatives are often frozen for extended storage. Since repeated freezing and thawing damages proteins, sera should be frozen in aliquots of the volume appropriate for individual use. Frozen sera should be thawed at 37 C and mixed thoroughly before use. Frozen-thawed reagents, like any other reagents that are not subjected to daily quality control surveillance, should be monitored at the time of use by testing against appropriately selected controls (ie, cells with a single dose of the relevant antigen and cells negative for that antigen).

Testing for Reactivity

Antisera must be tested each day of use, preferably before use or concomitantly with the first tests. Since cell and serum (direct and reverse) ABO grouping constitute a built-in check on specificity, it is not necessary to perform additional tests on these sera and cells, provided that an adequate number of consistent results have been observed with those reagent lots on the previous day, and that the observation and interpretation are suitably recorded. In small laboratories, it may not be possible to accumulate a sufficient number of test results, and direct testing of the antisera used for ABO testing should then be done.

All other antisera should be monitored with control cells at the time the test is performed. Positive and negative controls are usually employed, but controls should be used with discretion to preserve rare sera and cells. If several samples are being tested with antibody against a high-incidence antigen, a negative control is desirable because positive results are expected and would serve as their own control. Similarly, a positive control (but not a negative one) is indicated for antibodies against low-incidence antigens. Red cells with a weak expression of the antigen provide a better test of antibody potency and specificity than cells with a strong expression of the antigen. If control cells are selected from a pretested panel of group O cells, it is best to use cells with a single dose of the relevant antigen.

Reagent Red Cells

Red cells used for ABO grouping and for antibody identification may be obtained from commercial suppliers or may be prepared locally from selected donors of known red cell phenotypes. Cells used for antibody detection tests must meet or exceed FDA criteria. Selected cells used as an adjunct to antibody identification are not subject to specific criteria and, in many laboratories, locally available cells are used to confirm or amplify results obtained with commercially available cell panels.

Suspensions of reagent rbcs should be inspected visually for evidence of hemolysis each day of use. If the degree of hemolysis is such that a single wash removes the hemoglobin-stained supernatant fluid, the rbcs may be used satisfactorily as a freshly prepared saline suspension.

All reagent red cells should be refrigerated when not in use.

Red Cells for Antibody Detection and Identification

It is not feasible to test each cell each day for each antigen. Each cell used in the antibody detection test must be tested each day of use[5] for reactivity of one antigen. The test may be in any phase of the test procedure; use of actual serum specimens is ideal, but it may be necessary to use diluted reagent antisera. The expected reactivity should be 1+ to 2+. Antibodies that give stronger reactions will not detect minor changes in antigen reactivity. Maximal information can be obtained with minimal effort if at least one cell is tested with an antibody reactive only in the antiglobulin phase. This documents the reactivity of the antiglobulin serum as well as the integrity of the reagent cell. If antibody-containing serum from a donor or patient is used, it should be stored as small frozen aliquots for individual use.

Serum-to-Cell Ratio

Personnel in most blood banks use disposable Pasteur-type pipets to deliver serum in antibody screening, identification and compatibility testing. These pipets vary greatly in the size of the drop delivered due to the diameter of the orifice and the angle that the pipet is held at the time of delivery of the drop. One study[10] showed that the number of drops delivered per mL of serum varied from 21-43. The same study showed that the

droppers in commercial vials of reagent red cells delivered between 18-28 drops per mL. The ratio of serum to cells affects the sensitivity of antibody detection with the optimal ratio being approximately 80:1 or more.[10] (See Chapter 7 for a more detailed discussion of factors affecting agglutination.)

It is not necessary to test each pipet for volume delivered, but personnel in each laboratory should determine the average drop size and volume delivered by the transfer pipets and red cell droppers in local use. Once the average delivery volume has been determined, the directions for antibody detection and compatibility testing should designate volumes that approach the optimal 80:1 serum-to-cell ratio. Steps must be taken to ensure that the suspensions of red cell reagents prepared by a facility are produced to the same specifications on a lot-to-lot basis. Further, the suspensions of the different components of reagent red cell sets made within the facility (eg, serum grouping cells, antibody screening cells) should be standardized to the same red cell suspension parameters. When reagent red cell or antisera manufacturers are changed, the drop size should be checked and appropriate adjustments made in the number of drops of serum added from the disposable pipet that is in use.

Antiglobulin Testing

Most unexpected antibodies that cause red cell destruction are IgG; it is the anti-IgG in polyspecific antiglobulin serum that detects most clinically significant antibody activity in antibody detection tests and crossmatching. The anticomplement component of antiglobulin reagents is most useful in the direct antiglobulin test. Anticomplement may provide the only means of detecting occasional weakly reactive examples of complement-binding antibodies, especially in the Kidd blood group system. See Chapter 8.

Antiglobulin Serum

In daily QC testing it is sufficient to test antiglobulin serum for anti-IgG only. Anticomplement activity can be checked, if desired, against complement-coated rbcs but this need not be a routine procedure for polyspecific reagents. Standards[2] requires that IgG-coated cells be added as the final check on negative results obtained when antiglobulin serum is used in antibody screening tests or crossmatches. These cells should be lightly coated with antibody, to give no more than 2+ macroscopic reactions. In daily QC testing, adding antiglobulin serum to the IgG-coated rbcs provides a simultaneous check for both reagents. Heavily coated cells may not detect subtle loss of anti-IgG activity. For example, a difference in reactivity between 4+ macroscopically and 2+ macroscopically is not as readily apparent as a difference between 2+ macroscopically and a negative result.

Opened vials of antiglobulin serum must be tested each day of use to ensure their activity.[5] Loss of potency may result from inadvertent contamination with human serum or other reagents, or less often, from deterioration during storage.

Checking Negative Results

Negative results in antiglobulin procedures must be checked by adding rbcs lightly coated with IgG antibody, repeating centrifugation and reading. Agglutination at this point indicates that antiglobulin serum was present in the test, that it was not inactivated by unbound globulins or diluted by excess residual saline, that the antiglobulin phase of the test was done correctly and that all reagents were reactive. Using green antiglobulin serum does not substitute for this control. The presence of dye in the tube merely indicates that antiglobulin serum was added, and does not ensure antiglobulin activity.

Equipment

Properly functioning equipment is essential for accurate testing. All instruments must be properly maintained, cleaned and monitored. Temperature-regulated equipment must be checked daily[4] for correct temperature if used for blood component storage, or each day of use for other such equipment. The results and interpretations must be recorded and kept for the required record storage period. Corrective action must be documented when temperatures are outside prescribed ranges or instruments fail to function as expected.

Centrifuges for Serologic Testing

Two types of table-top centrifuges are in common use. One has fixed speed and variable time; the other has variable speed and time. The number of rotations per minute (rpm) must be checked at least every 6 months[4] with an optical or other device and the results recorded. The ARM recommends that this be upon receipt, after repair, and every 3-4 months. The time of centrifugation, which includes the time of acceleration but not deceleration, can be checked with a stopwatch.[5] For washing cell suspensions and for enhancing agglutination, centrifugation should bring the cells together in a well-defined button, but should not pack the cells so tightly that unagglutinated cells cannot be resuspended with gentle manipulation. A clearly delineated cell button is a small, round dot surrounded by clear supernatant fluid. The periphery of the cell button should be sharply defined, not fuzzy.

The best quality control mechanism is careful observation of all agglutination results obtained in daily testing. Each time the centrifuge is used, the technologist should observe red cell buttons for any departure from the usual pattern. If deterioration or inconsistencies are noted, the centrifuge may need recalibration or repair. See Method 11.4 for calibration of serologic centrifuge.

Many variables affect the results of centrifugation. The automatic timer may be poorly aligned or the set screw not tightened properly. The set screw can be tightened and the timer set correctly to match preexisting time intervals marked on the face of the timer, or timing can be checked with a stopwatch and the correction marked on the face of the timer. The time of acceleration varies from one centrifuge to another and depends on the load on the head.

Centrifuges for Component Preparation

Calibrating centrifuges for component preparation requires that the centrifuges should always be level. Special attention to leveling is necessary when centrifuges are installed at mobile drawing facilities. Each centrifuge must be calibrated to determine the optimal times and speeds of centrifugation for each component prepared.[5] See Method 11.5.

After the centrifuge has been calibrated, tachometer readings (rpm) at the selected speed setting should be recorded. The centrifuge lid should be closed during measurement. After initial calibration, revolutions per minute should be measured periodically to be certain that the final component meets the desired requirements.[5] If the reading does not vary and testing of the blood component is satisfactory, the centrifuge need not be recalibrated, but calibration must be performed after repairs. On each day of use, readings of the speed and temperature dials must be observed.[5] Records must be maintained of calibration data, tachometer readings, temperature, maintenance and repairs.

Waterbaths, Heat Blocks and Incubators

Tests to detect warm-reactive antibodies must be incubated at 37 C, unless appropriate and fully documented alternative methods have been adopted. Tubes may be incubated either in waterbaths or heat blocks. For most tests, the incubation time can be the same in waterbaths and heat blocks because the small volumes of sample used in serologic testing reach the appropriate temperatures rapidly. Time taken by a standard liquid volume to reach 37 C may be measured to determine if changes in volume or incubation time are needed. Incubation times may be posted on each incubation device used. Highly automated incubators have largely replaced waterbaths and heat blocks in viral serology testing laboratories in the donor centers.

Heat blocks occasionally show a difference in temperature between individual wells. This should be determined when the equipment is received and should be monitored thereafter. The functioning temperature of each piece of heat-regulated equipment must be tested in a single well each day of use. Systematic alternation of the heat block well or location in the waterbath at which the temperature is taken will allow all incubating sites to be tested periodically. These observations and any corrective action must be recorded.

Waterbaths used to thaw frozen blood components must have the temperature noted and recorded each day of use; immediately before each use, the technologist should check to ensure that temperatures are not unexpectedly high or low. Temperatures may drop if several frozen units are incubated in a small volume of water. *Standards*[2] requires FFP and CRYO to be thawed at temperatures between 30 and 37 C. If the same waterbath is used for thawing components and for incubating serologic tests, it is important to ensure that the temperature has returned to 37 C before tubes are incubated. A schedule for regular cleaning of the waterbath is recommended.

There must be a means to prevent contact of the entry ports of the blood container and the water, which may contain bacteria. The use of a waterproof overwrap or a device to keep the partially submerged bags in an upright position will accomplish this.

Thermometers

Thermometers should be checked on receipt for accuracy and consistency at the temperature of intended use. Either a thermometer certified by the National Institute of Standards and Technology (NIST) or one that has been tested against an NIST-certified thermometer should be used for comparison. Thermometers described as traceable to an NIST thermometer may be the only ones available. If this is the case, test such thermometers on receipt for consistent temperature indication, even if it is not possible to determine accuracy. The greatest amount of information can be obtained with the least effort if many thermometers are tested at once. See Method 11.7.

Blood Warmers

There must be surveillance of blood warmers used for transfusion. It is not necessary for transfusion service personnel to perform this testing; employees of a consulting service or personnel in the departments of anesthesia, surgery, mainte-nance or biomedical engineering may do the tests and record the results. However, the director of the blood bank or transfusion service must ensure that this is done, certify results of testing and ensure that the records are available. If this is not possible, there must be explicit written documentation from the responsible person in the hospital stating in writing that the transfusion service director is not to have responsibility for the operation and performance checks of the blood warmers.

Blood warmers must have a visible thermometer and should have an audible alarm that sounds if the temperature of the blood exceeds 38 C. The actual temperature of the warming unit should be checked with a thermometer applied to the warming surface or with a thermocouple probe, and the temperature reading on the built-in thermometer should be checked against the reading on the monitoring thermometer.

It is desirable to simulate a warmed transfusion by passing fluid through the instrument and measuring its temperature as it leaves the unit. At flow rates usually used for transfusion, refrigerated blood or even blood that has been at room temperature during the transfusion process seldom reaches 38 C. With a very slow flow or during a temporary interruption of transfusion, however, the blood may undergo prolonged contact with the warming surface. Allowing the test fluid to remain stationary in the unit for 10-15 minutes will give some idea of the maximal warming that could occur.

The alarm system is ordinarily activated by the temperature of the warming device, not by the temperature of the fluid; it is not possible or desirable to raise the temperature of the heating unit in order to test the alarm. In some units, the alarm can be checked by slowly running a fluid heated over 38 C through the unit.

Irradiators

If a device is used to irradiate blood or components, it must be monitored to ensure accurate and consistent delivery of the designated dose and to prevent radiation leakage. This testing is usually performed at approximately 6-month intervals by the institution's radiation safety department. The director of the blood bank or transfusion service should ensure that this testing is done, certify the results of testing and ensure that the records are available. *Standards*[2] states that the blood bank or transfusion service should participate in the development of blood component irradiation protocols.

Refrigerators and Freezers

There must be a system to continuously monitor the temperatures of blood bank refrigerators and freezers and an alarm system to warn personnel before storage temperatures reach unacceptable limits. Alarms must signal in an area that has adequate personnel coverage 24 hours a day to ensure that immediate corrective action can be taken. There must be continuous surveillance of temperature, but intermittent recording is permissible. With standard recorders, a continuous written record is generated, but electronic systems that generate periodic printouts are acceptable, provided temperatures are recorded at least every 4 hours. Temperature fluctuations that exceed regulatory requirements must be explained, in writing, on the record sheet (eg, "alarm check," "cleaned"). Readily available written procedures must contain directions on how to maintain blood and blood components within permissible temperature ranges.[5] These procedures must include instructions to be followed in the event of a power failure or other disruption of refrigeration. Chapter 3 presents a detailed discussion of storage requirements. See Methods 11.1 and 11.2.

Intraoperative Blood Collection Equipment

Maximal suction levels should be set with regulators to avoid excessive red cell destruction. Indicators should be established to monitor the quality of red blood cells collected and returned to the patient.[11] Relevant indicators might include the ratio of anticoagulant solution to the volume of blood collected, the volume of 0.9% NaCl used to wash the collected blood, the hematocrit of the final processed unit, the total volume of processed rbcs and periodic cultures.

Accreditation

The inspection and accreditation programs of the AABB and CAP provide a valuable mechanism for external peer review of operational policies and procedures. Accreditation ensures compliance with minimal standards established by professional peers. Unannounced inspections by the FDA monitor compliance of blood centers and hospital transfusion services with Federal regulations.

Proficiency Tests

External proficiency testing programs offer a valuable management tool since they enable laboratory personnel to compare the results obtained in their laboratory with those obtained in other laboratories when the same material is examined. All relevant laboratory staff members must participate on a rotating basis in the testing of these samples. Proficiency testing samples must be tested with the laboratory's regular patient workload using the routine testing methods. The Clinical Laboratory Improvement Amendments of 1988 (CLIA '88)[12] require that the laboratory participate in all proficiency tests for those procedures that are normally performed by the laboratory.[9] This may include ABO and D typing, unexpected antibody detection, compatibility testing, antibody identification, disease marker testing, hemoglobin determination, blood cell counts, etc. A score of 100% is required for ABO and D typing and compatibility testing. Unexpected antibody detection and antibody identification results must be at least 80% for satisfactory performance according to CLIA '88. Surveys that meet the CLIA requirements for blood centers and hospital transfusion services are available through the survey programs sponsored by the AABB and CAP. These external surveys help evaluate the procedures, equipment, materials and personnel of the individual blood bank or transfusion service. Specimens tested as part of proficiency testing should not receive special handling. There must be a record that supervisory personnel have reviewed the results and interpretations of these results, and that appropriate corrective actions, if needed, are taken. Periodic replicate, independent or blind testing may be helpful to ensure that all personnel adhere to testing standards and apply them uniformly.

Transfusion Practices

Standards[2] and regulations of other inspecting agencies require that transfusion services use a peer-review program that documents monitoring of transfusion practices. This is discussed in detail in Chapter 24. Appropriate topics for review include usage of blood and components, reports of adverse reactions and reports of disease transmission.

Adverse Reactions, Errors and Reporting

There must be a mechanism for detecting, reporting and evaluating suspected adverse reactions to transfusion. The ARM requires maintenance of an error or variance document.[5] (See also Chapter 23.) Documented posttransfusion hepatitis, HIV and other viral diseases must be reported to the facility that collected the transfused unit(s). Transfusion services should establish guidelines for identifying units implicated in posttransfusion hepatitis. Cases of transfusion-associated AIDS must be evaluated and confirmed cases must be reported to the blood collecting facility.[2] Fatalities resulting directly from transfusion must be reported within 24 hours to the Director, Center for Biologics Evaluation and Research (CBER) at (301) 295-8191 or 295-8994. A written report must be submitted to the Director, CBER (1401 Rockville Pike, Suite 200N, HFM-655, Rockville, MD 20852-1448) within 7 days.[1] Records of errors and accidents in collection, testing, distribution and administration of blood components are required by the FDA. Licensed facilities must comply with 21 CFR 610.12 in reporting errors that affect the safety, purity or potency of products.

Standards requires that a physician associated with the collecting facility shall establish the means to notify donors of any medically significant abnormality detected during the predonation evaluation or as a result of laboratory testing.[2(p 7)] Results of infectious disease testing are routinely communicated to the donors. The SOP manual of each blood center should include policy on what information is to be given to the donor or the donor's physician, and how the information is to be conveyed. Donor and patient information must not be given to unauthorized persons.

Donor Collection and Processing

Interview, physical examination and other screening of prospective donors should be performed in private conditions by skilled, well-trained personnel. Review of this activity could be performed as a QA monitor. Guidelines for conducting the donor screening and physical examination are described in Chapter 1. A system must be in place to identify deferred donors so that any blood units that might have been collected from them are discarded. Note that the AABB[2] and the FDA[4] have more stringent and comprehensive requirements for certain tests for donors participating in a serial plasmapheresis or cytapheresis program than they do for routine blood donors. Documentation of these tests for apheresis donors and the triannual review by a qualified licensed physician of this documentation is essential. In addition, the *ARM* requires that those facilities that collect autologous or patient directed blood should evaluate whether the program is satisfactory to the donor-patient, the ordering physician and the transfusing hospital. The level of autologous blood use by surgical services and by physicians can be instructive.

Hemoglobin or Hematocrit

Hemoglobin or hematocrit can be determined by a variety of standard methods. Estimation of acceptable hemoglobin by using copper sulfate solutions is imprecise but simple, quick and adequate. The microhematocrit is simple and accurate, but time-consuming, and requires special equipment. Recently, portable, quick-reading and display hemoglobin readers have been introduced.[13,14] The devices, using blood collected by fingerstick into specially designed collection-and-read samplers, produce accurate results in less than 1 minute. Although more costly to perform than either the copper sulfate or microhematocrit methods, these instruments offer increased accuracy in a timely manner and do so more quietly than is possible with the microhematocrit method. The instructions of the manufacturer should be followed regarding quality control and standards.

Copper Sulfate Procedure

Adequacy of a donor's hemoglobin level is often determined indirectly by demonstrating a minimum specific gravity of the donor's whole blood, tested with a copper sulfate solution. This procedure is subject to more variation and intrinsic error than the microhematocrit/hemoglobin method, but is widely used because large numbers of donors can be adequately processed in minimal time with very little equipment. Before use, the solutions must be mixed thoroughly and be at room temperature. Copper sulfate solutions should not be frozen or exposed to very high temperatures and stock solutions should be tightly sealed during storage. Specific gravity may change due to contamination or evaporation. Solutions should be changed daily and after every 25 tests if 50-mL volumes are used. The specific gravity should be checked periodically with a calibrated hydrometer or refractometer. A specific gravity of 1.053 corresponds to a hemoglobin of 125 g/L (12.5 g/dL). Copper sulfate screening is not a quantitative procedure. Therefore, unacceptably low values should be confirmed with a more accurate test for hemoglobin or hematocrit, where possible. Specific measurement of hemoglobin or hematocrit may indicate that a donor rejected by the copper sulfate procedure is, after all, acceptable.

Microhematocrit Centrifuge

The microhematocrit centrifuge calibration should be checked each day of use by testing with a control sample. The timer should be checked every 3 months.[4] A calibration method that provides quality surveillance and allows selection of optimal centrifugation times is to examine replicate specimens of red cell suspensions within, below and above the acceptable hematocrit range. The time selected for routine use should be the minimal time at which maximal packing occurs. Deviation of 1% between replicate tubes is acceptable (eg, 0.38 ± 0.01).

Volume of Blood Drawn

The volume of blood collected must be controlled to protect the donor from excessive loss of blood and to maintain the correct proportion of anticoagulant to blood in the prepared components. Several kinds of equipment may be used:

1. A trip balance that constricts the tubing to stop blood flow when the phlebotomy bag reaches the desired weight.
2. A mechanical agitator calibrated to shut off when the desired weight is achieved.
3. A platform scale that must be kept under observation so that the phlebotomist can stop the blood flow manually when sufficient blood has been collected.

Weight of Whole Blood

All these methods use weight to indicate the volume of blood collected. This is the weight of the final component, including bag, tubing and anticoagulant/preservative solution, as well as the blood. The volume of blood should be 450 ± 45 mL, but allowances may be made for special "low volume unit" collections and special collections into collecting bags containing an appropriately reduced volume of anticoagulant. One milliliter of blood weighs not less than 1.053 g, the weight of blood from a donor with a hemoglobin of 125 g/L (12.5 g/dL), so the final container should weigh no less than 426 g (1.053 g/mL × 405 mL) plus the weight of the container and its anticoagulant. It is recommended that this weight be determined by weighing at least 10 containers from the lot in use and posted for each manufacturer of bag in use, as products from different manufacturers and even different lots can vary considerably. Since anticoagulant effectiveness declines with increasing hematocrit and increasing volumes of blood, a practical maximum is 522 g (1.053 g/mL × 495 mL) plus the weight of the container and anticoagulant.

Workers using the new 800-mL collection bag for the Valeri[15,16] method of freezing red blood cells in the primary container must ensure that only 450 ± 45 mL are collected. Although balances must be recalibrated to accommodate this collection modification, folding over and clamping the bottom of the collection bag will give the bag an appearance more like the standard bag once it is full. Care must be taken, however, not to trap anticoagulant in the folded portion or to puncture the container.

Monitoring Weight

A simple method to determine if the equipment used in blood collection is functioning properly is to record the weight, determined on a scale or balance, of the first unit of blood collected each day with each scale or agitator.[4] This fulfills the requirement that donor scales or other such devices be checked each day of use. If a scale or agitator consistently overdraws, underdraws or produces units at one end of the allowable range, it should be recalibrated to bring it nearer to the mean acceptable drawing volume. The performance of platform scales and trip balances can be checked with prefilled bags (preferably sand) of known weight.

Donor Reactions

The number, type and severity of reactions before, during and after phlebotomy must be recorded and should be evaluated by supervisory personnel and the responsible physician. Any follow-up investigations and actions taken should also be made a part of the record. If a higher percentage of donor reactions is observed with one or two phlebotomists, it may be necessary to work with these persons individually to improve their techniques and/or confidence. All phlebotomists should receive some in-service training in postdonation reaction care and be knowledgeable in how to obtain required emergency care for a donor who needs it.

Infectious Disease Tests

As the requirements to rule out bloodborne infectious diseases increase, so does the level of expertise required to perform such tests. QACI is important in viral marker testing as in all other areas of the blood bank or transfusion service. It is especially critical that the test kit manufacturer's instructions for testing and recommendations for controls and cutoff values be followed exactly. The calculation used to determine cutoff values must be recorded and retained. Persons performing these tests within the blood bank may find the use of a "run control," as described by Nath et al,[17] an additional quality control measure that may be useful. In setting up tests, it is important to be sure the appropriate sample is added to each tube or well. In addition to usual inspection at various testing stages, unusually high or low results may indicate that the unknown was not added.[18] *Standards*[2] requires participation in a proficiency test program as part of quality assurance for these tests. The American Association of Blood Banks and the College of American Pathologists jointly sponsor such a program, which includes quarterly panels of unknown samples to be tested for ALT, anti-HCV, anti-HBc, anti-HIV-1/2, anti-HTLV-I/II, anti-CMV and HBsAg. Although both the AABB[2] and the FDA[4] allow qualified outside laboratories to perform required tests on behalf of the blood bank, the medical director must ensure that appropriate procedures and controls are being used within the testing laboratory.

Testing large numbers of individuals for an agent of low prevalence creates several problems that must be addressed. Even with a test that has good specificity, the incidence of false-positive results can be expected to be high. Because of the consequence of missing a true positive (disease in the recipient), the test used must be very sensitive. Generally, achieving a low rate of false negatives with a test system is done at the expense of specificity. To be useful in screening blood donors, the test needs to be in a format that makes automation possible: results should be available reasonably quickly; reagents must be safe; and a method to confirm positives is essential.

A system must be in place to locate and effectively quarantine all blood units and their components when positive test results are found during the processing of a donor unit.

Labeling

Among the most important steps in safe transfusion practice are the careful identification and proper labeling of the donor unit and its associated processing tubes. The crossmatch must be done on cells from the originally attached whole blood or component segment; however, blood samples in tubes numbered and filled at the time of phlebotomy may be used for ABO and Rh tests, for the detection of unexpected antibodies and for tests to detect disease markers. The laboratory that processes donor blood must ensure that the unique number assigned to the donor appears on the donor card, the primary collection bag, all satellite collection bags and all tubes used for processing. This allows prompt identification of the relevant specimen if any processing tests reveals abnormal or discrepant results.

Blood Components

Quality assurance of component preparation includes in-vitro assays to document the effective collection of specific elements or coagulation factors. Observations of posttransfusion effectiveness are often helpful, if available, but are not required. Considerations of donor selection, volume of blood drawn, accuracy of scales and anticoagulant volume apply to component preparation as well as to whole blood collection and processing.

Platelets

Facilities that regularly prepare platelets must evaluate at least four platelet preparations monthly for platelet count, pH and plasma volume.[2] Platelets should be selected from each centrifuge in use. This testing must be done when the platelets are at the end of the allowable storage period or at the time of use[2] and the container contents should be well-mixed before an aliquot is withdrawn. The temperature at which the pH is measured should be the same as that at which the platelets are stored. A statement of volume must be on the label and the actual volume by measurement must be ± 10% of that stated volume. Platelets stored at 20-24 C must be gently agitated. Although the Standards requires platelets to be stored at 20-24 C, the FDA also allows storage at 1-6 C. The number of platelets in each container equals:

Platelet count/μL $\times$ 1000 $\times$ volume (mL).

AABB Standards[2] requires that there be at least 5.5×10^{10} platelets in at least 75% of the units tested at the end of the allowable storage period. Platelets by apheresis must contain a minimum of 3 $\times 10^{11}$ platelets in at least 75% of units tested.[2] Platelets should be prepared within 8 hours of blood collection. The platelets must be suspended in a sufficient volume of plasma or approved solution to ensure that the pH determined at the temperature of storage is 6.0 or greater in all units tested at the end of the storage period. Units with grossly visible platelet aggregates after storage must not be selected for transfusion. The facility in which platelets are prepared, not that in which they are transfused, is responsible for measuring platelet numbers, volume and pH. The FDA[4] and AABB[2] require that both the preparing facility and the transfusing facility observe and record the temperature in the vicinity of storage. Standards requires that the temperature be recorded at least every 4 hours during platelet storage.

Excessive temperature fluctuations, low plasma volume or inadequate gas exchange during storage are the usual causes of pH values below 6.0. Consistently low pH determinations suggest the need to store platelets either in a part of the laboratory with better temperature control or in an environmental chamber manufactured especially for platelet storage. If temperature control is not the problem, and if stored units are kept in gentle movement with adequate exposure of container surfaces to air, it may be necessary to increase the volume of plasma in which the platelets are suspended.

Granulocytes

Facilities preparing granulocytes by apheresis must ensure that a minimum of 1.0×10^{10} granulocytes are present in at least 75% of all units tested.[2]

Fresh Frozen Plasma

Plasma that is separated from its rbcs and placed at −18 C or lower within 8 hours of collection can be stored for 1 year at −18 C.[2] It must be thawed at temperatures between 30 C and 37 C and transfused within 24 hours after thawing if it is given as a source of labile coagulation factors.

Cryoprecipitated AHF

In facilities that regularly prepare CRYO, in-vitro recovery of Factor VIII must be assayed on at least four bags of CRYO each month.[4] CRYO must be thawed at 37 C and used within 6 hours of thawing if it is being used for Factor VIII content.[2] The AABB[2] requires a minimum of 80 IU of Factor VIII per container in at least 75% of units tested. In tests performed on pooled components, at least 75% of pools tested shall have a minimum level of 80 IU times the number of components in the pool.[2(p 11)] The FDA[4] permits testing of the four samples pooled and requires that the average potency level be at least 80 IU of Factor VIII. Factor VIII assays are difficult to perform accurately and reproducibly. These tests should be performed in a coagulation laboratory that employs an established method for testing concentrated Factor VIII on a routine and regular basis. The results of these assays must be documented.

Red Blood Cells

RBCs prepared from WB collected in CPDA-1 and intended for 35-day storage should have a final hematocrit no higher than 0.80 (80%).[2] This is best achieved by removing a standard volume of plasma, usually 225-250 mL (232-258 g), from units that contain between 449 g and 522 g of blood. For units collected in CPDA-1, the hematocrit should be measured each month on a representative sample obtained during component preparation that month.

Red Blood Cells, Deglycerolized

The final wash solution should be tested periodically by colorimetric or spectrophotometric measurement to ensure acceptably low levels of free hemoglobin, and by osmometry to ensure that the residual glycerol is below 1%. See Chapter 5 for discussion of this requirement. If an osmometer is not available, a manual method to estimate unacceptable levels of residual glycerol should be employed. Although at least one other method to estimate glycerol manually has been published,[19] the "simplified method" of Silver et al[20] appears the easiest to use. In each facility there should be a standard, either in mg/mL or as a color comparator, to designate the allowable level of supernatant hemoglobin.

Standards[2] requires recovery of at least 80% of the original RBCs following deglycerolization and a 70% viability of the D-RBCs 24 hours after transfusion. Postthaw recovery of red cells can be calculated using the formula shown in Fig 22-1. Values less than those cited above require a review of the method used to determine if it follows the published reference method.

% RBC recovery =

$$\frac{\text{hematocrit after processing} \times \text{volume of final component after processing}}{\text{hematocrit before processing} \times \text{volume of initial component before processing}} \times 100$$

Note: Hematocrit before processing refers to that of the original unit, not after the addition of glycerol.

Figure 22-1. Formula for postthaw recovery of RBCs.

Leukocyte-Reduced Red Blood Cells (LR-RBCs)

Standards[2] requires that the methods used to prepare LR-RBCs be those that have been shown to retain 80% of the original RBCs. When intended to prevent febrile nonhemolytic transfusion reactions, the component shall be prepared by a method shown to reduce the leukocyte number to $< 5 \times 10^8$. When intended for other purposes, the component must contain $< 5 \times 10^6$ leukocytes. Specially designed leukocyte-reduction blood filters are available that are highly efficient at achieving significant leukocyte reduction of blood components when used properly. See Fig 22-2. Useful definitions and formulas for those interested in performing QC checks on these components are given in Appendix 22-1.

Transportation

A system must be in use to ensure that all blood and blood components shipped by or received into a blood bank or blood transfusion service have been maintained within the temperatures required by the Standards[2] for those components. All liquid red blood cell components must be kept at a temperature of 1-10 C during transport. All components routinely stored at 20-24 C should be kept at 20-24 C during shipment. All frozen components should be transported in a manner to maintain their frozen state, and the FDA requires that they be transported at −18 C or colder.

Periodic temperature checks of received components under all encountered environmental conditions, should be performed and documented to ensure shipping methods are adequate to meet these criteria. Blood components issued for infusion, if returned to the blood bank, must also meet these criteria or they must not be returned to inventory.

One method to test quickly the temperature of arriving units is to place a thermometer between a sandwich of two components that have been rubber-banded together and check the temperature after 60 seconds.

References

1. Accreditation manual for hospitals, Vol 1, Standards. Oakbrook Terrace, IL: Joint Commission on Accreditation of Healthcare Organizations, 1991:218.
2. Widmann FK, ed. Standards for blood banks and transfusion services. 15th ed. Bethesda, MD: American Association of Blood Banks, 1993.
3. Barr A, Muir W. Quality monitoring of blood and its components. Med Lab Sci 1983;40:253-6.
4. Code of federal regulations. Title 21 CFR 600-799. Washington, DC: US Government Printing Office, 1992 (revised annually).
5. Jones FS, ed. Accreditation requirements manual, 4th ed. Bethesda, MD: American Association of Blood Banks, 1992.
6. Bachner P et al. College of American Pathologists Conference XVII on Quality Assurance in Pathology and Laboratory Medicine. Arch Pathol Lab Med 1990;114:1112-77.
7. Linden JV, Paul B, Dressler KP. A report of 104 errors in New York state. Transfusion 1992;32:601-6.

Leukocyte Residual Counts (Per Unit)

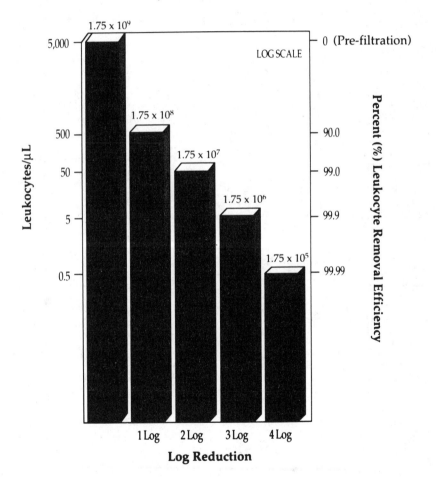

Figure 22-2. Logarithmic relationship between the number of leukocytes/μL and percent removal efficiency for leukocyte residual counts in a unit of Red Blood Cells. (Used with permission from Brandwein and Dickstein.[21])

8. Berte L. Developing performance standards for hospital personnel. Chicago, IL: American Society of Clinical Pathologists, 1989.
9. Ellinger P, South S. Proficiency/competency testing (teleconference). Bethesda, MD: American Association of Blood Banks, 1992.
10. Beattie KM. Control of the antigen-antibody ratio in antibody detection/compatibility tests. Transfusion 1980;20:227-84.
11. Guidelines for blood salvage and reinfusion in surgery and trauma. Arlington, VA: American Association of Blood Banks, 1990.
12. The Clinical Laboratory Improvement Amendments (CLIA). Federal Register 1992;57(40): 7002-288.
13. Von Schenck H, Falkensson M, Lundberg B. Evaluation of "HemoCue," a new device for determining hemoglobin. Clin Chem 1986;32: 526-9.
14. Neville R. Evaluation of portable haemoglobinometer in general practice. Br Med J [Clin Res] 1987;294:1263-5.
15. Valeri CR, Valeri DA, Anastasi J, et al. Freezing in the primary polyvinylchloride plastic collection bag: A new system for preparing and freezing nonrejuvenated and rejuvenated red blood cells. Transfusion 1981;21:138-48.
16. Kurtz SR, Valeri DA, Gray A, et al. A new approach to washing red blood cells frozen with a high concentration of glycerol in a special freezing container. Vox Sang 1982;43: 132-7.
17. Nath N, Wilkinson S, Dodd RY. Use of a control serum containing low level of HBsAg for monitoring proficiency in screening HBsAg. Transfusion 1986;26:519-24.
18. Wiltbank TB, McCarroll DR, Wartick MG. An undetectable source of technical error that could lead to false-negative results in enzyme-linked immunosorbent assay of antibodies to HIV-1. Transfusion 1989;29:75-7.
19. Meryman HT, Hornblower M. Quality control for deglycerolized red blood cells. Transfusion 1981;21:235-40.
20. Silver H, Umlas J, Kenney P, et al. A simplified method for quality control of deglycerolized erythrocytes. Transfusion 1982;22:254-6.
21. Brandwein H, Dickstein R. Leukocyte filtration: Understanding counting methods and their implications. East Hills, NY: Pall Biomedical, 1991.

Suggested Reading

Bozzo P. Implementing quality assurance. Chicago: American Society of Clinical Pathologists, 1991.

Clark G. Continuous quality improvement. Chicago: American Society of Clinical Pathologists, 1992.

Hoppe PA, Tourault MA. Quality control and regulatory requirements. In: Pittiglio D, ed. Modern blood banking and transfusion practices. Philadelphia: Davis Co, 1989:283-322.

Kurtz SR, Summers SH, Kruskall MS, et al. Improving transfusion practice: The role of quality assurance. Arlington, VA: American Association of Blood Banks, 1989.

National Committee for Clinical Laboratory Standards. Temperature monitoring and recording in blood banks. Tentative guideline. NCCLS document I16-T. Villanova, PA: NCCLS, 1987.

Otter J. Regulatory resource manual. Bethesda, MD: American Association of Blood Banks, 1992 (revised annually).

Taswell HF, Saeed SM, eds. Principles and practice of quality control in the blood bank. Washington, DC: American Association of Blook Banks, 1980.

Umiker W. The customer-oriented laboratory. Chicago: American Society of Clinical Pathologists, 1991.

Appendix 22-1. Leukocyte-Reduced Blood Components: Definitions, Formulas for Calculations, Presentation of Data and Calculation Example*

Definitions

Leukocytes/μL. The number of cells in a volume of 1 μL is determined by a direct microscopic counting method.

Leukocytes/mL. To determine leukocytes/mL, multiply the number of leukocytes/μL by 1000 (1000 μL = 1 mL).

Residual (Effluent) Content. The residual content is defined as the total number of leukocytes that remain in the unit following filtration. This is also referred to as the effluent content and can be calculated from the leukocytes/μL by multiplying this value × 1000 × unit volume (mL).

Log (Logarithm) Reduction. Log reduction is the reduction of leukocytes by filtration expressed in logarithmic form. Log is the power to which the number 10 must be raised in order to produce a given number. For example, log of 1000 = log 10^3 = 3; log of 10,000 = log 10^4 = 4.

Formula

Percent Leukocyte Removal Efficiency. For some time, the concepts of percent leukocyte removal efficiency and log reduction of leukocytes have been used to indicate the fraction or percentage of leukocytes that are removed during filtration. Having selected an appropriate counting method, the percent removal efficiency is calculated by the following formula:

$$\% \text{ Leukocyte Removal Efficiency} = \left[1 - \frac{(\text{effluent leukocytes/}\mu L)}{(\text{influent leukocytes/}\mu L)}\right] \times 100$$

Presentation of Data

Using the definitions and formulas, the following example of a unit of packed red cells is given:

Volume: 350 mL

Influent (prefiltration) Count:

1,750,000,000 (1.75 × 10^9) leukocytes/unit **or** 5,000,000 (5 × 10^6) leukocytes/mL **or** 5,000 (5 × 10^3) leukocytes/μL

Residual (Effluent) Count: 5 leukocytes/μL

Calculation Example

Percent (%) Leukocyte Removal Efficiency =

$$\left[1 - \frac{(\text{effluent leukocytes/}\mu L)}{(\text{influent leukocytes/}\mu L)}\right] \times 100 = \left[1 - \frac{(5)}{(5000)}\right] \times 100 = 99.9\%$$

$$\textbf{Log Reduction} = \text{Log}_{10} \frac{(\text{influent leukocytes/}\mu L)}{(\text{effluent leukocytes/}\mu L)} = \text{Log}_{10} \frac{(5000)}{(5)} = 3.00$$

Residual Content = Leukocytes/μL × 1000 × unit volume (mL) =

5 leukocytes/μL × 1000 × 350 mL/unit = 1.75 × 10^6 leukocytes/unit

*Modified from Brandwein H, Dickstein R.[21]

23

Records

Standard Operating Procedures

Perhaps the most important document that blood banks must maintain is the manual of standard operating procedures (SOPs). This manual describes the specific step-by-step procedures and techniques that the laboratory staff need for technical directions and use to fulfill the general requirements imposed by various standards and the federal regulations, "Current Good Manufacturing Practice for Blood and Blood Components" *Code of Federal Regulations* (21 CFR 606). The SOP manual interprets the meaning of all other policies and rules and must be clear, complete, concise, up to date and, most important, readily accessible to and consistently followed by the staff. For example, in approximately 20% of the transfusion fatalities reported to the FDA during the past 15 years, an adequate procedure for some critical step existed, but was not followed.

Standards and regulations usually define adequate performance while allowing choice of specific methods and procedures appropriate for each facility. If the AABB *Technical Manual* or another text serves as a part of the SOP manual, the facility's manual must define the edition and pages, and state exactly which procedures are to be used.

Elements of the SOP Manual

Procedural details, such as reagent volumes, times and temperatures of incubation or techniques, must be presented in a manner that will ensure that the processing records (worksheets, data cards, computer screens, etc) for the procedure are meaningful. For example, the processing record for antibody detection tests must include a record of reagent lots employed, the expiration dates, the positive or negative results observed, the controls used, the date and the operator's initials. These data are useless, however, without detailed instructions about how the test is performed.

The SOP manual should present, in an accessible and understandable fashion, the instructions and the indications for performing each test. An adequate SOP manual should provide enough information so that any trained person can perform all aspects of the SOPs used in that facility.[1] By combining the information in the SOP manual and the processing records, one should be able to reconstruct every test performed in the facility. It is preferable to use a uniform format for standard operating procedures.[2] (See Table 23-1.)

As an example, the following specific information might be included for a procedure such as "Pretransfusion Testing":

561

Table 23-1. Elements of a Written Technical Procedure*

1. NAME AND ADDRESS OF FACILITY: _____

_____

_____

2. NAME OF PROCEDURE—	all caps, bold letters, same for subheadings below
3. PRINCIPLE—	summarized in a few sentences
4. SPECIMEN—	type of specimen, labeling requirements, any special patient preparation, anticoagulant, volume, tube, storage requirements, etc.
5. REAGENTS AND EQUIPMENT—	includes purity requirements, standards, controls, special supplies and list of instruments used with calibration specifications
6. PROCEDURE—	step-by-step directions including use of quality controls and standards as appropriate
7. RESULTS—	includes calculations, reporting format, interpretations, frequency and tolerance of controls, the use of corrective action to be taken if tolerances are exceeded and "panic" values, which must be immediately communicated
8. NOTES—	includes precautions, validation, interfering substances, linearity graphs, limitations of method, etc.
9. REFERENCES—	includes source of procedure and/or relevant citations

10. REVIEW SCHEDULE—

Prepared by		
Adopted		
Reviewed		
Reviewed		
Reviewed		
Revised		
Supersedes		

*Modified from Summary of NCCLS Approved Guideline GP2-A2
Clinical Laboratory Technical Procedure Manuals—Second Edition, 1992 available from
National Committee for Clinical Laboratory Standards
    771 East Lancaster Avenue
    Villanova, PA 19085
    (215) 525-2435

1. The kinds of specimens needed and how they are to be obtained, including the directions for identifying patients and labeling samples.

2. Directions for documenting specimen receipt and identity of the personnel involved.

3. The steps necessary for comparing the request forms and the labels on specimen tubes to ensure accuracy of information before accepting the samples.

4. Description of reagents and equipment necessary to perform the tests.

5. Detailed instructions for performing and recording each test routinely performed, performing and evaluating control tests, and determining when additional tests are indicated.

6. The elements to be included in the required search for previous blood bank records for the patient.

7. Instructions for labeling the blood or component and for completing the necessary paperwork.

8. Instructions for retaining and storing tested samples.

The criteria for interpreting and recording observed results must be documented, and the directions for managing possible problems should be included in a readily accessible form. The limits of authority with respect to independent judgment and criteria for consulting a supervisor should be defined. The SOP manual should include definitions of symbols used in record-keeping and instructions to ensure uniform use of criteria and symbols. For example, agglutination reactions can be either graded or scored. Whichever system is adopted, it should be consistently used by all employees.

The SOP manual is also an appropriate place to maintain personnel information pertinent to the records. This should consist of a list of names, signatures and identifying initials or identifi- cation codes with inclusive dates of employment of personnel authorized to sign, initial or review reports and records. This list should include full-time and part-time personnel including phlebotomists and transfusionists, if appropriate.

Review and Revision

The SOP manual should be subject to ongoing review and revision. Whenever problems arise with a procedure, corrective measures or alternative techniques should be considered and, if approved, incorporated into the manual. Whenever a new procedure or policy is implemented, or a new regulation or standard becomes applicable, the existing manual should be reviewed and appropriate corrections made in accordance with the established policy for changes. Periodically, after publication of each new edition of AABB *Standards for Blood Banks and Transfusion Services,*[3] and upon receipt of any change in Food and Drug Administration (FDA), state or local requirements, the SOP manual should be examined page by page for conformance with requirements. The medical director must review the SOP manual at least annually and document the date of the review. If there is a schedule for review of several pages or sections at a time, the review will usually be more complete than if the responsible physician reviews the entire manual at one time.

Individuals who use the manuals, forms and labels should participate in their drafting and review. This involvement not only brings the results of their experience to bear on the instructions, but also heightens employee awareness of problems in writing instructions and keeping good records. Minor revisions may be noted with date and initials on the appropriate pages of the master copy; photocopies of amended pages may then be placed in other copies of the manual. For major revisions, a newly typed page, dated and initialed, should be inserted in the master manual and all copies. The number of SOPs in circulation should be controlled to ensure that some are not overlooked when changes are implemented. Pages removed from the master copy should be dated at the time of removal and be retained in a file for at least 5 years, or longer if required by local laws. This allows for documentation of the procedures used during the time covered by statutes of limitations for legal actions.

Obsolete computer software necessary to reconstruct or trace records must also be archived appropriately. New software should be implemented only in accordance with the documented change and validation procedures.

The SOP manual can most easily be revised or modified if it is in loose-leaf format. Revised pages and forms must be initialed and dated by the physician responsible for the facility. Alternatively, it is acceptable to list revisions and the approval dates on an index page signed by the responsible physician. Each copy of the SOP manual should contain the list of revisions. Records of changes should include documentation ensuring that all staff with a need to know have read or have been trained in the proper use of the revised or added procedure.

Categories of Records

Two categories of records deserve comment:

1. Processing records, which contain the observations and interpretations at the time of testing.
2. Statistical or summary records, which are analyses of the processing records.

Processing records document the many operations of the facility and include test results and interpretations, observations of temperatures, distribution of blood components and maintenance of schedules. Statistical records summarize one or more of these operations during a defined time span and provide information useful for evaluating service demands, production, adequacy of personnel, inventory control and other variables.

Professional and governmental organizations have historically placed primary emphasis on processing records, but current trends in evaluating and reviewing medical practice suggest that summary records will achieve increasing importance, especially as computerization makes it easier to prepare statistical summaries. Manual record-keeping systems designed for efficient and rapid summarization can also provide assembly and surveillance of data from records.

The Need for Records

The most frequently cited deficiencies in inspection or survey programs are record-keeping violations. This fact has created two widespread misconceptions:

1. The main reason for keeping records is to satisfy inspection programs.
2. The volume of required record-keeping interferes with the flow of work.

Do inspection programs lead to greater record-keeping demands? Probably so, especially in facilities in which maintaining records was never a priority. Inspections, by their very nature, require records as proof of satisfactory performance, because many procedures cannot be directly observed by the inspector and the nature of past performance can only be inspected through records.

Records reflect the history of operations and provide valuable insights about direction and supervision, as well as attitudes and work performance. Sloppy, inaccurate, illegible, incomplete or missing records suggest imprecision, haste, disorder and error; inadequate records of donor suitability threaten the safety of the blood supply.

Summary of General Requirements

Records must be made concurrently with performance. They must be legible and indelible; must identify the person immediately responsible for each significant step in collecting, processing, compatibility testing and distribution of blood or blood components; must include the dates of performance; and must be as detailed as necessary for clear understanding.[4] Records may be kept in handwritten or printed hard copy or may be retained entirely electronically, provided they can be easily retrieved for reference or review and adequate backup exists in case of system failure.[2] *Because these principles apply to every record, they will not be repeated as separate items in the following sections listing individual requirements.*

Many laboratory procedures are optional. However, if they are performed, there must be complete records of these procedures.

If it is necessary to alter or correct any record, the reason for change should be noted and the change must be identifiable by date and person responsible. The original recording must not be obliterated; it may be circled or crossed out in handwritten records, but it should remain legible. Computer records should permit tracking of both original and corrected data to include the date and the user identification of the person making the change.[2]

Rubber stamps, brackets or ditto marks are not acceptable means of identifying responsible personnel. Record formats should be designed to eliminate the need for repetitive signing by the same individual.

Use of Records

AABB *Standards* requires that results of each test must be recorded as observations are made. Interpretation, if separate from results, must be recorded upon completion of testing. If results and interpretation are synonymous, no additional record is needed. Records of each patient's blood type should be kept available for immediate reference for at least the current hospitalization; these records must be readily accessible for at least 12 months. In addition, *Standards* requires that records of difficulty in blood typing, clinically significant unexpected antibodies and severe adverse reactions to transfusion be kept for at least 5 years. These records should be reviewed before blood is issued for transfusion.

Reviewing previous records as part of pretransfusion testing provides some confirmation of the identity of the current sample. *Standards* requires that the results of previous ABO and Rh testing be compared to interpretations of the current tests before blood is issued for transfusion. It is highly desirable to keep permanent records on patients with unexpected antibodies readily available. Knowing whether unexpected antibodies have previously been noted and identified often speeds the procurement of compatible blood and may prevent delayed hemolytic reactions in patients whose antibodies are weak or undetectable at the time of subsequent testing.

Confidentiality

Blood bank records, like all medical information, must not be released or made available to unauthorized persons. Restricted access to computerized records must be ensured by an appropriately maintained computer access security system.

Record Design

To be effective, record systems must meet the needs of the institution and be used in a manner that satisfies this need. Interference with work flow generally results from imperfectly designed records and a poor understanding of their purpose. Each form should have a title that explains its intended use and includes the name of the facility and sufficient information, eg, address to distinguish it from other institutions with a similar name. Well-designed forms include as much preprinted information as possible, to minimize the number of manual entries needed.

One major concern in records is the identification, for legal or investigational purposes, of persons responsible for each significant process. For example, the component preparation log should have entries that correspond with each of the main procedural steps. In a large laboratory in which several persons may prepare components concurrently, the log should make it possible to identify the persons involved in preparation of each group of components. It is not required, however, that each person initial the log for each step of component preparation. The SOP manual may indicate that the supervisor assumes the overall responsibility by initialing or validating processing records. This obviously requires that the supervisor monitor the work area closely and have confidence that there is control in the processes being performed by staff.

Significant Steps

The number of records maintained varies according to the facility's methods of operation. Each significant step and critical point of a procedure must be recorded in a manner that permits tracing a blood component or patient specimen through all related procedures from the first step to final disposition. An adequate processing record is one that makes it possible for an auditor or reviewer to reconstruct, from the record alone, the procedures performed. Records of phlebotomy, for example, must include results of examining both arms for signs of illegal drug use, but need not include documentation of each step in the arm preparation. The arm preparation is a single significant step in blood collection; if fully described in the SOP manual, performance is adequately documented when the phlebotomist initials the donation record. Similarly, it is sufficient to record the identity of persons involved in preparing blood containers for use, without recording each step of the process. Assessing the quality of performance requires not only good training and supervision but also documentation of the critical points of a procedural step.

Errors in Processing

If a specific processing error could adversely affect patient safety or component purity, potency, safety or effectiveness, an investigation should be conducted and a record maintained to ensure fulfillment of the requirements of good manufacturing practice. For example, an inappropriately warm storage temperature may render Cryoprecipitated AHF useless for its intended purpose; consequently, records of storage temperature and any problems are essential. On the other hand, the volume of each red cell component prepared routinely in a standardized procedure is usually not critical, and no routine records of red cell volume are required.

Record-Keeping Requirements

In designing records systems it is helpful to scrutinize the inspection checklists used by the AABB, the FDA and any other inspecting agencies to determine whether the procedures and the records comply with published requirements. These checklists summarize the records that are considered necessary. In the component preparation sections of FDA inspection forms, for example, there are lists of critical steps for each blood component. Records must include personnel identification and the performance date of each critical step in preparation.

Retention of Records

The FDA requires that records be kept for at least 5 years or for 6 months after product expiration if the dating period exceeds 5 years. For frozen red cells or source plasma this means that records must be retained for 10 years and 6 months. Records must be kept indefinitely when there is no dating period for the component. *Standards*[3] requires that all records relevant to the operation of a blood bank or transfusion service be kept for a minimum of 5 years or as required by law [21 *CFR* 600.12(b)].[4] Records of a patient's ABO and Rh types should be readily available for 12 months for review and comparison to current test results, and must be retained for at least 5 years.

Other records required by *Standards* to be retained 5 years include:

- Donors' ABO and Rh types, and difficulty in determining patient or donor ABO and Rh types.
- Severe adverse reactions to donation or transfusion.

- Patients' therapeutic procedures and donor hemapheresis clinical records.
- Compatibility test interpretation and clinically significant unexpected antibodies found in patients.
- Blood component inspection during storage and prior to issue.
- Superseded procedures, manuals and publications.
- Storage temperatures, control testing and proficiency testing surveys and any resulting corrective actions taken.

In addition, the following records must be retained indefinitely:

- Donors' medical history, physical examination, consent, and interpretations of tests for disease markers, including deferral status, for each donation, including hemapheresis.
- Blood and components received from outside sources, including numeric or alphanumeric identification of blood units, and identification of the collecting facility. However, the information from an intermediate facility may be used if the intermediate facility retains the unit number and identification of the collecting facility.
- Information to identify facilities that carry out any part of the preparation of blood components and the function performed.
- Final disposition of each unit of blood or component.
- Names, signatures and initials or identification code, and inclusive dates of employment of those authorized to sign or initial or review reports and records.
- Notification to donors of permanent deferral.
- Notification to recipients of potential exposure to disease transmissible by blood.

Record Storage

As with record-keeping, the act of retention is not enough. The degree of accessibility of records of the facility's operation should be in direct proportion to frequency of their use.

The method and location of record storage depend on the volume of records and the amount of available storage space. Some large blood banks use microfilm or microfiche, not only to reduce storage costs but also to provide ready access to important documents. Such records legitimately replace original documents that may be stored elsewhere or destroyed, but there must be documentation that the transformed records are true copies of the material they replace. Magnetic media used to back up or archive computer records and databases must be stored in accordance with the manufacturer's recommendations and instructions. An archival copy of the computer operating system and applications software should be stored in the same manner. The facility must properly index and organize the records and must have a properly functioning viewer available on the premises. During inspection, the facility personnel must be able to produce, within a reasonable time, legible "hard copy" of the record, if requested.

A designated responsible person must review and, by means of a signed and dated certification record, ensure authenticity and completeness of each group of documents copied. If color-coded records lose meaning in black-and-white reproduction, or if the original document is altered (eg, by erasure or retyping), the original copies should also be retained.

Computers

For records maintained in a computer, there must be a method of verifying accuracy of data entry. Hardware and software security measures must prevent unintended deletion of data or access by unauthorized persons. A backup disk or tape should be maintained in the event of unexpected loss of information from the storage medium. While microfilm or microfiche may adequately fulfill requirements for retaining records, computer systems requiring transfer of results may not replace certain required original records. The FDA and the AABB accept magnetically coded employee badges and other computer-related identifying methods in lieu of written signatures, but controls must be established to prevent misuse. All recorded information must be available for hard-copy (paper) reproduction.

When records are maintained by electronic data processing, there must be a secure means of identifying changes or corrections made in the original records. The audit trail should identify the original data, the data entry person, the modifier, the modification and the date/time of change. If the records concern confidential medical data [eg, positive human immunodeficiency virus antibody (anti-HIV-1/2) test results] or cross-reference test results and personal data (ie, name and sample number), special attention to systems security is essential.

The following details should be considered in designing systems employing computers for required record-keeping:
1. The program specifications, procedures used to validate the program and the test results must be available for review.
2. The location and the means of access to the source code should be in the SOP manual.
3. There must be validated documentation of systems used to prevent unauthorized access and to prevent unintended deletion or addition of data. It

must be possible to identify data that have been altered, and to trace when and by whom the changes were made.

4. There must be a clear identification of the levels of access to confidential data and of the ways to ensure this confidentiality.
5. There must be a clear definition of the backup system(s) for computer downtime, and test records to show that the backup system works properly.
6. There must be records that personnel have received adequate training and that each employee has achieved adequate proficiency in using the system.
7. There should be periodic audits to ensure that stored data can be retrieved and made available within a reasonable time.
8. In multi-user systems, validated safeguards must be in place to ensure that a record can be edited by only one person at a time.
9. All changes to the software must be fully documented and validated. The record of change should be similar to an audit trail and include the name of the module changed (original data) and all modules affected by the change.

Summary Records

In general, summary records are not required. It is very useful, however, to review at least an annual summary of all blood bank error and accident records. Such a summary provides an overview of operations and may identify procedures that need clarification and personnel who need retraining. Summaries also contain useful information for internal audits. Advances in adapting automated data processing equipment to all phases of blood bank operations facilitate review of processing records and the compilation of statistical summaries. Strict adherence to the facility's SOP manual and uniform notation among staff are critical if useful data are to be obtained with a minimum of effort.

Specific Record Requirements

Minimum Requirements for Records of Laboratory Tests on Patient or Recipient Blood Specimens

1. First and last names and patient identification number. The specimen label should include the date of collection.
2. There must be a mechanism to identify the person who drew the blood.
3. Date of testing.
4. The test performed, results observed and final interpretation of results.
5. Results of ABO and Rh testing including control for autoagglutinins and weak D (D^u) testing, if performed.
6. Interpretation of ABO and Rh tests.
7. Results and interpretation of tests for unexpected antibodies.
8. Difficulty in blood grouping, clinically significant unexpected antibodies and serious adverse reactions to transfusion.

Minimum Requirements for Records of Compatibility Tests

1. Patient's ABO and Rh types.
2. Identification numbers for the patient and for donor unit(s).
3. ABO and Rh types of the donor unit(s).
4. Results and interpretation of compatibility tests.
5. Testing date.
6. Component being tested or prepared.

Minimum Requirements for Records of Transfusion Requests

1. Recipient's first and last name.
2. Recipient's identification number (hospital, admission, emergency room or other). Additional helpful information includes: age, diagnosis, hospital location, clinical history, including recent transfusions and pregnancy, drug therapy and name of requesting physician.
3. Number of units of blood or component required. The date and time units are to be available is not required but is recommended.

Minimum Requirements for Records of Blood Donations

At each blood donation, there must be a record that provides true identification of the donor and gives pertinent information; either single-use or multiple-donation forms are acceptable. These records may be filed either by donor name or donor unit number, with appropriate cross-references. Records required for laboratory tests on donor blood are considered in a later section. Information required in the donation record is as follows:

1. Donor unit number.
2. Donor's first and last name and middle initial.
3. Donor's address and phone number.
4. Donor's date of birth.
5. Donor's social security number or other equivalent unique permanent identifier that will ensure accurate maintenance of donor deferral registries.
6. Date of donation.
7. Date of last donation.
8. Record of physical examination (temperature, blood pressure, pulse, hemoglobin or hematocrit, arm examination) and identification of the examiner. In addition, the record must include documentation that the donor weighs at least 110 pounds or that a low volume unit was collected. (See Chapter 1.)
9. Medical history with answers recorded as "yes" or "no" for each question with any pertinent explanation.
10. Identification of the interviewer.
11. Record of whether the donor was accepted, and whether the phlebotomy was satisfactory or unsatisfactory. If the donor is deferred, the reason should be given, with notation about temporary, indefinite or permanent deferral. The names of donors who have been deferred or placed on indefinite surveillance for the protection of the potential recipient should be readily accessible.
12. Informed consent: Consent to have blood drawn and tested, an opportunity to exclude use for transfusion (if applicable), a statement that AIDS information educational material is understood and an accurate medical history has been given, permission for the blood bank to use blood as it deems fit if unsuitable for transfusion, and signatures of the donor and a witness. Legal advice may be helpful in designing this portion of the form.
13. Identification of the phlebotomist.
14. Record of any donor reaction; symptoms, treatment, condition of the donor upon release and notation about whether the donor can be accepted again; identification of person attending the donor, time released and notation if the donor refuses treatment or advice. This record may be kept on a separate form designed for this purpose.
15. Supplementary records: There are additional record requirements for donors in special categories. These

records may be included in the donor form, may be attached to it or may be filed separately.

a. Donors under age 17: Written permission from a parent or guardian if it is required by state law. Minors who are in the military or legally married are generally exempt from this requirement.

b. Therapeutic bleedings: A record that the patient's physician has ordered phlebotomy; records of the disease and whether or not the unit may be used for transfusion purposes; volume of blood drawn; and final disposition of unit.

c. Autologous donations: If all donor suitability criteria defined by the SOP for autologous donation are not met, written consent of the patient's physician, the blood bank physician and the patient (or, if indicated, the patient's parent or guardian). The FDA requires that a physician examine the donor and certify good health if the donation interval is less than 8 weeks.[4] The physician's written order requesting autologous collections is an acceptable alternative.

If the blood meets all requirements for release for allogeneic use, the date of release and any labeling changes must be recorded by the facility making the change. If hepatitis tests [hepatitis B surface antigen (HBsAg)] or anti-HIV-1/2 tests are positive, the identity of the physician requesting release of blood should be recorded. If the hepatitis C virus antibody (anti-HCV) test is positive, notification of the patient's physician should be documented. The destruction of blood not released should be doc-

umented. However, care should be taken throughout the process to protect the confidentiality of the donor-patient.

Helpful Donor Information That Is Not Required

1. Although not specifically required by federal regulations, identification (such as social security number, driver's license number or photograph identity card) is necessary to ensure accurate donor deferral registries. The donor's social security number is not required, but is recommended in case it becomes necessary to locate a donor with a positive anti-HIV-1/2 test.

2. Name of patient or donor group to be credited for the donation.

3. Results of tests for antibody detection, HBsAg, anti-HIV-1/2, anti-HCV, hepatitis B core antibody, human T-cell lymphotropic virus type I antibody, alanine aminotransferase and the serologic test for syphilis. These results are a required part of the processing record. A record of these results on the donor record is optional except for reasons for permanent deferral, such as confirmed positive results of anti-HIV-1/2, anti-HCV and HBsAg testing. Results of abnormal findings may be useful for reference at a future donation. It is strongly recommended that indefinite or permanent deferral be noted in donor records to help prevent errors in the release of an unsuitable donor's blood components if future donation occurs.

4. Disposition of the unit is required information that may be recorded on the donation form.

5. Race.

6. The name of the manufacturer and lot number of the container/antico-

agulant. Although this information is required, it is optional on the donation form.

Minimum Requirements for Records of Hemapheresis, Therapeutic Phlebotomy or Plasma Exchange

If no component is prepared, only those records necessary to ensure donor protection are necessary. If transfusion components are prepared, the records of these procedures must include all required information for blood donors and in addition must include the following as part of a separate file on each donor[3]:

1. All initial and periodic physical examinations by a physician, including medical history interviews. The physician's acceptance or rejection of the donor, based on the accumulated laboratory data. In the case of therapeutic procedures, the prescribing physician's order may substitute for all of the above.

2. The results of all laboratory tests to determine donor suitability.

3. The explanation of the procedures that will be performed and the patient's or donor's informed consent.

4. All test results for infectious disease markers.

5. A record of any whole blood, red cell, leukocyte or platelet reduction, including planned donations of those components.

6. For hemapheresis donors who are given medications or are immunized, there must be a separate informed consent as well as complete information on the drug or antigen source; the schedule, dosage and route of administration; adverse reactions; and response (eg, antibody titer) to the stimulating agent as measured by laboratory tests.

7. The name of the manufacturer and the lot numbers and volumes of all solutions, software and drugs used. This is a required record but it is optional in the individual donor record file.

8. The time the procedure begins and ends, the volume of blood processed, the volume of each component harvested, the estimated blood cell loss and any adverse reactions.

9. Disposition of any components collected or processed.

Laboratory Processing of Donor Blood

The type of test, the results observed and a final interpretation of results must be recorded for all tests.[3,4] Entries must be made as work is done, using symbols that clearly indicate positive or negative results. The symbols must be defined and used uniformly by all personnel. Most required records can be incorporated in one worksheet to facilitate labeling and the review of records before release of each batch of blood components. One of the most critical steps in processing donor blood is identification and quarantine of all units unsuitable for distribution. Because an error at this point may result in transfusion of anti-HIV-1/2 positive or HBsAg-reactive components, labeling procedures should include a double check of units to be quarantined before components from those units are released for distribution. Units not suitable for distribution must be destroyed and final disposition must be recorded.

Minimum Requirements for Records of Tests on Donor Blood Samples

1. Donor unit number.

2. Results of ABO and Rh testing, including the test for weak D (D^u) if indicated.

3. Results of serum or plasma tests for expected antibodies in the ABO system.
4. Interpretation of ABO and Rh tests.
5. Results and interpretations of tests for the detection of unexpected antibodies, if indicated, including use of IgG-coated control cells if used.
6. Results of serologic test for syphilis.
7. Results of tests for all infectious disease markers and surrogate tests. Relevant calculations to define positive results and control values must also be retained. The record of these calculations may be kept separately from the results on donor samples but must be readily associated with specific sample records.
8. Results of positive and negative controls run with the donor samples must be retained.
9. Reagents used, manufacturer, lot number, expiration date, control values and calculations if applicable, and evidence that reagents have been subjected to performance checks.
10. Equipment validation records.
11. Criteria for repeating positive samples, including the number of permissible retests.
12. Criteria for determining that a test or group of tests is invalid.
13. Results of tests performed by outside testing laboratories, with the name and location of the testing laboratory on the record.

Useful Laboratory Tests That Are Not Required

1. Control tests on anti-D serum, except as required to comply with the manufacturer's instructions.
2. Identification of unexpected antibodies if the plasma will not be transfused.

Minimum Requirements for Labeling

1. Documentation that verifies all records of test results are reviewed for completeness and accuracy prior to labeling. Frozen products may be prelabeled, provided they remain in quarantine until all test results are available and the batch is released.
2. Identity of each component in quarantine to prevent unsuitable units from being released. A system that provides a double check of correct selection of units quarantined is strongly recommended.
3. Documentation that ensures current, accurate donor deferral registries have been checked and necessary action has been taken to prevent distribution of unsuitable products.
4. Verification that units released have accurate blood group labels, expiration dates and component labels.

Minimum Requirements for Records of Component Preparation

1. Donor unit number.
2. Date and, if appropriate, time drawn and whether a manual or an automated collection method was used.
3. Name and volume of anticoagulant.
4. Name of component.
5. Date and time each component was prepared. If the preparation involves multiple steps such as separation, freezing and thawing, the time each step was taken must be documented.
6. Date and time of component expiration.
7. Volume of component, except for Cryoprecipitated AHF and Red Blood Cells (RBCs) prepared in a routine manner from 450 mL of Whole Blood. Similar records must be kept when separating and pooling recovered plasma for further manufacture. For any pooled product, records must indicate

the identity of each donor who contributed to the pool.

Minimum Requirements for Records of Blood and Components Received From Other Facilities

1. Name and address of shipping facility. It is not necessary to record the address with each unit if this information is readily available.
2. Name of blood component.
3. Donor unit number assigned by collecting facility.
4. Accession or inventory number, if any, assigned by receiving bank.
5. ABO and Rh types of components.
6. Component expiration date and time, if indicated.
7. Date component was received.
8. For blood that is received already crossmatched, the name and identification number of the intended recipient and interpretation of results of compatibility tests.
9. Results and interpretation of tests done by the receiving facility.

Minimum Requirements for Records of Storage and Inspection of Blood Components (See Also Chapter 3)

1. Recording charts for refrigerator, freezer and platelet incubator temperatures, with inclusive dates, explanation of abnormal temperatures and action taken, and initials of certifying personnel.
2. Records of periodic testing of alarm systems.
3. Records of temperatures observed daily and their comparison to automated temperature recordings. Centralized electronic temperature recording and alarm systems can replace records of daily observations but *Standards* requires that temperature results be printed at least every

4 hours. If components are stored in an open storage area, the ambient temperature must be recorded at least every 4 hours.
4. Notation of quarantine of unsatisfactory units, record of any tests performed and final disposition of each unit.

Disposition of Blood and Components

It must be possible to follow every unit of blood (including each of the components prepared from a unit) from records of the donor suitability and required testing to its disposition by transfusion, shipment or destruction. When destruction is necessary, the identification of each of the components destroyed, the reason for destruction, date and method of destruction must be recorded [21 *CFR* 600.12(a)]. When units are shipped, the shipping facility must record the following information:

1. Name and address of receiving facility.
2. Date and time of shipment.
3. A list of each donor unit number, blood group and expiration date.
4. Name of each blood component.
5. Final inspection of Whole Blood (WB) or RBC units.
6. Name of person filling order.
7. Periodic tests documenting that shipping containers maintain an acceptable storage temperature range.

Minimum Requirements for Records of Issue for Transfusion

1. Time and date of issue or reissue. For reissued WB or RBCs, a record that proper temperature has been maintained, that container and closure are intact and that inspection for abnormal color or appearance has been satisfactory.

2. Donor unit number of blood or component, or lot number of product.
3. Comparison of the patient's current ABO and Rh types with results of previous tests performed in preceding 12 months.

Minimum Requirements for Records of Transfusion

1. A signed statement that the information on the container label and the compatibility record has been matched with the wristband or other identification of intended recipient, item by item, prior to transfusion (Standard J2.100).
2. Useful, but optional information includes the time transfusion is started and completed, the volume transfused and the patient's condition.

Some or all of the compatibility, issue and transfusion records can be combined on one multipart form. After termination of transfusion, one copy of the form is attached to the patient's chart, a record is filed in the blood bank and another copy may be sent to accounting.

Emergency Issue of Blood or Components

Blood components may be issued before completion of routine tests in situations in which a delay in providing blood might unduly jeopardize the life of the patient.[1,3,4] The label or tie-tag must clearly identify those required tests that have not been completed. The records must contain a statement of the requesting physician indicating that the clinical situation is sufficiently urgent to require release of blood before completion of testing.

Many transfusion services no longer routinely perform antiglobulin crossmatches. The requesting physician's statement concerning the abbreviated testing is not required before issuing the blood in transfusion services where the SOP manual distinguishes between performing a full antiglobulin crossmatch and performing a Type and Screen. In these cases, the blood bank director assumes the responsibility for transfusion without an individual antiglobulin crossmatch. In all other cases, the compatibility label must clearly state that tests routinely performed in that facility have not been completed. All other record requirements apply as usual.

Minimum Requirements for Records of Quality Control and Quality Assessment

1. Dated and signed or initialed temperature recording charts for each refrigerator and freezer or central monitor record, temperature records of refrigerated centrifuges, heat-regulated devices (ie, blood warmers, incubators).
2. Record of quality control tests performed on reagents for infectious disease marker tests, antihuman globulin, blood grouping serum and reagent red blood cells as specified by the SOP manual.
3. Results of tests to evaluate the performance of other reagents (eg, copper sulfate) and equipment, as required by the AABB National Inspection and Accreditation Committee.
4. Results of equipment calibration, validation of equipment software (see also Computer Systems Requirements) and equipment maintenance logs.
5. Log of personnel signatures and inclusive dates of employment. If signature abbreviations or employee codes are used in record-keeping, these must be identified.
6. Record of quality control tests of components prepared.

7. Record of periodic checks on sterile technique if components are prepared in an open system, unless an equivalent method has been approved by the FDA.

8. Record of sterilization of supplies and reagents prepared within the facility, including date, time interval, temperature and mode. Records of biological indicator tests to determine the effectiveness of sterilization.

9. Record of disposition of rejected supplies or reagents used in collection, processing and compatibility testing of blood and blood components.

10. Record of supplies and reagents used, including manufacturer, lot numbers, date received, inclusive dates in use and expiration date.

11. Record of employee participation in job-related education or training with inclusive dates, subjects and evaluation, if appropriate.

12. Records of proficiency testing. The FDA and the Health Care Financing Administration both have additional proficiency testing requirements for blood banks and transfusion service laboratories.[5,6] It is recommended, therefore, that the following documentation be available:
   a. Sources of samples and expected answers.
   b. Frequency and number of tests related to each laboratory category.
   c. Identity of personnel performing the proficiency testing assays and relevance to their work assignments.
   d. System by which responsibility for proficiency testing assays is rotated or other assurance that the competence of all employees is ensured.
   e. Dates of testing and evaluation of performance.

f. Corrective action, if necessary, and monitoring to ensure effectiveness of corrective action, if indicated.
g. Training and retraining of personnel when indicated.
h. Notification of state or federal agency, if required.

13. Records of parallel studies performed.

Minimum Requirements for Computer Systems

1. Documentation of computer system to include:
   a. SOPs that reflect current standards and clearly explain system use as necessary.
   b. Program development and system modifications if done internally.
   c. Installation of the system.
   d. Validation of functionality and data integrity.
   e. Training of personnel.
   f. Policies and procedures for system maintenance and operation.
   g. All changes in operations or software, explained both in complete technical detail and in language understood by users.

2. Audit trails of the database to include:
   a. Identification number of sample or unit.
   b. Original value.
   c. New value.
   d. Originator identification, person or device that created the record.
   e. Modifier identification, person or device that changed the record.
   f. Date and time of change.
   g. Authorization identification.

3. Software record of change to include:
   a. System name.
   b. Version, release or model number.
   c. Module name.
   d. Change made.

e. Modules affected.

f. Modifier identification.

g. Modification date and time.

h. Authorization identification.

i. Verification date and time.

j. Reason for change.

The FDA has recommended that records for computer systems include: hardware configuration diagrams, software version logs, maintenance schedules (including preventive maintenance), software validation protocols, hardware validation protocols, system reliability logs, training records and master manual copies.

Errors, Accidents and Adverse Reactions

Quality assessment dictates that records be kept of errors, accidents and corrective actions made. *Standards* and the *Code of Federal Regulations* [21 *CFR* 606.170 (a)] require records of adverse reactions in donors or patients.[3,4]

Standards requires that each facility have a system for detecting, reporting and evaluating suspected adverse reactions to transfusion. Chapter 19 outlines the recommended tests for evaluating reported transfusion reactions. The report form and the results of all tests must be retained for at least 5 years, or as required by local statutes of limitations, whichever is longer. When an error or accident involving a blood component occurs, the following information is recommended for records required by the FDA [21 *CFR* 606.160 and 606.170]:

1. A description of the error or accident including whether all components involved were completely tracked.

2. The name of the blood component(s) or product(s) involved.

3. The donor unit number(s) of the blood component(s) or lot numbers of the blood product(s) implicated and the manufacturer (ie, collecting or processing facility if not the same as reporting facility).

4. The date of discovery.

5. The date of occurrence.

6. Whether or not the blood component or product was transfused.

7. Whether or not the patient's physician was made aware of the error or accident, if the blood or blood product was transfused. (Note: Federal regulations requiring notification in certain cases have been proposed and may be applicable after publication of this manual.)

8. The category of personnel responsible for the error or accident (eg, nurse, technologists, shipping personnel or others) and identity of the individual.

9. An explanation of how the error or accident occurred.

10. The actions taken to prevent a recurrence of the error or accident.

11. The name of the manufacturer, lot number and expiration date of the product if defective reagents or supplies were implicated.

12. A copy of the notification of appropriate authorities, when applicable. All licensed establishments are required to notify the FDA of errors or accidents in the manufacture of products that may affect the safety, purity or potency of any biological product (21 *CFR* 600.14). The FDA has requested voluntary reporting of errors and accidents[7] and has identified the following examples as reportable events if components or products are released for distribution:

- Units repeatedly reactive for viral marker testing.
- Units from donors for whom test results were improperly interpreted due to testing errors related to

improper use of equipment or failure to strictly follow the reagent manufacturer's directions for use.

- Units from donors who are (or should have been) either temporarily or permanently deferred due to medical history or a history of repeatedly reactive results for viral marker tests.
- Units released prior to completion of all tests.
- Incorrectly labeled blood components (eg, ABO, expiration date).
- Microbial contamination of blood components when the contamination is attributed to an error in manufacturing.

The record system should include a method for reporting cases of AIDS, suspected posttransfusion hepatitis or other diseases resulting from blood transfusion or errors and accidents in the manufacture of components or products that may affect their safety, purity or potency. It is imperative to make a careful and complete record of all investigations to ensure adequate care of patients, to prevent subsequent errors and to provide legal evidence if this is needed.

FDA Required Reports

Fatalities related to blood collection or transfusion must be reported promptly to the Director, Center for Biologics Evaluation and Research (CBER), 1401 Rockville Pike, Suite 200N, HFM-655, Rockville, MD 20852-1448. An immediate report should be made by telephone (301-295-8191) and a written report should be submitted within 7 days (21 *CFR* 606.170b).[4] The report should include a description of any new procedures implemented to avoid a recurrence of the error or accident.

If anti-HIV-1/2 positive, anti-HCV or HBsAg-reactive components are transfused, patient follow-up must be long enough to determine if infection occurred and the final report must indicate whether the patient(s) contracted the disease. If plasma from an anti-HIV-1/2 positive, anti-HCV or HBsAg-reactive unit is shipped for further manufacture, both the manufacturer and the CBER should be notified immediately. Reports concerning the transfusion of incorrectly identified red cells during a plasmapheresis procedure should also include the approximate volume of red cells transfused, the blood groups of the donor and the transfused cells, a description of the effect on the donor and the care given to the donor.

References

1. Clinical laboratory technical procedure manuals. Second Edition. GP2-A2, Vol 12, No 10. Villanova, PA: National Committee on Clinical Laboratory Standards, 1992.
2. Jones FS, ed. Accreditation requirements manual. 4th ed. Bethesda, MD: American Association of Blood Banks, 1992:211.
3. Widmann FK, ed. Standards for blood banks and transfusion services. 15th ed. Bethesda, MD: American Association of Blood Banks, 1993.
4. Code of federal regulations. Title 21, Parts 600-799. Washington, DC: US Government Printing Office, 1992 (revised annually).
5. Food and Drug Administration. Current good manufacturing practice for blood and blood components; proficiency testing requirements. Proposed rule. Fed Regist 1989;54(107):24296-301.
6. Health Care Financing Administration. Medicare, Medicaid and CLIA programs; revision of the Clinical Laboratory regulations for the Medicare, Medicaid and Clinical Laboratories Improvement Act of 1967 programs. Final rule with comment period. Fed Regist 1992;57(40):7002-186.
7. Food and Drug Administration. Memorandum: Responsibilities of blood establishments related to errors and accidents in the manufacture of blood and blood components. March 20, 1991.

24

Blood Usage Review

Requirements for Review

There are several justifications for transfusion practice quality assessment activities. The use of component therapy has made available to the clinician many choices. This situation has increased the potential for component misuse, particularly since the level of expertise in transfusion practice varies among clinicians. The risks of component misuse—including infectious disease transmission and alloimmunization—are well known to blood bankers. Choosing an inappropriate component can alter the transfusion risk/benefit ratio or fail to correct the patient's problem. The costs of blood and blood components justify transfusion monitoring in efforts to contain the increasing costs of health care.

Peer review of transfusion practice is required by the Joint Commission on Accreditation of Healthcare Organizations (JCAHO) as a prerequisite for hospital accreditation; by the *Code of Federal Regulations* for a hospital to qualify to receive Medicare reimbursement; by most states for Medicaid reimbursement; and by the College of American Pathologists (CAP) and the American Association of Blood Banks, as part of their inspection and accreditation processes.

The JCAHO standards state, in part, that "the medical staff performs blood usage review at least quarterly. Blood usage review includes the following[1]:

1. The review of usage of all categories of blood and blood components.

2. The evaluation of all confirmed transfusion reactions.

3. The development or approval of policies and procedures relating to the distribution, handling, use and administration of blood and blood components.

4. The review of the adequacy of transfusion services to meet the needs of patients.

5. The review of ordering practices for blood and blood products."

The JCAHO has defined a 10-step model for hospital quality assessment of blood use that can be applied to transfusion committee activities.[2] The 10 steps that should be utilized in blood usage review include:

1. Assign responsibility.
2. Delineate the scope of blood use.
3. Identify the important aspects of blood use.
4. Identify indicators.
5. Establish thresholds for indicators.
6. Monitor indicator data.
7. Evaluate blood use and problems.
8. Take actions to resolve problems.
9. Assess the actions and document improvement.
10. Communicate relevant information to the organization-wide quality assessment program.

Because the transfusion committee is typically assigned the responsibility for transfusion review in most hospitals, these procedures are relevant to the function of the transfusion committee.

24

More recently, the JCAHO has defined an "agenda for change" that places blood transfusion review into a reorganized program with emphasis upon continuous quality improvement.[2]

These regulations specify functions that can be met by mechanisms other than a hospital transfusion committee, such as a tissue committee or a laboratory utilization committee. Since the JCAHO also requires the medical staff of the hospital to perform surgical case review, drug usage evaluations, medical record review and pharmacy and therapeutic review, some large hospitals have organized their quality assessment programs by clinical departments whereby a department such as surgery may have a staff committee review all of these issues, including blood transfusion. However, the specified transfusion functions are so demanding that most hospitals have found it expedient to have a staff committee concerned solely with blood transfusion.

Results of Review

Many reports in the medical literature support the monitoring of transfusion practice. Several reports have suggested that many blood transfusions are given without valid indications. In 1962 a blood conservation program was described that is remarkably similar to current "model" peer review programs.[3] A hospital staff adopted in its bylaws "indications for blood transfusions," which were:

1. For replacement of needed whole blood volume.
2. For oxygen transport in either:
   a. An anemic patient with a hemoglobin of 70 g/L (7 g/dL) or less.
   b. An anemic patient with complications affecting oxygenation or undergoing anesthesia, who may be transfused if hemoglobin is less than 100 g/L (10 g/dL).

3. For exchange transfusion of infants.
4. For replacement of labile coagulation factors, a rare indication for use of fresh Whole Blood.

Emphasizing these simple indications, a hospital staff education program produced a drop in use factor (units of blood transfused divided by the number of patients hospitalized) from 0.237 to 0.110, a decrease of more than 50%.

A prospective study[4] of blood transfusion practice in a large general hospital during a 2-month period when 675 units of blood were transfused revealed that 17% of the units transfused on the surgical service, 25% on the medical service and 38% on the obstetric and gynecologic service did not meet criteria similar to those described above. Comparison of single-unit transfusions with multiple-unit transfusions showed far more single units than multiple units to be considered unnecessary.

A study[5] of patients admitted at 300 hospitals located throughout the United States analyzed 401 nonsurgical patients who had a diagnosis of anemia and a recorded hemoglobin $\geq$ 100 g/L (10 g/dL). These patients received a mean of 2.5 units of blood, yet most physicians would agree that most of these patients did not require transfusion. One possible exception might be severe coronary artery disease causing predisposition to angina at hemoglobin levels below 100 g/L (10 g/dL). However, 14% of these patients were women between the ages of 20 and 49 years, a group not known to have increased risk of coronary artery disease. This group received a mean of 2.4 units of blood transfused even though the diagnosis was iron deficiency anemia. The unnecessary transfusions exposed the recipients to the hazards of transfusion, increased the cost of therapy and imposed an extra burden on donor recruitment and blood collection.

The necessity for peer review of transfusion practice was obvious.

The National Institutes of Health has used the consensus conference format to present evidence to document the appropriate use and occasional misuse of blood components. Consensus conferences have suggested that many transfusions of FFP, PCs and RBCs are inappropriate. The publication of summary statements from these conferences and their supporting citations from the medical literature provide useful material to focus hospital transfusion practice review.[6-8]

The medical literature contains several examples of comprehensive transfusion quality assessment programs instituted by transfusion committees around the world. A comprehensive approach taken by a large general hospital in Israel showed that a large proportion of FFP, RBC and platelet transfusions had been prescribed inappropriately.[9] In the hospital studied, patients with end-stage renal disease and cancer patients receiving chemotherapy were most at risk for inappropriate transfusion. The study demonstrated that the medical staff was able to modify clinical practice as well as meet regulatory requirements that often appear to be a bureaucratic burden. Although the transfusion committee activities consume a major resource commitment, this study shows that local protocol modifications can result in medical benefit to patients, which can offset the time commitment required to perform these reviews.[9]

A study from Italy focused on blood usage in elective surgery. Using a multidisciplinary transfusion committee, key indicators were established to monitor transfusion practice. After implementation of the program, excessive transfusions in the surgical department were reduced by two-thirds and minimal progress was made in increasing autologous transfusions. The partial success led this hospital to continue its program in the expectation of increasing autologous utilization, decreasing excessive crossmatch requests and reducing the use of reconstituted whole blood.[10]

Transfusion committees have also begun to use new technologies or data collection systems to monitor transfusion practice. Computer systems have been shown to be a valuable tool in monitoring blood utilization and effecting change.[11] In the absence of computer systems, however, transfusion committees can still be effective in reducing unnecessary utilization of crossmatching in a type and screen program.[12] Finally, the use of diagnosis-related group data can be helpful in comparing utilization among different institutions, which can be persuasive in affecting local transfusion practices.[13]

Organization of the Transfusion Committee

The transfusion committee may be a standing committee, or its functions may be carried out by a hospital committee with a broader scope of responsibility, such as "tissue and transfusion."[14,15] The transfusion committee members and the chairman are generally appointed by the hospital chief of staff upon the recommendations of department chairmen. Representation should include all major medical departments that routinely order blood: surgery, anesthesiology, medicine, obstetrics and pediatrics. In addition, subspecialties that use large amounts of the blood supply should be represented, such as cardiovascular surgery, orthopedics, hemodialysis, oncology, hematology and neonatology. Other members are also desirable: a hospital administrator; nurses representing the services that administer most of the transfusions; a medical records department representative, since most reviews are done using patient records; and a blood bank technologist, to provide practical and technical information to the committee.

Members should be knowledgeable and experienced in one or more aspects of transfusion therapy and blood banking. Tenure on the committee should be long enough that skills acquired by new members can be used and shared. In small hospitals with few specialists on the staff, individual staff member interest and commitment may be the criteria for appointment. In such cases it may be useful to have a medical or technical representative from the supplying blood center as a consultant to the committee. Observers, such as SBB students or interested staff and residents, are usually welcome to attend committee meetings.

The medical director of the transfusion service should be a member of the committee but not necessarily its chairman. The transfusion service director already influences blood usage in the hospital on a daily basis, and a committee chairman who directs the transfusion service might be accused of having a conflict of interest if called upon to defend transfusion committee policies. In addition, the chairman is responsible for enforcement aspects of the committee functions. Responsibility for activities viewed as regulatory by staff members may invite resentment and impaired cooperation. Constructive criticism may be more acceptable to staff members when it comes from a clinician other than the medical director of the transfusion service.

Functions of the Transfusion Committee

The committee is required by the JCAHO to meet at least quarterly and as often as necessary to perform its functions. All committee activities should be documented, usually in the committee minutes. Reports should be made regularly to the hospital staff or its committee responsible for overall quality assessment activities. There are many aspects of hospital transfusion practice suitable for review by the transfusion committee. These include, but are not limited to, the use of blood and blood components; the indications for irradiated blood; and the appropriate use of various blood administration devices including filters, warmers, blood pumps and intraoperative autologous transfusion devices. The transfusion committee should monitor the use of cell separators for intraoperative recovery and the collection of plasma or cells from patients undergoing plasmapheresis or cytapheresis procedures. It may be appropriate for the transfusion committee to review the use of blood derivatives such as albumin, plasma protein fraction and immune serum globulins if they are dispensed by the blood bank. Other issues that could be considered are informed consent for transfusion and directed donor policies.

Guidelines for evaluating transfusion reactions should be reviewed by the transfusion committee to establish an overall hospital policy. In-service programs are an important function of hospital transfusion committees and provide a framework for educating all hospital personnel in the appropriate use of blood and blood components. In addition to audits of usage, the transfusion committee may find it useful to evaluate how blood components are ordered, including verification of the presence of written orders in the patient's chart and whether type of component, volume and rate of infusion are specified. These audits also provide the nursing service or the hospital IV team with information on compliance with requirements for recording the time the transfusion was started and stopped, the performance of appropriate identification checks and the occurrence of any adverse reactions. The committee can also note whether or not transfusion increments are monitored by posttransfusion laboratory tests or notations of clinical condition.

Outpatient transfusion practices including transfusion, phlebotomy and hemapheresis services should be evaluated by the transfusion committee when necessary; the availability of home transfusion facilities is an appropriate topic. The transfusion committee may wish to review and recommend special blood components for segments of the hospital population; eg, the suitability of providing CMV-seronegative blood for low-birth-weight infants born of CMV-seronegative mothers, or the use of irradiated blood components for patients at high risk for transfusion-associated graft-vs-host disease.

In some medical centers the transfusion service director may decide many of these issues. In hospitals without a full-time transfusion service director, these practices and questions would fall under the jurisdiction of the committee as a whole. Although the transfusion service director may make the decisions, it is appropriate for the transfusion committee to review these issues that affect the entire hospital staff. Valuable input from all sectors of the hospital population can thus be brought to bear on the appropriate use of blood components and transfusion practices in the institution.

Some of the specific functions of the hospital transfusion committee include the following objectives:

1. Establish broad policies for blood transfusion therapy.
2. Develop criteria audits of transfusion practice.
3. Enhance quality of patient care through objective assessment of ongoing blood and blood component therapy.
4. Review and analyze the statistical reports of the transfusion service.
5. Audit blood use, with particular attention to Whole Blood, components, reactions, the occurrence of posttransfusion infections and other adverse events. Audits of hemotherapy in specific circumstances are encouraged. The audit could include hospitalized patients, Emergency Room patients and outpatients, where indicated.
6. Reaudit previously identified problem areas to evaluate improvement.
7. Promote continuing education in transfusion practices for the hospital staff.
8. Assist the hospital or blood center, as appropriate, in blood procurement efforts.
9. Assess adequacy and safety of the blood supply.
10. Ensure that written policies and procedures for the blood transfusion service conform to the AABB *Standards* and review these annually.
11. Report to that committee of the hospital charged with the responsibility for overall quality assessment activities and recommend corrective action when indicated.

Monitoring Hospital Transfusion Practice

The need to encourage appropriate blood utilization underlies all the functions of the transfusion committee. The committee can perform two broad categories of review: 1) statistical, or systems, data derived from records of the blood bank (retrospective review) and 2) medical practice data generated by analysis of patients' hospital charts (retrospective review and concurrent review). The JCAHO allows the review of blood utilization by screening and/or intensive evaluation. Screening refers to the use of predetermined criteria applied to individual cases to determine if an individual case or group of cases should be evaluated more intensively. Intensive evaluation involves a specific group of cases such as cardiac surgery or joint replacement where statistical techniques may be used to uncover practice trends; specific practices such as autologous blood transfusion or intraoperative blood recovery can also be subjected to intensive evaluation.

Formerly, the JCAHO required that all blood components transfused be reviewed by the medical staff. For components used in low volume or to establish a baseline of practice, every case may require review. For high volume blood components, a sample of cases can be studied; a minimum sample is 5% of cases or 30 total cases, whichever is larger.[2]

Statistical Data—Retrospective Review

Transfusion services should record certain statistics to monitor workload and for inspection and accreditation purposes: blood component usage; outdate rate for each component; number of each type of transfusion reaction; number of hepatitis cases; crossmatch/transfusion ratio; and transfusion service workload and productivity. A more complete list of systems indicators is given in Appendix 24-1.[15] Which variables should be measured and how frequently must be determined by the transfusion committee and the transfusion director. Computerization of transfusion service record-keeping makes a greater variety of statistical data available and makes it

more current. The labor-intensive nature of manual record-keeping systems limits generation of such data by this method.

When possible, some critical systems data should be monitored continuously because spot checks are subject to sampling errors, which could prompt a policy change to correct a nonexistent problem. Once a hospital has accurate statistics on its own transfusion data base, it is possible to measure the effects of instituting any new policy or procedure.

Medical Practice Data—Retrospective Review

In most hospitals these data are extracted by medical audit analysts from reviews of patients' charts. The transfusion committee should draft the audit criteria in an open and participatory manner. All clinical department chairmen should be informed in writing of the purpose and method of the audit process. Most departments will have representation on the transfusion committee. For those that do not, the department chairman may be asked to attend and participate or send a delegate. The committee minutes of the developmental meetings should be distributed to all concerned departments so the staff will be informed that criteria are being drafted.

Development of audit criteria by a group of physicians provides credibility among the clinical staff. It is helpful to have medical records or quality assessment personnel participate in the drafting process because the criteria will be used by nonphysician reviewers to select patient charts for study.

Medical Practice Data—Concurrent Review

Hospitals with effective computer and technical support should consider concurrent review of transfusion practices. Such a program could be appropriate for transfusion of PCs and FFP. The blood bank technologist could access the patient's platelet count or coagulation studies prior to issue of components. If these test results are not within a previously approved acceptable range, the medical director should consult with the ordering physician before blood components are issued for transfusion. Concurrent review systems have been successfully implemented at several hospitals.[16] The use of concurrent review mechanisms has been shown to be effective in ensuring appropriate platelet transfusion and reducing fresh frozen plasma utilization.[17-19] For example, the use of concurrent review mechanisms has reduced FFP use by as much as 77% and platelet transfusions by 14-55% at university hospitals.[17]

Concurrent review has the additional advantage of addressing the potential problem of undertransfusion. With the increased awareness of the risks of transfusions, some patients may be jeopardized by the use of inadequate doses of blood components or replacement factors. A concurrent review system can ensure that adequate therapy is provided at the time of transfusion.

Audit Criteria

Audit criteria are guidelines used by medical audit personnel to select charts that the transfusion committee physicians will review. The criteria serve as a filter that eliminates those charts that reflect acceptable transfusion practice and selects a few charts that are most likely to reveal practices in need of scrutiny. The criteria should not attempt to define a comprehensive standard of practice. Nonphysician reviewers are not expected to apply complex instructions to the screening process; comprehensive

medical evaluation is the function of the physician reviewers.

Audit criteria have three parts:

1. *Elements* that are the indications for transfusion. Documentation of these exempt a chart from further review.

2. *Exceptions* describe situations that also exempt a chart from further review even though it does not comply with the indications in the Elements. These should be kept to a minimum to facilitate the audit.

3. *Instructions and Definitions* contain detailed directions to records personnel about where to locate information in the chart (in the laboratory report, anesthesia records or doctor's notes, etc) and information about terminology and intent of the Elements.

The transfusion committee should develop criteria that are appropriate for its own hospital and/or clinical departments. Variable local conditions may make a criterion applicable in one hospital and invalid in another. For example, use of WB to treat patients who have suffered acute trauma and massive blood loss may be justified at one hospital, but WB simply may not be available at another hospital. Examples of audit criteria are available in the literature.[1,20] Additional criteria should be formulated for auditing patient records of a particular clinical department; eg, the number of trauma service patients who received uncrossmatched blood transfusions.

Published examples of standards appropriate for pediatric transfusion monitoring are available.[21,22]

Performing Audits

Complete charts and thorough documentation are essential for medical audits. Criteria may be debated, but basic criteria appropriate for every audit must include documentation of: 1) reason for the transfusion and 2) effect of the transfusion. There are other justifications for requiring that such information always be in the chart. If an adverse reaction occurs, the legal position of the physician and the hospital is strengthened. Also, when the ordering physician justifies the transfusion in writing, he or she is likely to think through the decision carefully. Finally, the documentation of effect serves as a quality control check both for the decision to transfuse and for the choice of blood components transfused.[20,23]

Corrective Actions

After criteria have been developed and agreed upon, but before any formal audits are conducted, the transfusion committee should agree upon actions that will be taken after chart reviews are completed. Options include:

1. The patient's name and the name of the involved physician can be recorded; or anonymous statistical summary reports can be generated.
2. The committee can send a letter or other written notice of variance in practice to the responsible physician, the department chairman, the chief of professional services, the hospital risk management office, the hospital credentials committee or a combination of these.
3. The name of the transfusion committee members who reviewed the chart should not be made known to the involved clinician.
4. The involved physician may respond in writing or may be requested to meet with the transfusion committee or the department chairman to clarify apparently inappropriate therapy.

These issues should be discussed with the hospital's administration and legal office and decided prior to the first audit. In most cases, these issues and corrective actions should be outlined in the medical staff bylaws. The hospital staff must be informed of the criteria, the audit process and the mechanisms that the committee intends to use for documentation and corrective action.

It is essential to remember at all times that the fundamental process of the audit is educational and not punitive, because the goal is to improve the practice of blood transfusion.[24]

References

1. Medical staff monitoring functions: Blood usage review. Chicago: Joint Commission on Accreditation of Hospitals, 1988:128.
2. Accreditation manual for hospitals, vol 1, Standards. Oakbrook Terrace, IL: Joint Commission on Accreditation of Healthcare Organizations, 1991:218.
3. McCoy KL. The Providence Hospital blood conservation program. Transfusion 1962;2:3-6.
4. Diethrich EB. Evaluation of blood transfusion. Transfusion 1965;5:82-8.
5. Friedman BA. Patterns of blood utilization by physicians: Transfusion of non-operated anemic patients. Transfusion 1978;18:193-8.
6. NIH Consensus Conference. Fresh frozen plasma. Indications and risks. JAMA 1985; 253:551-3.
7. NIH Consensus Conference. Platelet transfusion therapy. JAMA 1987;257:1777-80.
8. NIH Consensus Conference. Perioperative red blood cell transfusion. JAMA 1988;260:2700-3.
9. Mozes B, Epstein M, Ben-Bassat I, et al. Evaluation of the appropriateness of blood and blood product transfusion using preset criteria. Transfusion 1989;29:473-6.
10. Giovanetti AM, Parravicini A, Baroni L, et al. Quality assessment of transfusion practice in elective surgery. Transfusion 1988;28:166-9.
11. Hoeltge GA, Brown JC, Herzig RH, et al. Computer-assisted audits of blood component transfusion. Cleve Clin J Med 1989;56:267-72.
12. Davis SP, Barrasso C, Ness PM. Maximizing the benefits of type and screen by continued surveillance of transfusion practice. Am J Med Technol 1983;49:579-82.
13. Surgenor DM, Wallace EL, Churchill WH, et al. Utility of DRG and ICD-9-CM classification codes for the study of transfusion issues. Transfusions in patients with digestive diseases. Transfusion 1989;29:761-7.

14. Grindon AJ, Tomasulo PS, Bergin JJ, et al. The hospital transfusion committee. JAMA 1985;253:540-3.

15. Hoeltge GA. Peer review of transfusion practices. In: Summer SH, Smith DM Jr, Agranenko VA, eds. Transfusion therapy: Guidelines for practice. Arlington, VA: American Association of Blood Banks, 1990:157-75.

16. Toy PTCY. Monitoring transfusion practice. In: Kolins J, McCarthy LJ, eds. Contemporary transfusion practice. Arlington, VA: American Association of Blood Banks, 1987:85-90.

17. Simpson MB. Prospective-concurrent audit and medical consultation for platelet transfusion. Transfusion 1987;27:192-5.

18. McCullough J, Steeper TA, Connelly DP, et al. Platelet utilization in a university hospital. JAMA 1988;259:2414-18.

19. Shanberge JN. Reduction of fresh frozen plasma use through a daily survey and education program. Transfusion 1987;27:226-7.

20. Simpson MB. Audit criteria for transfusion practices. In: Wallas CH, Muller VH, eds. The hospital transfusion committee. Arlington, VA: American Association of Blood Banks, 1982:21-60.

21. Blanchette VS, Hume HL, Levy GJ, et al. Guidelines for auditing pediatric blood transfusion practices. Am J Dis Child 1991;145:787-98.

22. Sacher RA, Luban NLC, Strauss RG. Current practice and guidelines for the transfusion of cellular components in the newborn. Transfus Med Rev 1989;3:39-54.

23. Myhre BA. Quality control of clinical transfusion practices. In: Myhre BA, ed. Quality control in blood banking. New York: John Wiley & Sons, 1974.

24. Smith DE. Utilization review. In: Wallas CH, Muller VH, eds. The hospital transfusion committee. Arlington, VA: American Association of Blood Banks, 1982:61-85.

Appendix 24-1. Key Indicators for Systems Audits[20]

1. UNITS TRANSFUSED—Total number of units of WB, RBCs, PCs, apheresis platelets (SD-PCs), granulocyte apheresis units, FFP, CRYO, Factor VIII and IX concentrates, Rh Immune Globulin (RhIG), cryopreserved red cells (D-RBCs), washed red cells (W-RBCs), leukocyte-reduced red cells (LR-RBCs) and reconstituted red cells for exchange transfusion.

2. PATIENTS TRANSFUSED—Total number of patients receiving each component or product listed in item 1 above.

3. UNITS TRANSFUSED PER PATIENT TRANSFUSED—The average number of units of each component or product given to patients receiving that component. In some situations, it may be useful to analyze on the basis of diagnosis or surgical or medical procedure.

4. RELATIVE PERCENT OF LR-RBCs VS RBCs TRANSFUSED

5. CROSSMATCH-TO-TRANSFUSION RATIO (C:T)—The number of units crossmatched divided by the number of units transfused. This analysis may be applied to the total operations of the transfusion service or to the operating room, specific floors, particular surgical procedures, individual physicians, various clinical services or specialties and emergency versus routine requests.

6. OUTDATE RATE—The total number of units outdated divided by the sum of the units received. This should be monitored for all blood, components and derivatives; in some instances, analysis by ABO and Rh type may prove informative.

7. TRANSFUSION REACTIONS—The number and percent of various types of reported transfusion reactions, including posttransfusion hepatitis.

8. WORKLOAD AND PRODUCTIVITY—Workload and productivity data may be useful to evaluate the activities and efficiency of the lab; this may be analyzed by day of week and by shift in some situations; workload per unit transfused may be valuable as an efficiency measure.

9. HOURS WORKED PER UNIT TRANSFUSED OR PATIENT TRANSFUSED—In many transfusion services, this variable may be a more valid indicator of the efficiency of operations than the value obtained from traditional workload productivity figures.

10. UNCROSSMATCHED UNITS—The number and percent of units issued uncrossmatched or with abbreviated pretransfusion testing; analysis by floor, service or physician may be useful.

11. FRESH UNIT REQUESTS—The number and percent of requests for "freshest" or "fresh" units, analyzed by floor, service, physician and diagnosis.

12. TURNAROUND TIME—The total time required between receipt of transfusion request and availability of the unit for transfusion to the patient. This may be examined for emergency, routine and operative requests.

13. EMERGENCY REQUESTS—The number and percent may be analyzed by floor, service, requesting physician and diagnosis; distribution of requests by day or week, shift and hour may be revealing in some situations; the C:T ratio should be measured for appropriateness of request.

14. UNITS RETURNED UNUSED—The number and percent of units that are signed out from the transfusion service and later returned unused; ana

ysis by floor, clinical service and requesting physician may be informative.

15. AGE DISTRIBUTION OF UNITS— Analysis by statistical methods and/or frequency histograms for the age of inventory units and crossmatched units by ABO and Rh; the age at the time of receipt from the supplier; the age at the time of transfusion; the age when returned to the supplier.

16. SURGICAL CANCELLATIONS DUE TO UNAVAILABILITY OF BLOOD— The number and percent of cases that were delayed due to unavailability of blood; analysis by number of hours or days delayed, by surgical procedure and by cause (ie, antibody vs shortage of particular ABO and Rh type).

25

Blood Inventory Management

Blood from volunteer donors is a precious resource and should be used in the most efficient and effective way. Medical directors of hospital transfusion services, in conjunction with their transfusion committees and regional blood centers, can accomplish this goal by regularly conducting both a systems audit and a medical practice audit.

In the systems audit, managerial and operational data are reviewed to determine the efficiency of the transfusion service. Considerations include, but are not limited to, the rate of outdating, the ratio of blood crossmatched to that transfused (C:T ratio) and the adequacy of observation and reporting of transfusion reactions.

The medical practice audit is an important function of the transfusion committee. This committee should monitor whether blood components are used for recognized indications with expected results and whether blood is transfused in accordance with accepted medical practice. See Chapter 24 for more details.

Because hospital transfusion services and regional blood centers face different inventory control problems, they will be considered separately in this chapter.

Hospital Transfusion Services

Hospital blood inventories have a direct impact on the balance between outdating and shortages. In a hospital with low transfusion activity, the greater the number of units in inventory, the higher the potential for outdating. Conversely, the fewer the units in inventory, the more frequent the shortages and the greater the need for expensive emergency deliveries from the blood supplier. The optimal number of units to be kept in the hospital inventory can be derived by using complicated mathematical formulas,[1] a relatively simple computer simulation[2,3] or an empirical calculation as shown below.

Calculation of Optimal Inventory

1. Collect weekly blood and component usage data over a 6-month period.
2. Determine usage by ABO and Rh type for each week.
3. To correct for unusual week-to-week variation (eg, a large volume used for an emergency), the single highest usage for each type should not be used in calculating the average weekly blood usage.
4. Total the number of units of each ABO and Rh type, omitting the highest week in each column.
5. Divide each total by 25 (total number of weeks minus the highest week), as shown in Table 25-1.
6. This gives an estimate of the average weekly blood usage of each ABO and Rh type.

Alternatively, Fig 25-1 gives a formula for estimating the minimum inventory for a hospital blood bank.[4]

Table 25-1. Whole Blood and Packed Cells Transfused by Week and by Blood Group (Small Hospital Example)

Week	O+	A+	B+	AB+	O−	A−	B−	AB−
1	4	2	−	−	2	−	−	−
2	−	6	6	−	−	2	−	−
3	10	−	−	−	2	−	1	−
4	−	2	−	−	4	2	1	−
5	4	2	−	−	9	−	−	−
6	−	5	2	−	−	−	−	−
7	1	13	−	−	1	2	2	−
8	20	9	−	−	5	2	−	−
9	2	12	2	−	−	−	−	−
10	−	8	−	−	−	−	1	−
11	−	−	−	−	−	2	1	−
12	4	3	2	−	1	−	−	−
13	2	4	−	−	2	−	−	−
14	2	9	3	−	−	2	2	−
15	7	−	−	−	1	−	−	−
16	3	2	−	−	−	−	−	−
17	−	2	1	2	1	2	1	−
18	11	1	1	2	1	1	1	−
19	3	3	4	−	2	−	1	−
20	3	3	4	−	−	1	1	−
21	2	1	−	−	2	1	−	−
22	4	−	1	−	−	−	−	−
23	2	5	1	−	−	1	2	−
24	4	−	1	−	−	2	−	−
25	9	4	1	−	6	8	−	−
26	5	−	−	−	4	−	2	−
Total used	102	96	29	4	43	28	16	0
Highest week (subtract)	20	13	6	2	9	8	2	0
Subtotal	82	83	23	2	34	20	14	0
Divided by 25 = average weekly blood usage	3.3	3.3	0.9	0	1.4	0.8	0.6	0

The choice of how much blood should be kept in inventory depends on many factors. Practical aspects such as the amount of refrigerator space and distance from the blood supplier must be considered. As an arbitrary starting point, a remote hospital with fewer than 150 beds might want to keep a 2-week inventory on hand, while a hospital with 150-500 beds might want to keep a 1-week supply on hand. Large hospitals (over 500 beds) may be limited by refrig erator space to a 2 or 3 days' supply i inventory.

After a suitable trial period (eg, 6-weeks), an evaluation of inventory prac tices should consider such variables a the outdate rate, the frequency of emer gency blood shipments, the frequency o switching from ABO-specific to ABO compatible blood, delay in scheduling elective surgery and other practica

(Average no. of units issued per month/30) × Fractional distribution of type

+ predetermined minimum for emergency = Daily inventory needs

Example: 400 units of RBCs were issued in a 30-day month. What is the estimated daily minimum inventory of group O Rh− units, assuming that 3 units are necessary at all times for emergencies?

400/30 (RBC/month/30) × 0.06 (proportion of O negs) + 3* = 3.8 (4 units 0 neg) units per day.

*Minimum number will vary depending on distance from supplier and type of services offered—ie, trauma vs elective only.

Figure 25-1. Formula to estimate daily minimal inventory for a hospital blood bank.[4]

problems. Following this evaluation, optimal inventory levels can be adjusted. The addition of more beds, new surgical procedures or specialties such as oncology, transplantation, neonatology or cardiac surgery may increase special blood component needs and require re-evaluation of the optimal inventory.

Considerations in Blood Usage

The outdate rate is affected by factors other than inventory level. These include:

Size of the hospital. An acute care hospital with a large surgical load and/or an active emergency service often receives and uses blood nearing outdate simply because large volumes of blood are transfused daily. Blood centers often ship short-dated blood to large hospitals because the likelihood of transfusion there is much greater than at a small hospital.[3]

The distance between a hospital and the blood supplier, and the frequency with which shipments are delivered. The hospital that is a great distance from the supplier or that receives infrequent shipments must maintain enough blood to cover most emergencies. The larger the blood inventory compared to the amount of blood actually used, the greater the outdate rate. Proximity to other hospitals that can supply blood in an emergency can reduce the need for large inventories.

Policy of using the oldest blood first. Good inventory management demands transfusing the oldest blood first (first in, first out) in order to reduce outdating. However, the policy of stock rotation should be flexible when good clinical indications exist for fresher blood (eg, neonates).

Average dating of components received from blood supplier. In general, the shorter the remaining shelf life upon receipt, the less likely it is that a unit will be used within the dating period. This varies, of course, with daily usage patterns.

Ordering policies. If many technologists on all shifts order blood, duplication of orders occurs more frequently than if the responsibility for ordering is centralized and based on established policies. For large users, one technologist on each shift may order blood components to bring the inventory to a pre-established level. In contrast, small hospitals may require only one person to rotate stock back to the blood center, by expiration date. Standing orders can be helpful for planning ease, both for the hospital and the blood center.

Services provided by the hospital. Hospitals that perform many surgical procedures may require large inventories of blood to fill requests. Because blood is frequently ordered in large amounts to cover potential problems, all units crossmatched may not be used. These units may subsequently outdate. If a service C:T ratio is high (≥3), a more aggressive type and screen or maximum surgical blood order schedule (MSBOS) policy may help to reduce waste.

Presence of a frozen blood program. Freezing units of blood when it appears that an excess number of units will be available can reduce outdating and provide an extra source during shortages. Some centers with a frozen blood program routinely freeze all group A and O units from donors with unexpected antibodies. Others have found it useful to rejuvenate and freeze only selected units prior to outdating. However, freezing adds considerable cost to preparing a unit of blood and the length of time needed to thaw and deglycerolize these units limits their use for rapidly bleeding patients.

Freezing is an excellent strategy for use with blood of rare or uncommon phenotype, and may be helpful in some autologous transfusion programs. Given the current status of rapidly changing requirements and test methods for infectious disease testing, it would be prudent to save and store multiple donor serum aliquots for ease of new test implementation.

Crossmatch-to-transfusion ratio. Hospitals with inexperienced house staff may place larger than usual blood orders, increasing the possibility of outdating. A C:T ratio >2 usually indicates excessive requests for crossmatches.[5] If units are held in reserve for 24-48 hours for patients who will not use the blood, the available shelf life of these units diminishes by 24-48 hours each time they are held. Establishing guidelines for transfusion therapy[5,6] or a MSBOS[7,8] can decrease the C:T ratio, since data about past blood usage are used to recommend how much blood should be crossmatched for use in future procedures.

Suggested Ordering Policies

The transfusion guidelines in Table 25-2 are average transfusion levels derived by reviewing blood usage over several months.[9] Data are collected for each procedure performed in the hospital. This should include the number of patients for whom blood was requested, number of patients who received blood, number of units crossmatched, number of units transfused, the average number of units transfused per patient crossmatched and the C:T ratio. Conclusions can then be drawn about likelihood of transfusion and probable blood usage for each surgical procedure. The use of type and screen (T & S, see p 315) is recommended for procedures for which blood usage is 0.5 unit or below.[10,11] The guidelines developed should reflect local patterns of surgical practice and patient population. These should be compared to published guidelines to be sure local practice does not markedly deviate from generally accepted standards of care.

Once a MSBOS is put into place the size of the routine inventory can be reduced.[12] A blood order schedule is intended for typical circumstances. The surgeon or anesthesiologist may individualize specific requests to accommodate special needs. For the patient with a positive antibody screen, the antibody should be identified. If clinical significance is determined, a sufficient number of antigen-negative units should be identified (often at least two), even if the original order was a type and screen. Antiglobulin crossmatches must be performed before the blood is administered.

Table 25-2. Maximum Surgical Blood Order Schedule

Procedure	Units
General Surgery	
Aneurysm Resection	6
Breast Biopsy	T/S
Colon Resection	2
Exploratory Laparotomy	4
Femoropopliteal Bypass	T/S
Hernias	T/S
Mastectomy-Radical	1
Pancreatectomy	4
Splenectomy	2
Thyroidectomy	T/S
GYN	
AP Repair	1
D & C	T/S
Hysterectomy Abdominal	T/S
Radical	2
OB	
C-Section Hysterectomy	2
C-Section	T/S
L & D Admission	HOLD
Thoracic-Cardiac	
Bypass Procedures	
Adult	6
Children	4
Vascular	
Aortic Bypass	6
Endarterectomy	1
Renal Artery Repair	6
Orthopedics	
Arthroscopy	T/S
Laminectomy	3
Spinal Fusion	8
Total Hip	5
Total Knee	T/S
Urology	
Prostatectomy	
Perineal	2
Transurethral (TURP)	T/S
Renal Transplant	2

(Modified from Sharpe.[9])

Regional Blood Centers

Recruiting and drawing blood donors are functions that are commonly concentrated in regional blood centers, which today provide 85% of allogeneic blood donations. In some hospitals, donors are still regularly drawn; in others, donors are drawn only rarely, in times of acute shortage. When there is a consignment arrangement between a regional blood center and a transfusion service, blood remains under the control of the blood center until it is transfused. The hospital is billed for the processing fee only if the unit is transfused. Using this approach, hospitals at a greater distance can be stocked with units having 28 days or more remaining before expiration. The blood can then be returned to the blood center for full credit with 10 days left before expiration to be redistributed to the large volume hospital users. This helps keep total regional outdating to a minimum. The blood center usually absorbs the cost of outdated blood. If hospitals have a direct reimbursement arrangement with the supplier, the hospital absorbs the cost for outdated blood and the blood center has little control of the blood after delivery.

To overcome anticipated seasonal shortages, blood centers and those transfusion services that draw donors develop recruitment plans several months to a year in advance. When possible, large draws are scheduled in advance of holiday periods. Using blood additives, the shelf life of Red Blood Cells is 42 days. This increase in shelf life is helpful in adding flexibility to planning donor drives and helps to decrease the rate of outdating of available blood supplies.

During acute shortages, due either to decreased donations or increased usage, regional blood centers may request blood from other blood centers, either directly or through various blood organizations (eg, AABB, CCBC, ARC). It is also common practice to share excess inventory through various blood exchange programs. Finally, blood centers depend on the media—TV, radio and newspapers—to make the public aware of the community's low blood inventories.

Managing Platelet Inventories

There are few articles describing the inventory management of platelets.[13,14] It is difficult to keep an inventory of platelets in anticipation of use because demand is episodic and the shelf life of platelets is only 5 days (often 3 days, in practice) less one for testing and another for travel. Many patients on long-term platelet support need special components such as cytomegalovirus-seronegative or irradiated platelets, apheresis platelets, leukocyte-reduced platelets or HLA-matched platelets. Thus, inventory management requires coordination of anticipated clinical needs with selection of appropriate donors. Often, platelets ordered for one patient and not used can still be used by another patient.

It may be advisable to predict an increase in platelet usage the day after a holiday for delayed elective surgery and oncology transfusion. Planning to stock and use single-donor apheresis platelets may ease the post-holiday demand. Communication and cooperation among hospitals and regional blood centers improve management of inventories when platelets are ordered for specific patients. Knowing the diagnosis and the expected schedule of platelet transfusions helps the blood center plan how many platelet concentrates to produce daily.

Inventory Control of Frozen Plasma Derivatives

Since Fresh Frozen Plasma and Cryoprecipitated AHF can be stored for 1 year, little has been published about how to manage inventories. Inventories of these components should be determined by patient population and review of usage. Many centers preferentially make these components from group AB and A donors since this practice allows transfusion to any potential recipient.

Components From Selected Donors

With units from autologous and directed donors making up a larger fraction of the inventory, it is very important to develop policies to manage these components. It is essential that if autologous blood is available it be used before allogeneic units. Directed donations should be used after autologous and before allogeneic blood. Blood for autologous use only must be labeled clearly and stored separately from the allogeneic supply to avoid inadvertent crossover. It is also important to have a policy on the release of autologous and directed units for other recipients.

References

1. Brodheim E, Hirsch R, Prostacos G. Setting inventory levels for hospital blood banks. Transfusion 1976;16:63-70.
2. Friedman BA, Abbott RD, Williams GW. A blood ordering strategy for hospital blood banks derived from a computer simulation. Am J Clin Pathol 1982;78:154-60.
3. Abbott RD, Friedman BA, Williams GW. Recycling older blood by integration into the inventory of a single large hospital blood bank: A computer simulation application. Transfusion 1976;16:709-15.
4. Butch SH. Blood inventory management. Laboratory Medicine 1985;16:17-20.

5. Mintz PD, Nordine RB, Henry JB, et al. Expected hemotherapy in elective surgery. NY State J Med 1976;76:532-7.
6. Boral LI, Dannemiller FJ, Stanford W, et al. A guideline for anticipated blood usage during elective surgical procedures. Am J Clin Pathol 1979;71:680-4.
7. Friedman BA, Oberman HA, Chadwick AR, et al. The maximum surgical blood order schedule and surgical blood use in the United States. Transfusion 1976;16:380-7.
8. Friedman BA. The maximum surgical blood order schedule. In: Polesky HF, Walker RH, eds. Safety in transfusion practices. Skokie, IL: College of American Pathologists, 1982:169-88.
9. Sharpe MA. Inventory management. In: Treacy M, Bertsch JA, eds. Selecting policies and procedures for the transfusion service. Arlington,

VA: American Association of Blood Banks, 1982:85-99.
10. Boral LI, Henry JB. The type and screen: A safe alternative and supplement in selected surgical procedures. Transfusion 1977;17:163.
11. Boral LI, Hill SS, Apollon CJ, Folland J. The type and antibody screen, revisited. Am J Clin Pathol 1979;71:578-81.
12. Rouault C, Gruenhagen J. Reorganization of blood ordering practices. Transfusion 1978;18:448-53.
13. Katz AJ, Carter CW, Saxton P, et al. Simulation analysis of platelet production and inventory management. Vox Sang 1983;44:31-6.
14. McCullough J, Undis J, Allen JW Jr. Platelet production and inventory management in platelet physiology and transfusion. Washington, DC: American Association of Blood Banks, 1978:17-38.

Methods

The methods that follow are in a format based on a modification of the *Guidelines for Clinical Laboratory Procedure Manuals*, 2nd edition, (NCCLS Document GP2-A2, Vol. 12, No. 10, July 1992) of the National Committee for Clinical Laboratory Standards. Their inclusion in this edition of the *Technical Manual* is a subjective decision of the Technical Manual Committee. Readers are encouraged to refer to previous editions of the manual for methods not appearing in this edition, as exclusion from the current edition is not intended as a prohibition against their use.

There are often many different ways to perform the same test procedure. Although some workers may prefer other methods, those given here are reliable, straightforward and of proven value. Although the investigation of unusual serologic problems often requires flexibility in thought and methodology, adoption of uniform methods for routine procedures in the laboratory is imperative. In order for laboratory personnel to have reproducible and comparable results in a test procedure, it is essential that everyone in the laboratory perform the same test in the same manner.

General Laboratory Methods

Introduction

The methods outlined in the following sections are examples of acceptable procedures. To the greatest extent possible, the written procedures conform to the *Guidelines for Clinical Laboratory Procedure Manuals* developed by the National Committee for Clinical Laboratory Standards.

Reagent Preparation

Many procedures include formulas for reagent preparation. When prepared in-house, the reagent label must contain the following information:
1. Name of solution.
2. Date of preparation.
3. Expiration date (if known).
4. Storage temperature.
5. Initials of person preparing solution.

Temperatures

Whenever specific incubation or storage temperatures are given, the following ranges are considered satisfactory:

Stated Temperature	Acceptable Range
4 C	2-8 C
Room temperature	20-24 C
37 C	36-38 C
56 C	54-58 C

Incubation Times

Whenever specific incubation times are given, it is not acceptable to shorten the stated time. Immediate-spin tests should be read without deliberate delay. Extending the incubation times to twice those stated for serologic tests is usually not deleterious to the detection of antigen-antibody interactions, except when indicated by the reagent manufacturer. However, any deviation from the manufacturer's stated directions should be approved by the medical director on a case-by-case basis. An increase in the number of unwanted (false) positive tests may occur with extended incubation. Moreover, stated incubation times should not be extended when treating rbcs with proteolytic enzymes.

Stated Incubation Time	Acceptable Range
Immediate-spin	Without deliberate delay
1-5 minutes	1-10 minutes
5-30 minutes	5-60 minutes
30-120 minutes	30-180 minutes

Centrifugation Parameters

Centrifugation speeds (relative centrifugal force) and times should be standardized for equipment in use (see Chapter 22).

Reference

Guidelines for clinical laboratory procedure manuals, 2nd ed. (NCCLS Document GP2-A2, Vol. 12, No. 10). Villanova, PA: National Committee for Clinical Laboratory Standards, 1992.

601

Method 1.1. Shipment of Blood Specimens

Principle

The US Postal Service regulations for mailing blood samples, sharps and other medical devices are frequently updated.[1,2] The Department of Health and Human Services (DHHS) and the Department of Transportation (DOT) have also revised 42 CFR 72 and 49 CFR 173, respectively, but some uncertainties still exist concerning interpretations of overlapping regulations pertinent to shipments.[3,4] The shipping specifications described here are consistent with the latest Centers for Disease Control and Prevention (CDC) revision to 42 CFR 72, "Interstate Shipment of Biological Materials That Contain or May Contain Etiologic Agents." DOT regulations do not apply to biologic products under the jurisdiction of the US Food and Drug Administration. If the product may transmit infectious diseases, procedures consistent with Biosafety Level 2 are appropriate. See Chapter 21.

The procedure for clinical specimen packaging is applicable to samples containing animal material known or presumed to contain an etiologic agent and to all human material including (but not limited to) excreta, secreta, blood and its components, body fluids, tissue and tissue fluid. Samples known to be positive for disease markers including HBsAg and anti-HIV-1, and samples shipped for confirmatory testing of initially reactive screening test results, require the more stringent packaging procedure applicable to shipment of etiologic agents. An etiologic agent is defined as a microbiological agent or its toxin that causes, or may cause, human disease. Blood samples known to be positive for HBsAg or anti-HIV are in this category and should be packaged in accordance with the procedures described below.

Because requirements have been in transition, the resources provided in Table 21-1 should be consulted if questions arise. Although the current federal requirements allow the shipper to determine the shipment classification, it is particularly important that unsuspecting transportation or postal workers not be exposed to infectious materials as a result of inadequate packaging. It is strongly recommended, therefore, that double the calculated amount of absorbent material necessary to absorb all potentially infectious material in the event of breakage or spillage be used. The package integrity should be ensured by use of only tested, approved materials such as rigid metal canisters. Persons receiving inadequately packaged samples are encouraged to document the incident and follow up appropriately to ensure correction of unsafe practices. Packages should always be opened by trained staff who are wearing latex gloves.

Materials

1. Dry ice (solid carbon dioxide): If dry ice is used, place the dry ice outside the secondary container and consult 39 CFR 124.386(d) for restrictions. Precautions must be taken to avoid both pressure buildup and loosening of secondary containers as sublimation of the dry ice occurs. If more than 5 pounds of dry ice is used, the weight must be on the package label; no more than 30 pounds of dry ice is permitted per shipment.

2. Clinical Specimens
   a. Packaging:
      1) Sealed primary container(s) (eg, test tube), with total volume not larger than 1 L or 1 kg, in a leak-proof secondary container with sufficient nonparticulate absorbent material to absorb the entire contents in case of leakage.

PACKAGING FOR A CLINICAL SPECIMEN
(VOLUME >50 mL AND <4000 mL)

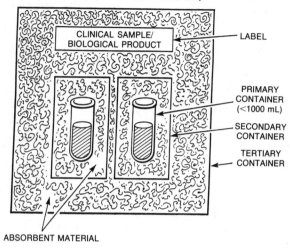

Figure 1.1-1. Appropriate packaging of clinical specimen material.

2) For total shipment volumes exceeding 50 mL: a tertiary or third container of fiberboard or equivalent DOT-approved material (200-lb burst strength). See Fig 1.1-1. Each package is limited to a total volume of 4000 mL or 4 kg.

b. Labels: The package must identify the content as "Clinical Specimen." Affix the Clinical Speci-

mens/ Biological Products label required by 42 CFR 72.3(a)(3). The label except for size must be as shown in Fig 1.1-2.

1) The color of material on which the label is printed shall be fluorescent orange or orange-red and the symbol and the printing in black.

2) The label shall be a rectangle measuring 51 mm (2 inches)

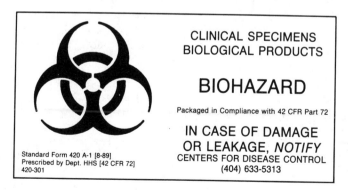

Figure 1.1-2. Label for clinical specimen material.

high by 102.5 mm (4 inches) long.

3) The symbol, measuring 35 mm (1.375 inches) in diameter, shall be centered on a fluorescent orange or orange-red square measuring 51 mm (2 inches) on each side.

4) The size of the letters on the label shall be as follows:

Clinical specimens/Biological products
- 10 pt.

Biohazard - 18 pt.

Packaged in compliance with 42 CFR part 72 - 6 pt.

In case of damage or leakage, notify
- 10 pt.

Centers for Disease Control - 8 pt.

(404) 633-5313 - 8 pt.

At least one inner container and the outer shipping container shall bear a label with the name, address and telephone number of the shipper.

3. Etiologic Specimen:
   a. Packaging:
      1) Sealed primary and durable, watertight secondary (sturdy metal containers are ideal) containers with absorbent material as described for clinical specimens. The primary container must provide sufficient space for liquid expansion so that it is not full at 130 F (55 C).
      2) A tertiary container constructed of 200 pound burst strength corrugated cardboard, wood or other material of equivalent strength. Shipments of etiologic agents may contain multiple secondary containers, but the total volume as for clinical samples may not exceed 4 L or 4 kg for the shipment. Place the

label shown in Fig 1.1-3 on the outer shipping container.

   b. Labels: The label for Etiologic Agents/Biohazard, except for size and color, must be as shown in Fig 1.1-3.
      1) The color of material on which the label is printed shall be white, the symbol red, and the printing in red on white or white on red (reversed).
      2) The label shall be a rectangle measuring 51 mm (2 inches) high by 102.5 mm (4 inches) long.
      3) The red symbol, measuring 35 mm (1.375 inches) in diameter shall be centered on a white square measuring 51 mm (2 inches) on each side.
      4) Size of the letters on the label shall be as follows:

Etiologic agents - 10 pt.

Biohazard - 18 pt.

Packaged in compliance with 42 CFR Part 72 - 6 pt.

In case of damage or leakage, *notify*
- 10 pt. rev.

Centers for Disease Control - 8 pt. rev.

(404) 633-5313 - 8 pt. rev.

The secondary container(s) and the outer shipping container shall bear, in addition to the label in Fig 1.1-3, labels with the name, address and telephone number of the shipper.

Procedure

1. Place the primary container in the secondary container. Add sufficient nonparticulate absorbent material to cover all sides of the primary container to absorb the entire contents in case of breakage (eg, paper towel, disposable diaper). Seal securely.

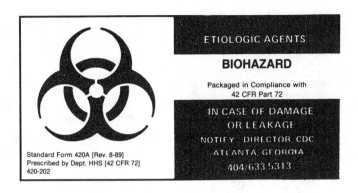

Figure 1.1-3. Label for etiologic agents/biomedical material.

2. For clinical specimens >50 mL and all etiologic agents, place the secondary container in a tertiary or outer shipping container.

3. Apply as appropriate, clinical specimen or etiologic agent labels that conform to 42 CFR 72.3 and 72.4.

4. If the US Postal Service is used, only First Class Mail, Priority Mail or Express Mail may be selected. Etiologic agents must be tendered to air carriers as "outsides," which means that they are not to be enclosed in mailbags.

5. When transporting etiologic agents >50 mL by air, attach the infectious substances label (135.4, International Mail Manual), proper shipping name and UN number (2814). Complete a "Shippers Declaration for Dangerous Goods" and attach labeling for "Cargo Aircraft Only."

6. Attach a return address label that includes the sender's telephone number to provide notification in case of damage. It is recommended that the consignee's phone number also be included with the address.

7. The consignee should be notified of shipment of etiologic agents so that the CDC can be notified and tracing can be initiated if the shipment is not received within 5 days of the expected arrival date.

Notes

1. Damaged or leaking packages. The carrier, the receiver or anyone handling these packages that are damaged or leaking shall, upon discovery of damage or leakage, isolate the package and, immediately or within 24 hours, notify the Centers for Disease Control by telephone at (404) 633-5313 and provide a description of the condition of the package, the name and address of the shipper, and other pertinent information.

2. If breakage occurs during shipment, extreme caution is warranted and the entire package should be autoclaved before it is discarded. Supervisory personnel should be notified if contents have been lost in transit or if the damage appears related to inadequate packaging by the sender.

3. Etiologic agents cannot be imported unless in conformance with 42 CFR 71 (Foreign Quarantine Regulations) and accompanied by a permit issued by the Director, CDC. Contact the CDC at (404) 639-3883.

References

1. Code of federal regulations. Title 39, Parts 111 and 124. Mailability of etiologic agents. Wash-

ington, DC: US Government Printing Office, 1992 (revised annually).
2. Federal register. 57 FR 55112. Mailability of sharps and other medical devices. Washington, DC: US Government Printing Office, 1992.
3. Code of federal regulations. Title 42, part 72. Interstate shipment of etiologic agents. Washington, DC: US Government Printing Office, 1992 (revised annually).
4. Code of federal regulations. Title 49, part 173. Etiologic agents. Washington, DC: US Government Printing Office, 1992 (revised annually).

Method 1.2. Treatment of Incompletely Clotted Specimens

Principle

Fibrin may continue to be generated in serum separated from incompletely clotted blood, especially during incubation at 37 C. This produces shreds and strands of protein that entrap rbcs and make it difficult to evaluate agglutination. Blood from patients who have received heparin may not clot at all, and blood from patients with excessive fibrinolytic activity may reliquefy, or contain protein fragments that interfere with examination for agglutination.

Materials

1. Thrombin: dry human/bovine thrombin or thrombin solution (50 units/mL in saline).
2. Glass beads.
3. Protamine sulfate: 10 mg/mL in saline.
4. Epsilon aminocaproic acid (EACA): 0.25 g/mL in saline.

Procedure

1. To accelerate clotting, either of the following techniques may be used:
   a. Add to whole blood or the separated serum the amount of dry thrombin that adheres to the tip of an applica-

tor stick, or one drop of thrombin solution per mL of blood.
   b. Gently agitate separated serum with small glass beads, at 37 C, for several minutes. Then centrifuge and use supernatant serum.
2. To neutralize heparin, add one or more drops of 1% solution of protamine sulfate (10 mg/mL) in saline to 4 mL of whole blood.
3. To inhibit fibrinolytic activity, add 0.1 mL of EACA to 4 mL of freshly drawn whole blood.

Notes

1. Use protamine sparingly. Excess protamine promotes rouleaux formation and, in great excess, will itself inhibit clotting.
2. Human thrombin may be contaminated with anti-A and anti-B.

Method 1.3. Solution Preparation—General Instructions

Principles

The basic definitions, calculations and instructions given below serve as a review of simple principles necessary for solution preparation.

1. Mole, gram-molecular weight: Weight, in grams, of a substance so that the number of grams is numerically equal to the molecular weight of the substance.
2. Molar solution: A one molar (1 M) solution contains one mole of solute in a liter of solution. The solvent should always be assumed to be distilled or deionized water unless otherwise indicated.
3. Gram-equivalent weight: Weight, in grams, of a substance that will produce or react with 1 mole of hydrogen ion.

4. Normal solution: A one normal (1 N) solution contains one gram-equivalent weight of solute in a liter of solution.

5. Percentage solutions: The percent of a solution gives the weight or volume of solute present in 100 units of total solution. Percent can be expressed as:

    a. Weight/weight (w/w), giving grams of solute in 100 g of solution.
    b. Volume/volume (v/v), giving milliliters of solute present in 100 mL of solution.
    c. Weight/volume (w/v) giving grams of solute in 100 mL of solution. Unless otherwise specified, a solution expressed in percentage can be assumed to be w/v.

6. Water of crystallization, water of hydration: Molecules of water that form an integral part of the crystalline structure of a substance. A given substance may have several crystalline forms, with several different numbers of water molecules intrinsic to the entire molecule. The weight of this water must be included in calculating molecular weight of the hydrated substance.

7. Anhydrous: The salt form of a substance with no water of crystallization.

8. Atomic weights (rounded to whole numbers):

    H, 1; O, 16; Na, 23; P, 31; S, 32; Cl, 35; K, 39

9. Molecular weights:

    HCl: $1 + 35 = 36$; $NaCl$: $23 + 35 = 58$; KCl: $39 + 35 = 74$
    H_2O: $(2 \times 1) + 16 = 18$
    NaH_2PO_4: $23 + (2 \times 1) + 31 + (4 \times 16) = 120$
    $NaH_2PO_4 \cdot H_2O$: $23 + (2 \times 1) + 31 + (4 \times 16) + (2 \times 1) + 16 = 138$
    KH_2PO_4: $39 + (2 \times 1) + 31 + (4 \times 16) = 136$
    H_2SO_4: $(2 \times 1) + 32 + (4 \times 16) = 98$

Examples

1. Molar solutions:

    $1 M KH_2PO_4 = 136$ g solute made up to 1 L
    $0.15 M KH_2PO_4 = (136 \times 0.15) = 20.4$ g solute made up to 1 L
    $0.5 M NaH_2PO_4 = (120 \times 0.5) = 60$ g solute made up to 1 L

2. Molar solution with hydrated salt:

    $0.5 M NaH_2PO_4 \cdot H_2O = (138 \times 0.5) = 69$ g of the monohydrate crystals made up to 1 L

3. Normal solutions:

    $1 N HCl = 36$ g solute made up to 1 L. One mole HCl dissociates into one mole H^+, so gram-equivalent weight and gram-molecular weight are the same.
    $12 N HCl = (36 \times 12) = 432$ g solute made up to 1 L
    $1 N H_2SO_4 = (98 \div 2) = 49$ g solute made up to 1 L. One mole H_2SO_4 dissociates to give two moles of H^+, so the gram-molecular weight is double the gram-equivalent weight.

4. Percent solution:

    $0.9\% NaCl$ (w/v) $= 0.9$ g solute made up to 100 mL solution

Notes

Accurate results require accurate preparation of reagents. It is important to read all instructions and labels carefully, and to follow instructions carefully.

1. Know the accuracy of the weighing equipment; the instruction manual includes this in the specifications. Weigh quantities appropriate for the accuracy of the equipment.

2. Prepare the largest volume that is practicable, because there is greater accuracy in measuring larger volumes than smaller volumes. If a re-

agent balance is accurate to ± 0.01 g, the potential error in weighing 0.05 g (50 mg) will be 20%, whereas the potential error of weighing 0.25 g (250 mg) will be only 4%.

If the solution retains its activity when stored appropriately, it is usually preferable to prepare a large volume. If the solution deteriorates rapidly, considerations of accuracy must be weighed against cost and convenience.

3. Note whether a substance is in the hydrated or anhydrous form. If the instructions give solute weight for one form, and the available reagent is in another form, be sure to adjust the measurements appropriately. For example, if instructions for 0.5 M NaH_2PO_4 call for 60 g, and the reagent is $NaH_2PO_4 \cdot H_2O$, find the ratio between the weights of the two forms:

$$\left(\frac{NaH_2PO_4 \cdot H_2O}{NaH_2PO_4} = \frac{138}{120} = 1.15 \right)$$

and multiply the designated weight by that figure (60 g × 1.15 = 69 g).

4. Dissolve the solute completely before making the solution to the final volume. This is especially important for substances, such as phosphates, that dissolve slowly. For example, to make 500 mL of 0.15 M KH_2PO_4:
   a. Weigh 10.2 g solute in a weighing boat or glass [(0.15 × 136) ÷ 2, since only 500 mL will be made].
   b. Place 350 mL water in a 500-mL volumetric flask on a magnetic stirrer. Add the stirring bar and adjust the speed of stirring.
   c. Add 10.2 g salt, then rinse the boat with several aliquots of water until no salt remains. Numerous small-volume rinses remove adherent material more effectively than a few larger volumes. Add the rinse water to the material in the flask

and stir until the salt is completely dissolved.
   d. Add water to the 500-mL mark, adjusting the volume for the stirring bar, and mix thoroughly.

5. Adjust the pH of the solution before bringing it to final volume so that addition of water (or other solvent) does not markedly change the adjusted pH. For example, to bring 500 mL of 0.1 M glycine to pH 3.0:
   a. Add 3.75 grams of glycine (H_2NCH_2COOH: molecular weight, 75) to 400-475 mL water in a beaker. Dissolve completely, using magnetic stirrer.
   b. Add a few drops of concentrated (12 N) HCl and measure pH after acid is thoroughly mixed. Continue adding HCl until pH is 3.0.
   c. Transfer the solution to a 500-mL volumetric flask; rinse beaker and stirring bar with aliquots of water, adding the rinse water to the flask. Use the rinses to contribute to the total 500-mL volume.
   d. Measure the pH of the solution at final volume.

References

1. Remson ST, Ackerman PG. Calculations for the medical laboratory. Boston, MA: Little, Brown & Co., 1977.
2. Henry JB, ed. Clinical diagnosis and management by laboratory methods. 18th ed. Philadelphia: WB Saunders, 1991.

Method 1.4. Serum Dilution

Principle

In serologic tests, serum is frequently diluted in a diluent (such as saline) to determine antibody concentration. It is customary to express the volume of diluted serum in terms of the unit 1, which means 1 part of serum *contained in the total number of parts of the dilution*. For example, if it is desired to test the serum in one-tenth its original concentration, a dilution of 1 part in 10 may be made by mixing 1 mL of serum with 9 mL of saline. Thus, it is 1 in 10 (not 1 + 10) so that the *final volume consists of 10*. Each of the 10 parts of the dilution will then contain one-tenth (1/10 or 0.1) of the serum diluted.

Procedure

1. Dilution of Existing Dilution
   a. A higher new dilution can readily be made from a lower dilution by adding the proper amount of diluent. The formula for calculating the new higher final dilution or the amount of diluent to add to obtain a desired new higher final dilution is:

$$= \frac{\frac{\text{reciprocal of present serum dilution}}{\text{volume of serum dilution used}}}{\frac{\text{reciprocal of new final dilution}}{\text{total final volume}}}$$

   b. Example:
      Serum dilution is one in two and volume of serum dilution is 1.0 mL. If 4.0 mL of saline is added, what will be the new final dilution?

$$\frac{2}{1} = \frac{X}{5} \qquad X = 10 \text{ or } 1 \text{ in } 10 \text{ dilution}$$

2. Diluting a Dilution to a Specified Volume
   a. The formula for calculating the volume of diluent to add to a dilution to achieve a certain quantity of a new higher final dilution is:

$$= \frac{\frac{\text{reciprocal of present dilution}}{\text{volume of present dilution needed}}}{\frac{\text{reciprocal of final dilution}}{\text{total final volume required}}}$$

   b. Example:
      Present serum dilution is one in two, total final volume is 100 mL,

new final serum dilution is 1 in 10. How much serum (diluted one in two) will have to be added to make up a final volume of 100 mL of a 1 in 10 dilution?

$$\frac{2}{X} = \frac{10}{100}$$ X = 20 or 20 mL of serum (dilution of one in two) must be added to 80 mL of diluent to obtain 100 mL of a 1 in 10 dilution.

Method 1.5. Dilution of % Solutions

Procedure

1. Dilutions can be prepared from more concentrated solutions by the use of the following formula:

   $$(\text{Volume}_1 \times \text{Concentration}_1) = (\text{Volume}_2 \times \text{Concentration}_2)$$

   $$V_1 \times C_1 = V_2 \times C_2$$

   Where V_1 and C_1 represent original volume and concentration, and V_2 and C_2 represent final desired volume and concentration.

2. Example:
   30% albumin is available but 2 mL of 6% albumin is needed. How should the albumin be diluted?

   $$V_1 \times 30 = 2 \times 6$$
   $$30V_1 = 12$$
   $$V_1 = 12 \div 30 = 0.4$$

   Therefore, mix 0.4 mL of 30% albumin with 1.6 mL saline to obtain 2.0 mL of 6% albumin, or for small volume use, mix 4 drops 30% albumin with 16 drops saline to obtain 20 drops of 6% albumin.

Method 1.6. Preparation and Use of Phosphate Buffer

Principle

Mixtures of acids and bases can be prepared at specific pH values and used to buffer (render) other solutions to that pH. The following procedure includes a method to prepare phosphate-buffered saline (PBS) at a neutral pH, which can then be used as a diluent in serologic tests.

Reagents

1. Prepare acidic stock solution (solution A) by dissolving 22.07 g of $NaH_2PO_4 \cdot H_2O$ in 1 liter of distilled water. This 0.16 M solution of the monobasic phosphate salt (monohydrate) has a pH of 5.0.
2. Prepare alkaline stock solution (solution B) by dissolving 22.7 g of NaH_2PO_4 in 1 L of distilled water. This 0.16 M solution of the dibasic phosphate salt (anhydrous) has a pH of 9.0.

Procedure

1. Prepare working buffer solutions of the desired pH by mixing appropriate volumes of the two solutions. A few examples are:

pH	Solution A	Solution B
5.5	94 mL	6 mL
7.3	16 mL	84 mL
7.7	7 mL	93 mL

2. Check pH of working solution before using it. Add small volumes of acid solution A or alkaline solution B to achieve desired pH.
3. To prepare PBS of a desired pH, add one volume of phosphate buffer at that pH to nine volumes of normal saline.

Reference

Hendry EB. Osmolarity of human serum and of chemical solutions of biologic importance. Clin Chem 1961;7:156-64.

Method 1.7. Preparation of EDTA-Saline for Use in the Immediate-Spin Crossmatch

Principle

Anti-A and anti-B cause direct agglutination and/or lysis of rbcs. Direct agglutination of incompatible rbcs usually is readily observed following centrifugation of rbc-serum mixtures. However, with high-titer IgG anti-A and/or anti-B that fix complement to rbcs, the first component of human complement (C1) may sterically hinder agglutination when tests are performed by immediate-spin technique; hence, the use of saline containing EDTA, which chelates the Ca^{++} ions that are essential for the integrity of the C1 molecule.

Reagents

1. Ethylenediaminetetraacetic acid, dipotassium salt dihydrate ($K_2EDTA \cdot 2H_2O$), 500 g (eg, Aldrich Chemical Co, Milwaukee, WI).
2. Sodium hydroxide (NaOH) pellets, 40 g.
3. Normal saline: 0.85% or 0.9% (w/v) sodium chloride, 20 L.

Procedure

1. Add the contents of a 500 g bottle of K_2EDTA to 20 L saline; mix well.
2. Pour a little of the solution into a 1 L container and to this add 40 g NaOH.
3. Dissolve the NaOH pellets using a magnetic stirrer; and add to the 20 L container.
4. Mix well and allow to stand overnight (to ensure that all chemicals are completely dissolved).

5. Mix again and perform quality control tests as described below. Keep a permanent record of the data for each batch.

Notes

1. Before use, each batch of EDTA-saline should be shown to inhibit lysis of sheep rbcs (available in most immunology laboratories) and human serum, or should inhibit lysis between hemolytic anti-A or anti-B and A or B rbcs, respectively.
2. The osmolarity of the EDTA saline should be 450 mOsm/kg and the pH should be 6.7 ± 0.2.

Reference

Judd WJ, Steiner EA, O'Donnell DB, Oberman HA. Discrepancies in ABO typing due to prozone: How safe is the immediate-spin crossmatch? Transfusion 1988;28:334-8.

7. Trisodium citrate: $C_6H_5Na_3O_7 \cdot 2H_2O$, 8.0 g.

Procedure

1. Dissolve citric acid, dextrose, sodium chloride and trisodium citrate in approximately 600 mL of distilled water.
2. Add chloramphenicol, inosine and neomycin sulphate; mix well.
3. Dilute to 1 L with distilled water.
4. Store at 4 C.

Note

For use, mix one volume Alsever's solution with one volume of whole blood. Alternatively, prepare 3-5% suspensions of rbcs in Alsever's solution; store at 4 C.

Reference

Collins R. Personal communication, 1992.

Method 1.8. Modified Alsever's Solution

Principle

Alsever's solution contains the necessary nutrients for in-vitro storage of rbcs for reagent use. The following formulation includes antibiotics to retard bacterial growth. Rbcs stored in Alsever's solution at 4 C maintain their viability for several weeks.

Reagents

1. Chloramphenicol: 0.33 g.
2. Citric acid - monohydrate: $C_6H_8O_7 \cdot H_2O$, 0.55 g.
3. Dextrose: $C_6H_{12}O_6$, 20.5 g.
4. Inosine: 2.0 g.
5. Neomycin sulphate: 0.5 g.
6. Sodium chloride: NaCl, 4.2 g.

Method 1.9. Grading of Test Results

Principle

The grading of agglutination reactions should be standardized among the members of the blood bank staff in the interest of uniformity and reproducibility of test results. Many workers assign numerical values (scores) to the observed reactions, as described by Marsh.[1]

Materials

1. Centrifuged serologic tests for agglutination.
2. Agglutination viewer.

Procedure

1. Gently shake the tube and disrupt the rbc button in the tube.

Table 1.9-1. Interpretation of Agglutination Reactions

Strength of Reaction	Grade	Score Value	Appearance
4+	"Complete"	12	A single agglutinate. No free rbcs detected.
3-1/2+	4+^{w} or 3+^{s}	11	
3+	3+	10	Strong reaction. A number of large agglutinates.
2-1/2+	3+^{w} or 2+^{s}	9	
2+	2+	8	Large agglutinates in a sea of smaller clumps, no free rbcs.
2+^{w}	2+^{w}	7	Many agglutinates—medium and small, no free rbcs.
1-1/2+	1+^{s}	6	Many medium and small agglutinates, and free rbcs in the background.
1+	1+	5	Many small agglutinates and a background of free rbcs.
1+^{w}	1+^{w}	4	Many very small agglutinates with a lot of free rbcs.
1/2+ or −	± Macro	3	Weak granularity in the rbc suspension. A few macroscopic agglutinates but numerous agglutinates microscopically.
Trace or micro	(+) Micro	2	Appears negative macroscopically. A few agglutinates of 6–8 rbcs in most fields.
Questionable	(0^R) Rough	1	Rare agglutinates observed microscopically.
0	0	0	An even rbc suspension. No agglutinates detected.

2. Observe the way the rbcs leave the rbc button.
3. Record the reactivity by comparing the agglutinates to Table 1.9-1.

Interpretation

Refer to Table 1.9-1.

Notes

1. Serum surrounding the centrifuged rbc button must be inspected for hemolysis. Hemolysis must be regarded as a positive sign of an antigen-antibody reaction if the pretest serum was *not* hemolyzed and no hemolytic agent was added to the test.
2. The character of the agglutination should be noted and recorded. Loose, "stringy," mixed field or refractile agglutinates should be noted, as they provide valuable clues in the investigation of aberrant findings.

Reference

Marsh WL. Scoring of hemagglutination reactions. Transfusion 1972;12:352-3.

Method 1.10. Microplate Techniques Applied to Routine Blood Bank Procedures

Principle

Microplate methods were adapted to blood bank use in the late 1960's and have gained popularity for routine blood processing in blood banks too small for cost-effective automation. Advantages of microplate techniques include enhanced sensitivity of reactions; savings in reagents, supplies and equipment; and reduced requirements for laboratory space and technologist time.

Microplate techniques can be used to test for antigens on rbcs and for antibodies in serum. A microplate can be considered as a matrix of 96 "short" test tubes. Thus, the principles that apply to hemagglutination tube tests also apply to microplates.

Microplates may be rigid or flexible, with either U-shaped or V-shaped bottoms. U-bottom plates are more widely used because results can be read by observing the characteristics of resuspended rbcs or the streaming pattern of rbcs when the plate is placed at an angle. (See section on Interpretation.) Agglutination strength can be estimated using either reading technique.

Equipment

1. Dispensers: Semiautomated devices are available for dispensing equal volumes to a row of wells. Serial dilution titrations can be automated or performed with the specially calibrated Takatsky loops. Special plate carriers can be purchased to fit common table-top centrifuges.

2. Washers: Semiautomated washers are normally used to wash specimens before adding antiglobulin serum. U-bottom plates are preferred for washing rbcs because the samples resuspend more easily.

3. Microplate Readers: Automated devices are available that read microplate results by photometry; differentiation between positive and negative tests is accomplished by measuring light absorbance in U-bottom wells. Ninety-six absorbance values can be processed in less than 1 minute and the results interfaced with a microprocessor. The automated reader passes light beams through the bottoms of the microplate wells. Negative results produce high optical density readings because the rbcs dispersed over the well bottom absorb more light than the concentrated button of cells obtained in a positive result. The microprocessor component of the reader interprets the reactions and the blood group results are printed on the laboratory record.

Rbc controls must be run with automated readers to enable the reader to differentiate false-positive reactions due to nonspecific aggregation. Serum or plasma controls must also be run that will enable the machine to differentiate falsely high absorbance readings due to bilirubin or hemoglobin. For accurate results, the rbc concentrations of routine test samples must be carefully controlled (0.5 to 2% give the best sensitivity) and centrifugation and resuspension must be performed in a very uniform manner. Clotted blood samples are not suitable for use with automated microplate readers.

4. Centrifuges: Appropriate centrifugation conditions must be established for each centrifuge. The following times and relative centrifugal forces, expressed as g are suggested as guidelines to determining the appropriate times and forces. Consult the manufacturer's directions for specific information.

   For flexible U-bottom (U) microplate:
   a. $700 \times g$ for 5 seconds for rbc testing, serum grouping and immediate-spin phase of antibody screening
   b. $700 \times g$ for 20 seconds for washing rbcs for the AHG test
   c. $700 \times g$ for 5 seconds after addition of AHG

   For rigid U microplate:
   a. $400 \times g$ for 30 seconds for rbc testing, serum grouping and immedi-

ate-spin phase of antibody screening
b. $400 \times g$ for 3 minutes for washing the AHG test
c. $400 \times g$ for 30 seconds after addition of AHG

For flexible V-bottom (V) microplate:
a. $700 \times g$ for 10 seconds for rbc testing, serum grouping and immediate-spin phase of antibody screening
b. $700 \times g$ for 20 seconds for washing rbcs for the AHG test
c. $700 \times g$ for 10 seconds after addition of AHG

For rigid V microplate:
a. $900 \times g$ for 40 seconds for rbc testing, serum grouping and optional immediate-spin phase of antibody screening
b. $900 \times g$ for 40 seconds for washing rbcs for the AHG test
c. $900 \times g$ for 10 seconds after addition of AHG

Reagents

1. FDA Requirements for Microplate Use. Many manufacturers supply ABO or Rh typing reagents that are licensed for use as undiluted reagents in microplate tests. Most reagent rbcs licensed for use in tube tests can be used in U-bottom plates without additional preparation other than dilution. If an FDA-licensed laboratory wishes to employ the reagents in a manner not specified by the manufacturer (ie, diluting the reagent before use), the laboratory must submit a description of their procedure to the Office of Biologics Evaluation and Research. The user who changes the test conditions assumes responsibility for appropriate reagent evaluation. Unlicensed blood banks do not need FDA approval for microplate use. The following testing is recommended before adopting the new procedure:

a. After personnel have had sufficient training, the microplate procedure should be run in parallel with the standard procedure using large numbers of specimens, to show that the microplate procedure is at least as accurate as the standard procedure. All discrepant results obtained in the parallel evaluation should be recorded, with a summary of the investigations undertaken to resolve each discrepancy.

b. The standard operating procedures (SOP) manual should describe laboratory procedures used to evaluate each lot of reagent not specifically labeled for microplate use. There should be documentation that each lot of reagent is potent and specific when used according to the SOP. Control testing should include weakly reactive examples of the appropriate phenotypes wherever possible [eg, weak D (D^u) rbcs for anti-D and A_2B rbcs for anti-A]. Control samples may be fresh or frozen-thawed rbcs. If reagents are used at varying dilutions, the protocol should clearly indicate how the correct dilution is selected for use with a new lot.

c. The SOP should describe routine test performance, including daily quality control procedures. At least one positive and one negative control sample should be used daily to verify that each reagent is giving the expected results. Clotted blood samples are not suitable for use with the automated microplate reader.

2. Reagent Testing. If a blood grouping reagent is not specifically labeled for microplate use, the FDA requires that each licensed blood bank test each lot of the reagent with a panel of reagent

rbcs. Such testing helps ensure, with a minimum of effort, that the laboratory's routine procedures will provide appropriate positive and negative results. Appropriate controls to detect nonspecific reactivity are especially important when using procedures employing enzymes. Such specificity testing does not ensure reactivity with weak examples of the antigen, nor does it exclude antibodies to low-incidence antigens not represented on the test panel.

Daily performance checks are recommended to demonstrate appropriate reactivity and specificity of each reagent as well as proper application of the test system. In the ABO system, the serum grouping serves as a control for rbc grouping results; additional ABO controls are not required.

3. Reagent Requirements
   a. Use only licensed anti-A, anti-B, anti-D and antihuman globulin reagents.
   b. Reagent RBCs for ABO Grouping. Commercially available rbcs can be used, or A_1, A_2 and B rbcs can be prepared from anticoagulated donor samples. Rbcs prepared from tubes or sealed donor segments may be used for up to 5 days after the specimen is first entered.
   c. Licensed Reagent RBCs for Antibody Screening. To test donor blood samples but not patients' samples, rbcs may be pooled; the vials of a single lot of screening rbcs may be pooled or a commercially prepared rbc pool may be used.
   d. Diluent for Blood Grouping Reagents. A suggested diluent is: 3% (± 0.5%) bovine albumin in saline prepared by adding nine volumes of normal saline to one volume of commercially available 30% albumin (or 6.3 volumes of normal saline to one volume of 22% albu-

min). The addition of 0.1% sodium azide permits extended storage. Please note: If the manufacturer does not address reagent dilution in the product insert, the user must assume responsibility for the performance of diluted reagents. This diluent may not be suitable for monoclonal blood grouping reagents. Contact manufacturers for further information.
   e. Wash Solution. Use either 0.1% albumin prepared by adding 2 mL of 30% albumin to 500 mL of normal saline or use saline with Tween 20 (0.2 mL/L). These solutions must be prepared fresh daily or purchased ready to use.
   f. Enzyme Solution. Bromelain solutions may be used for microplate procedures. Appropriate working dilutions must be prepared daily. A pH 5.5 phosphate-buffered saline (p 610) is used as the diluent for preparing the 1% stock bromelain. This diluent ensures stability of the frozen product.
   g. Antihuman Globulin (AHG). Commercially available reagents may be adapted to microplate procedures, but many AHG reagents licensed for the blood bank may cause rbcs to adhere to the bottom of wells. Each lot of AHG reagent must be evaluated to determine the dilution that will eliminate prozoning and false-positive reactions while maintaining a system at least as sensitive as manual tube methods (see p 640). (See also note to item 4a.)
   h. Sodium Azide. Use a 0.1% solution prepared from a 2% stock solution in distilled or deionized water. Add 1 mL of stock solution to 19 mL of 3% bovine albumin in order to achieve a final concentration of 0.1% sodium azide. Take appropriate pre-

cautions when using and discarding sodium azide (see p 526 and Method 1.11).

i. Normal saline. 0.9% with or without sodium azide.

4. Preparation of Diluted Reagents

a. Because the sensitivity of blood grouping reagents may be enhanced in microplate tests, some workers choose to dilute the reagents before use. For each new lot of reagent, the appropriate dilution must be established. Reagents diluted in 3% bovine serum albumin or other suitable diluent may be used for as long as 1 week if stored at 1-6 C when not in use. Note: The user assumes responsibility for the performance of diluted reagents, if dilution of reagents is not described in the manufacturer's product insert.

b. Records must be maintained of all reagent evaluation for 5 years. Records should include the following:

1) Date of testing.

2) Initials of technologist performing procedure.

3) Manufacturer, lot number, expiration date and specificity of reagent tested.

4) Identification number and source of rbcs tested, lot number and working dilution of reagent tested.

5) Record of endpoint and working dilution used.

6) Worksheets showing titration format.

c. Any containers other than the original reagent vial should be labeled with the following information:

1) Specificity of reagent.

2) Manufacturer's lot number.

3) Dilution (if applicable).

4) Date of preparation.

5) Initials of technologist.

6) Date and hour at which diluted reagent expires.

d. To establish the appropriate dilution, the serum should be tested against rbcs with a weak expression of the antigen, eg, A_2B for anti-A, weak D (D^u) for anti-D. Deglycerolized frozen rbcs may be used.

e. Rbc suspensions must be accurately prepared. For V-bottom (V) plates, 0.2% cell suspensions are used. For U-bottom (U) plates, use 2-4% suspensions. A 0.2% suspension for use in V plates can be made by diluting to 1 in 10 a 2% suspension made by adding 0.04 mL packed rbcs to 1.96 mL of saline. The rbc concentration is particularly important if streaming is the endpoint. If the suspension is too light, streaming may not occur for negative reactions; if the suspension is too heavy, streaming may occur for positive reactions.

f. Comparison standards are useful, especially while personnel are achieving proficiency.

5. Enzymes

If enzymes are used in routine testing, enzyme-treated rbcs must be used in determining the appropriate reagent dilution according to the testing protocol.

Rbcs should be mixed with enzymes and allowed to stand at room temperature for at least 10 minutes before use. To avoid overtreatment, rbc samples suspended in enzyme solutions should be discarded 4 hours after preparation.

6. Quality Control

Once the working dilution of a reagent has been established, daily quality control should include testing the diluted serum against positive and negative controls.

The working dilution established for each new lot must be tested against a panel of reagent rbcs. If enzymes are used in testing, the panel should be treated in the same manner as routine rbc samples. For diluted anti-D to be used in tests for weak D (D^u), this testing includes an antiglobulin phase using AHG at the optimal working dilution; a negative control using 3% bovine albumin must be run in parallel. Use of the rbc panel will confirm the specificity of anti-D and, if the tests with the group O panel rbcs are negative, will confirm the absence of unexpected antibodies in the anti-A, anti-B and anti-A,B reagents under test conditions.

Procedures

See Methods 2.3, 2.8 and 3.4 for specific examples of microplate techniques.

Interpretation

1. U-Plates. Antigen-antibody reactions can be detected in U-bottom microplate systems by several different modes of interpretation.
   a. For rbc testing, serum grouping and the optional immediate-spin phase of antibody screening, use either of the following methods:
      1) Gently agitate the plate by hand or use a mechanical device to resuspend the rbcs completely. Examine the pattern of the resuspended rbcs by using the ceiling lights as a light source or by supporting the microplate over a magnifying mirror. A positive reaction is the presence of small or large agglutinates, comparable to those seen in tube testing. A negative reaction is a smooth rbc suspension in the bottom of the well.
      2) Observe the streaming pattern of the rbc button, as described in (b.) below.
   b. For weak D (D^u) testing and the AHG phase of antibody screening, interpret the reactions by examining the streaming pattern. Leave the centrifuged microplate on a microplate reader or a support device that is at a 60-degree angle to the bench top for 3-5 minutes. A positive reaction is persistence of an rbc button at the bottom of the well. The edge of the rbc button may be smooth or jagged. Negative reactions show streaming of the rbcs down the well.
   c. To verify weak reactions in any procedure, interpret the settled rbc pattern as follows: Gently agitate the microplate to resuspend the rbcs completely. Place the microplate on a support platform over a magnifying mirror. Allow rbc suspensions to settle completely, a minimum of 20-30 minutes. The settle pattern is then read by observing the underside of the well through the magnifying mirror. Negative reactions appear as smooth round rbc buttons. Strong positive reactions will appear as jagged clumps of rbcs. A weak positive reaction appears as an rbc button with a "halo" surrounding it.
2. V-Plates
   a. Interpretations on all testing procedures (including antibody screening) are recorded as positive or negative. Because of increased sensitivity, the usual grading scale applied to agglutination reactions cannot be used for reactions in the V-bottom microplate.
   b. Negative reaction = No visible button; a distinct streaming tail is apparent. Positive reaction = Firm button in center of well. Some sera produce positive reactions that are variations of the typical pattern. These are described according to

the shape or size of the button and the degree of streaming noted. Several of the forms seen are illustrated in Fig 1.10-1.

3. Resolution of Discrepancies or Unexpected Results
   a. Check to see if results of rbc tests and serum or plasma tests are in agreement. All discrepancies must be resolved. Resolve unexpected results by repeating the tests, using microplate and standard tube methods. The repeat tests should be done on the sample originally examined and also, if available, on a segment. Record results and interpretations of repeat testing on a separate laboratory recording sheet.
   b. Positive results on the rbc control invalidate the results of the rbc grouping.
      1) Prepare a new suspension of enzyme-treated, twice-washed donor rbcs and repeat microplate testing.
      2) If microplate testing again gives invalid results, perform rbc grouping using standard tube methods.

Notes

1. Protein concentration, antibody strength and viscosity of the reagent system must be monitored. Excessively low or high protein concentrations can impair results. Diluting some reagent anti-D with 3% bovine serum albumin will decrease reagent viscosity, thus enabling tests to be read more easily. Other antibodies may perform better with other diluents. Chemically modified reagents may not withstand dilution in diluents other than those used by the manufacturer. If the manufacturer does not certify that the reagent in question is suited to microplate testing, the reagent must be evaluated by the testing facility before use.
2. Both volume and concentration of rbc suspensions and reagent preparations must be carefully standardized.
3. Centrifugation conditions and resuspension techniques must be carefully standardized.
4. Enzymes can be used to enhance reactivity; however, they can also in-

TYPICAL REACTIONS

Negative

Positive

Variant appearances of positive reactions

"Fangs"

"Wings"

"Teardrop"

"Fan"

"Halo"

Figure 1.10-1. Tests done in V-bottom microplates usually present one of the above appearances.

crease the likelihood that nonspecific reactions will be obtained. Suitable controls must be included in enzyme tests.

5. Fibrin present in plasma often interferes with test interpretations. Serum may be preferred to plasma in antibody detection tests.

6. Before use, new plates should be treated to reduce nonspecific binding of test components to the plastic. Pretreatment with 0.1% bovine albumin in saline or human serum prevents the nonspecific adsorption of antibody or nonspecific adherence of rbcs. Static electricity can be reduced by flaming the plate or by washing or wiping the bottom of the plate with a wet towel.

7. Evaporation can be a problem if small volumes of fluid are incubated in plate wells at 37 C or for long periods. Plates can be covered during incubation to prevent evaporation.

8. Plates may be reused, but must be carefully washed.

9. Accurate sample identification may be difficult if microplate tests are performed and read manually. Using microplates eliminates the labeling process associated with tube tests. However, laboratories employing microplate methods must establish a uniform convention for sample placement that must be adhered to by all laboratory personnel. Semiautomated equipment has been designed for sample placement that can provide positive sample identification.

10. Reagents should be added precisely in the center of wells to prevent cross-contamination between wells.

11. Antibodies diluted for use in microplate tests may lose stability in solutions with low protein concentration; such dilutions should not be frozen. If the diluents are not sterile,

bacterial contamination may cause antibody deterioration. Diluted antisera should be stored at 1-6 C for no more than 7 days.

Method 1.11.
Decontamination of Metallic Azides

Principle

Chemically, sodium azide can react slowly with both copper and lead to produce explosive metal azides. Brass or copper drain pipes or cast iron pipes with lead joints may form copper or lead azides. The explosive azides may be detonated directly by shock, friction, heat, electrical discharges and other energy sources such as concussion from hammers, chisels and wrenches.

All laboratory sink traps and drains that have not been converted to glass or plastic, or are not routinely flushed, are potentially contaminated. Therefore, they should be chemically treated. The following procedure is appropriate for use in preventive maintenance and decontamination of laboratory drain systems used to dispose of wastes containing sodium azide. However, the rigorous process may damage older plumbing and professionals should be consulted before the start of any such procedure.

Materials

1. 10% (w/v) sodium hydroxide: slowly add 200 g NaOH to approximately 2 L of water; mix to dissolve NaOH pellets.
2. Soft rubber or plastic hose for syphoning.
3. Plastic bucket for waste.
4. Protective clothing (rubber gloves, gown and goggles).

Procedure

1. Syphon all liquid from the trap and drain using a soft rubber or plastic hose. Use proper precautions against any hazardous chemical that may be present.
2. Pour the sodium hydroxide slowly into the trap. CAUTION: This solution is caustic: wear gloves and goggles.
3. Tape a Chemical Hazard warning sign to the sink. Write "Do Not Use Sink" on the sign.
4. Allow the solution to remain in the trap a minimum of 16 hours.
5. Flush the drain with water for a minimum of 15 minutes. If the drain will not flow, the sodium hydroxide should be removed by syphoning, if possible, then diluted with water. Maintenance personnel should be advised that the drain contains caustic material.

Notes

1. Where it is not possible for a drain line to remain filled with sodium hydroxide solution for at least 16 hours:

   a. Pour five gallons of sodium hydroxide solution into the piping rapidly enough to simulate the flushing action of a toilet.
   b. Flush with copious amounts of water.
   c. Repeat steps 1, 2 and 3 two more times at intervals of a week or so.
2. Because the possibility of residual sodium hydroxide will always exist, personnel should wear gloves and face shields when breaking the drain line or trap for maintenance. Protective equipment should be worn when breaking any laboratory drain, as the presence of hazardous chemicals should always be suspected. Extreme caution should be exercised when unplugging a drain line potentially contaminated with heavy metal azides.
3. Formation of metallic azides can be minimized by thoroughly flushing drains with water when discarding solutions containing sodium azide.

Blood Grouping and Typing

Method 2.1. Slide Test for Determination of ABO Group of Red Cells

Principle

See Chapter 10 for a discussion of the principles of ABO grouping.

Specimen

The reagent manufacturer's instructions should be consulted before performing slide tests since some manufacturers recommend performing slide tests with whole blood, while others specify the use of rbc suspensions of lighter concentrations prepared in saline, serum or plasma.

Materials

1. FDA-licensed monoclonal or polyclonal anti-A.
2. FDA-licensed monoclonal or polyclonal anti-B.
3. FDA-licensed anti-A,B. Note: Use of this reagent is optional.
4. Glass microscope slides.
5. Applicator sticks.

Procedure

1. Place one drop of anti-A on a clean, labeled glass slide.
2. Place one drop of anti-B on a second clean, labeled glass slide.
3. Place one drop of anti-A,B on a third slide, if parallel tests are to be performed with this reagent.
4. Add to each drop of reagent on the slides one drop of well mixed suspension (in saline, serum or plasma) of the rbcs to be tested. (Consult reagent manufacturer's instructions to determine the correct rbc concentration to be used.)
5. Mix the reagents and rbcs thoroughly, using a clean applicator stick for each reagent. The mixture should be spread over an area of approximately 20 mm × 40 mm.
6. Gently tilt the slide continuously for up to 2 minutes. Do not place the slide over a heated surface such as an Rh viewbox during this period. *Do not allow the serum/cell mixture to come into contact with the hands because of the risk of exposure to infectious agents.*
7. Read, interpret and record the results of the reactions on all slides.

Interpretation

1. Strong agglutination of rbcs in the presence of any ABO grouping reagent constitutes a positive result.
2. A smooth suspension of rbcs at the end of 2 minutes is a negative result.
3. Samples that give weak or doubtful reactions should be retested using Method 2.2.

Note

ABO serum groups cannot be accurately determined by slide tests.

Method 2.2. Tube Tests for Determination of ABO Group of Rbcs and Serum

Principle

See Chapter 10 for discussion of principles of ABO grouping. The following procedure is representative of methods in use.

Specimen

Clotted or anticoagulated blood samples may be used for ABO grouping. The test rbcs may be suspended in native serum/plasma or saline, or may be washed and resuspended in saline.

Reagents

1. FDA-licensed monoclonal or polyclonal anti-A.
2. FDA-licensed monoclonal or polyclonal anti-B.
3. FDA-licensed anti-A,B. Note: Use of this reagent is optional.
4. Group A_1 and B rbcs. These can be obtained commercially or prepared by the testing laboratory on each day of use as a 2-5% suspension.

Procedures

Rbc Testing

1. Place one drop of anti-A serum in a clean, labeled test tube.
2. Place one drop of anti-B in a second clean, labeled tube.
3. Place one drop of anti-A,B into a third tube, if parallel tests are to be performed with this reagent.

4. Add to each tube one drop of a 2-5% suspension (in saline, serum or plasma) of the rbcs to be tested. Alternatively, the equivalent amount of rbcs can be transferred to each tube with clean applicator sticks.
5. Mix the contents of the tubes gently and centrifuge for 15-30 seconds at approximately $900\text{-}1000 \times g$.
6. Gently resuspend the rbc buttons and examine for agglutination.
7. Read, interpret and record test results. Confirm rbc test results with those obtained in ABO serum tests (see below).

Serum Testing

1. Label two clean test tubes (A_1 and B). (Note: Label additional tubes if optional tests with A_2 and O rbcs are to be performed.)
2. Add two or three drops of serum to both tubes.
3. Add one drop of A_1 reagent rbcs to the tube labeled A_1.
4. Add one drop of B reagent rbcs to the tube labeled B.
5. Add A_2 and/or O rbcs to the appropriate tube(s). (Note: Tests with A_2 and O rbcs are optional.)
6. Mix the contents of the tubes gently and centrifuge the tubes for 15-30 seconds at approximately $900\text{-}1000 \times g$.
7. Examine the tubes for evidence of hemolysis. Gently resuspend the rbc buttons and examine them for agglutination.
8. Read, interpret and record test results. Confirm serum test results with those obtained in ABO rbc tests (see above).
9. Incubate tubes at room temperature for 5-15 minutes to enhance weak serum reactions.

Interpretation

1. Agglutination in any tube of rbc tests or hemolysis or agglutination in

serum tests constitutes positive test results.

2. A smooth suspension of rbcs after re-suspension of an rbc button is a negative test result.

3. The interpretation of ABO rbc and serum tests is given in Table 10-1 of Chapter 10.

4. Discrepancies between rbc and serum typing tests should be resolved before the patient's or donor's ABO group is interpreted. See Chapter 10.

Note

The expected reactions for positive tests are 3+ to 4+. See Chapter 10 for discussion of weakly reactive samples.

Method 2.3. Microplate Test for Determination of ABO Group of Rbcs and Serum

Principle

See Method 1.10 and Chapter 10 for discussion of microplate testing and principles of ABO grouping.

Specimen

Clotted or anticoagulated blood samples may be used for ABO grouping. However, clotted samples should not be used when utilizing semiautomated microplate readers. See Method 1.10 for preparation of test rbcs.

Reagents

1. FDA-licensed monoclonal or polyclonal anti-A.

2. FDA-licensed monoclonal or polyclonal anti-B.

3. FDA-licensed anti-A,B. Note: Use of this reagent is optional.

4. Group A_1 and B rbcs. These can be obtained commercially or prepared by the testing laboratory on each day of use as a 2% suspension.

Procedures

Rbc Testing

1. Place one drop of anti-A and anti-B in separate clean wells of the microtiter plate. If tests with anti-A,B are to be performed, add this reagent to a third well.

2. Add one drop of a 2% saline suspension of rbcs to each well containing blood grouping reagent.

3. Mix the contents of the wells by gently tapping the sides of the plate.

4. Centrifuge the plate for 30-60 seconds at approximately $200 \times g$.

5. Resuspend the rbc buttons by manually tapping the plate or with aid of a mechanical shaker.

6. Read, interpret and record results. Confirm rbc test results with those obtained in ABO serum tests.

Serum Testing

1. Add one drop of a 2% suspension of reagent A_1 and B cells to separate clean wells of a U-bottom microtiter plate. (Note: If A_2 rbcs are to be tested add them to a third well. Tests with A_2 rbcs are optional.)

2. Add one drop of serum or plasma under test to the wells.

3. Mix the contents of the wells by gently tapping the edges of the plate.

4. Centrifuge the plate for 30-60 seconds at approximately $200 \times g$.

5. Resuspend the rbc buttons by manually tapping the plate or with the aid of a mechanical shaker.

6. Read, interpret and record results. Confirm rbc test results with those obtained in ABO serum tests.

7. Incubate plates at room temperature for 5-10 minutes to enhance weak serum reactions.

Interpretation

1. Agglutination in any well of rbc tests or hemolysis or agglutination in any well of a serum test constitutes a positive result.
2. A smooth suspension of rbcs after resuspension of an rbc button is a negative test.
3. The interpretation of ABO rbc and serum tests is given in Table 10-1 of Chapter 10.
4. Discrepancies between rbc and serum results should be resolved before the patient's or donor's ABO group is interpreted. See Chapter 10.

Method 2.4. Confirmation of Weak A or B Subgroup by Adsorption and Elution

Principle

Red cells having weak A or B antigens may not be agglutinated by anti-A or anti-B but may adsorb the specific antibody. Removing the adsorbed antibody by elution makes it possible to identify the presence of antigenically active material capable of reacting with antibody of known specificity.

Reagents

1. Human (polyclonal) anti-A and/or anti-B. Note: Some monoclonal ABO grouping reagents are sensitive to changes in pH and osmolarity and, thus, may not be suitable for use in adsorption/elution tests.
2. Eluting solution/organic solvent: see Methods Section 5.

Procedure

1. Wash 1 mL of the rbcs to be tested at least three times with saline. Remove and discard the supernatant saline after the last wash.
2. To the rbcs add 1 mL of reagent anti-A if a weak variant of A is suspected or 1 mL of anti-B if a weak variant of B is suspected.
3. Mix the rbcs with the reagent and incubate at 4 C for 1 hour.
4. Centrifuge the mixture to pack the rbcs. Remove the supernatant reagent.
5. Transfer the rbcs to a clean test tube.
6. Wash the rbcs at least eight times with large volumes (10 mL or more) of cold (4 C) saline. Save an aliquot of the final wash supernatant and test for free antibody.
7. Add an equal volume of saline to the washed packed rbcs. Mix well.
8. Elute the adsorbed antibody by a method shown suitable for the recovery of ABO antibodies. See Methods Section 5.
9. Centrifuge to pack the rbcs.
10. Transfer the supernatant eluate to a clean test tube.
11. If anti-A was used, test the eluate against three different group A_1 and three different group O rbc samples at room temperature, at 37 C and by the indirect antiglobulin test.
12. If anti-B was used, similarly test the eluate against three different group B and three different group O rbc samples.
13. Test the supernatant from the final wash (step 6, above) in the same manner to show that washing removed all antibody not bound to the rbcs.

Interpretation

1. If the eluate agglutinates or reacts in antiglobulin testing with specific A or B rbcs and does not react with O rbcs, the rbcs must have active A or B antigen on their surfaces capable of binding specific antibody.

2. If the eluate also reacts with O rbcs, it indicates antibody other than anti-A or anti-B was recovered in the eluate.
3. If the eluate does not react with the A or B rbcs, it indicates the patient or donor's rbcs will not adsorb and elute antibody. It could also indicate the antibody would not bind to specific antigen under the test conditions. If the eluate is nonreactive, it may mean the rbcs under evaluation did not carry weakened A or B antigens. Alternatively, failure to recover antibody may indicate failure to prepare the eluate correctly.
4. If the saline wash material is reactive with A or B rbcs, the results of tests made with the eluate are not valid: the red cells were either not washed adequately, and unbound antibody was not completely removed before elution, or bound antibody dissociated from the rbcs during the washing process.

Reference

Beattie KM. Identifying the causes of weak or "missing" antigens in ABO grouping tests. In: The investigation of typing and compatibility problems caused by red blood cells. Washington, DC: American Association of Blood Banks, 1975:15-37.

Method 2.5. Saliva Testing for A, B, H, Le^a and Le^b

Principle

Some 78% of individuals possess the *Se* gene that governs the secretion of water-soluble ABH antigens into all body fluids with the exception of cerebrospinal fluid. These secreted antigens can be demonstrated in saliva by inhibition tests with ABH and Lewis antisera. See Chapter 10.

Specimen

1. Collect 5-10 mL saliva in a small beaker or wide-mouthed test tube. Most people can accumulate this much in several minutes. To encourage salivation, the subject can chew wax, paraffin or a rubber band, but not gum or anything else that contains sugar or protein.
2. Centrifuge saliva at high speed for 10 minutes.
3. Transfer supernatant to a clean test tube and place in boiling waterbath for 8-10 minutes to inactivate salivary enzymes.
4. Remove clear or slightly opalescent supernatant and dilute with an equal volume of saline. Discard the opaque or semisolid material.
5. Refrigerate if testing is to be done within several hours. If testing will not be done on the day of collection, store the sample in the freezer. Frozen samples retain activity for several years.

Reagents

1. Human (polyclonal) anti-A and anti-B. Note: False inhibition of monoclonal reagents has been observed.
2. Anti-H lectin from *Ulex europaeus*: Obtained commercially or prepared by saline extraction of *Ulex europaeus* seeds.
3. Polyclonal (rabbit/goat) anti-Le^a. There are no published data on the suitability of monoclonal Lewis antibodies.
4. A$_1$ and B rbcs, as used in Method 2.2.
5. Group O, Le(a+b−) rbcs, as used for antibody detection. See Chapter 14.

Procedures

Selection of Blood Grouping Reagent Dilution

1. Prepare doubling dilutions of the appropriate blood grouping reagent.
2. To one drop of each reagent dilution add one drop of 2-5% saline suspen-

sion of rbcs. Use A, B or O rbcs for A, B or H secretor status determination, respectively. Use Le(a+b–) rbcs for Lewis secretor status determination.
3. Centrifuge each tube and examine macroscopically for agglutination.
4. Select the highest reagent dilution that gives 2+ agglutination.

Test for Secretor Status

1. Add one drop of appropriately diluted blood grouping reagent to each of four tubes. For ABH secretor studies, these should be labeled "Secretor," "Nonsecretor," "Saline" and "Unknown." For Lewis studies, these are "Lewis-positive," "Lewis-negative," "Saline" and "Unknown."
2. Add one drop of the appropriate saliva to the "Secretor," "Nonsecretor" and "Unknown" tubes, and one drop of saline to the tube marked "Saline."
3. Mix the tube contents. Incubate for 10 minutes at room temperature.
4. Add one drop of 2-5% saline suspension of washed indicator rbcs to each tube [group A, B or O for ABH secretor status, as appropriate, or Le(a+) for Lewis testing].

5. Mix the tube contents. Incubate for 30-60 minutes at room temperature.
6. Centrifuge each tube. Inspect each rbc button macroscopically for agglutination.

Interpretation

1. Agglutination of indicator rbcs by antibody in tests containing saliva indicates absence of the corresponding antigen in the saliva.
2. No agglutination of indicator rbcs by antibody in tests containing saliva indicates presence of the corresponding antigen in the saliva.
3. Absence of agglutination in control tests containing dilute antibody, indicator rbcs and saline invalidates the results of saliva tests and is due to use of reagents that are too dilute. Redetermine the appropriate reagent dilution as described above.
4. For further interpretation see Table 2.5-1.

Notes

1. Include known secretor and nonsecretor salivas as controls. For ABH secretor status, use saliva from previously tested *Se* and *sese* persons. For

Table 2.5-1 Interpretation of Saliva Testing

| | Testing With Anti-H | | | |
Unknown Saliva	Se Saliva (H Substance Present)	Non-Se Saliva (H Substance not Present)	Saline (Dilution Control)	Interpretation
2+	0	2+	2+	Nonsecretor of H
0	0	2+	2+	Secretor of H

| | Testing With Anti-Le^a | | | |
Unknown Saliva	Le-positive Saliva	Le-negative Saliva	Saline (Dilution Control)	Interpretation
2+	0	2+	2+	Lewis-negative
0	0	2+	2+	Lewis-positive*

*A Lewis-positive person shown to be a secretor of ABH can be assumed to have Le^b as well as Le^a in saliva. A Le(a+) person who is *sese* and does not secrete ABH substance will have only Le^a in saliva.

Lewis testing, use saliva from a person whose rbcs are Le(a+b−) or Le(a−b+) and from a Le(a−b−) person. Freeze aliquots of saliva from persons of known secretor status for later use.

2. This screening procedure can be adapted for the semiquantitation of blood group activity by testing serial saline dilutions of saliva. The higher the dilution needed to remove inhibitory activity, the more salivary blood group substance is present. Saliva should be diluted before incubation with antibody. To detect or to measure salivary A or B substance in addition to H substance, the same procedure can be used with diluted anti-A and anti-B reagents. The appropriate dilution of anti-A or anti-B is obtained by titrating the reagent against A or B rbcs, respectively.

3. A Lewis-positive person shown to be a secretor of A, B and H can be assumed to have Le^b as well as Le^a in the saliva. An Le(a+) person, who is *sese* and does not secrete A, B or H substances, will have only Le^a in the saliva.

Method 2.6. Slide Test for Rh Testing

Principle

See Chapter 11 for a discussion of the principles of Rh typing.

Materials

1. Reagent anti-D: Polyclonal high-protein, chemically modified low-protein or blended IgM/IgG monoclonal/polyclonal low-protein reagents are suitable. Consult the direction circular of the anti-D in use before performing slide tests, since the manufacturer's instructions may be different from the method presented here.
2. Glass microscope slides.
3. Applicator sticks.
4. Rh viewbox.

Procedure

The following is representative of methods in current use.

1. Place one drop of anti-D serum on a clean, labeled slide.
2. Place one drop of the appropriate control reagent on a second labeled slide. (Manufacturer's direction circular will indicate type of control, if needed.)
3. To each slide add two drops of a well-mixed 40-50% suspension (in their own or group-compatible serum or plasma) of the rbcs to be tested.
4. Thoroughly mix the rbc suspension and reagent, using a clean applicator stick for each test, and spread the reaction mixture over an area of each slide of approximately 20 mm × 40 mm.
5. Place the slides on the view box simultaneously and tilt them gently and continuously to observe for agglutination (see note 1). Most manufacturers stipulate that the test must be read within 2 minutes because drying of the reaction mixture may cause formation of rouleaux, which may be mistaken for agglutination.
6. Interpret and record the results of the reactions on both slides.

Interpretation

1. Agglutination with anti-D and a smooth suspension on the control slide constitute a positive test result and indicate the rbcs under test are D+.
2. No agglutination with anti-D and Rh control suggests the rbcs are D−. Testing by the antiglobulin procedure will show if rbcs that type as D−

on slide tests carry a weak D (D^u) antigen.

3. Drying around the edges of the reaction mixture must not be confused with agglutination.

4. If there is agglutination on the control slide, the anti-D test must not be interpreted as positive without further testing.

Notes

1. Do not allow the rbc/serum mixture to come into contact with the hands, because of risk of exposure to infectious agents.

2. A negative test with anti-A and/or anti-B serves as a control test for low protein anti-D.

Method 2.7. Tube Test for Rh Testing

Principle

See Chapter 11 for a discussion of the principles of Rh typing.

Reagents

1. Reagent anti-D: Polyclonal high-protein, chemically modified low-protein or blended IgM/IgG monoclonal/polyclonal low protein reagents are suitable. Consult the direction circular of the anti-D in use before performing slide tests, since the manufacturer's instructions may be different from the method presented here.

2. Rh control reagent: manufacturer's direction circular will indicate type of control, if needed.

Procedure

The following is representative of methods in current use.

1. Place one drop of anti-D serum in a clean, labeled test tube.

2. Place one drop of the appropriate control reagent in a second labeled tube.

3. Add to each tube one drop of a 2-5% suspension (in saline, serum or plasma) of the rbcs to be tested; alternatively, use separate clean applicator sticks to transfer the equivalent amount of rbcs to each tube.

4. Mix gently and centrifuge for the time and speed specified by the manufacturer.

5. Gently resuspend the rbc button and examine for agglutination. If a stick was used to transfer the rbcs, adding one drop of saline to each tube before resuspending the rbc button will provide more fluid to aid resuspension.

6. Grade reactions, and record test and control results.

Interpretation

1. Agglutination $\geq$2+ in the anti-D tube and a nonreactive control constitute a valid test and indicate the rbcs under investigation are D+.

2. If there is agglutination in the control tube, or if the agglutination in the anti-D tube is <2+, the Rh type must not be interpreted as positive without further testing [see weak D (D^u) test, Method 2.9].

3. A smooth suspension of rbcs in both the anti-D and control tubes is a negative test result. Although blood from patients may be designated as D– at this point, donor blood must be further tested by the weak D (D^u) test (or equally sensitive method) for weakened forms of the D antigen. The original test mixture may be used for weak D testing, providing the manufacturer's directions state that the reagent is suitable for the test for weak D.

Note

A negative test with anti-A and/or anti-B serves as a valid control when using low protein reagents.

Method 2.8. Microplate Test for Determination of Rh Type of Rbcs

Principle

See Chapter 11 for a discussion of the principles of Rh typing and Method 1.10 for a discussion of microplate tests.

Specimen

Clotted or anticoagulated samples may be used for Rh testing. However, clotted samples should not be used when using semiautomated microplate readers. See Method 1.10 for preparation of test rbcs.

Reagents

Use only reagents approved for use in microplate tests.

Procedure

The following is representative of methods in use.
1. Place one drop of the Rh reagent to be used in a clean well of the microtitration plate. If the reagent requires the use of an Rh control, add one drop of the control to a second well.
2. Add one drop of a 2% saline suspension of rbcs to each well.
3. Mix the contents of the wells by gently tapping the sides of the plate.
4. Centrifuge the plate for 30-90 seconds at approximately $200 \times g$.
5. Resuspend the rbc buttons by manually tapping the plate or with the aid of a mechanical shaker.
6. Read, interpret and record results.

7. Incubate negative tests at 37 C for 15 minutes.
8. Centrifuge the plate for 30-90 seconds at approximately $200 \times g$.
9. Resuspend the rbc buttons by manually tapping the plate or with the aid of a mechanical shaker.
10. Read, interpret and record results.

Interpretation

Agglutination with Rh reagent following the immediate-spin or 37 C incubation phase indicates a positive test, provided there is no agglutination with the applicable control reagent. See Table 11-3 of Chapter 11 for interpretation of reactions obtained with Rh blood typing reagents.

Method 2.9. Test for Weak D (D^u Test)

Principle

Some rbcs carry a D antigen that is expressed so weakly that the cells are not directly agglutinated by most anti-D reagents. Weak expression of D antigen can be recognized most reliably by the IAT after incubating the test rbcs with anti-D.

Reagents

1. Reagent anti-D: Polyclonal high-protein, chemically modified low-protein or blended IgM/IgG monoclonal/polyclonal low protein reagents may be used. Not every anti-D reagent is suitable for the weak D test, either because testing by the manufacturer has not shown reliable reactions with weak D+ rbcs, or because the reagent contains other antibodies reactive by the AHG test. The manufacturer's package insert will state whether the reagent may be used for weak D testing.

Note: If the original, direct test with anti-D was performed by the tube test technique, the same tube may be used directly for the weak D test, providing the manufacturer's directions so state. In this case, proceed directly to step 4 of the following procedure, after recording the original anti-D tube test as negative.

2. Anti-IgG.
3. IgG-coated rbcs.

Procedure

1. Place one drop of anti-D serum in a clean, labeled test tube.
2. Place one drop of the appropriate control reagent in a second labeled test tube.
3. To both tubes add one drop of a 2-5% suspension in saline of the rbcs to be tested. A DAT may be performed on the rbcs being tested instead of the control test, if desired, but it is better to perform an IAT with the control reagent, as this ensures that all the components of the reagent that might cause a false-positive result are represented.
4. Mix and incubate both tubes for 15-30 minutes at 37 C, according to manufacturer's directions.
5. Centrifuge for 15-45 seconds at 900-1000 × g.
6. Gently resuspend the rbc buttons and examine for agglutination. If strong agglutination of the test cells is observed at this point with anti-D, but not with the control, record the test sample as D+. There is no need to proceed with the antiglobulin phase of the test.
7. If the test rbcs are not agglutinated, or show doubtful agglutination, wash the rbcs three or four times with large volumes of saline.
8. After the final wash, decant the saline completely and blot the rims of the tubes dry.

9. Add one or two drops of anti-IgG, according to manufacturer's directions.
10. Mix gently and centrifuge for 15-30 seconds at 900-1000 × g.
11. Gently resuspend each rbc button, examine for agglutination, grade and record the test result.
12. If the test result is negative, the reaction may be confirmed by adding known IgG-sensitized rbcs, recentrifuging and reexamining for agglutination. The development of agglutination at this point confirms the presence of active AHG in the test mixture.

Interpretation

1. Either a diluent control test or a direct antiglobulin test must accompany the weak D test procedure. Agglutination in the anti-D tube and none in the control tube constitutes a positive test result. The blood must be classified as D+. It is incorrect to report such rbcs as being "D−, D^u+."
2. A negative result is absence of agglutination in the test with anti-D. This means that the rbcs do not have D activity and are to be classified as D−.
3. If the control test is positive, no valid interpretation of the weak D test can be made. In this situation, Rh− blood should be given if the test rbcs are from a patient; if the rbcs are from a donor the rbcs should not be used for transfusion.
4. Causes of false-positive and false-negative antiglobulin tests are discussed in Chapter 8.

Method 2.10. Capillary Testing for Rh

Principle

Although not as widely used as slide and tube tests for D, the capillary Rh testing method[1] is very convenient when many blood units are being processed. This procedure utilizes a saline-active anti-D.

To use this method one must make sure, by adequate testing, that the reagent gives satisfactory results in capillary tubes, and become familiar with the vagaries of reading test results in capillary tubes.

The following procedure is given only in brief outline; the interested reader is advised to consult the original literature as well as the more detailed discussion in Moore, Humphreys and Lovett-Moseley.[2]

Materials

1. Glass capillary tubes, approximately 7.5 cm long and 0.4 mm (ID) in diameter.
2. Saline active (low-protein) IgM anti-D. Blended reagents containing monoclonal IgM anti-D may be suitable for use by this method.

Procedure

1. Place a capillary tube into anti-D reagent. Allow a column of reagent about 2 cm long to enter the capillary tube. Wipe the outside of the capillary tube.
2. Prepare a 20-30% saline suspension of twice-washed rbcs.
3. Allow about 2 cm of the rbc suspension to flow into the capillary tube at the same end as the serum. Hold the capillary tube in a vertical position until after the addition of the blood in order to prevent a bubble from forming at the blood-serum interface. Wipe the outer surface of the tube.
4. Invert the capillary tube, so that the rbcs are above the anti-D, thus enabling the rbcs to fall into and through the reagent. Stand the capillary tube in plasticine at a 45-degree angle.

5. Inspect the rbc column macroscopically after 5-10 minutes. Interpret and record results.

Interpretation

1. Agglutination in the form of a rough and beaded thread inside the capillary tube indicates that the blood is D+.
2. A long smooth line indicates that the blood is D-.

References

1. Chown B, Lewis M. The slanted capillary method of Rhesus blood-grouping. Clin Pathol 1951;4: 464.
2. Moore BPL, Humphreys P, Lovett-Moseley CA. Serological and immunological methods, 6th ed. Toronto: Canadian Red Cross Society, 1968: 36-9.

Method 2.11. Low-Ionic Polybrene® Microplate Technique

Principle

Cationic polymers such as Polybrene® cause aggregation of normal rbcs that can be dispersed with sodium citrate. However, sodium citrate does not disperse Polybrene®-induced aggregation of antibody-coated rbcs. In the low-ionic Polybrene® procedure, rbcs are first incubated with serum under low-ionic conditions to facilitate antibody uptake. Aggregation of rbcs is induced by Polybrene®; if antibody has coated the rbcs, immunoglobulin molecules form bridges between adjacent rbcs that persist after sodium citrate is added. This procedure permits detection of IgG antibodies without use of the indirect antiglobulin technique.

Materials

1. Low-ionic medium: dextrose, 50 g; disodium EDTA, 2 g; distilled water

to 1 L; adjust to pH 6.4 with 3 N NaOH (120 g/L); store at 2-6 C.

2. Neutralizing agent: trisodium citrate, 3.53 g; dextrose, 2 g; distilled water to 100 mL; store at 2-6 C.

3. Polybrene®—10% w/v stock solution: Polybrene® (Aldrich Chemicals, Milwaukee, WI) 5 g; saline, 50 mL; store in plastic at 2-6 C.

4. Polybrene®—aggregating solution: stock polybrene solution, 1 mL; saline 199 mL; store in plastic at 2-6 C.

5. Reagent antibody: from clotted or anticoagulated whole blood centrifuged at 1000 × g for 5 minutes. Note: Not all antibodies that react by IAT are suitable for use with cationic polymers; however, examples of most specificities can be found that react by this method, making antiglobulin testing unnecessary.

6. Test rbcs: from clotted or anticoagulated blood samples, washed once and resuspended to a 1% concentration with saline.

7. U-bottom microplates.

Procedure

1. For each sample to be tested, dispense 25 µL of antibody and 100 µL of low-ionic medium into a microplate well.

2. Add 25 µL of 1% test rbcs and mix on a plate shaker for 15-30 seconds.

3. Incubate at room temperature for 1 minute.

4. Add 25 µL of aggregating solution to each well and mix.

5. Incubate for 15 seconds at room temperature.

6. Centrifuge at 300 × g for 1 minute.

7. Decant the supernatant and add 25 µL of resuspending solution to each well.

8. Agitate the plate by hand to resuspend the rbcs.

9. Examine the rbcs macroscopically for agglutination; grade and record the results.

Interpretation

1. Agglutination usually indicates that the rbcs carry the antigen detected by the test sera. However, false-positive results may occur with rbcs with a positive DAT.

2. Absence of agglutination usually indicates that the rbcs lack the antigen detected by the test sera.

Note

Reagents selected for antigen typing must be shown to be specific for the relevant antigen(s) by this method.

Reference

Malde R, Redman M. Low-ionic Polybrene® technique. In: Knight R, Poole G, eds. The use of microplate technology in the UK. Manchester: British Society of Blood Transfusion, 1987:42-3.

Method 2.12. Preparation and Use of Lectins

Principle

Saline extracts of seeds make useful typing reagents, and are highly specific at appropriate dilutions. Diluted *Dolichos biflorus* extract agglutinates A_1 but not A_2 rbcs. *Ulex europaeus* extract reacts with the H determinant; it agglutinates in a manner proportional to the amount of H present ($O > A_2 > B > A_2B > A_1 > A_1B$). Other lectins useful for special purposes include *Arachis hypogaea* (anti-T), *Glycine max* (*soja*) and the *Salvia* lectins (*S. horminum*, anti-Tn/Cad; *S. sclarea*, anti-Tn).

Materials

1. Seeds: *Arachis hypogaea* (peanuts) and *Glycine max* (soy beans) may be obtained from health-food stores. Oth-

ers may be obtained from commercial seed companies.

2. Electric blender or pestle and mortar.

Procedure

1. Grind seeds in a blender until the particles look like coarse sand. Mortar and pestle may be used, or seeds can be used whole.
2. In a large test tube or small beaker, place ground seeds and three to four times their volume of saline. (Seeds vary in the quantity of saline they absorb.)
3. Incubate at room temperature for 4-12 hours, stirring occasionally.
4. Transfer supernatant fluid to a centrifuge tube and centrifuge for 5 minutes, to obtain clear supernatant. Collect, then filter the supernatant fluid.
5. Determine activity of extract with appropriate rbcs.

   For *Dolichos biflorus*:
   a. Add one drop of 2-5% saline suspension of known A_1, A_2, A_1B, A_2B, B and O rbcs to appropriately labeled tubes.
   b. Add one drop of extract to each tube.
   c. Centrifuge 15 seconds.
   d. Inspect for agglutination and record results.
   e. Lectin should agglutinate A_1 and A_1B rbcs and not A_2, A_2B, B or O rbcs. Often, the native extract agglutinates all rbcs tested. To make the product useful for reagent purposes, add enough saline to the extract so there is 3+ or 4+ agglutination of A_1 rbcs. The diluted extract should also agglutinate A_1B rbcs but not A_2, A_2B, B or O rbcs.

   For *Ulex europaeus*:
   a. Add one drop of 2-5% saline suspension of known A_1, A_2, A_1B, B

and O rbcs to each of five appropriately labeled tubes.
   b. Add one drop of extract to each tube.
   c. Centrifuge 15 seconds.
   d. Inspect for agglutination and record results.
   e. Strength of agglutination should be in the order $O > A_2 > B > A_2B > A_1 > A_1B$.
   f. Dilute extract with saline if necessary, to a point that O rbcs show 3 or 4+ agglutination, A_2 cells show less, and A_1 or A_1B cells are not agglutinated.
6. Store extract in refrigerator for several days, or in freezer for longer period (may be stored indefinitely if frozen).
7. To use for testing, include known positive and negative controls each time. Follow the procedure given in step 5.

Note

To investigate rbc polyagglutination, prepare and test the rbcs with *Arachis*, *Glycine*, *Salvia* and *Dolichos* lectins. The anticipated reactions with various types of polyagglutinable rbcs are as shown in Table 2.12-1.

Table 2.12-1. Reactions Between Lectins and Rbcs

	T	Th	Tk	Tn	Cad
Arachis hypogaea*	+	+	+	0	0
Dolichos biflorus†	0	0	0	+	+
Glycine max (soja)	+	0	0	+	+
Salvia sclarea	0	0	0	+	0
Salvia horminum	0	0	0	+	+

*T and Th rbcs give weaker reactions with *Arachis* after protease treatment; Tk reactivity is enhanced after protease treatment.
†A and AB rbcs may react due to anti-A reactivity of *Dolichos* lectin.

Method 2.13. Use of Thiol Reagents To Disperse Autoagglutination

Principle

Thiol reagents, which cleave the intersubunit disulfide bonds of pentameric IgM molecules, can be used to disperse agglutination caused by cold-reactive autoantibodies. Treating spontaneously agglutinated rbcs with thiol reagents provides a nonagglutinated specimen suitable for use in blood grouping tests.

Reagents

1. 0.01 M dithiothreitol (DTT) or 0.1 M 2-mercaptoethanol (2-ME).
2. Phosphate-buffered saline (PBS) at pH 7.3.
3. Packed washed rbcs to be treated.

Procedure

1. Dilute rbcs to a 50% concentration in PBS.
2. Add an equal quantity of 0.01 M DTT in PBS, or 0.1 M 2-ME in PBS, to the rbcs.
3. Incubate at 37 C for 10 minutes (2-ME) or 15 minutes (DTT).
4. Wash rbcs three times.
5. Dilute the treated rbcs to a 3-5% concentration in saline and use in blood grouping tests.

Reference

Reid ME. Autoagglutination dispersal utilizing sulphydryl compounds. Transfusion 1978;18:353-5.

Method 2.14. Testing DAT Positive Rbcs for Rh Antigens

Principle

When rbcs are heavily coated with IgG, testing with antiglobulin-reactive sera is difficult and tests with high-protein agglutinating reagents are impractical. It may be necessary to dissociate antibody from the rbcs by elution without damaging rbc membrane integrity or altering antigen expression. The elution procedure employed to prepare antibody-free rbcs differs from those intended to recover active antibody. To demonstrate that elution has not damaged antigen reactivity of the test rbcs, it is desirable to treat in parallel an aliquot of uncoated, normal rbcs of the appropriate phenotype.

Reagents

1. Low-protein Rh typing reagents with matched inert control reagent.
2. Antigen-positive rbcs (single-dose expression) to serve as controls.

Procedure

1. Place one volume of washed, packed antibody-coated rbcs and three volumes of normal saline in a test tube of an appropriate size. In another tube, place an equal volume of saline and washed, packed rbcs positive for the antigen thought to be present, usually D. This will provide a check that the elution technique did not destroy the antigen reactivity.
2. Incubate the contents of both tubes at approximately 45 C for 10-30 minutes. The tubes should be agitated frequently. The time of incubation should be roughly proportional to the degree of antibody coating, as indicated by strength of antiglobulin reactivity.
3. Centrifuge the tubes to separate the rbcs and saline. Discard the supernatant saline.
4. Test the formerly antibody-coated rbcs for degree of antibody removal by comparing a direct antiglobulin test on the eluted rbcs with the antiglobulin results on untreated rbcs. If the anti-

body coating is reduced but still present, repeat steps 1 through 3.

5. Test the treated rbcs with low-protein anti-D by Method 2.7.

Notes

1. If there is no agglutination when the rbcs are tested with blood grouping reagents (eg, anti-D), it is desirable to demonstrate that the eluted rbcs have not lost all antigenic reactivity. Seemingly D– rbcs should be tested with anti-c and anti-e in parallel with a diluent control. If the rbcs are not agglutinated by either reagent, the negative results on D testing become suspect.

2. An alternative heat elution technique is to maintain the rbcs and saline at 56 C for 3 minutes. Incubation at this temperature for longer periods will damage antigenic reactivity. Short exposure to a high temperature (56 C) may more effectively dissociate antibody than longer incubation at a moderate temperature (45 C).

Method 2.15. Dissociation of IgG by Chloroquine

Principle

Rbcs with a positive DAT cannot be used directly for blood grouping with reagents, such as anti-Fy^a, that require use of an indirect antiglobulin technique. Under controlled conditions, chloroquine diphosphate dissociates IgG from antibody-coated rbcs with little or no damage to the integrity of the rbc membrane. Use of this procedure permits complete phenotyping of rbcs coated with warm-reactive autoantibody, including tests with reagents solely reactive by indirect antiglobulin techniques.

Reagents

1. Chloroquine diphosphate solution prepared by dissolving 20 g of chloroquine diphosphate in 100 mL saline. Adjust to pH 5.1 with 1 N NaOH, and store at 2-6 C.

2. Test rbcs with a positive DAT due to IgG coating.

3. Control rbcs, carrying a single-dose expression of antigens for which the test samples are to be phenotyped.

4. Anti-IgG antiglobulin reagent (need not be specific for heavy chains).

Procedure

1. To 0.2 mL of washed packed IgG-coated test rbcs add 0.8 mL of chloroquine diphosphate solution. Similarly treat the control sample.

2. Mix, and incubate at room temperature for 30 minutes.

3. Remove a small aliquot (eg, one drop) of the treated test rbcs, and wash four times with saline.

4. Test the washed rbcs with anti-IgG.

5. If nonreactive with anti-IgG, wash the total sample of treated test rbcs and the control sample three times in saline, and use for phenotyping with antiglobulin-reactive blood grouping reagents. Use an anti-IgG reagent when performing these studies.

6. If the treated rbcs react with anti-IgG after 30 minutes of incubation in chloroquine diphosphate, steps 3 and 4 should be repeated at 30-minute intervals (for a maximum incubation period of 2 hours), until the rbcs are nonreactive with anti-IgG. Then proceed as described in step 5.

Notes

1. Chloroquine diphosphate does not dissociate complement components from rbcs. If rbcs are coated with both IgG and C3 in vivo, tests performed after

chloroquine treatment should be performed with anti-IgG.

2. Incubation of rbcs in chloroquine diphosphate should not be extended beyond 2 hours. Prolonged incubation at room temperature, or incubation at 37 C may result in hemolysis and loss of rbc antigens.

3. Some denaturation of Rh antigens may occur. This is most often noted when rbcs have hemolyzed following incubation with chloroquine diphosphate, or when saline-reactive or chemically modified anti-Rh typing reagents are used. Use high-protein reagents and controls when Rh typing chloroquine-treated rbcs.

4. Include an inert control reagent when typing chloroquine-treated rbcs for antigens other than Rh.

5. Chloroquine diphosphate may not remove all antibody from sensitized rbcs. The strength of the DAT of rbcs of some patients, particularly those with strongly positive DATs when untreated, may only be diminished in strength.

6. This method can be used to remove Bg (HLA)-related antigens from rbcs.

References

1. Edwards JM, Moulds JJ, Judd WJ. Chloroquine diphosphate dissociation of antigen-antibody complexes: A new technique for phenotyping rbcs with a positive direct antiglobulin test. Transfusion 1982;22:59-61.

2. Swanson JL, Sastomoinen R. Chloroquine stripping of the HLA-A,B antigens from red cells (letter). Transfusion 1985;25:439.

Method 2.16. Acid Glycine/EDTA Method To Remove Antibodies From Rbcs

Principle

Acid glycine/EDTA can be used to dissociate antibody molecules from rbc mem-branes. The procedure has been used with some success for the preparation of eluates. More frequently, the procedure has been employed to dissociate IgG from rbcs that are then to be used in blood grouping tests or adsorption procedures. All common rbc antigens can be detected on acid glycine/EDTA-treated rbcs with the exception of Kell system antigens. Thus, rbcs treated with acid glycine/EDTA cannot be used to determine Kell antigen status. Acid glycine/EDTA-treated rbcs can be used for adsorption procedures in the investigation of serologic problems due to autoimmune antibodies. Rbcs treated with acid glycine/EDTA can be further treated with dilute solutions of enzymes to enhance antibody uptake.

Reagents

1. 10% EDTA prepared by dissolving 2 g disodium ethylenediaminetetraacetic acid (Na_2EDTA) in 20 mL distilled or deionized water.

2. 0.1 M glycine-HCl buffer (pH 1.5) prepared by diluting 0.75 g glycine to 100 mL with isotonic (unbuffered) saline. Adjust the pH to 1.5 using concentrated HCl.

3. 1.0 M TRIS-NaCl prepared by dissolving 12.1 g tris(hydroxymethyl)aminomethane hydrochloride (TRIS) and 5.25 g sodium chloride (NaCl) to 100 mL with distilled or deionized water.

Procedure

1. Wash the rbcs to be treated six times with isotonic saline.

2. In a test tube mix together 20 volumes of 0.1 M acid glycine-HCl (pH 1.5) with five volumes of 10% EDTA. This is the acid glycine/EDTA reagent.

3. Place 10 volumes of washed packed rbcs in a clean tube.

4. Add 20 volumes of acid glycine-HCl.

5. Mix the contents of the tube thoroughly.

6. Incubate the mixture at room temperature for no more than 2-3 minutes.
7. Add one volume of 1.0 M TRIS-NaCl and mix the contents of the tube.
8. Centrifuge at 900-1000 × g for 1-2 minutes to separate rbcs from fluids.
9. Aspirate the supernatant fluid and discard.
10. Wash the rbcs four times with saline.
11. Test the washed rbcs with anti-IgG.
12. If nonreactive with anti-IgG, the rbcs are ready to be used in blood grouping or adsorption procedures.

Notes

1. Overincubation of rbcs in acid glycine/EDTA causes irreversible damage to rbc membranes.
2. Include an inert control reagent when typing treated rbcs.

References

1. Louie JE, Jiang AF, Zaroulis CG. Preparation of intact antibody-free red cells in autoimmune hemolytic anemia. Transfusion 1986;26:550.
2. Byrne PC. Use of a modified acid/EDTA elution technique. Immunohematology 1991;7:46-7.

Method 2.17. Separation of Transfused From Autologous Rbcs by Simple Centrifugation

Principle

Newly formed autologous rbcs, having a lower specific gravity than transfused rbcs, may be separated from the transfused population by simple centrifugation in microhematocrit tubes. The newly formed autologous rbcs concentrate at the top of the column of red cells in a centrifuged microhematocrit tube. Microhematocrit centrifugation provides a simple method for recovering autologous rbcs in blood samples from recently transfused patients and can be performed in any clinical laboratory. Note: Rbcs from patients with hemoglobin S or spherocytic disorders are not effectively separated by this method. See Method 2.18 for an alternative procedure.

Specimen

Rbcs from a recently transfused patient. Blood samples should be collected into EDTA.

Materials

1. Microhematocrit equipment: centrifuge, plain (not heparinized) glass hematocrit tubes and sealant such as Seal-ease®.
2. 2-mL syringe and 23-gauge needle.

Procedure

1. Wash the rbcs three times in saline. For the last wash, centrifuge at 900-1000 × g for 5-15 minutes. Remove as much of the supernatant fluid as possible without disturbing the buffy coat. Mix thoroughly.
2. Fill 10 microhematocrit tubes to the 60-mm mark with packed rbcs.
3. Seal the ends of the tubes by heat, or with sealant.
4. Centrifuge all tubes in a microhematocrit centrifuge for 15 minutes.
5. Cut the microhematocrit tubes 5 mm below the top of the centrifuged rbc column.
6. Flush the upper layer of rbcs from the cut hematocrit tubes into a clean test tube using a saline-filled syringe and 23-gauge needle. Alternatively, place the cut microhematocrit tubes into 10 or 12 × 75 mm test tubes and centrifuge at 1000 × g for 1 minute. Remove the glass hematocrit tubes.
7. Wash the separated rbcs three times in saline before testing.

Notes

1. Separation is better when blood samples are obtained 3 or more days after transfusion.
2. The packed rbcs should be mixed continuously during the filling of microhematocrit tubes.
3. Conditions that result in decreased bone marrow production, eg, aplastic anemia, will preclude effective use of this method due to decreased reticulocyte formation.
4. Separation techniques are only effective if the patient is producing normal or greater than normal amounts of reticulocytes.
5. The expression of some rbc antigens may not be as strong on reticulocytes as on older rbcs.

Reference

Reid ME, Toy P. Simplified method for recovery of autologous red blood cells from transfused patients. Am J Clin Pathol 1983;79:364-6.

Method 2.18. Separation of Transfused From Autologous Rbcs in Patients With Hemoglobin S Disease

Principle

Rbcs from patients with hemoglobin S or sickle cell (SC) disease are resistant to lysis by hypotonic saline, in contrast to normal donor rbcs and donors with hemoglobin S trait. Use of this procedure permits serologic testing of autologous rbcs from recently transfused patients with hemoglobin S or SC disease.

Reagents

1. Hypotonic saline - 0.3% w/v NaCl: NaCl, 3 g; distilled water to 1 L.
2. Normal saline - 0.9% w/v NaCl: NaCl, 9 g; distilled water to 1 L.
3. Whole blood: freshly collected (ie, within past 24 hours) and anticoagulated with EDTA/ACD/CPD/CPDA-1, 7 mL (more if patient is anemic).

Procedure

1. Place four or five drops of rbcs into a 10 or 12 × 75-mm test tube.
2. Wash the rbcs six times with 0.3% NaCl, or until gross hemolysis is no longer apparent; use centrifugation at 1000 × g for 1 minute per wash.
3. Wash the rbcs twice with 0.9% NaCl to restore tonicity; use centrifugation at 200 × g for 2 minutes per wash to facilitate removal of residual stroma.
4. Resuspend the rbcs to a 5% concentration for phenotyping or use packed rbcs in microautoadsorption tests.

Note

Larger volumes, for use in adsorption studies, can be processed in a 16 × 100-mm test tube.

Reference

Brown D. A rapid method for harvesting autologous red cells from patients with hemoglobin S disease. Transfusion 1988;28:21-3.

Antibody Detection and Compatibility Testing

Method 3.1. Antiglobulin Tests

Principle

The saline, albumin, low-ionic strength saline (LISS), polyethylene glycol (PEG) and low-ionic Polybrene® (LIP) procedures described below are suitable for use in pretransfusion testing. The enzyme techniques described later in this section are best reserved for antibody identification. With the exception of the LIP technique, detailed discussions of the merits and pitfalls of these procedures are to be found in Chapters 14 and 15.

In the LIP procedure, Polybrene®, a highly cationic quaternary ammonium polymer, causes reversible aggregation of normal rbcs. If rbcs sensitized with antibody are brought together by Polybrene®, irreversible agglutination occurs. Rbcs are first incubated with serum in a medium of low-ionic-strength, to facilitate attachment of antibody to rbcs. Polybrene® is then added to aggregate the cells. After centrifugation, the aggregating effect of Polybrene® is neutralized by the addition of sodium citrate. Antibody-mediated agglutination will persist after addition of citrate, but nonagglutinated cells will be dispersed. If the rbcs are subsequently to be tested with antiglobulin serum, additional citrate is used in the washing process.

Specimen

Serum or plasma may be used. If used for pretransfusion testing, specimens should be collected within 3 days of scheduled transfusion if the patient has not been transfused or pregnant within the last 3 months.

Materials

1. Normal saline.
2. Bovine albumin (22% or 30%) or LISS additive.
3. LISS:
   a. Add 1.75 g NaCl and 18 g glycine to a 1-L volumetric flask.
   b. Add 20 mL of phosphate buffer prepared by combining 11.3 mL of 0.15 M KH_2PO_4 and 8.7 mL of 0.15 M Na_2HPO_4.
   c. Add distilled water to the 1-L mark.
   d. Adjust pH to 6.7 with NaOH.
   e. Add 0.5 g sodium azide as a preservative.
      Note: Adding sodium azide at this concentration raises the ionic strength from 0.0355 to 0.043. This does not make any practical difference in terms of serologic reactivity.
4. PEG: 20% w/v; 3350 MW PEG, (SIGMA Chemicals, St. Louis, MO), 20 g; pH 7.3 PBS (see Method 1.6) to 100 mL.
5. LIP Reagents:
   a. Low ionic medium (LIM): To a 500-mL volumetric flask, add 25 g dextrose and 1 g $Na_2EDTA \cdot 2H_2O$. Fill

Section 3

flask to 500-mL mark with distilled water.

b. Polybrene®: *Stock solution*: Prepare 10% Polybrene® by adding 5 g Polybrene® to 50 mL normal saline. Store in plastic container. *Working solution*: Make a 0.05% solution by mixing 0.1 mL of stock solution with 19.9 mL normal saline.

c. Resuspending solution: *0.2 M trisodium citrate*: Add 5.88 g $Na_3C_6H_5O_7 \cdot 2H_2O$ to a 100-mL volumetric flask; fill to mark with distilled water. *5% dextrose*: Add 5 g dextrose to 100 mL of distilled water. *Working solution*: Mix 60 mL of trisodium citrate with 40 mL of 5% dextrose.

d. Washing solution (for antiglobulin testing): *10 mM sodium citrate*: Make a 1 in 20 dilution of 0.2 M trisodium citrate (see above) in normal saline, eg, add 50 mL of 0.2 M trisodium citrate to 950 mL of saline.

6. Antihuman globulin (AHG) reagent. Polyspecific or anti-IgG may be used unless otherwise indicated. Anti-IgG need not be heavy-chain specific.

7. IgG-coated rbcs, to confirm the validity of negative tests.

8. 10 or 12 × 75-mm test tubes.

Method 3.1.1. Saline IAT

Procedure

1. Add two or three drops of serum to properly labeled tubes.
2. Add one drop of 2-4% saline-suspended rbcs (reagent or donor) to each tube and mix.
3. Centrifuge and observe for hemolysis and agglutination. Grade and record the results.
4. Incubate at 37 C for 30-60 minutes.

5. Centrifuge and observe for hemolysis and agglutination. Grade and record the results.
6. Wash the rbcs three or four times with saline and completely decant the final wash.
7. Add AHG according to the manufacturer's directions to the dry rbc button. Mix well.
8. Centrifuge and observe for reaction. Grade and record the results.
9. Confirm the validity of negative tests with IgG-coated rbcs.

Method 3.1.2. Albumin IAT (or LISS-Additive IAT)

Procedure

1. Add two or three drops of serum (use volumes specified by manufacturer for LISS additives) to properly labeled tubes.
2. Add 22% or 30% bovine albumin, or LISS additive, according to the manufacturer's directions.
3. Add one drop of 2-4% saline-suspended rbcs (reagent or donor) to each tube and mix.
4. Incubate at 37 C for 30 minutes. For LISS additives, follow the manufacturer's directions.
5. Centrifuge and observe for hemolysis and agglutination. Grade and record the results.
6. Perform the IAT described in Method 3.1.1, steps 6-9.

Method 3.1.3. LISS IAT

Procedure

1. Wash rbcs three times in normal saline.
2. Completely decant saline.

3. Resuspend the rbcs to a 2% suspension in LISS.
4. Add two drops of serum to properly labeled tube.
5. Add two drops of LISS-suspended rbcs.
6. Mix and incubate 10-15 minutes at 37 C.
7. Centrifuge and observe for hemolysis and agglutination by gently resuspending the cell button. Grade and record results.
8. Perform the IAT described in Method 3.1.1, steps 6-9.

Method 3.1.4. PEG IAT

Procedure

1. For each rbc sample to be tested, mix two drops of test serum, four drops of 20% PEG in phosphate-buffered saline (PBS) and one drop of rbcs.
2. Incubate at 37 C for 15 minutes.
3. DO NOT CENTRIFUGE.
4. Wash the rbcs four times with saline; completely decant the final wash supernatant.
5. Perform the IAT, using anti-IgG, described in Method 3.1.1, steps 6-9.

Reference

Nance S, Garratty G. Polyethylene glycol: A new potentiator of red blood cell antigen-reactions. Am J Clin Pathol 1987;87:633-5.

Method 3.1.5. LIP IAT

Procedure

1. Make a 1% saline suspension of rbcs. This can be done as follows: Wash one drop of a 3-5% suspension. Decant, shake lightly. Resuspend. Decant forcefully.
2. Add 0.1 mL serum to each tube.

3. Add 1.0 mL LIM solution. Mix and incubate for one minute at room temperature.
4. Add 0.1 mL 0.05% Polybrene® to each tube. Mix.
5. Centrifuge for 10 seconds at 900-1000 × g and decant supernatant. DO NOT RESUSPEND BUTTON.
6. Add 0.1 mL resuspending solution. Observe for persistence of agglutination after gently shaking. Note: If strength of agglutination is weak, compare the test with negative control microscopically. DO NOT RECENTRIFUGE.
7. If desired, the antiglobulin test may be performed as follows:
   a. Add 0.05 mL (50 μL) of resuspending solution to each tube. Mix.
   b. Wash the cells three times with 10 mM sodium citrate solution.
   c. Add two drops of anti-IgG to the dry button. Mix.
   d. Centrifuge for 15 seconds. Read and record results.
   e. Add IgG-coated rbcs to each negative tube.

Reference

Lalezari P, Jiang AF. The manual Polybrene® test: A simple and rapid procedure for detection of red cell antibodies. Transfusion 1980;20:206-11.

Interpretation (for antiglobulin tests above)

1. The presence of agglutination/hemolysis after incubation at 37 C constitutes a positive test.
2. The presence of agglutination after addition of AHG constitutes a positive test.
3. Antiglobulin tests are negative when no agglutination is observed, providing the IgG-coated rbcs are reactive. If they are not agglutinated, the negative result is invalid and the test must be repeated.

4. For the LIP procedure, the presence of persistent agglutination after addition of resuspending solution constitutes a positive test.

Controls

1. When used for the detection of unexpected antibodies in pretransfusion testing, the method in use should be checked daily with weak examples of antibody (eg, weak human IgG anti-C and weak human IgG anti-E, prepared from reagent grade typing sera by dilution with 6% bovine albumin such that the expected reaction by IAT is 2+).
2. For testing an unknown serum against reagent rbcs by the LIP technique, an inert serum should be tested against a random rbc sample for comparative purposes.
3. When testing a known blood grouping reagent against unknown rbcs, an rbc sample with single-dose expression of the antigen (ie, from a heterozygote) and a sample negative for the antigen should be tested.

Notes

1. The incubation times and the volume and concentration of rbcs used are those given in the references cited. Individual laboratories may choose to standardize techniques with somewhat different values. See Chapter 8 for other limitations when modifying procedures.
2. For the PEG procedure:
   a. Omit centrifugation after 37 C incubation as rbcs will not resuspend readily.
   b. Use anti-IgG, rather than polyspecific AHG, to avoid unwanted positive reactions due to C3-binding autoantibodies.

Method 3.2. Prewarmed Technique for Antibody Detection and Crossmatching

Principle

The prewarmed technique may be useful in the detection and identification of those red cell antibodies that are able to bind to rbcs only at 37 C. It may be helpful in testing sera of patients with a history or current evidence of potent cold-reactive autoantibody, the reactivity of which may mask clinically significant antibodies.

This technique should be used with some caution, as there are anecdotal reports of loss of reactivity of some examples of clinically significant antibodies.

Reagents

As for Method 3.1.

Procedure

1. Prewarm a bottle of saline to 37 C.
2. Label one tube for each reagent or donor sample to be tested.
3. Add one drop of 2-4% saline-suspended rbcs to each tube.
4. Place the tubes containing rbcs and a tube containing a small volume of the patient's serum at 37 C; incubate for 5-10 minutes.
5. Using a prewarmed pipet, transfer two drops of prewarmed serum to each tube containing prewarmed rbcs. Mix without removing tubes from the incubator.
6. Incubate at 37 C for 30-60 minutes.
7. Without removing the tubes from the incubator, fill each tube with prewarmed (37 C) saline. Centrifuge and wash 3-4 times with 37 C saline.
8. Add anti-IgG according to the manufacturer's directions, and complete the antiglobulin test described in Method 3.1.1, steps 6-9.

Note

The prewarmed procedure described above does not allow for the detection of alloantibodies that agglutinate at 37 C or lower and are not also reactive in the antiglobulin phase. To demonstrate them, testing (including centrifugation) may have to be done at 37 C. If time permits, a tube containing a prewarmed mixture of serum and rbcs can be incubated at 37 C for 60-120 minutes to allow the rbcs to settle. The rbcs can be examined for agglutination by resuspending the button without centrifugation.

Method 3.3. Saline Replacement To Demonstrate Alloantibody in the Presence of Rouleaux

Principle

When rouleaux are present, a saline replacement technique is sometimes useful. Rouleaux can be identified by microscopic examination of rbcs in serum. The rbcs adhere to one another on their flat surface, giving the classic "stack of coins" appearance. In assessing rouleaux formation, knowledge of the patient's clinical diagnosis and the protein content and proportions in the serum are helpful; globulins are usually elevated such that the 2:1 albumin:globulin ratio is reversed.

Procedure

After routine incubation and resuspension, proceed with the following steps:
1. Recentrifuge the serum/rbc mixture when rouleaux formation is suspected.
2. Remove the serum.
3. Replace the serum with an equal volume of saline (two drops) and gently mix.
4. Spin the saline/rbc mixture.

5. Resuspend the saline/rbc mixture and observe for agglutination. Rouleaux will disperse when suspended in saline, whereas true agglutination will remain.

Reference

Issitt PD. Applied blood group serology. 3rd ed. Miami: Montgomery Scientific Publications, 1985:605.

Method 3.4. Microplate Method for Antibody Detection Using LISS

Principle

This procedure is especially useful for screening large numbers of sera for unexpected antibodies.

Materials

1. AHG: polyspecific or anti-IgG.
2. IgG-coated rbcs: obtain commercially; dilute to a 0.5% concentration with saline before use.
3. LISS solution: see Method 3.1.
4. Microplate equipment: V-bottom microplates.
5. Rbcs: allogeneic homologous group O, R_1 and R_2 rbc samples, washed once with LISS and resuspended to a 0.5% concentration with LISS; use within 6 hours of preparation.
6. Test serum or plasma: collected within the previous 3 days if to be used for pretransfusion testing.
7. Wash solution: 30% bovine serum albumin (BSA), 6 mL (or 22% BSA, 8 mL); Tween 20, 0.2 mL; normal saline to 1 L.

Procedure

1. For each sample to be tested, dispense one drop (0.35 µL) of serum/plasma into each of two microplate wells.

2. To one well of each serum sample add an equal volume of 0.5% R_1 rbcs in LISS; similarly, set up tests with R_2 rbcs.
3. Mix and incubate at 37 C for 15-20 minutes.
4. Wash the rbcs 4 times with albumin-Tween-saline wash solution. Note: Use 0.2 mL volume for each wash; centrifuge at 180 × g for 2 minutes; decant the supernatant following each centrifugation.
5. Add one drop of AHG to each test well.
6. Mix, and centrifuge at 50 × g for 1 minute.
7. Stand the microplates at a 45 (± 15) degree angle for 3-5 minutes and observe for agglutination; record the results.
8. Confirm negative reactions with IgG-coated rbcs.

Interpretation

NEGATIVE: A distinct streaming tail of rbcs is apparent with no visible rbc button.

POSITIVE: A firm button persists in the center of the well; a variable degree of streaming may be present.

Note

Test results can be recorded as positive or negative only; due to the sensitivity of tests in V-bottom microplates, the normal grading system (see Method 1.9) should not be used.

Reference

Ball M. Methods for blood grouping, antibody screening and rare phenotype screening in microplates. In: Knight R, Poole G, eds. The use of microplates in blood group serology: A review of microplate technology in the UK. Manchester, England: British Society of Blood Transfusion, 1987: 33-41.

Method 3.5. Enzyme Techniques

Proteolytic enzymes modify rbc antigens in ways that enhance the reactivity of some antigen-antibody systems (notably Rh and Kidd) and abolish antigenic configurations of others (notably M, N, Fy^a and Fy^b). Enzyme modification also alters physical properties of the rbc suspension and can cause spontaneous aggregation of rbcs in an immunologically inert system.

Method 3.5.1. Preparation of Enzymes

Principle

The preparations used in blood banking differ from lot to lot, so each time a stock enzyme solution is prepared, its reactivity should be tested and incubation periods standardized for optimal effectiveness.

Materials

1. Dry enzyme powder (papain, ficin, etc).
2. Phosphate-buffered saline (as indicated): see Method 1.6.
3. L-cysteine hydrochloride.
4. Protective clothing (as indicated).
5. Glassware (as indicated).
6. Magnetic stirrer or flask agitator.

Procedure

A. Ficin
   1. Place 1 g powdered ficin in a 100-mL volumetric flask. Handle ficin carefully because it is harmful if inhaled or if it gets in the eyes. Wearing gloves, mask and apron or working under a hood is desirable.

2. Add PBS, pH 7.3 to 100 mL, to dissolve ficin. Agitate vigorously by inversion, rotate for 15 minutes, or mix with a magnetic stirrer until mostly dissolved. The powder will not dissolve completely.
3. Collect clear fluid, either by filtration or centrifugation, and prepare small aliquots. Store aliquots at –20 C or below. Do not refreeze thawed solution.

B. Löw's Activated Papain
1. Grind 0.5 g papain in a mortar with a few milliliters of PBS, pH 5.5.
2. Wash the papain suspension into a 250-mL flask with 190 mL PBS, pH 5.5.
3. Add 0.6 g L-cysteine hydrochloride dissolved in 10 mL distilled water and neutralized with 1N NaOH.
4. Incubate at 37 C for 1 hour. Incubation time should begin when the solution reaches 37 C.
5. Centrifuge the solution. Keep the supernatant fluid and discard undissolved papain.
6. Store activated papain solution at –20 C or below in small aliquots. Activated papain is not stable at 4 C. Once the solution is thawed, the unused portion must be discarded at the end of the day.

Method 3.5.2. Standardization of Enzyme Procedures

Principle

For a two-stage enzyme procedure, the optimal dilution and incubation conditions must be determined for each new lot of stock solution. The technique given below for ficin can be modified for use with other enzymes.

Reagents

1. Stock solution of ficin in PBS, pH 7.3.
2. Several sera that contain no unexpected antibodies.
3. Anti-D that agglutinates only enzyme-treated Rh+ rbcs and does not agglutinate untreated Rh+ rbcs.
4. Anti-Fy^a of moderate or strong reactivity.
5. Rbcs positive for D and Fy^a.

Procedure

1. Dilute one volume of stock ficin solution with nine volumes of PBS, pH 7.3.
2. Label three tubes: 5 minutes, 10 minutes and 15 minutes.
3. Add equal volumes of washed rbcs and 0.1% ficin to each tube.
4. Mix and incubate at 37 C for the time designated. Incubation time is easily controlled if the 15-minute tube is prepared first, followed by the 10- and 5-minute tubes at 5-minute intervals. Incubation will be complete for all three tubes at the same time.
5. Immediately wash the rbcs three times with large volumes of saline.
6. Resuspend treated rbcs to 2-5% in saline.
7. Label four tubes for each serum to be tested: untreated, 5 minutes, 10 minutes, 15 minutes.
8. Add two drops of the appropriate serum to each of the four tubes.
9. Add one drop of the appropriate rbc suspension to the labeled tubes.
10. Mix and incubate at 37 C for 15 minutes.
11. Centrifuge, and examine for agglutination by gently resuspending button.
12. Wash rbcs three or four times with saline and test by the IAT.

Table 3.5.2-1. Hypothetical Results With D +, Fy(a +) Cells

Rbcs + Enzyme		Inert Serum	Anti-D	Anti-Fy^a
Untreated	37 C inc.	0	0	0
	AHG	0	1+	3+
5 minutes	37 C inc.	0	1+	0
	AHG	0	2+	1+
10 minutes	37 C inc.	0	2+	0
	AHG	0	2+	0
15 minutes	37 C inc.	0	2+	0
	AHG	w+	2+	w+

Interpretation

Table 3.5.2-1 shows the hypothetical results with D+, Fy(a+) cells. The optimal incubation time would be 10 minutes. Incubation for only 5 minutes does not completely abolish Fy^a activity or maximally enhance anti-D reactivity. Incubation for 15 minutes causes false-positive antiglobulin reactivity with sera that should not have reacted immunologically.

If incubation for 5 minutes proves to overtreat the rbcs, it is better to use a more dilute working solution of enzyme than to reduce incubation time, because it is difficult to determine and then to monitor very short incubation times with sufficient accuracy. In additional tests, a single dilution can be selected and studied for different incubation times, or a single time can be selected and the effects of different dilutions studied.

Method 3.5.3. Evaluating Treated Rbcs

Principle

After optimal incubation conditions have been determined for a new lot of enzyme solution, treated rbcs should be evaluated before use to demonstrate that they are adequately, but not excessively, mod-

ified. Satisfactory treatment produces cells that are agglutinable by an antibody that gives only antiglobulin reactions with unmodified rbcs, and are not agglutinated or aggregated in the presence of inert serum.

Procedure

1. Select an antibody that agglutinates antigen-positive enzyme-treated rbcs but gives only AHG reactions with unmodified rbcs. Many examples of anti-D in sera from patients behave in this way.
2. Add two drops of the selected antibody-containing serum to a tube labeled "positive."
3. Add two drops of a serum free of unexpected antibodies to a tube labeled "negative."
4. Add one drop of 2-5% suspension of enzyme-treated rbcs to each tube.
5. Mix and incubate 15 minutes at 37 C.
6. Centrifuge and resuspend the rbcs by gentle shaking.
7. Examine macroscopically for the presence of agglutination.

Interpretation

There should be agglutination in the "positive" tube and no agglutination in the "negative" tube. If agglutination occurs in the "negative" tube, the rbcs have been overtreated; if agglutination does not occur in the "positive" tube, treatment has been inadequate.

Method 3.5.4. One-Stage Enzyme Technique

Procedure

1. Add two drops of serum to a properly labeled tube.
2. Add two drop of a 2-5% saline suspension of rbcs.

3. Add two drops of papain solution and mix well.
4. Incubate at 37 C for 30 minutes.
5. Centrifuge; gently resuspend the rbcs and observe for agglutination. Grade and record the results.
6. Proceed with the antiglobulin procedure described in Method 3.1.1, steps 6-9.

Method 3.5.5. Two-Stage Enzyme Technique

Procedure

1. Prepare a diluted enzyme solution (papain or ficin) by adding 9 mL PBS, pH 7.3 to 1 mL of stock enzyme.
2. Add one volume of diluted enzyme to one volume of packed, washed rbcs.
3. Incubate at 37 C for the time determined to be optimum for that enzyme solution.
4. Wash treated rbcs at least three times with large volumes of saline.
5. Resuspend rbcs to 2-5% concentration in saline.
6. Add two drops of serum to be tested to properly labeled tube.
7. Add one drop of 2-5% suspension of enzyme-treated rbcs.
8. Mix and incubate for 30 minutes at 37 C.
9. Centrifuge; gently resuspend the rbcs and observe for agglutination. Grade and record the results.
10. Proceed with the antiglobulin procedure described in Method 3.1.1, steps 6-9.

Notes

1. An alternative method for steps 4 and 5 (Method 3.5.4) or steps 8 and 9 (Method 3.5.5) is to incubate the serum and enzyme-treated cells at 37 C for 60 minutes and then to examine the settled rbcs for agglutination without centrifugation. This can be useful for serum with strong cold-reactive agglutinins and can sometimes prevent problems with false-positive results.
2. Microscopic examinations are not recommended for routine use and are particularly inappropriate with enzyme enhanced tests due to an increased rate of false-positive reactions detected.
3. Either papain or ficin may be used in a two-stage procedure.

References

1. Issitt PD. Applied blood group serology. 3rd ed. Miami: Montgomery Scientific, 1985.
2. Löw B. A practical method using papain and incomplete Rh-antibodies in routine Rh blood-grouping. Vox Sang 1955;5:94-8.

Method 3.6. Direct Antiglobulin Test

Principle

The DAT is used to demonstrate in-vivo coating of rbcs with globulins, in particular IgG and C3dg. Washed rbcs from a patient or donor are tested directly with AHG reagents.

Reagents

1. AHG: The following procedure is for direct testing with polyspecific AHG, but all AHG reagents may be used in this manner.
2. Rbcs from a blood sample anticoagulated with EDTA, to avoid in-vitro uptake of complement that may occur to rbcs from clotted samples (see p 183).

Procedure

1. Wash one drop of a 2-5% suspension of rbcs four times with saline. Com-

pletely decant the final supernatant wash solution, and immediately add one or two drops of polyspecific AHG, as specified by the manufacturer.

2. Mix, centrifuge and examine the rbcs for agglutination. Grade and record the reaction. The manner in which rbcs are dislodged from the bottom of the test tube is critical. The tube should be gently tilted back and forth until an even suspension of rbcs or agglutinates is observed, and all rbcs are resuspended.

3. If using polyspecific AHG or anti-C3d, leave apparently nonreactive tests at room temperature for 5 minutes, recentrifuge and read again. This achieves maximal sensitivity for complement detection, as in the investigation of immune hemolysis (see Chapter 16). This additional reading should never be substituted for an immediate reading because reactions due to IgG coating may become weaker after incubation.

4. Add one drop of IgG-coated rbcs to any tests that are nonreactive. If monospecific anticomplement reagents are used, complement-coated rbcs should be substituted for IgG-coated rbcs. Centrifuge, examine the rbcs for agglutination and grade and record the results. If the rbcs were not adequately washed, residual unbound globulins from the original serum will neutralize AHG reagents. This important test is the only way to monitor the efficacy of the washing process and demonstrate that reactive AHG was added.

Interpretation

1. The DAT is positive when agglutination is observed either after immediate centrifugation or after centrifugation following room temperature incubation. Immediate reactions are seen with IgG-coated rbcs; complement coating may be more easily demonstrable after incubation.[1,2] This distinction cannot be used for reliable determination of immunoglobulin type. Monospecific AHG reagents are needed to confirm the types of globulins present.

2. The DAT is negative when no agglutination is observed at either test phase, providing the IgG-coated rbcs added in step 4 above are reactive. If the globulin-coated rbcs are not agglutinated, the negative DAT result is considered invalid and the test must be repeated. A negative DAT does not necessarily mean absence of coating globulins. Polyspecific and anti-IgG reagents detect approximately 200-500 molecules of IgG per rbc,[1] but autoimmune hemolytic anemia has been reported with IgG coating below this level.[2]

References

1. Mollison PL, Engelfriet CP, Contreras M, eds. Blood transfusion in clinical medicine. 9th ed. Oxford: Blackwell Scientific Publications, 1993.
2. Petz LD, Garratty G. Acquired immune hemolytic anemia. New York: Churchill-Livingstone, 1980.

Alloantibody Identification and Titration

Method 4.1. Calculating Probability Levels

Principle

Probability levels for antibody identification (see p 339-40) are calculated by constructing 2 × 2 tables in which the presence and absence of serum reactivity are correlated with the presence and absence of a particular antigen among the red cell samples tested.

Procedure

A 2 × 2 table is constructed as follows:

Serum Reactions	Red Cells		Total
	Antigen Present	Antigen Absent	
Positive	A	B	A + B
Negative	C	D	C + D
Total	A + C	B + D	N

A = number of positive reactions observed with antigen-positive rbc samples

B = number of positive reactions observed with antigen-negative rbc samples

C = number of negative reactions observed with antigen-positive rbc samples

D = number of negative reactions observed with antigen-negative rbc samples

N = total number of rbc samples tested

The formula for calculating probability (p) from a 2 × 2 table is as follows:

$$\frac{(A+B)! \times (C+D)! \times (A+C)! \times (B+D)!}{N! \times A! \times B! \times C! \times D!}$$

Note: ! = the symbol for factorial, the product of all the whole numbers from 1 to the number involved. For example:

$6! = 6 \times 5 \times 4 \times 3 \times 2 \times 1 = 720$
$3! = 3 \times 2 \times 1 = 6$
$1! = 1$
$0! = 1$

Interpretation (examples)

Clearly Defined Results

For a serum reactive with three E+ rbc samples and nonreactive with three E− samples, the 2 × 2 table is:

Serum Reactions	Red Cells		Total
	E+	E−	
Positive	3	0	3
Negative	0	3	3
Total	3	3	6

$$p = \frac{3! \times 3! \times 3! \times 3!}{6! \times 3! \times 0! \times 0! \times 3!} = \frac{36}{720} = \frac{1}{20} = 0.050$$

This means there is a 1 in 20 likelihood that an antibody other than anti-E could, by chance, have given the observed reactions. This level of probability is the minimum acceptable for statistical significance. Testing the serum against 10 rbc samples, six E– and four E+, dramatically improves the probability level of anti-E.

Serum Reactions	Red Cells		Total
	E +	E –	
Positive	4	0	4
Negative	0	6	6
Total	4	6	10

$$p = \frac{4! \times 6! \times 4! \times 6!}{10! \times 4! \times 0! \times 0! \times 6!} = \frac{1}{210} = 0.005$$

Ambiguous Results

This formula is also useful in determining the significance of discrepant results. For example, a reagent rbc panel has eight e+ samples and two e– samples, and a serum reacts with only seven of the e+ samples:

Serum Reactions	Red Cells		Total
	e +	e –	
Positive	7	0	7
Negative	1	2	3
Total	8	2	10

$$p = \frac{7! \times 3! \times 8! \times 2!}{10! \times 7! \times 0! \times 1! \times 2!} = \frac{1}{15} = 0.067$$

These results indicate that a serum that does not contain anti-e would, by chance, give these reactions once in 15 trials; this is an unacceptable level for identification. To confirm the presence of anti-e, tests with additional rbc samples are required. The final probability level obtained may be influenced by the phenotypes of the additional rbc samples used. For example, if two additional e+ samples were tested and found to be reactive, the probability level is improved only modestly:

Serum Reactions	Red Cells		Total
	e +	e –	
Positive	9	0	9
Negative	1	2	3
Total	10	2	12

$$p = \frac{9! \times 3! \times 10! \times 2!}{12! \times 9! \times 0! \times 1! \times 2!} = \frac{1}{22} = 0.045$$

A more convincing p value could be obtained by testing an additional e+ and another e– sample, if the reactions were as anticipated:

Serum Reactions	Red Cells		Total
	e +	e –	
Positive	8	0	8
Negative	1	3	4
Total	9	3	12

$$p = \frac{8! \times 4! \times 9! \times 3!}{12! \times 8! \times 0! \times 1! \times 3!} = \frac{1}{55} = 0.018$$

The probability level could be improved still further by using two additional e– samples and finding both nonreactive:

Serum Reactions	Red Cells		Total
	e +	e –	
Positive	7	0	7
Negative	1	4	5
Total	8	4	12

$$p = \frac{7! \times 5! \times 8! \times 4!}{12! \times 7! \times 0! \times 1! \times 4!} = \frac{1}{99} = 0.010$$

Recommended Reading

1. Moore BPL. Serological and immunological methods of the Canadian Red Cross Blood Transfusion Service. 8th ed. Toronto: The Canadian Red Cross Society, 1980:200-2.
2. Race RR, Sanger R. Blood groups in man. 6th ed. Oxford: Blackwell Scientific Publications, 1975:480-1.

Method 4.2. Using the AABB Rare Donor File

Principle

The AABB Rare Donor File helps locate blood for patients requiring rare or unusual blood. The File has inventories of all AABB-accredited Immunohematology Reference Laboratories. The File maintains information regarding those donors and units representing either high-incidence antigen-negative or multiple antigen-negative phenotypes of rare (<1 in 5000) or uncommon (<1 in 1000) frequencies.

All requests for assistance from the File are to be made by an AABB-accredited Immunohematology Reference Laboratory. Fees have not been established for services provided through the File. All charges are established by the shipping institution.

Procedure

1. A hospital blood bank or transfusion service discovers a need for rare blood.
2. The request is referred to the nearest AABB-accredited Immunohematology Reference Laboratory. See the listing in the front of the AABB *Membership Directory* or contact the AABB National Office.
3. The AABB reference laboratory will supply blood if available. The AABB reference laboratory may request a sample to verify antibody identification.
4. If the local reference laboratory cannot supply blood, *that reference laboratory* contacts AABB Rare Donor File. To prevent confusion, *all* requests to the AABB Rare Donor File *must* be made by the local AABB-accredited reference laboratory (or another rare donor file). Requests that are received directly from a hospital or transfusion service are referred to an AABB-accredited Immunohematology Reference Laboratory located near the requesting hospital or transfusion service.
5. AABB Rare Donor File personnel search records for AABB reference laboratories that may be able to supply appropriate units. In the event that no suitable blood is available in the AABB Rare Donor File, other rare donor files will be contacted (American Red Cross, World Health Organization, etc). The requesting AABB-accredited reference laboratory will be notified of potential suppliers.
6. The requesting reference laboratory contacts potential suppliers regarding availability of units and coordinates contact with the potential supplier. It is the prerogative of the supplying institution to request a patient's sample, if deemed necessary. It is strongly recommended that charges be discussed and that the hospital or transfusion service be notified of all costs *before* units are shipped.
7. The institution supplying the rare blood completes and mails a postcard to the AABB Rare Donor File indicating that rare units have been shipped so that inventory records can be adjusted.

Method 4.3. Antibody Titration

Principle

Titration is a semiquantitative method of determining the antibody content (titer) of a given serum sample, or it may be used to compare the antigen expression (dosage) of different rbc samples. The primary applications of titration studies are: 1) determining antibody levels in alloimmunized pregnancies when the results will be used to decide when to monitor the fetus for hemolytic disease of the newborn by other methods such as amniocentesis (see Chapter 18); 2) in the elucidation of autoantibody specificity (see Chapter 16); 3) in the recognition of antibodies with high-titer, low-avidity reaction characteristics (see Chapter 12); and 4) studying the effect of thiol reagents on antibodies to determine their immunoglobulin class (IgG or IgM).

Materials

1. Transfer pipets to deliver 50 μL, 100 μL and 0.2-1.0 mL.
2. Serum (antibody) to be titrated.
3. Rbcs that carry the antigen(s) to which the serum contains antibody(ies). Prepare rbcs in saline; uniform suspensions (eg, 4%) of each rbc sample should be prepared.

Procedure

The master dilution technique for titration studies is as follows:

1. Label 10 test tubes according to the serum dilution (eg, 1 in 1, 1 in 2, etc). A 1 in 1 dilution means one volume of serum undiluted; a 1 in 2 dilution means one volume of serum in a final volume of two, or a 50% solution of serum in the diluent. See Methods 1.4 and 1.5.
2. Deliver one volume of saline to all test tubes except the first tube (1 in 1).
3. Add an equal volume of serum to each of the first two tubes (1 in 1, 1 in 2).
4. Using a clean pipet, mix the contents of the 1 in 2 dilution several times, and transfer one volume into the next tube (1 in 4 dilution).
5. Continue the same process for all dilutions, using a clean pipet for each transfer of diluted serum. Remove one volume of diluted serum from the final tube, and save for use if further dilutions are required.

6. Using separate pipets for each dilution, transfer 100 μL of diluted serum into appropriately labeled test tubes. For each dilution to be tested, add 50 μL of the appropriate reagent rbc sample.
7. Mix well, and test by the appropriate technique.
8. Examine test results macroscopically, and grade and record the reactions. Since the prozone phenomenon (see p 165) may cause the reactions to be weaker with low serum dilutions than with the higher dilutions, it may be preferable to begin reading the tube containing the most dilute serum, and proceed to the most concentrated sample.

Interpretation

1. Report the results as the reciprocal of the highest dilution that produces 1+ macroscopic agglutination. A titer is reported as 32, not 1 in 32 (see Table 4.3-1 for an example). If there is agglutination in the tube containing the most dilute serum, the titration endpoint has not been reached, and it is necessary to prepare and test additional dilutions.
2. In comparative studies, a difference in titer of at least three dilutions can be considered a significant difference.
3. Variations in technique, and inherent variability can cause results of duplicate tests to differ by as much as plus or minus one dilution.
4. Titer values alone can be misleading. Titration results can also be expressed by assigning a number to each reaction based on the observed strength of agglutination. The sum of these values represents the score, which is another semiquantitative measurement of antibody reactivity. A difference of 10 or more between different test samples has arbitrarily

Table 4.3-1. Examples of Antibody Titers, Endpoints and Scores

		Reciprocal of Serum Dilution										
		1	2	4	8	16	32	64	128	256	512	Titer*	Score
Sample 1	Strength:	3+	3+	3+	2+	2+	2+	1+	±	±	0	64(256)	
	Score:	10	10	10	8	8	8	5	3	2	0		64
Sample 2	Strength:	4+	4+	4+	3+	3+	2+	2+	1+	±	0	128(256)	
	Score:	12	12	12	10	10	8	8	5	3	0		80
Sample 3	Strength:	1+	1+	1+	1+	±	±	±	±	±	0	8(256)	
	Score:	5	5	5	5	3	3	3	2	2	0		33

*In prenatal testing, or for reagent evaluation, the titer is usually determined from the highest dilution of serum that gives a reaction ≥1 + (score 5). This may differ significantly from the titration endpoint (shown in parentheses), as with the reactions of an HTLA antibody with high-titer, low-avidity characteristics, manifested by Sample #3.

been deemed significant. In many laboratories, a scoring system similar to that described in Method 1.9 is used.

5. Table 4.3-1 shows the results of titration studies on three sera, each with an endpoint of 256. The differences in score values, however, indicate that the sera vary in their strength of reactivity. The results with sample 3 are characteristic of antibodies with high-titer, yet low-avidity characteristics (eg, endpoint as high as 256, score only 33).

Notes

Titration is a semiquantitative technique. Technical variables can greatly influence the results. For reliable results, the following technical variables must be kept to a minimum.

1. A careful pipetting technique is essential. Eppendorf or similar pipets with disposable tips that can be changed after each dilution are recommended.

2. Optimal incubation time, incubation temperature and centrifugation times must be used consistently.

3. The age, phenotype and concentration of the test rbcs may affect the results. When the titers of several different examples of an antibody are to be compared, all sera should be tested against rbcs (preferably freshly collected) from the same donor. If this is not possible, the sera should be tested against a pool of reagent rbcs from donors of the same phenotype. When a single serum is to be tested against different rbc samples, the samples should be collected and preserved in the same manner, and diluted to the same concentration before use.

4. Completely reproducible results are virtually impossible to achieve. Comparisons are valid only when specimens are tested concurrently. In prenatal testing, when sequential serum samples are tested for changing antibody titer, samples should be frozen for comparison with subsequent specimens. Each new sample should be tested in parallel with the imme-

diately preceding sample. In tests with a single serum against different reagent rbc samples, the same specimen of diluted serum must be used for all tests.

5. Measurements are more accurate with large volumes than with small volumes, and a master dilution technique (see below) gives more reliable results than individual dilutions for a single set of tests. If serum dilutions are to be tested against several reagent rbc samples, a sufficient volume of each dilution must be prepared to permit the same dilution to be tested against each test rbc sample.

Method 4.4. Use of Thiol (Sulfhydryl) Reagents To Distinguish IgM From IgG Antibodies

Principle

IgM immunoglobulin molecules consist of five radially arranged subunits linked by disulfide bonds called intersubunit bonds. Each subunit consists of two μ heavy chains and two κ or λ light chains, which are linked by disulfide bonds known as interchain bonds. Thiol reagents can cleave disulfide bonds; intersubunit bonds are cleaved far more readily than interchain bonds. The interchain bonds of IgG and IgA monomers, which have a structure similar to that of IgM subunits, are not readily cleaved by thiol reagents.

Treating IgM antibodies with thiol reagents abolishes both agglutinating and complement-binding activities. Thiol treatment is useful in determining the immunoglobulin class of antibodies known to be present in a serum. It can also be used to abolish activity of IgM antibodies to permit detection of coexisting IgG antibodies.

Reagents

1. PBS at pH 8.0.
2. Dithiothreitol (DTT), prepared by dissolving 0.154 g of DTT in 100 mL of pH 8.0 PBS. Store at 2-6 C.
3. 2 mL of serum to be treated.

Procedure

1. Dispense 1 mL of serum into each of two test tubes.
2. To one tube, labeled control, add 1 mL of pH 8.0 PBS.
3. To the other tube, labeled test, add 1 mL of 0.01 M DTT.
4. Mix and incubate at 37 C for 30 minutes to 1 hour.
5. Test the antibody activity in each sample by titration.

Interpretation

See Table 4.4-1.

Table 4.4-1. Effect of Dithiothreitol on Blood Group Antibodies

	Dilution					
Test Sample	1/2	1/4	1/8	1/16	1/32	Interpretation
Serum + DTT	3+	2+	2+	1+	0	IgG
Serum + PBS	3+	2+	2+	1+	0	
Serum + DTT	0	0	0	0	0	IgM
Serum + PBS	3+	2+	2+	1+	0	
Serum + DTT	2+	1+	0	0	0	IgG + IgM*
Serum + PBS	3+	2+	2+	1+	0	

*May also indicate only partial inactivation of IgM.

Notes

1. 2-mercaptoethanol can also be used for this purpose.
2. Thiol reagents used at low concentration may weaken certain antigens within the Kell system.
3. Alkylation using iodoacetic acid, followed by dialysis, may be necessary when investigating antibodies in the Kell system.
4. Gelling of a serum or plasma sample may be observed during treatment with DTT. This can occur if 0.01 M DTT solutions are prepared incorrectly, and are actually of concentrations above 0.01 M. Alternatively, gelling may occur on extended serum incubation in the presence of DTT. Samples undergoing treatment can be inspected after 30 minutes and again after 60 minutes of treatment to determine if gelling has occurred. Gelled samples cannot be tested for antibody activity since overtreatment with DTT has led to the denaturation of all serum proteins.
5. Test an aliquot of DTT-treated serum/plasma after 30 minutes of treatment. If tests with the aliquot indicate that suspected IgM antibody activity has been destroyed, there is no need to incubate further.

Reference

Mollison PL, Engelfriet CP, Contreras M, eds. Blood transfusion in clinical medicine, 9th ed. Oxford: Blackwell Scientific Publications, 1993.

Method 4.5. Demonstration of Antibodies Reacting With High-Titer, Low-Avidity (HTLA) Characteristics

Principle

Some antibodies are known to react to a high titer, yet with low avidity (HTLA). They react at high dilutions in antiglobulin tests but the reactions are not strong (2+ or less, even with undiluted serum). In contrast, other undiluted alloantibodies (such as anti-D, anti-Fy^a and anti-K) that react 2+ or less in antiglobulin tests usually have titers less than 8.

Antibodies of this group include anti-Kn^a, -McC^a, -Cs^a, -Yk^a, -Ch, -Rg and -JMH. Occasional examples of anti-Hy and antibodies to Lutheran system antigens may also display HTLA characteristics, as do antibodies to leukocyte antigens such as Bg^a.

Reagents

1. Reactive rbc samples, selected from previously tested samples. More than one sample may be selected based on the strength of observed reactions (eg, 2+, 1+ and ±); however, some antibodies with HTLA characteristics react consistently with all rbcs tested, and only one test sample need be used.
2. Serum under investigation.
3. Anti-IgG.

Procedure

1. Prepare serial two-fold dilutions of test serum in saline. The dilution range should be from 1 in 2 to at least 1 in 512 (9 tubes), and the volumes prepared should be not less than 0.6 mL.
2. Place two drops of each dilution into each labeled 10 or 12 × 75-mm test tube. (Three drops of dilute serum may be used, if preferred.)
3. Add one drop of a 2-5% suspension of rbcs to each labeled dilution (or series of dilutions).
4. Mix the contents of each tube and incubate at 37 C for 30-60 minutes.
5. Wash the rbcs four times in saline and test with AHG reagent.
6. Examine the rbcs for agglutination; confirm all nonreactive tests micro-

scopically. Grade and record the results.

Interpretation

1. Sera that continue to react at four dilutions beyond the first tube that gives a 1+ reaction can be considered to contain an antibody with high-titer, low-avidity characteristics.
2. Rbcs that react at varying strengths with undiluted serum should be tested to determine whether dilution exerts the same effect on all reactions. If some rbcs react only or preferentially with low serum dilutions, the serum may also contain non-HTLA antibodies such as anti-E or anti-K.

Method 4.6. Rapid Identification of Anti-Ch and -Rg

Principle

Anti-Ch and anti-Rg are directed toward the C4d fragment of human complement. These antibodies usually react only weakly in antiglobulin tests with the trace amount of C4d present on normal rbcs. However, they may cause direct agglutination of rbcs coated in vitro with excess C4d. Such rbcs are prepared by incubation of Ch+, Rg+ plasma in a low-ionic medium containing EDTA. Under these conditions, C4b is bound non-immunologically to rbcs. The bound C4b can be converted to C4d by trypsin.

Reagents

1. Anti-IgG: need not be heavy-chain-specific.
2. Phosphate buffer: 0.1 M at pH 7.7 (see Method 1.6); KH_2PO_4 (13.6 g/L), 10 mL; Na_2HPO_4 (14.2 g/L), 90 mL.
3. Trypsin—1% w/v: trypsin, 1:250 (Difco Laboratories, Detroit, MI), 1 g; 0.05 N

HCl, 100 mL; agitate at room temperature for 15 minutes; leave overnight at 4 C; store at 4 C. Centrifuge to remove insoluble materials before use.
4. Sucrose/EDTA: sucrose, 10 g; K_3EDTA, 0.15 g; distilled water to 100 mL.
5. Whole blood: group O, D–, from a known Ch+ or Rg+ individual; collected within the previous 7 days and anticoagulated with ACD, CPD or CPDA-1.

Procedure

Preparation of C4d-Coated Rbcs

1. Mix 1 mL of WB with 10 mL of sucrose/EDTA.
2. Incubate at 37 C for 15 minutes.
3. Wash the rbcs three times with saline; the rbcs are now coated with C4b.
4. Dilute one part of trypsin with nine parts of pH 7.7 phosphate buffer.
5. Mix 0.1 mL of C4b-coated rbcs with 0.1 mL of dilute trypsin.
6. Similarly, prepare non-C4d-coated control rbcs by trypsin-treating an aliquot of washed rbcs from the WB sample (without exposure to sucrose/EDTA).
7. Incubate test and control cells at 37 C for 30 minutes.
8. Wash rbcs three times with saline.
9. Resuspend to a 5% concentration with Alsever's solution (see Method 1.8); store at 4 C.

Testing for Anti-Ch/Anti-Rg

1. Mix two drops of test serum with one drop of C4d-coated rbcs.
2. Similarly, test the non-C4-coated trypsin-treated (control) rbcs.
3. Incubate at room temperature for 5 minutes.
4. Centrifuge at $1000 \times g$ for 15 seconds.
5. Examine the rbcs macroscopically; grade and record the results.

6. Wash the rbcs four times with saline; completely decant the final wash supernatant.
7. To the dry rbc buttons, add anti-IgG according to the manufacturer's directions.
8. Centrifuge at $1000 \times g$ for 15 seconds.
9. Examine the rbcs macroscopically; grade and record the results.

Interpretation

1. Agglutination of C4d-coated rbcs, but not trypsin-treated control rbcs, is indicative of either anti-Ch or anti-Rg.
2. Equal agglutination of both C4d-coated and control rbcs is an invalid test result, due either to the presence of trypsin-dependent panagglutinins or an alloantibody unrelated to anti-Ch or -Rg.
3. With anti-IgG (step 9), there may be weak reactivity with trypsin-treated control rbcs; if the C4d-coated rbcs are strongly reactive and the control rbcs are weakly reactive, this is also indicative of anti-Ch or anti-Rg.

Notes

1. There is no need to incubate tests at 37 C before testing with anti-IgG.
2. The exact amount of K_3EDTA required for preparing 10 mL of sucrose-EDTA is present in a 16×100-mm (10 mL) Vacutainer® tube (B2991-54, from American Scientific Products, McGaw Park, IL).

References

1. Judd WJ, Kraemer K, Moulds JJ. Rapid identification of Chido and Rodgers antibodies using C4d-coated red cells. Transfusion 1981;21:189-92.
2. Judd WJ. Methods in immunohematology. Miami: Montgomery Scientific Publications, 1989.

Method 4.7. Plasma Inhibition To Distinguish Anti-Ch and -Rg From Other Antibodies With HTLA Characteristics

Principle

Anti-Ch and anti-Rg antibodies, directed against the fourth component of human complement (C4), are inhibited by incubation with plasma containing C4 from Ch+, Rg+ individuals. Demonstrating inhibition may help in differentiating anti-Ch and anti-Rg from other antibodies with HTLA characteristics.

Reagents

1. Reactive rbc samples, similar to those used to demonstrate HTLA antibodies (see Method 4.5).
2. A pool of six or more normal plasma samples.
3. Serum under investigation.
4. 6% bovine albumin, prepared from stock 22% or 30% bovine albumin by dilution with saline.
5. Anti-IgG.

Procedure

1. Prepare serial two-fold dilutions of test serum in saline. The dilution range should be from 1 in 2 to 1 in 512, or to one tube beyond the known titer as determined above. The volume prepared should be not less than 0.3 mL for each red cell sample to be tested.
2. For each rbc sample to be tested, place two drops of each serum dilution into each of two appropriately labeled 10 or 12×75-mm test tubes.
3. To one tube add two drops of pooled plasma.
4. To the other tube add two drops of 6% albumin.
5. Gently agitate the contents of each tube and incubate at room temperature for at least 30 minutes.

6. Add one drop of a 2-5% suspension of rbcs to each tube.
7. Gently agitate the contents of each tube and incubate at 37 C for 1 hour.
8. Wash the rbcs four times in saline and test with AHG reagent.
9. Examine the rbcs for agglutination; confirm all nonreactive tests microscopically. Grade and record the results.

Notes

1. Diluted bovine albumin is used as the negative control because it provides a protein concentration in the incubated serum similar to that in the tube containing serum and pooled plasma.
2. Inhibition of antibody activity by plasma suggests anti-Ch or anti-Rg specificity. This inhibition is often complete. The presence of partial inhibition may suggest the presence of additional alloantibodies. In such situations, a large volume of inhibited serum can be tested against a reagent red cell panel to see if the nonneutralizable antibodies display specificity.
3. Antibodies to white cell antigens (eg, anti-Bg^a) may also be subject to partial inhibition by plasma.
4. Alternatively, adsorption of anti-Ch/-Rg may be preferred. See reference.

Reference

Ellisor SS, Shoemaker MM, Reid ME. Adsorption of anti-Chido from serum using autologous red blood cells coated with homologous C4. Transfusion 1982;22:243-5.

Method 4.8. Dithiothreitol (DTT) Treatment of Red Cells

Principle

DTT is one of the most efficient reducing agents known.[1] It can irreversibly reduce protein disulfide bonds to free sulfhydryl groups, resulting in the disruption of protein tertiary structure. Without tertiary structure, protein-containing antigens can no longer bind with specific antibodies and serologic reactivity is abolished.

Rbcs treated with DTT will not react with antibodies in the Kell blood group system, nor with most examples of anti-LW, -Yt^a, -Yt^b, -Do^a, -Do^b and most antibodies with HTLA characteristics.[2] This technique may be helpful in identifying some of these antibodies, or used to determine if additional underlying alloantibodies are present.

Reagents

1. 0.2 M DTT at pH 8.0.
2. PBS at pH 7.3, see Method 1.6.

Procedure

1. Wash one volume of rbcs with PBS. After decanting, add four volumes of 0.2 M DTT, pH 8.0. Also treat a k+ rbc sample as a control.
2. Incubate at 37 C for 30-45 minutes.
3. Wash four times with PBS. Slight hemolysis may occur. If excessive, use fresh rbcs and decrease the concentration of DTT.
4. Resuspend rbcs to a 3-5% suspension in PBS.
5. Test DTT-treated rbcs with the appropriate sera. Test k+ rbcs with anti-k.

Interpretation

1. The control k+ rbcs should give negative reactions when tested with anti-k. If not, the rbcs have not been treated adequately. Other Kell antigens can also serve as the control.
2. If the test serum reactivity is eliminated, the suspected antibody reactivity has been abolished. Test enough

rbcs to exclude most other clinically significant alloantibodies.

Note

Treatment of rbcs with 0.2 M DTT, pH 8.0 is optimal for denaturation of all antigens of the Kell, Cartwright, LW and Dombrock systems, and most HTLA antigens. Lower concentrations of DTT may selectively denature particular blood group antigens (ie, 0.002 M DTT will only denature Js^a and Js^b antigens). This property may aid in certain antibody investigations.

References

1. Cleland WW. Dithiothreitol, a new protective reagent for SH groups. Biochem 1964;3:480-2.
2. Branch DR, Muensch HA, Sy Siok Hian S, Petz LD. Disulfide bonds are a requirement for Kell and Cartwright (Yt^a) blood group antigen integrity. Br J Haematol 1983;54:573-8.

Method 4.9. Urine Neutralization of Anti-Sd^a

Principle

Sd^a substance is present in large amounts in the urine of Sd(a+) individuals. It is useful in the neutralization of suspected anti-Sd^a, the presence of which may mask concomitant nonneutralizable blood group antibodies.

Specimen

Urine from an Sd(a+) individual.

Reagents

1. PBS, pH 7.3. See Method 1.6.
2. Dialysis membrane.
3. Heating apparatus.
4. Polyspecific antihuman globulin.

Procedure

Preparation of Stock Urine

1. Collect urine. Immediately boil for 10 minutes.
2. Dialyze in PBS, pH 7.3 at 4 C for 48 hours. Change PBS several times.
3. Centrifuge.
4. Dispense supernatant into aliquots.
5. Store at –20 C. Thaw as needed.

Test for Neutralization

1. Mix equal volumes of thawed urine and test serum. (0.2-mL volumes are required to test three rbc samples.)
2. Prepare a control tube containing equal volumes of serum and PBS.
3. Prepare a negative urine control by mixing equal volumes of thawed urine and PBS.
4. Incubate all tubes at room temperature for 30 minutes.
5. Mix one drop of each test rbc sample with two or three drops of neutralized serum.
6. Mix one drop of each test rbc sample with two or three drops of control serum.
7. Mix one drop of each test rbc sample with two or three drops of distilled urine.
8. Incubate all tubes for 20-30 minutes at 22 ± 2 C.
9. Wash three times.
10. Add polyspecific antiglobulin reagent.
11. Centrifuge, read and record results. It may be helpful to examine microscopically.

Interpretation

1. Persistent agglutination in the test samples means either that partial or no neutralization was achieved or that underlying antibodies were detected. The microscopic examination may be helpful in distinguishing these outcomes. Reactions due to anti-Sd^a

often have a refractile mixed-field appearance under the microscope.

2. No agglutination in the tests with persistent agglutination in the control tubes means that the antibody has been neutralized.

3. No agglutination in the control tubes means that the dilution in the neutralization step was too great for the antibody present. The results of the test are invalid.

Note

Urine may also contain ABO and Lewis blood group substances according to the ABO, Lewis and secretor status of the donor.

Reference

Judd WJ. Methods in immunohematology. Miami: Montgomery Scientific Publications, 1988.

Elution

Method 5.1. Chloroform Elution

Principle

The objective of all elution techniques is to interfere with the noncovalent binding forces that hold antibody-antigen complexes together on the rbc surface. Physical disruption of the rbc membrane using heat, ultrasound, freeze-thawing, detergents or organic solvents, or direct chemical interference of the binding forces of antigen-antibody complexes using alterations in pH or salt concentration have all been used.

The reader should refer to Chapter 21 for the proper handling of hazardous chemicals.

The chloroform elution method is suitable for the investigation of a positive DAT associated with warm-reactive (IgG) auto- or alloantibodies and, in conjunction with adsorption techniques, the separation of mixtures of IgG rbc antibodies.

Reagents

1. Spectrophometric grade chloroform (the chloroform used must be of very high grade).
2. 6% bovine albumin, prepared by diluting 22% or 30% bovine albumin with saline.
3. Packed rbcs, washed six times in saline.
4. Supernatant saline from final wash.

Procedure

1. Prepare a 50% suspension of well washed rbcs in saline or LISS in a 13 × 100-mm test tube. Use 6% bovine albumin as diluent for increased stability of eluted antibody if it is to be frozen.
2. Add an equal volume of chloroform.
3. Stopper the tube with a cork, and shake the tube vigorously for 10-15 seconds. Mix further by inversion for approximately 1 minute.
4. Carefully remove the cork, and place the tube in a 56 C waterbath for exactly 5 minutes **(Do not exceed 5 minutes at 56 C.)** Vigorously stir the contents of the tube with an applicator stick periodically during this time.
5. Centrifuge the tube at 900-1000 × g for 4-5 minutes.
6. Transfer the supernatant eluate into a clean test tube, and test in parallel with the supernatant saline from the final wash.

Note

The use of LISS as the elution diluent and LISS-suspended reagent rbcs in the detection system can greatly facilitate the detection of eluted antibody.

Reference

Branch DR, Sy Siok Hian AL, Petz LD. A new elution procedure using chloroform, a nonflammable organic solvent. Vox Sang 1982;42:46-53.

Method 5.2. Citric Acid Elution

Principle

See Method 5.1.

Reagents

1. Eluting solution: citric acid (monohydrate), 1.3 g; KH_2PO_4, 0.65 g; saline to 100 mL; store at 4 C.
2. Neutralizing solution: Na_3PO_4, 13.0 g: distilled water to 100 mL; store at 4 C.
3. Packed rbcs, washed six times in saline.
4. Supernatant saline from final wash.

Procedure

1. Chill all reagents to 4 C before use (use an ice bath).
2. Place 1 mL of packed rbcs in a 13 × 100-mm test tube.
3. Add 1 mL of eluting solution and note the time.
4. Stopper the tube and mix by inversion for exactly 90 seconds.
5. Remove stopper and promptly centrifuge the tube at 900-1000 × g for exactly 45 seconds.
6. Transfer supernatant fluid to a clean test tube and add 5-6 drops of neutralizing solution; save rbcs for adsorption studies if needed.
7. Check pH; adjust, if necessary, to pH 7.0 by adding more neutralizing solution.
8. Centrifuge at 900-1000 × g for 2-3 minutes to remove precipitate that forms after neutralization; harvest the supernatant eluate and test in parallel with the supernatant saline from the final wash.

Notes

1. Except for Kell system antigens, rbcs obtained in step 6 above may be used in tests to determine phenotype if the DAT is negative; Kell system antigen expression is markedly weakened after citric acid treatment.
2. Citric acid-modified rbcs may also be protease-treated and used in autologous adsorption studies.

Reference

Burich MA, AuBuchon JP, Anderson HJ. Antibody elution using citric acid (letter). Transfusion 1986;26:116-7.

Method 5.3. Cold-Acid Elution

Principle

See Method 5.1.

Reagents

1. Glycine-HCl (0.1 M, pH 3.0), prepared by dissolving 3.75 g of glycine and 2.992 g of sodium chloride in 500 mL of distilled water. Adjust pH to 3.0 with 12 N HCl. Store at 4 C.
2. Phosphate buffer (0.8 M, pH 8.2), prepared by dissolving 109.6 g of Na_2HPO_4 and 3.8 g of KH_2PO_4 in approximately 600 mL of distilled water. Adjust pH, if necessary, with either 1N NaOH or 1N HCl. Dilute to a final volume of 1 L with distilled water. Store at 4 C (see note 2).
3. Isotonic saline, at 4 C.
4. Packed rbcs, washed six times in saline.
5. Supernatant saline from final wash.

Procedure

1. In a 13 × 100-mm test tube, chill the rbcs in an ice bath for 5 minutes before adding the glycine-HCl.
2. Add 1 mL of chilled saline and 2 mL of chilled glycine-HCl to 1 mL of washed rbcs.
3. Mix and incubate the tube in an ice bath for 1 minute.

4. Quickly centrifuge the tube at 900-1000 × *g* for 2-3 minutes.
5. Transfer the supernatant eluate into a clean test tube, and add 0.1 mL of pH 8.2 phosphate buffer for each 1 mL of eluate (see note 3).
6. Mix and centrifuge at 900-1000 × *g* for 2-3 minutes.
7. Transfer the supernatant eluate into a clean test tube, and test in parallel with the supernatant saline from the final wash.

Notes

1. Keep glycine in an ice bath during use, to maintain correct pH.
2. Phosphate buffer will crystallize during storage at 4 C. Redissolve at 37 C before use.
3. Addition of phosphate buffer restores neutrality to the acidic eluate. Some persistence of acidity may result in hemolysis of reagent rbcs. The addition of 22% bovine albumin (one part to four parts of eluate) may reduce such hemolysis.

References

1. Rekvig OP, Hannestad K. Acid elution of blood group antibodies from intact erythrocytes. Vox Sang 1977;33:280-5.
2. Judd WJ. Methods in immunohematology. Miami: Montgomery Scientific Publications, 1988.

Method 5.4.
Glycine-HCl/EDTA Elution

Principle

See Method 5.1.

Reagents

1. Disodium EDTA - 10% w/v: Na$_2$EDTA •2H$_2$O, 10 g; distilled water to 100 mL.

2. Glycine-HCl - 0.1 M at pH 1.5: glycine 3.754 g; NaCl, 2.922 g; distilled water to 500 mL; adjust to pH 1.5 with 12 N HCl; store at 4 C.
3. TRIS Base - 1 M: TRIZMA® BASE (SIGMA Chemicals, St. Louis, MO), 12.1 g; distilled water to 100 mL.
4. Packed rbcs, washed six times in saline.
5. Supernatant saline from final wash.

Procedure

1. Mix 4 mL of glycine-HCl and 1 mL of EDTA in a 16 × 100-mm test tube.
2. Immediately add 1 mL of washed rbcs and mix well.
3. Incubate at room temperature for 1-2 minutes.
4. Centrifuge the tube at 900-1000 × *g* for 2-3 minutes.
5. Transfer the supernatant eluate into a clean test tube, and adjust to pH 7.5 with 1 M TRIS base.
6. Mix and centrifuge at 900-1000 × *g* for 2-3 minutes.
7. Transfer the supernatant eluate into a clean test tube, and test in parallel with the supernatant saline from the final wash.

Notes

1. Except for Kell system antigens, rbcs obtained in step 5 above may be used in tests to determine phenotype if the DAT is negative. Kell system antigens are denatured after glycine-HCl/EDTA treatment.
2. Glycine-HCl/EDTA-modified rbcs may also be protease-treated and used in autologous adsorption studies.

Reference

Byrne PC. Use of a modified acid/EDTA elution technique. Immunohematology 1991;7:46-7.

Method 5.5. Heat Elution

Principle

See Method 5.1. This procedure is best suited for the investigation of ABO hemolytic disease of the newborn, and the elution of IgM antibodies from rbcs. It should not be routinely used for the investigation of immune rbc destruction by IgG auto- or alloantibodies.

Reagents

1. 6% bovine albumin, prepared by diluting 22% or 30% bovine albumin with saline.
2. Packed rbcs, washed six times in saline.
3. Supernatant saline from final wash.

Procedure

1. Mix equal volumes of washed packed rbcs and 6% bovine albumin in a 13 × 100-mm test tube.
2. Place the tube at 56 C for 10 minutes. Agitate the tube periodically during this time.
3. Centrifuge the tube at 900-1000 ×g for 2-3 minutes, preferably in a heated centrifuge.
4. Immediately transfer the supernatant eluate into a clean test tube, and test in parallel with the supernatant saline from the final wash.

Reference

Landsteiner K, Miller CP. Serological studies on the blood of primates. II. The blood groups in anthropoid apes. J Exp Med 1925;42:853-62.

Method 5.6. Xylene Elution

Principle

See Method 5.1.

Reagents

1. Reagent grade xylene.
2. Packed rbcs, washed six times in saline.
3. Supernatant saline from final wash.

Procedure

1. Mix equal volumes of rbcs, normal saline and xylene in a 13 × 100-mm test tube.
2. Stopper the tube with a cork, and agitate the tube vigorously for 1-2 minutes. Remove the cork.
3. Place the tube at 56 C for 10-15 minutes. Stir the contents of the tube with applicator sticks during this time.
4. Centrifuge the tube at 900-1000 × g for at least 10 minutes.
5. Carefully remove and discard the upper layer of xylene and the stroma by vacuum aspiration (see note below).
6. Transfer the eluate into a clean test tube, and test in parallel with the supernatant saline from the final wash.
7. Add 30% albumin (two drops) to the test system to prevent rbc lysis by residual xylene.

Note

Care should be taken not to contaminate the eluate with stroma. Do not use a Pasteur pipet during step 5. If contamination does occur, recentrifuge the eluate at 900-1000 × g for at least 10 minutes.

References

1. Chan-Shu SA, Blair O. A new method of antibody elution from red blood cells. Transfusion 1979;19:182-5.
2. Bueno R, Garratty G, Postaway N. Elution of antibody from red blood cells using xylene—a superior method. Transfusion 1981;21:157-62.
3. Garratty G, O'Neill P, Smith R. Overcoming lysis of test cells following xylene elution (letter). Transfusion 1986;26:487.

Immune Hemolysis, Autoantibodies and Drugs

Method 6.1. Cold Autoadsorption

Principle

Potent cold-reactive autoantibodies may mask the presence of concomitant clinically significant alloantibodies in a serum. Adsorbing the serum in the cold with autologous rbcs can remove autoantibody, permitting detection of underlying alloantibodies. Circulating autologous rbcs, however, are already coated with IgM autoantibody and complement. ZZAP reagent can remove both immunoglobulins and complement from coated rbcs. Thus, ZZAP-treatment of autologous rbcs will remove IgM and complement and uncover antigen sites, which are then capable of binding free autoantibody in the serum.

This method is used to detect clinically significant alloantibodies in the presence of cold-reactive autoantibodies.

Reagents

1. 1% cysteine-activated papain or 1% ficin (see Method 3.5.1).
2. PBS at pH 6.5 and pH 8.0 (see Method 1.6).
3. 0.2 M DTT prepared by dissolving 1 g of DTT in 32.4 mL of pH 8.0 PBS. Dispense into 3 mL aliquots and store at or below –20 C.
4. 2 mL of serum or plasma to be adsorbed.
5. 2 mL of packed autologous rbcs.

Procedure

1. Prepare ZZAP reagent by mixing 0.5 mL of 1% cysteine-activated papain with 2.5 mL of DTT and 2 mL of pH 6.5 PBS. Alternatively, use 1 mL of ficin, 2.5 mL of DTT and 1.5 mL of pH 6.5 PBS. Adjust the pH to 6.5.
2. Add 2 mL of ZZAP reagent to 2 mL of packed autologous rbcs.
3. Mix, and incubate at 37 C for 20-30 minutes.
4. Wash the rbcs three times in saline. Centrifuge the last wash for 3-5 minutes at 900-1000 $\times g$, and remove as much of the supernatant saline as possible (see note below).
5. To the tube of ZZAP-treated rbcs add 2 mL of the autologous serum.
6. Mix, and incubate at 4 C for 30-40 minutes.
7. Centrifuge at 900-1000 $\times g$ for 4-5 minutes, and transfer the serum into a clean tube.
8. Steps 2 through 7 may need to be repeated for a second autoadsorption.
9. Following the final adsorption, test the serum for alloantibody activity.

Note

To avoid dilution of the serum and possible loss of weak alloantibody activity during the adsorption process, it is important to remove as much of the residual saline as possible in step 4. Placing a narrow strip of filter paper into the packed rbcs helps remove saline that surrounds the rbcs.

Reference

Branch DR. Blood transfusion in autoimmune hemolytic anemias. Lab Med 1984;15:402-8.

Method 6.2. Demonstration of High-Titer Cold-Reactive Autoagglutinins

Principle

Serum is diluted serially in order to determine the strength of the cold-reactive autoagglutinin. The strength, expressed as titer, is of diagnostic usefulness.

Reagents

1. Serum or plasma to be tested; separate serum at 37 C from sample allowed to clot at 37 C; or plasma from an anticoagulated sample that is inverted several times at 37 C for approximately 15 minutes.
2. 1% saline suspension of washed group O, I+ rbcs; rbcs should be from a sample anticoagulated with ACD and CPD, collected within the preceding 7 days.
3. PBS at pH 7.3 (see Method 1.6).

Procedure

1. Dilute the serum or plasma 1 in 5 with saline.
2. Prepare serial two-fold dilutions of diluted serum or plasma in saline. Use 0.5 mL volumes when making these dilutions. The final dilution range should be from 1 in 10 to 1 in 20,480 (12 tubes).
3. Add to each tube 0.5 mL of a 1% saline suspension of freshly collected, washed group O, I+ rbcs.
4. Mix, and incubate overnight at 4 C.
5. Do not centrifuge the test mixtures. Examine the rbcs macroscopically for agglutination. Grade and record the results.

Interpretation

The reciprocal of the highest dilution of serum at which agglutination is observed is reported as the titer. With this technique, titers above 40 are considered elevated. However, hemolytic anemia due to cold-reactive autoagglutinins is not usually seen unless the titer is above 640. Titers below 640 may be obtained when the autoantibody has anti-i specificity. In this situation, I– (i_{cord} or i_{adult}) rbcs may be substituted for the I+ rbcs. Alternatively, Method 6.3, which follows, may be used to determine the titer.

Notes

1. It is important to use separate pipets for each tube when preparing serum dilutions. If a single pipet is used throughout, falsely high titration endpoints may be obtained due to serum carried from one tube to the next. The difference can be as great as an apparent titer of 100,000 using a single pipet, and a true titer of 4000 when separate pipets are used.
2. Serum dilutions can be prepared more accurately when large volumes (eg, 0.5 mL) are used.

Reference

Henry JB, ed. Clinical diagnosis and management by laboratory methods. 18th ed. Philadelphia: WB Saunders, 1991:667.

Method 6.3. Determining the Specificity of Cold-Reactive Autoagglutinins

Principle

Serologic specificity of cold-reactive autoagglutinins can be determined by testing the serum against target rbcs selected for antigens relevant to these antibodies. Serologic specificity depends upon the resulting patterns of reactions.

Reagents

1. Serum or plasma to be studied. Serum should be separated at 37 C from a blood sample allowed to clot at 37 C. Plasma should be separated from an anticoagulated sample after periodic inversion at 37 C for approximately 15 minutes.
2. Test rbcs; the following are required:
   a. Two adult group O, I+ samples, ordinarily reagent rbcs used for alloantibody detection.
   b. The patient's own (autologous) rbcs.
   c. Red cells of the same ABO phenotype as the patient, if the patient is not group O. Use rbcs of different A subtype (ie, A_1 and A_2) if the patient is group A or AB.
   d. Ficin or papain-treated group O, I+ rbcs.
   e. Group O, I– cord blood or adult I– rbcs, or both.

Procedure

1. Prepare serial two-fold dilutions of the serum or plasma in saline. The dilution range should be from 1 in 2 to 1 in 4096 (12 tubes), and the volumes prepared should not be less than 1 mL.
2. Mix three drops of each dilution with one drop of a 5% saline suspension of each test rbc sample.
3. Incubate at room temperature for 15 minutes. Centrifuge, and examine the rbcs macroscopically for agglutination. Grade and record the results.
4. Transfer the tubes to 4 C, and incubate at this temperature for 1 hour. Centrifuge, and examine the rbcs for agglutination. Grade and record the results.

Interpretation

Table 6.3-1 summarizes the reactions of some commonly encountered cold-reactive autoantibodies. Anti-I is seen frequently in cold agglutinin syndrome, but anti-i and anti-Pr specificities may also be encountered. Some examples of anti-I display a preference for rbcs that have a strong expression of H antigen (eg, O and A_2); such antibodies are called anti-IH. The reactivity of all autoantibodies with specificity related to the I system is enhanced in tests with protease-treated rbcs. In contrast, anti-Pr antibodies react weakly (if at all) with enzyme-treated rbcs, and react with all

Table 6.3-1. Comparative Reactions To Demonstrate Specificity of Cold-Reactive Autoantibodies

Rbcs	Anti-I	Anti-i	Antibody Specificity Anti-H*	Anti-IH*	Anti-Pr
Oi (adult)	NR/ ↓	↑	≡	↓	≡
Oi (cord)	NR/ ↓	↑	<	↓	≡
A_1I	≡	≡	↓	↓	≡
OI (enzyme-treated)	↑	↑	↑	↑	NR/ ↓
Autologous	≡	≡	↓	↓	≡

NR = nonreactive   ≡ = equal to OI rbcs
↑ = stronger than OI rbcs   < = equal to or weaker than OI rbcs
↓ = weaker than OI rbcs
*anti-H and anti-IH antibodies are seen predominantly in A_1 and A_1B individuals

untreated rbcs to the same degree regardless of their I/i status.

Notes

1. With potent examples of cold-reactive autoantibodies, specificity may not be apparent when titration studies are performed at room temperature or 4 C. In such circumstances, incubation of tests at 30-37 C should be undertaken (see reference). Also, specificity may be more readily ascertained if incubation times are prolonged and agglutination is evaluated after settling, without centrifugation.
2. Some workers use this procedure for determining both titer and specificity. If multiple readings are taken following incubation at different temperatures, the specificity, titer and thermal amplitude of the autoantibody can be determined with a single set of serum dilutions.

Reference

Petz LD, Branch DR. Serological tests for the diagnosis of immune hemolytic anemias. In: McMillan R, ed. Methods in hematology: Immune cytopenias. New York: Churchill Livingstone, 1983:2-48.

Method 6.4. Autologous Adsorption of Warm-Reactive Autoantibodies

Principle

Warm-reactive autoantibodies may mask the presence of concomitant clinically significant alloantibodies in a serum. Adsorbing the serum with autologous rbcs can remove autoantibody from the serum, permitting detection of underlying alloantibodies. Circulating autologous rbcs, however, are already coated with autoantibody.

Autologous adsorption of warm-reactive autoantibodies can be achieved most effectively by removing the autoantibody and then pretreating the rbcs with a proteolytic enzyme. Removal of coating antibody uncovers antigen sites, which are then capable of binding free autoantibody in the serum. Enzyme treatment enhances the adsorption process by removing rbc membrane structures that otherwise hinder the association between antigen and antibody.

The best procedure involves the use of ZZAP reagent, a mixture of a proteolytic enzyme and a thiol reagent. Treatment of IgG molecules with a thiol reagent increases their susceptibility to digestion by proteases. When IgG-coated rbcs are treated with ZZAP reagent, the immunoglobulin molecules lose their integrity and dissociate from the rbc surface. Simultaneously, the rbcs are subjected to the action of a proteolytic enzyme to increase their adsorbing capacity.

Autoadsorption should not be performed on rbcs from a recently transfused patient because the circulating transfused rbcs may adsorb the alloantibodies that are being sought.

Reagents

1. 1% cysteine-activated papain or 1% ficin (see Method 3.5.1).
2. PBS at pH 6.5 and pH 8.0 (see Method 1.6).
3. 0.2 M DTT prepared by dissolving 1 g of DTT in 32.4 mL of pH 8.0 PBS. Dispense into 3 mL aliquots and store at or below −20 C.
4. Blood samples containing warm-reactive autoantibodies.

Procedure

1. Prepare ZZAP reagent by mixing 0.5 mL 1% cysteine-activated papain with 2.5 mL of DTT and 2 mL of pH 6.5

PBS. Alternatively, use 1 mL of ficin, 2.5 mL of DTT and 1.5 mL of pH 6.5 PBS. Check pH and adjust to 6.5 if necessary.

2. To two tubes, each containing 1 mL of packed rbcs, add 2 mL of ZZAP reagent. Mix, and incubate at 37 C for 20-30 minutes with periodic mixing.
3. Wash the rbcs three times in saline. Centrifuge the last wash for at least 5 minutes at 900-1000 × g. Use suction to remove as much of the supernatant as practical.
4. Add patient's serum to an equal volume of ZZAP-treated rbcs.
5. Incubate at 37 C for approximately 20-45 minutes.
6. Centrifuge and carefully remove serum.
7. Steps 4 through 6 should be repeated once more using the once-adsorbed patient's serum and a different aliquot of ZZAP-treated cells.

Interpretation

Two adsorptions ordinarily remove sufficient autoantibody from the serum that alloantibody reactivity is readily apparent. Test the twice-autoadsorbed serum for activity using group O reagent rbcs. If positive, determine specificity by testing against a small panel of reagent rbcs. If all panel cells are positive, additional autoadsorptions may be necessary, or the serum contains an antibody (eg, anti-Ge) that does not react with ZZAP-treated rbcs and, therefore, cannot be adsorbed by this method. To confirm this possibility, test the reactive autoadsorbed serum against reagent screening cells that have been pretreated with the ZZAP reagent.

Notes

1. ZZAP treatment destroys all Kell system antigens, and other antigens that are destroyed by proteases, including M, N, Fy^a, Fy^b, S. In addition, ZZAP

reagent denatures the s antigen and antigens of the LW, Gerbich, Cartwright and Dombrock systems. Also, some of the antigens defined by HTLA antibodies may be denatured.
2. There is no need to wash rbcs before treatment with ZZAP.
3. Rarely, ZZAP treatment will cause rbcs to gel. This is suspected to be related somehow to abnormally high white cell counts.

Reference

Branch DR, Petz LD. A new reagent (ZZAP) having multiple applications in immunohematology. Am J Clin Pathol 1982;78:161-7.

Method 6.5. Differential Warm Adsorption Using ZZAP-Treated Allogeneic (Homologous) Rbcs

Principle

ZZAP treatment of rbcs results in rbcs lacking all Kell, MNSs, Duffy and Gerbich antigens; most LW, Cartwright and Dombrock antigens; and other antigens destroyed by enzymes. Adsorption of serum with selected rbcs having known phenotypes will remove autoantibody and leave antibodies to most blood group systems. Specificity of the antibodies that remain following adsorption can be confirmed by testing with a panel of reagent rbcs.

This method is used to remove autoantibody from the serum of an individual with warm autoantibodies in order to determine if clinically significant alloantibodies are present. This procedure is used if the patient has been recently transfused, or insufficient autologous rbcs are available, and the patient's phenotype is unknown.

Reagents

1. 1% cysteine-activated papain or 1% ficin (see Method 3.5.1).
2. PBS at pH 6.5 and pH 8.0 (see Method 1.6).
3. 0.2 M DTT prepared by dissolving 1 g of DTT in 32.4 mL of pH 8.0 PBS. Dispense into 3 mL aliquots and store at or below −20 C.
4. R_1, R_2 and r cells.
5. Blood samples containing warm-reactive autoantibodies.

Procedure

1. Prepare ZZAP reagent by mixing 0.5 mL cysteine-activated papain with 2.5 mL of DTT and 2 mL of pH 6.5 PBS. Alternatively, use 1 mL of ficin, 2.5 mL of DTT and 1.5 mL of pH 6.5 PBS. Check pH and adjust to 6.5 if necessary.
2. Select R_1, R_2 and r rbcs.
3. Wash 1 mL of rbcs once in a large volume of saline.
4. To each aliquot of washed packed cells, add 2 mL of working ZZAP reagent. Invert several times to mix.
5. Incubate at 37 C for 20-30 minutes. Mix periodically throughout incubation.
6. Remove from 37 C and wash the rbcs three times with large volumes of saline. Remove last wash as completely as possible to prevent serum dilution.
7. To one volume of ZZAP-treated rbcs, add an equal volume of patient's serum.
8. Mix. Incubate at 37 C for 30-60 minutes, mixing occasionally.
9. Centrifuge at 900-1000 × g for approximately 5 minutes and harvest supernatant serum.
10. Test adsorbed serum with its respective adsorbing rbcs. If positive, repeat steps 7 through 9 with a fresh aliquot of ZZAP-treated red cells until negative. The adsorbed serum may then be used for antibody identification and for crossmatching.

Notes

1. If the autoantibody is very strong, three or more aliquots of adsorbing rbcs should be prepared.
2. An excess of rbcs in relation to the amount of serum/eluate to be adsorbed will greatly facilitate the removal of antibody.
3. The adsorbing rbcs should be tightly packed to remove any residual saline that could result in dilution of the antibodies remaining in the serum.
4. Agitate the rbc/serum mixture during incubation to allow for maximum surface contact.
5. If the antibody does not appear to be adsorbing, non-ZZAP-treated rbcs may be tried.

References

1. Branch DR, Petz LD. A new reagent (ZZAP) having multiple applications in immunohematology. Am J Clin Pathol 1982;78:161-7.
2. Judd WJ. Methods in immunohematology. Miami: Montgomery Scientific Publications, 1988.

Method 6.6. One-Cell Sample ZZAP Allogeneic (Homologous) Adsorption

Principle

If a recently transfused patient's Rh and Kidd phenotypes are known or can be determined, then alloantibodies contained in the presence of autoantibodies can be evaluated using serum adsorbed onto only one allogeneic rbc sample. The source of the rbcs is selected to be matched with the patient for Rh and Kidd phenotypes and then ZZAP-treated to denature Kell, Duffy and MNSs antigens (and others; see Method 6.4).

This method is used to detect clinically significant alloantibodies in the presence of warm-reactive autoantibodies in patients who have been recently transfused, where the Rh and Kidd phenotypes are known.

Reagents

1. ZZAP reagent (see Method 6.4).
2. Rbcs matched with the patient's Rh and Kidd phenotypes.

Procedure

1. Wash selected allogeneic rbcs once in a large volume of saline.
2. To one volume of these packed rbcs, add two volumes of ZZAP reagent.
3. Incubate at 37 C for 20-30 minutes with periodic mixing.
4. Remove from 37 C and wash the rbcs three times with saline. Remove last wash as completely as possible to prevent serum dilution.
5. To one volume of ZZAP-treated rbcs add an equal volume of patient's serum.
6. Mix. Incubate at 37 C for 30-60 minutes, mixing occasionally.
7. Centrifuge at 900-1000 × g for approximately 5 minutes and harvest supernatant serum.
8. Test adsorbed serum with its respective adsorbing rbcs. If positive, repeat steps 5 through 7 with a fresh aliquot of ZZAP-treated rbcs until negative.

References

1. Shulman IA, Branch DR. Strategies for the safe transfusion of crossmatch-incompatible blood. Paper presented at Fall Meeting of the American Society of Clinical Pathologists, Orlando, FL, September 27 to October 3, 1986.
2. Shulman IA. Personal communication.

Method 6.7. The Donath-Landsteiner Test

Principle

For a detailed discussion of the principle of the Donath-Landsteiner test, see Chapter 16. The primary application of this test is in the differential diagnosis of immune hemolysis and diagnosis of paroxysmal cold hemoglobinuria (PCH). In particular, this procedure should be considered when cold-reactive autoantibodies are absent from the serum, C3 alone is present on the rbcs, the eluate is nonreactive and the patient has hemoglobinemia or hemoglobinuria, or both.

Reagents

1. Serum to be tested, separated from a freshly collected blood sample maintained at 37 C.
2. Freshly collected normal serum as a source of complement.
3. 50% suspension of washed group O, P+ rbcs (P_1 or P_2 phenotype).

Procedure

1. Label three sets of three 10 × 75-mm test tubes as follows: A1-A2-A3; B1-B2-B3; C1-C2-C3.
2. To tubes 1 and 2 of each set, add 10 volumes of the patient's serum.
3. To tubes 2 and 3 of each set, add 10 volumes of fresh normal serum.
4. To all tubes, add one volume of washed 50% P+ rbcs and mix well.
5. Place the three "A" tubes first in a bath of melting ice for 30 minutes, and then at 37 C for 1 hour.
6. Place the three "B" tubes in a bath of melting ice, and keep them in melting ice for 90 minutes.
7. Place the three "C" tubes at 37 C, and keep them at 37 C for 90 minutes.
8. Centrifuge all tubes, and examine the supernatant fluids for hemolysis.

Interpretation

The Donath-Landsteiner test is considered positive when the patient's serum, with or without added complement, causes hemolysis only in those tubes that have been incubated first in melting ice and then at 37 C (ie, tubes A1 and A2). No hemolysis should be seen in any of the tubes maintained strictly at 37 C or in melting ice, or in which complement alone is present.

Notes

1. To demonstrate the biphasic hemolysin associated with PCH, it is necessary to incubate the serum with rbcs first at or below 4 C, then at 37 C.
2. Active complement is essential to demonstrate the antibody. Since patients with PCH often have low levels of serum complement, fresh normal serum should be included in the reaction medium as a source of complement.
3. To avoid loss of antibody by autoadsorption before testing, the patient's blood should be allowed to clot at 37 C, and the serum separated from the clot at 37 C.

Reference

Dacie JV, Lewis, SM. Practical hematology, 4th ed. London: Churchill, 1968.

Method 6.8. Detection of Antibodies to Penicillin or Cephalothin

Principle

This method is used in the investigation of drug-induced positive DATs associated with β-lactam antibiotics (ie, penicillin or cephalothin). See Chapter 16 for discussion of the mechanisms by which drugs cause a positive DAT.

Reagents

1. Barbital-buffered saline (BBS) at pH 9.6, prepared by dissolving 20.6 g of sodium barbital in 1 L of saline. Adjust to pH 9.6 with 0.1 N HCl. Store at 4 C.
2. PBS, pH 6.0 (see Method 1.6). Adjust pH to 6.0 with NaOH; store at 4 C.
3. Penicillin (approximately 1×10^6 units per 600 mg).
4. Cephalothin sodium (Keflin).
5. Washed, packed group O rbcs.
6. Serum or eluate to be studied.

Procedure

1. Prepare penicillin-coated rbcs by incubating 1 mL of rbcs with 600 mg of penicillin in 15 mL of BBS for 1 hour at room temperature. Wash three times in saline and store in Alsever's solution (see Method 1.8) at 4 C. Cephalosporins other than cephalothin can also be coated onto rbcs using this method.
2. Prepare cephalothin-coated rbcs by incubating 1 mL of rbcs with 300 mg of cephalothin sodium in 10 mL of PBS, pH 6.0 for 1 hour at 37 C with frequent mixing. Wash three times in saline and store in Alsever's solution at 4 C.
3. Mix two or three drops of serum or eluate with one drop of 5% saline suspension of drug-coated rbcs.
4. Test in parallel, uncoated rbcs from the same donor.
5. Incubate the tests at 37 C for 30-60 minutes. Centrifuge, and examine the rbcs macroscopically for agglutination. Grade and record the results.
6. Wash the rbcs four times in saline, and test by an indirect antiglobulin technique using polyspecific or anti-IgG reagents.

Interpretation

Antibodies to penicillins or cephalosporins will react with the drug-coated rbcs but not with uncoated rbcs. Antibodies to either drug may cross-react with rbcs coated with the other drug (ie, anti-penicillin antibodies cross-react with cephalothin-coated rbcs and vice versa). Furthermore, most anticephalosporins will cross-react with cephalothin.

Notes

1. Normal sera may react with cephalothin-coated rbcs, since such rbcs may adsorb all proteins nonimmunologically. However, this reactivity does not often occur when using a low pH method to couple cephalothin to rbcs (see reference).
2. If gross lysis occurs with pH 6.0 cephalothin-coated rbcs, recheck the pH and make sure it is not below 6.0.
3. Reactivity of an eluate with cephalothin-coated rbcs, and not untreated rbcs, indicates antibody to cephalosporins, which may also cross-react with penicillin-coated rbcs.
4. Once prepared, the drug-coated rbcs may be kept in Alsever's solution (see Method 1.8) at 4 C for up to 1 week.

Reference

Petz LD, Branch DR. Drug-induced immune hemolytic anemia. In: Chaplin H, ed. Methods in hematology: Immune hemolytic anemias. New York: Churchill Livingstone, 1985:47-94.

Method 6.9. Demonstration of Immune Complex Formation Involving Drugs

Principle

Immune complexes formed between certain drugs and their respective antibodies may attach weakly to rbcs. The bound immune complex activates complement, which may lead to hemolysis in vivo. This procedure provides an in-vitro means to demonstrate immune complex formation

associated with drug/anti-drug interactions.

Reagents

1. Drug under investigation, in the same form (tablet, solution, capsules) that the patient is receiving.
2. PBS at pH 7.0-7.4 (see Method 1.6).
3. Patient's serum.
4. Fresh, normal serum known to lack unexpected antibodies, as a source of complement.
5. Group O reagent rbcs, both untreated and treated with a proteolytic enzyme (see Method 3.5.5).

Procedure

1. Prepare a 1 mg/mL suspension solution of the drug in PBS. Centrifuge, and adjust the pH of the supernatant fluid to 7.0 with either 1 N NaOH or 1 N HCl, as required.
2. Using 0.2 mL of each reactant, prepare the following test mixtures.
   a. Patient's serum + drug
   b. Patient's serum + complement (normal serum) + drug
   c. Patient's serum + complement (normal serum) + PBS
   d. Normal serum + drug
   e. Normal serum + PBS
3. To three drops of each test mixture, add one drop of a 5% saline suspension of group O reagent rbcs. To another three drops of each test mixture add one drop of a 5% saline suspension of enzyme-treated group O reagent rbcs.
4. Mix, and incubate at 37 C for 1-2 hours, with periodic gentle mixing.
5. Wash the rbcs four times in saline, and test with a polyspecific antiglobulin reagent.

Interpretation

Hemolysis, agglutination or coating can occur. Such reactivity in any of the tests containing patient's serum to which the drug was added, and absence of reactivity in the corresponding control tests containing PBS instead of the drug, indicates a drug/anti-drug interaction.

Notes

1. The use of a pestle and mortar (if the drug is in tablet form), incubation at 37 C and vigorous shaking of the solution may help dissolve the drug.
2. Many drugs will not dissolve completely, but enough may be dissolved to react in serologic tests. Other methods, obtained from the manufacturer or other publications, may be needed to dissolve adequate quantities of some drugs.

References

1. Garratty G. Laboratory investigation of drug-induced immune hemolytic anemia. Supplement to: Bell CA, ed. A seminar on laboratory management of hemolysis. Washington, DC: American Association of Blood Banks, 1979.
2. Petz LD, Branch DR. Drug-induced immune hemolytic anemia. In: Chaplin H, ed. Methods in hematology: Immune hemolytic anemias. New York: Churchill Livingstone, 1985:47-94.

Method 6.10. Demonstration of Drug/Anti-Drug Complexes—Ex-Vivo Method

Principle

Immune complexes formed between certain drugs and their respective antibodies can activate complement, which may lead to hemolysis in vivo. The detection of these immune complexes can be accomplished by serologic testing in the presence of the drug; however, with some drugs (notably nomifensine), antibodies are formed against metabolites of the drug rather than epitopes on the native drug. Serum and/or urine from volunteers who have ingested therapeutic levels of the drug are required as a source of these metabolites.

This method is used in the investigation of drug-induced immune hemolysis, particularly when the results of tests by the preceding methods are not informative.

Reagents

1. AHG: polyspecific.
2. Drug metabolites:
   a. Serum samples from volunteer drug recipients: separate at 37 C from blood clotted at 37 C. Obtain samples immediately before (VS$_0$) and at 1 hour (VS$_1$) and 6 hours (VS$_6$) after drug administration; 1 mL serum per sample; keep on ice or aliquot and store below –20 C until required.
   b. Urine from the above volunteers: obtained immediately before (VU$_0$) and at 1 hour (VU$_1$), 3.5 hours (VU$_{3.5}$), 7 hours (VU$_7$) and 16 hours (VU$_{16}$) after drug administration; 1 mL per sample; keep on ice or aliquot and store below –20 C until required.
3. Human complement: freshly collected normal human serum known to lack unexpected antibodies, 1 mL.
4. PBS at pH 7.3 (see Method 1.6).
5. Rbcs: pooled group O reagent rbcs; washed three times with saline and resuspended to a 5% concentration with PBS.
6. Rbcs—ficin-treated: pooled group O rbcs; 5% suspension in PBS.
7. Test serum: separated at 37 C from blood clotted at 37 C, 3 mL.

Procedure

1. For each serum (VS) and/or urine (VU) sample collected from volunteer drug recipients, prepare two sets of the following test mixtures using 0.1 mL volumes of each reactant:
   a. Test serum + VS (or VU)
   b. Test serum + VS (or VU) + complement

c. Complement + VS (or VU)
2. Using 0.1 mL volumes, prepare duplicate control tubes of:
   a. Test serum + PBS
   b. Test serum + complement
   c. Complement + PBS
3. To one set of test mixtures, add one drop of untreated rbcs.
4. To the other set add one drop of ficin-treated rbcs.
5. Similarly, add rbcs to the control mixtures.
6. Agitate the contents of each tube and incubate at 37 C for 1 or 2 hours; agitate the contents of each tube periodically.
7. Centrifuge at $900\text{-}1000 \times g$ for 10-20 seconds.
8. Examine the red cells macroscopically; grade and record the results.
9. Wash the rbcs four times with saline; completely decant the final supernatant fluid.
10. Add polyspecific AHG according to the manufacturer's directions.
11. Centrifuge at $900\text{-}1000 \times g$ for 10-20 seconds.
12. Examine the rbcs macroscopically; grade and record the results.

Interpretation

Reactivity (hemolysis, direct or indirect agglutination) in any of the tests containing test serum to which VS or VU was added, and absence of reactivity among controls, indicates presence of a metabolite-specific antibody.

Notes

1. Complement may be omitted from step 1b, above, providing the VS samples are kept on ice and tested within 8 hours of collection.
2. The sample collection times are those used in the detection of antibodies to nomifensine metabolites; different

times may be required for different drugs.

Reference

Salama A, Mueller-Eckhardt C. The role of metabolite-specific antibodies in nomifensine-dependent immune hemolytic anemia. N Engl J Med 1985; 313:469-74.

Method 6.11. Treatment of Antiglobulin Reagents for Tests on Samples From Patients Receiving Antilymphocyte or Antithymocyte Globulin Preparations

Principle

Equine (horse) preparations of antilymphocyte globulin (ALG) and antithymocyte globulin (ATG) contain heterophile antibodies that coat recipient rbcs. Thus, patients receiving ALG/ATG develop a positive DAT within a few days. Rabbit antihuman globulin (AHG) reagents contain antibodies that react with the equine immunoglobulin. This reactivity can be removed from AHG by adsorption with rbcs coated with ALG/ATG, or by neutralization with equine serum.

This method is used to perform serologic tests, particularly the detection of alloantibodies to human rbc antigens, in samples from recipients of ALG/ATG.

Reagents

1. AHG: polyspecific or anti-IgG (rabbit), 10 mL.
2. Equine serum: sterile, mycoplasma-free, nonhemolyzed (PelFreez, Rogers, AR).
3. IgG-coated rbcs: available commercially.
4. Reagent rbcs: 5% suspensions of O, R_1 and R_2 rbcs.

Procedure

1. Mix 0.2 mL of equine serum with 10 mL of AHG.
2. Incubate at room temperature for 20-45 minutes.
3. Label appropriately; confirm reactivity with rbcs coated with human IgG; store at 4 C.
4. Use in antibody detection and identification tests.

Notes

1. Problems associated with ALG/ATG therapy are not usually encountered by the LIP technique described in Method 3.1.5. LIP tests may, therefore, be used to screen for unexpected alloantibodies in ALG/ATG recipients.
2. ALG/ATG preparations may exhibit a Lutheran-related specificity. If available, Lu(a–b–) rbcs can be used to detect concomitant alloantibodies.
3. To avoid ALG/ATG problems, the medical staff should be advised to submit samples for pretransfusion testing before giving ALG/ATG.

References

1. Swanson JL, Issitt CH, Mann EW, et al. Resolution of red cell compatibility testing problems in patients receiving anti-lymphoblast or anti-thymocyte globulin. Transfusion 1984;24:141-3.
2. Anderson HJ, AuBuchon JP, Draper EK, Ballas SK. Transfusion problems in renal allograft recipients: Anti-lymphocyte globulin showing Lutheran system specificity. Transfusion 1985;25:47-50.

Method 6.12. Mononuclear Phagocyte Assay (MPA)

Principle

Antibody- and/or complement-coated rbcs are incubated in vitro with peripheral blood monocytes over a short-term culture period. The recognition by receptors on the monocyte-macrophages of the rbcs with their subsequent phagocytosis or adherence is an index of the antibody's potential to decrease the in-vivo survival of the patient's rbcs or, after incubation with the patient's serum, donor rbcs for transfusion.

This method is used to predict the in-vivo clinical significance of auto- and alloantibodies.

Materials

1. Lymphocyte separation medium (ie, Ficoll-Hypaque).
2. Heparinized whole blood kept at room temperature (sample good for 24 hours).
3. Medium: RPMI-1640 supplemented with 10% (v/v) fetal bovine serum and 20 mM Hepes buffer.
4. 35-mm Petri dishes.
5. 22 × 22-mm glass coverslips.
6. ABO-compatible, fresh frozen serum.
7. 37 C incubator containing 5% CO_2 in air.
8. Methanol.
9. Hematological stain (ie, Wright/Giemsa).
10. Phosphate-buffered saline (PBS), pH 7.3 (see Method 1.6).
11. Test rbcs:
    a. In-vivo sensitized rbcs
       1) The rbcs under investigation, washed four times in saline and resuspended to 2.5% in saline.
       2) Mix one volume of the 2.5% rbc suspension with one volume of medium (approximately 10^8 rbc/mL).
       3) The rbcs are now ready for layering over the monocyte-macrophage monolayer.
    b. In-vitro sensitized rbcs
       1) Reagent or donor rbcs, washed two times in saline then once in LISS and resuspended to 5% in LISS.

2) Mix 1 mL of 5% LISS-suspended rbcs with 1 mL of test serum, with and without added ABO-compatible serum as a source of complement.
3) Incubate at 37 C for 30 minutes.
4) Wash rbcs three times in saline, then resuspend to 2.5% in saline.
5) Perform an antiglobulin test (see Method 3.1.1) to estimate the degree of sensitization.
6) Mix one volume of 2.5% sensitized rbcs with one volume of medium (approximately 10^8 rbc/mL).
7) The rbcs are now ready for layering over the monocyte-macrophage monolayer.

Procedure

1. Isolate mononuclear cells from heparinized whole blood using density gradient centrifugation over lymphocyte separation medium.
2. Wash mononuclear cells three times in PBS, pH 7.3.
3. Resuspend mononuclear cells in medium.
4. Count and adjust concentration to 10^6 cells/mL.
5. Place 1 mL (10^6 cells) per 35-mm Petri dish containing a 22 × 22-mm coverslip.
6. Incubate for 1 hour at 37 C and 5% CO_2.
7. Remove coverslips and rinse vigorously with PBS to remove nonadherent cells.
8. Place coverslips with adherent cells (>85% monocytes) in new Petri dishes (side that was facing up in step 5 above should now also be facing up).
9. Overlay with the red cell population to be tested (10^8 rbcs/mL in medium; see above).
10. Incubate for 2 hours at 37 C and 5% CO_2.

11. Remove coverslips and rinse gently with PBS to remove unassociated red cells.
12. Fix (methanol, 1 minute), stain and observe coverslips for associated (rosetted) and phagocytosed rbcs.

Interpretation

The number of phagocytosed rbcs per 100 monocyte-macrophages counted is the usual readout. When low numbers of phagocytosed rbcs are seen, 200-500 monocyte-macrophages should be counted. Using this system, levels >2 phagocytosed rbcs per 100 monocyte-macrophages are considered significantly elevated. However, each laboratory must establish its own conditions so that the assay correlates with in-vivo rbc destruction (see notes).

Notes

1. The mononuclear cells can be from normal volunteers or from the patient.
2. The coverslip method can be replaced with a Titertek method (see reference 4) but conditions of the assay need to be restandardized.
3. Normal ranges are established by observing the interaction of the mononuclear phagocytes with rbcs from normal individuals or patients without hemolytic anemia having a negative DAT.
4. Positive control samples are usually single donor R_1 or R_1R_2 rbcs that have been sensitized with varying concentrations of commercial anti-D to give high and low indices of interaction.
5. Normal ranges and positive control ranges should be established in each laboratory. Clinically significant ranges should be established using rbcs from DAT-positive patients with and without hemolytic anemia.

References

1. Gallagher MT, Branch DR, Mison A, Petz LD. Evaluation of reticuloendothelial function in autoimmune hemolytic anemia using an in vitro assay of monocyte-macrophage interaction with erythrocytes. Exp Hematol 1983;11:82-9.
2. Branch DR, Gallagher MT, Mison AP, et al. In vitro determination of red cell alloantibody significance using an assay of monocyte-macrophage interaction with sensitized erythrocytes. Br J Haematol 1984;56:19-29.
3. Schanfield MS. The role of mononuclear phagocytes in RBC destruction: In vitro test systems. In: Chaplin H, ed. Methods in hematology: Immune hemolytic anemias, vol. 12. New York: Churchill Livingstone, 1985:135-53.
4. Nance SJ, Arndt P, Garratty G. Predicting the clinical significance of red cell alloantibodies using a monocyte monolayer assay. Transfusion 1987;27:449-52.

Method 6.13. In-Vivo Crossmatch With ^{51}Cr-Labeled Rbcs

Principle

Donor rbcs are tagged with ^{51}Cr and their rbc survival in the recipient's circulation is measured by counting radioactivity in recipient blood samples. This "in-vivo crossmatch" can be very useful when: 1) the patient is serologically incompatible with all or most donor units and the antibody(ies) cannot be characterized, 2) the antibody is known and of relatively high incidence but the clinical significance is unknown or questionable or 3) the rbc survival of transfused units is markedly shortened but there is no serologic evidence of antibody.

There are many variations on the basic technique employing different doses of ^{51}Cr, different tagging methods and different schedules to draw blood for testing. This method is simple and allows a quick assessment of short-term survival. One mL is used for the initial test dose to minimize the risk to the recipient from clinically significant hemolysis.

Procedure

1. Select the donor unit to be studied. For demonstrable antibodies the least compatible unit can be selected, so that the rbc survival test will show the worst case. A 5-10 mL aliquot of rbcs is withdrawn from the unit to be tagged with ^{51}Cr. If the unit is entered, it should be transfused or discarded within 24 hours. Ideally, the aliquot can be taken off into an integrally connected satellite bag, or a sterile connecting device may be used, so that the expiration date of the unit does not change. The storage date of the unit selected for study should also be considered since units that are at or near the end of their shelf life will normally have about 70% survival 24 hours posttransfusion. For long-term survival studies, the age of the unit would have to be considered when evaluating the results of a ^{51}Cr study.

2. Sterile technique should be followed since the tagged rbcs will be injected into the recipient. Ten to 20 µCi of ^{51}Cr is added per one mL of rbcs, mixed, and incubated in a 37 C waterbath for 30 minutes. Mix the sample several times during incubation.

3. After incubation, wash the rbcs in saline. For short-term studies 1 mL is taken off into a syringe to be injected. Save the remaining mixture for a dilutional control.

4. Inject 1 mL of tagged rbcs into the patient. Preferably, the injection site should be different from the site used to collect samples. Start a stopwatch at the midpoint of the injection of the 1 mL of rbcs. The first sample should be taken at 3 minutes, with subsequent samples at 10 minutes and 60 minutes. A heparin lock at the sample withdrawal site allows for timely and easy withdrawal of samples.

5. The 3-minute sample is considered 100% or baseline. In-vivo mixing

should be complete at 3 minutes with little or no rbc destruction. If there is destruction within the first 3 minutes, then this sample would have plasma radioactivity. In addition, the first sample should be used to calculate the patient's total blood volume and this figure should then be compared to the expected blood volume. If destruction has occurred before withdrawal of the 3-minute sample, then the blood volume calculated from this first sample will appear to be greater than the expected blood volume. Additionally, an aliquot of tagged rbcs that have not been injected can be diluted to represent the dilution that injected rbcs have undergone in the patient. This sample can then be counted and compared to the counts from the 3-minute sample.

6. The subsequent sample counts taken at 10 minutes and 60 minutes are compared to the 3-minute count and expressed as a percentage. For example:

3-minute count = 1000 CPM
10-minute count = 950 CPM
60-minute count = 930 CPM

$$\frac{\text{10-minute CPM}}{\text{3-minute CPM}} \times 100 = \frac{\text{950 CPM}}{\text{1000 CPM}}$$
$$\times\ 100 = 95\% \ (10 \text{ minutes})$$

$$\frac{\text{60-minute CPM}}{\text{3-minute CPM}} \times 100 = \frac{\text{930 CPM}}{\text{1000 CPM}}$$
$$\times\ 100 = 93\% \ (60 \text{ minutes})$$

Separated plasma should also be counted.

Interpretation

If the rbc survival at 1 hour is 70% or higher, and there is less than 5% activity in the plasma, then it can be assumed that a whole unit of red cells will not undergo rapid intravascular destruction, or cause a severe adverse effect. However, it should be remembered that even though the 1-hour survival value is a good indication of immediate transfusion outcome, it does not predict as reliably the long-term survival. Studies listed in the references provide examples of acceptable 1-hour survival with poor long-term survival, when measured at 24 hours or days after infusion. If time is critical, a 1-hour test can be informative; however, the best information is gained from additional samples taken after injection of the test dose. It should also be recognized that an incompatible unit that survives well for several days or weeks may still provide the patient with a therapeutic benefit in the short term when serologically compatible blood is unavailable.

Long-term survival may also be measured with infusion of a unit of rbcs. After a successful 1 mL test, then 3-5 mL of tagged rbcs may be injected immediately before infusion of the unit of rbcs. Mixing this larger aliquot of tagged rbcs with the unit of rbcs is not as efficient since some of the tagged rbcs may not be infused (trapped in the filter, or left as residual in the bag). A 3-minute sample can be taken as a baseline and then samples taken hours and days after infusion of the unit. The patient's condition in long-term studies must also be considered. If the patient has any bleeding during the study period, the measured survival may be adversely affected. Additionally, the patient's own rbcs may be tagged with a different isotope (^{99}Tc) and autologous survival compared to allogeneic survival.

^{51}Cr-tagged rbcs may also be used to evaluate cases when an alloantibody is suspected of causing shortened rbc survival, but an antibody cannot be demonstrated serologically. In these cases, 1 mL tagged test doses of donor rbcs that have an antigen that the patient lacks are infused and the survival measured. The references below review several of these unusual cases.

If any of these studies are to be undertaken, it is best to work with a nuclear medicine department that has experience with in-vivo isotope studies for safe handling, proper counting and valid interpretation.

References

1. International Committee for Standardization in Haematology. Recommended method for radioisotope red-cell survival studies. Br J Haematol 1980;45:659-66.
2. Baldwin ML, Ness PM, Barrasso C, et al. In vivo studies of the long-term ^{51}Cr red-cell survival of serologically incompatible red cell units. Transfusion 1985;25:34-8.
3. Wallace ME, Davey RJ, eds. Diagnostic and investigational uses of radiolabeled blood elements. Arlington, VA: American Association of Blood Banks, 1987.

Hemolytic Disease of the Newborn

Method 7.1. Indicator Cell Rosette Test for Fetomaternal Hemorrhage

Principle

This test detects D+ rbcs in the blood of a D– woman who has given birth to a D+ infant. The small amount of D+ fetal blood present is never enough to undergo direct agglutination when anti-D is added to the mother's blood sample. The D+ cells do, however, become coated with anti-D when the blood is incubated with reagent antibody. Mixed-field agglutination occurs when antiglobulin serum is used to demonstrate coating antibody, but the mixed-field positive result may be difficult to detect. This test uses D+ rbcs as the indicator to demonstrate antibody coating. The indicator rbcs combine with the anti-D present on the coated rbcs, and form easily visible rosettes of several cells clustered around each antibody-coated D+ cell in the mixed population.

Although the number of rosettes is roughly proportional to the number of D+ rbcs present in the mixture, this test provides only qualitative information about fetal-maternal admixture. Specimens giving a positive result should be tested with an acid-elution procedure, or other acceptable methods such as ELAT or flow cytometry, to quantify the number of fetal rbcs present.

Reagents

1. 3-4% saline suspension of washed rbcs from the mother's postdelivery blood sample.
2. Negative control: 3-4% saline suspension of washed rbcs known to be D–.
3. Positive control: 3-4% saline suspension of a mixture of rbcs containing approximately 0.6% D+ rbcs and 99.4% D– rbcs (see note).
4. Indicator rbcs: 0.2-0.5% saline suspension of group O, R_2R_2 rbcs. Either enzyme-treated or untreated cells in an enhancing medium can be used.
5. Chemically modified or high-protein reagent anti-D serum. Monoclonal/polyclonal blended reagents are unsuitable for use in this method.

Procedure

1. To each of three 12×75 mm test tubes, add 1 drop (or follow manufacturer's instructions) of reagent anti-D.
2. Add 1 drop of maternal rbcs, negative control rbcs and positive control rbcs to the appropriately labeled tubes.
3. Incubate at 37 C for 15-30 minutes, or as specified by manufacturer's instructions.
4. Wash rbc suspensions at least four times with large volumes of saline to remove all unbound reagent anti-D. Decant saline completely after last wash.

5. To the dry rbc button left after the last wash, add 1 drop of indicator cells and mix thoroughly to resuspend. Add enhancing medium if appropriate.
6. Centrifuge tubes for 15 seconds at approximately 1000 × *g*.
7. Resuspend rbc button and examine rbc suspension microscopically at 100-150 × magnification.
8. Examine at least 10 fields and count the number of rbc rosettes in each field.

Interpretation

Absence of rosettes is a negative result. With enzyme-treated indicator rbcs, up to one rosette per three fields may be seen as a negative result; using untreated rbcs and an enhancement medium, there may be up to six rosettes per five fields in a negative test. The presence of more rosettes than the allowable minimum constitutes a positive result and the specimen should be examined with a quantitative test for the amount of fetal blood present.

The presence of rosettes or agglutination in the negative control tube indicates inadequate washing after incubation, such that residual anti-D is present to agglutinate the D+ indicator rbcs.

Blood from a woman whose Rh phenotype is weak D (D^u) rather than D− will give a strongly positive result. A massive fetomaternal hemorrhage may produce an appearance difficult to distinguish from results seen with individuals with a weak D (D^u) phenotype. A quantitative test for fetal rbcs in the mother's blood should be performed. One must be cautious in interpreting a negative result if the infant is shown to be weak D (D^u).

Note

A control mixture containing 0.6% D+ rbcs can be prepared from 3% saline suspensions of washed D+ and D− rbcs as follows:

1. Add 1 drop of a 3% suspension of D+ rbcs to 15 drops of a 3% suspension of D− rbcs. Mix well.
2. Add 1 drop of the suspension from step 1 to 9 drops of the 3% suspension of D− rbcs. Mix well.

Reference

Sebring ES, Polesky HF. Detection of fetal maternal hemorrhage in Rh immune globulin candidates. Transfusion 1982;22:468-71.

Method 7.2. Acid Elution Stain (Modified Kleihauer-Betke)

Principle

This technique utilizes the fact that fetal hemoglobin is resistant to acid elution, whereas adult hemoglobin is not. When a thin blood smear is exposed to an acid buffer, the adult rbcs lose their hemoglobin into the buffer so that only the stroma remains. Fetal rbcs are unaffected and retain their hemoglobin. The percentage of fetal rbcs in the maternal blood film is used to calculate the approximate volume of fetomaternal hemorrhage. Either clotted blood or anticoagulated blood may be used.

Reagents

1. Stock Solution A. 0.1M citric acid, MW 210. (21.0 g $C_6H_8O_7 \cdot H_2O$ diluted to 1 liter with distilled water). Keep in refrigerator.
2. Stock Solution B. 0.2M sodium phosphate, MW 268. (53.6 g; $Na_2HPO_4 \cdot 7H_2O$ diluted to 1 liter with distilled water). Keep in refrigerator.
3. McIlvaine's buffer, pH 3.2, prepared by adding 75-mL stock solution A to 21-mL stock solution B. Prepare fresh mixture for each test. The temperature

of this final buffer mixture should be approximately 25 C (room temperature), or 37 C.
4. Erythrosin B—0.5% in water.
5. Harris hematoxylin (filtered).
6. 80% ethyl alcohol.

Controls

1. Positive: 10 parts adult blood, 1 part cord blood (ABO compatible).
2. Negative: adult blood.

Procedure

1. Prepare very thin blood smears, diluting blood with an equal volume of saline. Air-dry.
2. Fix smears in 80% ethyl alcohol for 5 minutes.
3. Wash smears with distilled water.
4. Immerse smears in McIlvaine's buffer, pH 3.2, for 11 minutes at room temperature or 5 minutes at 37 C. This reaction is temperature-sensitive.
5. Wash smears in distilled water.
6. Immerse smears in Erythrocin B for 5 minutes.
7. Wash smears completely in distilled water.
8. Immerse smears in Harris hematoxylin for 5 minutes.
9. Wash smears in running tap water for 1 minute.
10. Observe under oil immersion.
11. Count a total of 2000 rbcs and record the number of fetal rbcs observed during this count.
12. Calculate percent fetal rbcs in the total counted.

Interpretation

1. Normal adult rbcs appear as very pale ghosts. Fetal rbcs appear as bright pink refractile bodies.
2. Volume of fetomaternal hemorrhage in mL of whole blood = percent fetal rbcs × 50.

Note

This test has poor accuracy and precision. Therefore, allowance for this should be made in determining the approximate dose of RhIG in massive fetomaternal hemorrhage. See p 465.

Reference

Sebring ES. Fetomaternal hemorrhage—incidence and methods of detection and quantitation. In: Garratty G, ed. Hemolytic disease of the newborn. Arlington, VA: American Association of Blood Banks, 1984:87-118.

Method 7.3.
Spectrophotometric Analysis of Amniotic Fluid

Principle

Scanning normal amniotic fluid with a continuous-recording spectrophotometer between 350-700 nm of the visible-light wavelength spectrum gives a smooth curvilinear tracing with higher absorbance at the shorter wavelengths. Bilirubin has a characteristic absorption peak at 450-455 nm.

Scanning clarified undiluted amniotic fluid in this visible range reveals bilirubin as a peak at 450 nm above a baseline drawn to simulate a normal curve. The height of the bilirubin peak is expressed as the ΔA_{450}.[1-5]

Reagents

1. Recording spectrophotometer.
2. Square cuvettes with 1 cm light path (glass or plastic acceptable).
3. No. 42 or No. 1 Whatman filter paper.
4. Suitable filtering apparatus.
5. Beckman airfuge or similar microcentrifuge.

Sample

A minimum of 5 mL is usually requested, since the cuvette typically requires 3 mL, and filtering may reduce the volume. If smaller cuvettes are available, the volume may be reduced accordingly.

Exposure to light will invalidate readings; wrap aluminum foil around the tube immediately after collection.

Procedure

1. Centrifuge the amniotic fluid at about 2000 × g for 5 minutes.
2. If the fluid is turbid, first filter by gravity through Whatman No. 1 filter paper. Alternatively, the fluid may be filtered by suction through Whatman No. 42 filter paper using a millipore apparatus.
3. Fill cuvette with undiluted amniotic fluid.
4. Zero the spectrophotometer with water.
5. Scan between 350 and 650 nm. For a manual spectrophotometer take absorbance readings against water at the following wavelengths: 350, 365, 380, 390, 400, 410, 415, 420, 430, 440, 450, 460, 470, 480, 500, 530, 550, 600, 630 and 650. Plot the absorbance values against the wavelengths on semilog paper with increasing wavelength on the linear horizontal axis.
6. Draw a tangential straight line from the linear portion of the 350-365 nm region to the linear portion of the 530-600 nm region as shown in Fig 7.3-1.

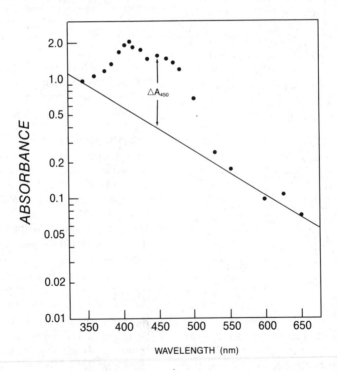

Figure 7.3-1. Visible absorption spectrums of amniotic fluid—absorbance plotted against wavelength. A tangent drawn to the curve serves as the baseline. The peak at 450 nm above background (ΔA_{450}) is directly related to the severity of the disease of the fetus in utero.

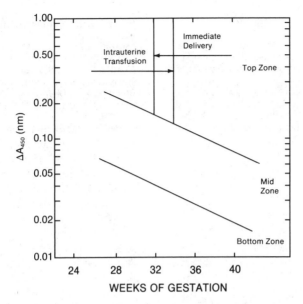

Figure 7.3-2. Liley graph for collecting data from amniotic fluid studies. Intrauterine transfusion should be done if the ΔA_{450} value is in the top zone prior to 32 weeks' gestation. After 34 weeks, top zone values indicate immediate delivery. Either intrauterine transfusion or immediate delivery may be indicated for top zone ΔA_{450} between 32 and 34 weeks, depending on studies of fetal maturity. Modified from Liley.[3]

7. Construct a vertical line from the absorbance at 450 nm to the straight line drawn in step 6 above. This represents the ΔA_{450}. (Fig 7.3-2.)

8. Construct a similar line from the absorbance at 410 nm to the baseline. This represents the absorbance of oxyhemoglobin which may contribute to the ΔA_{450} value.

9. Correct for oxyhemoglobin by subtracting 5% of the change in absorbance at 410 nm from the ΔA_{450}.

Notes

1. If the fluid remains turbid after filtration, centrifuge in a Beckman airfuge using the test tube rotor and repeat scan.

2. This method cannot be used if the 410-nm peak exceeds 1.0 absorbance units due to oxyhemoglobin or meconium, or if there is a significant methemoglobin peak (>0.05 absorbance units above constructed baseline) at 630 nm.

3. An alternative procedure utilizing the photodegradation method of Dubin[4] measures the rate of decrease in absorbance at 464 nm in amniotic fluid exposed to an intense light source such as that available from a conventional slide projector.

4. If the fluid cannot be analyzed immediately after collection, it may be held for later analysis up to 24 hours at room temperature if protected from light. Sunlight causes pigment to disappear. Storage at room temperature for 3 days may result in losses of 20% or more of the pigment.[1] This is an important consideration in mailing samples.

5. Samples may be preserved in the frozen state with little or no change in the ΔA_{450}.

References

1. Nelson GH, Talledo OE. Amniotic fluid spectral analysis in the management of patients with rhesus sensitization. Am J Clin Pathol 1961; 52:363-9.
2. Alperin WM. Spectrophotometric analysis of amniotic fluid. In: Charles AG, Friedman EA, eds. Rh isoimmunization and erythroblastosis fetalis. New York: Appleton-Century-Crofts, 1969:118.
3. Liley AW. Liquor amnii analysis in the management of the pregnancy complicated by rhesus sensitization. Am J Obstet Gynecol 1961;82:1359-70.
4. Dubin SB, Wardlaw S, Jatlow P. Kinetics of bilirubin photodegradation with application to amniotic fluid. Clin Chem Acta 1980;101:193-207.
5. Greene MF, Fencl M de M, Tulchinsky D. In: Tietz NW, ed. Textbook of clinical chemistry. Philadelphia: WB Saunders Co, 1986:1769-71.

HLA Typing

Method 8.1. Isolation of Mononuclear Cells (MNCs)

Principle

Peripheral blood lymphocytes (PBLs) are commonly used as target cells for HLA typing of Class I and Class II antigens, for crossmatching and for the mixed lymphocyte culture (MLC). The lymphocytes must be isolated from freshly drawn blood since good viability is essential.

Sample

Fresh heparinized blood (20 units preservative-free sodium heparin per mL of blood or use green-top Vacutainer tubes).
1. 10 mL is needed for typing Class I (HLA-A, -B, -C) antigens alone.
2. 20 mL is needed for typing Class II (HLA-DR, -DQ) antigens with *or* without simultaneous Class I typing.
3. 30 mL or more is needed for MLC tests.
4. 20 mL is needed for cell surface phenotyping.

Reagents

1. Hanks' balanced salt solution (HBSS).
2. RPMI-1640 culture media (commercially available) containing (per 100 mL RPMI):
   a. 10,000 units penicillin.
   b. 1.0 mL glutamine (2 mMol).
   c. 5 mb streptomycin.

d. 2.5 mL Hepes buffer (25 mM).
3. Ficoll-Hypaque (FH) solution. FH solution and other solutions suitable for isolation of lymphocytes are commercially available from several sources. To prepare 500 mL of FH solution:
   a. Weigh 30.2 g Ficoll 400.
   b. Dissolve in approximately 300 mL of double-distilled H_2O, using a magnetic stirrer on low.
   c. When dissolved, bring to final volume of 400 mL with double-distilled water.
   d. Add 100 mL 50% Hypaque. Mix well.
   e. Determine specific gravity with hydrometer (density = 1.077-1.076), adjusting with water or Hypaque as necessary.
   f. Filter through Nalgene 0.20 filter and store at 4 C. Good for 6 months.

Procedure

1. Dilute blood with an equal volume of either HBSS or RPMI.
   a. HBSS is suitable if the cells are to be isolated within a few hours of collection.
   b. Use RPMI if the blood will be held over for isolation at a later time; keep blood at room temperature.
2. Using red-top siliconized test tubes or plastic conical tubes (or equivalent), layer diluted blood over FH using ap-

proximately twice as much diluted blood as FH.

In an alternative approach, the FH solution may be layered under the diluted blood using 9-1/4" long Pasteur pipets and plastic conical tubes. Typical volumes are: 10 mL of diluted blood layered over 5 mL of FH solution in a 15-mL siliconized red-top tube or in a 25-mL plastic conical tube; or 30 mL of diluted blood layered over 15-20 mL of FH solution in a 50-mL conical plastic tube.

3. Centrifuge layered blood at about 700 $\times g$ at room temperature. Centrifuge for 20 minutes if using the 15-mL red-top tubes or 25-mL plastic tubes. Centrifuge for 30 minutes if using the 50 mL conical tubes.
   a. Do not use brakes on the centrifuge.
   b. Remember to balance the carriers and tubes before spinning.

4. Collect the mononuclear cells (MNCs), which appear as a grayish-white cloud floating at the interface of the FH and diluted plasma. These can be collected using a Pasteur pipet taking care not to disturb the interface. Transfer these cells to clean plastic (or siliconized glass) test tubes.

5. Collect isolated cells into a pellet by centrifugation for 5 minutes at room temperature at about $700 \times g$.

6. Decant supernatant fluid; resuspend and combine the pellets. Wash the cells in HBSS, as follows: Add HBSS to the tube containing the pellet, centrifuge for 5 minutes at 700 $\times g$, decant the supernatant fluid and proceed to step 9. If excess platelets are noted when the cell suspension is examined, go to step 7.

7. Remove excess platelets by slow centrifugation as follows: Resuspend pellet in HBSS or other medium. Centrifuge for 1 minute at $1000 \times g$. Carefully decant and discard the supernatant fluid.

8. Resuspend pellet in 5 mL of HBSS, RPMI, or other appropriate medium. Count cells and check viability (see Methods 8.3 and 8.4). If too many platelets are still present, spin again as in step 7.

9. Proceed to use MNCs, which contain PBLs, according to other relevant test procedure(s).

Note

Although up to 30% of the cells harvested may be monocytes, over 70% of the cells are PBLs. The PBLs can be used directly for Class I HLA typing or they can be separated into T and B cells as required for the test procedure involved. There are numerous minor variations of the procedure found referenced in texts on HLA testing.

Reference

Nisperos B. Density gradient isolation of peripheral blood lymphocytes. In: Zachary AA, Teresi GA, eds. ASHI laboratory manual, 2nd edition. Lenexa, KS: The American Society of Histocompatibility and Immunogenetics, 1990:23-7.

Method 8.2. Nylon Wool Separation of T and B Lymphocytes

Principle

The nylon wool separation of T and B lymphocytes is based on the empirical observation that B lymphocytes adhere preferentially to nylon wool from which they can be eluted, whereas T lymphocytes do not adhere to the nylon. B-cell adherence to nylon is an active process and is reduced at room temperature or 4 C and by the presence of sodium azide or EDTA.

The main advantages of the nylon column separation of B and T lymphocytes lie in the simplicity of the technique and the short time necessary to obtain the two cell populations. Compared to other separation techniques, B cells eluted from nylon columns have excellent viability (95%) and are virtually free of monocytes. Since the technique does not require any agent that could interfere with the cell surface, the lymphocytes are not exposed to any antigens, enzymes or antisera.

Reagents

1. Flexible, transparent drinking straws.
2. Scrubbed, nylon wool.
3. Hanks' balanced salt solution (HBSS).
4. Phosphate-buffered saline (PBS) adjusted to pH 7.0. (See Method 1.6.)
5. RPMI-1640 or McCoy's medium containing 5% heat-inactivated fetal calf serum (FCS). FCS is commercially available. Inactivate the FCS by heating at 56 C for 30 minutes. Then dilute the FCS with RPMI-1640 or McCoy's medium by adding 95 mL of medium to 5 mL of heat-inactivated FCS to obtain the working dilution.

Procedure

Preparation of Nylon Columns

1. By heating, seal one end of a flexible, transparent drinking straw (0.6 × 12-14 cm) at a 45-degree angle.
2. Thoroughly tease 0.1 g of scrubbed nylon wool and soak in HBSS or PBS in a Petri dish.
3. Fill 3/4 of the straw with HBSS or PBS, then gradually and evenly pack the nylon into the straw to a height of approximately 6 cm. At this stage, the column can be stored overnight at 4 C. The straw can be packed using a Pasteur pipet.

Separation of T and B Cells

1. Cut or puncture the sealed end of the straw to make an opening of approximately 2 mm.

2. Allow medium to drip through and wash the nylon with 5 mL HBSS or PBS and then with 5 mL of medium containing 5% heat-inactivated FCS.
3. When the medium just covers the nylon wool, turn the straw to a horizontal position and incubate 30 minutes at 37 C. (Alternatively, use prewarmed medium.)
4. Add 0.5 mL of a purified lymphocyte suspension in medium with 5% heat-inactivated FCS to the top of the column and allow the cells to move all the way into the wool. A good T- and B-cell separation depends on the purity of the initial lymphocyte preparation; therefore, the suspension should be as free of granulocytes and platelets as possible.
5. Lay the column flat, add approximately 0.2 mL of medium to prevent drying and incubate 30 minutes at 37 C.
6. To recover T cells, allow two washes (8 mL each) at 37 C of medium to drip through the column held vertically. The effluent contains nonadherent T cells.
7. To recover the adherent B cells, add 1.5 mL of medium to the column and repeatedly squeeze the straw. Repeat this step until 4.5-5.0 mL of the medium has been used.
8. Centrifuge both T- and B-cell suspensions 5 minutes at $1000 \times g$ and wash once with 1 mL of medium with 5% heat-inactivated FCS.
9. Resuspend cells in a minimum amount of medium (eg, 0.5 mL), check viability and adjust concentration to 2×10^6 cells/mL. On the average, this procedure should provide recovery of 80-90% of the cells.

Note

The two most common problems encountered are contamination of the B-cell suspension with granulocytes and poor lymphocyte viability. The granulocytes and dead lymphocytes must be removed from the B-cell suspension in order to obtain accurate typing results.

Reference

Fotino M. Nylon wool separation of T and B lymphocytes. In: Zachary AA, Teresi GA, eds. The ASHI laboratory manual, 2nd edition. Lenexa, KS: American Society for Histocompatibility and Immunogenetics, 1990:65-70.

Method 8.3. Lymphocyte Viability

Principle

Good viability of lymphocytes used as targets in lymphocytotoxicity tests is essential for optimal results since the endpoint for a positive test is cell death. Viable cells are able to exclude trypan blue dye.

Reagents

1. Suspension of lymphocytes isolated from whole blood or lymph nodes.
2. Trypan blue solution, 0.4%, in phosphate-buffered saline.

Procedure

1. Mix one drop of the cell suspension with one drop of 0.4% trypan blue.
2. Place the mixture on a slide, cover with a cover slip and incubate at room temperature for 4-5 minutes.
3. Examine the mixture using phase-contrast microscopy. Viable cells will refract light and appear bright. Dead cells, penetrated by the dye, will appear large and stained blue.
4. Viability = (the number of live cells/number of total cells) × 100. Viability is expressed in percent.

Interpretation

A 90% viability is required for the lymphocytes used in crossmatching tests. For antigen identification, viability should exceed 80%.

Reference

Leffell MS. Assessment of purity and viability. In: Zachary AA, Teresi GA, eds. ASHI laboratory manual, 2nd edition. Lenexa, KS: American Society for Histocompatibility and Immunogenetics, 1990:38-48.

Method 8.4. Evaluation of Lymphocyte Suspension for Purity and Cell Concentration

Principle

Lymphocytes used as target cells in lymphocytotoxicity tests must be relatively pure since contamination with platelets, granulocytes and rbcs may cause false-positive or false-negative results. The cell concentration must be adjusted to 1000-2000 per 0.001 mL (1-2 × 10⁶/mL) for optimal results.

Reagents

1. Hemocytometer and phase-contrast microscope.
2. Hanks' buffered salt solution (HBSS).
3. Thrombin—100 NIH Units of thrombin per mL of PBS (pH 7.2-7.4).
4. TRIS-NH₄Cl lysing solution.
   a. Solution A. Use 20.6 g TRIS per 100 mL of distilled water. Adjust pH to 7.2-7.4 with concentrated HCl.
   b. Solution B. Use 0.83 g NH₄Cl per 100 mL distilled water.
   c. Mix one part of solution A with nine parts of solution B. If stored at 4 C, the lysing solution may be used for several weeks.

Procedure

1. Examine the lymphocyte cell preparation on a slide with a cover slip using a phase-contrast microscope.
2. If purity is unacceptable (appreciable contamination with platelets, granulocytes or rbcs) then proceed as follows:
   a. Platelet contamination.
      1) Centrifugation method: Remove platelets by 1 minute centrifugation at $1000 \times g$. Discard the supernatant and resuspend the lymphocyte pellet in HBSS.
      2) Thrombin method (alternative method to remove platelets):
         a) Add thrombin (100 U/mL) to the lymphocyte suspension ($4\text{-}8 \times 10^6$ cells/mL) to a final volume ratio of approximately 1:10 thrombin to lymphocyte suspension.
         b) Mix by inverting until platelet clumping occurs. Mix no longer than 2 minutes.
         c) Dispense into as many small volume conical centrifuge tubes (microfuge tubes) as required for the entire volume of lymphocyte/thrombin suspension.
         d) Centrifuge the tubes for 2 seconds (on/off) at $2000 \times g$ in a microcentrifuge to pellet the clumps of adherent cells and platelets. KEEP THE SUPERNATANT.
         e) Transfer the supernatant to another set of small microfuge tubes and centrifuge for 1 minute at $1000 \times g$ at room temperature to pellet the lymphocytes.
         f) Discard the supernatant fluid and resuspend the cell pellets in the desired medium.
   b. Granulocyte contamination.

Centrifuge the cell suspension at $4500 \times g$ for 45 seconds. Gently resuspend the pellet without breaking up the clumps and centrifuge at $1000 \times g$ for 3 seconds to sediment the clumps. Since the granulocytes are denser than the lymphocytes, most of the granulocytes will be in the pellet. Collect the supernatant fluid and examine for cell purity.
   c. Rbc contamination.
      1) Centrifugation method: Remove rbcs by quick on/off (3-second) spins in a small tabletop centrifuge.
      2) Hypotonic lysis method:
         a) Warm the NH_4Cl lysing solution to 37 C.
         b) Centrifuge the lymphocyte preparation for 10 minutes at $450 \times g$ in a 15-mL conical centrifuge tube.
         c) Completely remove the supernatant fluid from the cell button; resuspend the cells in 2-3 mL prewarmed lysing solution. Incubate at 37 C for 10 minutes.
         d) Centrifuge at $1000 \times g$ for 2 minutes and immediately remove the supernatant fluid.
         e) Wash the cells with medium. The procedure may be repeated if rbc contamination is still present.
         f) CAUTION: Multiple rbc lysing steps may cause decreased viability of lymphocytes. If lysing solution was used to prepare lymphocyte preparations that are to be separated into B and T cells by nylon wool separation, the cells MUST first be incubated in RPMI with 20% fetal calf serum prior to loading the cells on the nylon wool. This

incubation period allows the cells to "repair" any damage incurred during the lysing procedure.

   d. If the above methods do not clear the contaminating cells, consult a detailed laboratory procedure manual such as the *ASHI Laboratory Manual* for other techniques.

3. If purity is acceptable:

   a. Fill the space beneath the cover glass of a hemocytometer by touching the tip of a pipet to the angle of the floor piece with the cover glass. The space must be entirely filled but not run over.

   b. Using the central red cell area, count two rows out of the five. Count row number 2 and row number 4.

   c. Divide the total cell count by 40 (or 1 row by 20).

   d. The quotient equals cell count $\times$ 10^6/mL.

4. Adjust the concentration by dilution or centrifugation with removal of some supernatant fluid in order to achieve a final cell concentration of $1\text{-}2 \times 10^6$/mL.

Note

Attention to cell purity and proper cell concentration of the lymphocyte suspension (cell preparation) is absolutely critical to optimal test results.

References

1. Kadushin JM. Resolution of purity problems. In: Zachary AA, Teresi GA, eds. ASHI Laboratory Manual, 2nd edition. Lenexa, KS: American Society for Histocompatibility and Immunogenetics, 1990:81-6.
2. Leffell MS. Assessment of purity and viability. In: Zachary AA, Teresi GA, eds. ASHI laboratory manual, 2nd edition. Lenexa, KS: American Society for Histocompatibility and Immunogenetics, 1990:38-48.

Method 8.5. Quality Control of Complement

Principle

Each new lot of complement is tested to determine that it induces cytotoxicity in the presence of specific antibody, but that it is not cytotoxic in the absence of specific antibody. The testing procedure involves serial two-fold dilutions of complement to ensure that it is maximally active at least one dilution beyond that intended for use. Undiluted complement (full strength) is usually used routinely in all test procedures.

The complement titration is carried out with at least two different antibody specificities that react with two different test cells and with at least one cell that lacks the corresponding antigen. If possible, a strong-reacting antibody and a weak-reacting antibody are selected for the test.

Reagents

1. All new lots of rabbit serum (complement—commercial or local sources) received in the laboratory. Note: Different specifications or lots of complement may be required for Class II tests.
2. Two samples that contain HLA cytotoxic antibodies.
3. Antigen-positive and -negative target test cells.

Procedure

1. Prepare serial two-fold dilutions of the reconstituted complement in saline from 1 in 2 to 1 in 32.
2. Test the activity of the complement by performing crossmatches using the Class I crossmatch procedures (see Method 8.6) and the antigen-positive and antigen-negative target test cells with each serum. To check the comple-

ment used for Class II testing, test the activity of the serial dilutions of complement according to Method 8.9.

3. Record results on form.

Note

Acceptable limits are from a score of 8 at 1 in 2 dilution to a score of 6 at 1 in 4 dilution.

Reference

Tardif GN. Complement quality control. In: Zachary AA, Teresi GA, eds. ASHI laboratory manual, 2nd edition. Lenexa, KS: American Society for Histocompatibility and Immunogenetics, 1990:632-40.

Method 8.6. The HLA Crossmatch—Standard

Principle

Some patients have preformed antibodies to HLA Class I or Class II antigens. Such antibodies are due to prior alloimmunization secondary to pregnancy, transfusion or transplantation. If organs that possess the corresponding antigens are transplanted into these patients, they usually undergo hyperacute rejection if a Class I incompatibility exists or delayed rejection if a Class II incompatibility exists. The objective of the crossmatch is to detect such incompatibilities prior to transplantation and transplant only organs from crossmatch-compatible donors.

Samples

1. Recipient specimens
   a. Recipient serum collected within 1 month of the transplant and stored frozen. For patients who are sensitized [panel reactive antibody (PRA) > 15%] or have had a recent sensitizing event, or whose history is uncertain or unavailable, crossmatches should be done with a serum sample collected within 2 days of the transplant.
   b. Unique (frozen stored) specimens in which the PRA against panel lymphocytes was maximal.
   c. Recipient lymphocytes isolated from peripheral blood. The cells should be purified from other residual blood cells. See Method 8.4.
   d. For Class I crossmatches, use either unseparated peripheral blood lymphocytes (PBLs) or T cells. See Method 8.2.
   e. For Class II crossmatches, use B cells. See Method 8.2.
2. Donor specimens
   a. Use fresh heparinized or ACD whole blood from the donor.
   b. Use lymphocytes isolated from the donor's blood or lymph nodes. The cells should be purified from other contaminating blood cells. See Methods 8.1 and 8.4. Cells must have over 90% viability. See Method 8.3.
   c. For Class I crossmatching, use either unseparated PBLs or T cells. See Method 8.2.
   d. For Class II crossmatches, use B cells. See Method 8.2.
3. Labeling standards
   a. Blood samples must be individually labeled with the name or other unique identification of the donor.
   b. Vials containing lymph nodes or spleen must also be individually labeled.
   c. Multiple tubes bridged with one label or taped together with one label affixed are unacceptable.
   d. Unlabeled tubes placed in a labeled container are unacceptable.

Reagents

1. The same materials and reagents are needed as listed for Class I and Class II typing except for preloaded antisera typing trays.
2. Microdroplet test trays.
3. Anti-A, anti-B, A and B rbcs for ABO grouping of patient and donor.
4. Antilymphocyte serum (ALS) diluted 1 in 10 with HBSS or other suitable positive control.
5. Normal human serum (NHS) devoid of cytotoxic HLA antibody (negative control).
6. White mineral oil.

Procedure

1. Perform ABO grouping on blood specimens from the donor and the recipient. The organ donor must be ABO-compatible with the recipient.
2. Place 3-8 µL of mineral oil in each well of an unused microdroplet test plate.
3. Completely and thoroughly thaw all unique sera to be tested. Prepare the current serum specimen and the positive and negative control sera (ALS and NHS).
4. Add 1 µL of control sera to the first six wells of the microdroplet test tray as follows:

Well No.	Serum To Be Added
1	ALS 1/10
2	ALS 1/10
3	NHS
4	NHS
5	HBSS
6	HBSS

5. Prepare a 1 in 2 dilution of each serum sample to be crossmatched. Use HBSS for the diluent.
6. Use the next six wells for each recipient's serum specimen to be tested and add sera as follows:

Well No.	Serum To Be Added
7	1 µL undiluted serum
8	1 µL undiluted serum
9	3 µL undiluted serum
10	3 µL undiluted serum
11	1 µL of 1 in 2 dilution of serum in HBSS
12	1 µL of 1 in 2 dilution of serum in HBSS

7. Set up in a like manner a second tray for the autocrossmatch. In the autocrossmatch tray, the recipient serum is incubated with the recipient cells. Be sure the two trays are properly labeled.
8. Add 1 µL of the donor lymphocyte suspension to each well of the controls and recipient's serum in the crossmatch tray. Use donor T cells or donor PBLs for Class I crossmatches. Add 1 µL of the recipient lymphocyte suspension to each well of the controls and recipient's serum in the autocrossmatch tray.
9. Incubate each tray at room temperature for 30 minutes.
10. Add 5 µL of rabbit complement to each well and incubate at room temperature for 1 hour.
11. Add 3 µL of 5% eosin-Y to each well and incubate for 3 minutes.
12. Add 5-8 µL of 37% formaldehyde, pH 7.2-7.4.
13. Add coverslip, allow cells to settle for approximately 30 minutes and read.

Interpretation

See Method 8.7.

Note

In addition to the standard major crossmatch, an autocrossmatch is usually included in pretransplant crossmatching. Transplantation is permissible in the presence of a positive autocrossmatch. If the autocrossmatch is positive, further testing should be done to determine whether autoantibodies alone or a combination of auto- and alloreactivity are responsible for the positive results.

Reference

Noreen HJ. Crossmatch tests. In: Zachary AA, Teresi GA, eds. ASHI laboratory manual, 2nd edition. Lenexa, KS: American Society for Histocompatibility and Immunogenetics, 1990:307-20.

Method 8.7. The HLA Crossmatch—Alternative Methods

Principle

Several alternative methods for performing an HLA crossmatch have been developed. Detailed below are those methods most commonly used. The first three methods are more sensitive than the standard HLA crossmatch (Method 8.6). The extended incubation procedure allows more time for the reactants to be exposed to each other. The AMOS crossmatch employs a wash step prior to the addition of complement. Washing removes serum factors that inhibit complement reactivity and removes any soluble antigen-antibody complexes that compete with the target cell for complement. The antiglobulin crossmatch involves the addition of an antiglobulin reagent prior to the addition of complement. This reagent increases the number of complement binding sites on the target cell thus enhancing the cytotoxicity of the procedure. A method for a Class II crossmatch is also given.

Reagents

1. See Method 8.6.
2. The AMOS method requires a buffered salt solution (HBSS).

3. The antiglobulin method requires an anti-Kappa reagent that is commercially available.

Procedure

Extended Incubation Method

Perform tests as described in Method 8.6, except for the following:
1. Incubate recipient's serum with donor's lymphocytes for 45 minutes at room temperature.
2. Following addition of rabbit complement to each well, incubate for 1.5 hours at room temperature.

AMOS Method

Perform tests as described in Method 8.6, except for the following:
1. After incubation of serum with cells, add 5-10 µL of buffer (HBSS) to each well.
2. Allow cells to settle for 5-10 minutes or centrifuge the trays for 1 minute at $1000 \times g$.
3. Remove the supernatant buffer from the wells by flicking the trays with a sharp wrist motion.
4. Repeat wash steps 1 through 3 above two additional times.

Antiglobulin Method

1. Follow the AMOS modification of the crossmatch, including the three wash steps.
2. Prior to the addition of complement, add 1 µL of antiglobulin reagent to each well of the crossmatch trays. Note: The optimal dilution of the antiglobulin reagent must be determined by testing serial dilutions of the reagent against serial dilutions of at least one known alloantibody. The highest dilution of the antiglobulin reagent used should provide a maximum strength reaction with the highest dilution of the alloantibody.

3. Incubate 1 minute at room temperature.
4. At the end of the 1-minute incubation, add 5 µL of complement and proceed as described in Method 8.6.

Class II Crossmatch Method

1. Isolate, purify and adjust the cell concentration of B cells from the intended recipient to use as auto controls for the B-cell crossmatch.
2. Isolate, purify and adjust the cell concentration of B cells from the donor to use as targets for the B-cell crossmatch.
3. Prepare an appropriate dilution of the antiserum against B cells to be used as a positive control.
4. The remainder of the procedure is the same as that described for the Class I crossmatch with the following exceptions:
   a. B cells isolated from both the donor and recipient are used as targets.
   b. Duplicate trays are prepared for incubation of the crossmatch at two different temperatures.
   c. Incubate major crossmatch tray (recipient serum vs donor cells) and autocrossmatch tray (recipient serum vs recipient cells) at 4 C for 1 hour. Incubate an identical pair of trays at 37 C for 1 hour.
   d. The complement incubation is at room temperature for 2 hours.

Interpretation

1. The percent lysis of donor and recipient cells in the presence of recipient sera must be evaluated in comparison to the lysis of the cells in the presence of appropriate control sera.
2. The crossmatch results are interpreted according to Table 8.7-1:
3. Invalid crossmatch results include the following:
   a. Negative controls have more than 10% dead cells.
      or
   b. Positive controls are negative and no other positive reactions occur on that specific crossmatch tray.
4. Crossmatch results are valid when:
   a. Negative controls have less than 10% dead cells.
      and
   b. Positive controls are over 50% dead or positive controls are negative but expected positive reactions are present elsewhere on the crossmatch tray.
5. When reporting negative crossmatch results for recipients of cadaver organs, every dilution (1 in 1, 1 in 2 and 3 in 1) on every serum sample crossmatched must be read as negative (score of 1-2).
6. When reporting positive crossmatch results for recipients of cadaver organs:
   a. A positive reading (score of 2 or greater) at any dilution of any serum sample crossmatched denotes a positive crossmatch.
   b. Any well reported as a "no read" (NR, score of 0) for whatever rea-

Table 8.7-1. Interpretation of Class II Crossmatch Results

Score	Interpretation	%Dead Cells
1	Negative	Up to 10% > negative control
2	Positive	11–20% > negative control
4	Positive	21–50% > negative control
6	Positive	51–80% > negative control
8	Positive	81–100% > negative control
0	Not readable	

son (bubble, no cells, petrolatum in the well, defective well, etc) invalidates the crossmatch of that serum and will be recorded as a "NR" for the series (current or unique) where the serum appears.

7. Interpretation of current and unique crossmatch results must be defined by the laboratory and/or transplant director.

Notes

1. The clinical significance of preformed antibodies in the serum of transplant candidates against Class II antigens is controversial. These antibodies have been classified into "warm" and "cold" depending upon their optimal temperature for reactivity. The crossmatch is designed to detect both types of antibodies. Since autoantibodies against Class II antigens are frequently present in the serum of patients, it is important to include autocontrols in the procedure.

2. Rabbit complement optimized for DR typing and Class II crossmatching must be used in this procedure.

References

1. Cadaver donor crossmatching procedure. In: Procedure manual. Ann Arbor, MI: Transplantation Society of Michigan,1987:58-63.
2. Noreen HJ. Crossmatch tests. In: Zachary AA, Teresi GA, eds. ASHI laboratory manual, 2nd ed. Lenexa, KS: American Society for Histocompatibility and Immunogenetics, 1990:307-10.
3. Johnson AH. Antiglobulin microcytotoxicity test. In: Ray GR, ed. NIAID manual of tissue typing techniques. Bethesda, MD: National Institute of Allergy and Infectious Diseases, 1979:178-80.
4. Esquenazi V, Genco P. Cytotoxicity crossmatching. In: Tissue typing reference manual. Richmond, VA: Southeast Organ Procurement Foundation, 1987:19.1-19.15.
5. Lorentzen D. Quality control of reagents. In: Zachary AA, Teresi GA, eds. ASHI laboratory manual, 2nd edition. Lenexa, KS: American Society for Histocompatibility and Immunogenetics, 1990:646-52.

Method 8.8. HLA Class I (HLA-A, -B, -C) Antigen Typing

Principle

The basis of the procedure is cytolysis mediated by specific antibody in the presence of complement. Phenotyping for HLA Class I antigens involves a reaction between the lymphocytes to be typed with HLA antisera of known specificity in the presence of complement. Cell lysis is detected by phase microscopy. Either T lymphocytes or unseparated peripheral blood lymphocytes (PBLs) can be used as targets. Class I phenotypes are important in transplantation, disease association studies, parentage testing and transfusion practices.

Materials

1. Heparinized or citrated blood samples less than 48 hours old from which either T cells or PBLs have been isolated, purified and adjusted for cell concentration. See Methods 8.1 through 8.4.

2. HLA Class I antigen typing trays preloaded with specific HLA antisera, positive and negative controls. Commercially available typing trays specifically designed for HLA-A, -B, -C testing are widely available.

3. Fresh or lyophilized rabbit serum, suitable for HLA-A, -B, -C use.

4. Buffered formaldehyde, 37%, pH 7.2 to 7.4: add 2 mL of 5% phenol red to 500 mL of 37% reagent-grade formaldehyde. Add 1 N KOH or NaOH dropwise to achieve desired pH (salmon color). Store at room temperature and adjust pH as needed.

5. Eosin Y: dissolve 1 g eosin in 19 mL of distilled water, filter and store in the dark at 4 C. Check for precipitation, which may occur during stor-

age. Refilter if necessary to remove precipitate.

6. Liquid petrolatum (paraffin oil, light mineral oil).
7. Coverslip for typing tray.
8. Repeating syringe dispensers, 50 µL and 250 µL.
9. Jet pipet.
10. Phase microscope.

Controls

1. Most laboratories use fetal calf serum or normal serum from a nontransfused, group AB male screened and found to be negative for cytotoxic activity as the negative control serum, which is rendered free of complement activity by heat inactivation. Do not use buffer or saline as a negative control. The reactivity of the negative control defines the background cytotoxicity on the individual tray.
2. Several positive control sera are used including antilymphocyte serum, mixtures of anti-T- and anti-B-cell antibodies, or pooled serum from highly immunized individuals. The reactivity of the positive control establishes the expected outcome of positive cytotoxic reactions. Wells containing monoclonal anti-T and anti-B positive controls define the relative numbers of each cell type in the cell suspension.

Procedure

1. Prepare cells to yield a lymphocyte suspension that has maximal viability and is free of residual granulocytes, rbcs and platelets. See Methods 8.1 through 8.4.
2. Adjust the cell concentration to 2×10^6 cells/mL and mix.
3. Thaw typing trays immediately before using. Place the frozen trays on the light box and examine for empty wells while the trays are still frozen.

4. Before adding the cells to the typing trays make sure the repeating dispenser is rinsed 8 to 10 times with media or buffer. This rinsing procedure must be repeated between addition of different cells and before putting the syringe away.
5. Using a 50- or 80-µL repeating dispenser, add 1 µL of the thoroughly mixed cell suspension to each well. To avoid carryover, take care not to touch the antisera with the needle tip.
6. Either of the two techniques described below may be used to mix any wells where the cells and antisera do not initially mix:
   a. Take a fine wire and carefully mix the cells and antisera.
   b. Pass the wand of the high-frequency generator over the top of the typing tray with the lid off in a back-and-forth motion.
7. Incubate the trays at room temperature for 30 minutes.
8. Thaw the appropriate lot of complement optimized for the particular HLA-A, -B, -C typing tray. Allow the complement to thaw at room temperature and then place it at 4 C once it has completely thawed.
9. Add 5 µL of pretested HLA-A, -B, -C rabbit complement and incubate at room temperature for 1 hour.
10. Add 2-5 µL of 5% eosin to each well. Mix if necessary. Incubate for 2-3 minutes at room temperature to allow dead cells to take up the stain.
11. Add 5-10 µL of pH-adjusted formaldehyde to each well. Add enough to make a well-rounded meniscus. Mix if necessary.
12. Allow cells to settle for at least 10 minutes.
13. Lower a 50 × 75-mm microscope slide slowly until it rests on top of the wells in the tray. Avoid formation of bubbles.

14. Seal the tray by adding warm petrolatum around and under the microscope slide.
15. Trays should sit a minimum of 30 minutes before being read in order to allow the cells to settle sufficiently.
16. Examine each well microscopically using the inverted or upright phase-contrast microscope with the 10× objective and 10× or 15× eyepieces. Living cells exclude dye and are small and refractile; dead lymphocytes contain dye and are larger, flatter and stained darkly.
17. Score reaction by establishing the percentage of viable lymphocytes in the negative control and positive control wells as the baseline, and by establishing whether or not a distinct increased killing (staining) of lymphocytes occurs in the test serum wells.

Interpretation

1. Record the results according to the following scale:

Score	Interpretation	% Dead Cells
1	Negative	0-10
2	Doubtful Negative	11-20
4	Weak Positive	21-50
6	Positive	51-80
8	Strongly Positive	81-100
0	Not Readable	

2. Troubleshooting:
   a. High background reactivity. Cells have been damaged during collection, isolation, storage or transport.
   b. Cell viability is good, but cells die on plates. Cells may be killed by toxic substances (detergents, solvents, microbial products) in the reagents/equipment, or by exposure to reagents with a pH outside the physiologic range. Cell death caused by any of the above can be differentiated from complement-mediated cytotoxicity by using a complement control that substitutes heat-inactivated complement for normal complement.
   c. No cells visible on tray. Cells may have undergone lysis or disintegration. Look for cellular membrane debris in the wells.
   d. No strong positive reactions (including positive control). Absence of complement-dependent, antibody-mediated cytolysis may be due to:
      1) No serum or complement added.
      2) Inactivation/denaturation of antibody or complement prior to addition to the tray.
      3) Improper incubation temperature.
      4) Antigen excess caused by excessive number of cells expressing HLA antigens (usually platelets, monocytes).
      5) Exposure of cells to fixative prior to complement.
      6) Incomplete staining.

Notes

1. Each HLA-A, -B, -C antigen should be defined by at least one of the following:
   a. At least two different sera if both are operationally monospecific.
   b. One monospecific and two multispecific antisera.
   c. At least three multispecific antisera if only multispecific sera are used.
2. Fluorescent dyes can also be used to great advantage in staining cells. Live cells can be stained to fluoresce a different color than dead cells, allowing the observer ease of discrimination. B cells can be tagged with an antiglobu-

lin fluorescein dye, negating the need for B-cell separation prior to testing.

3. Commercially available magnetic beads coated with monoclonal anti-T-cell or anti-B-cell antibodies can be used to separate cells using a magnet applied to the test tube.

References

1. Ray JG Jr, ed. NIAID manual of tissue typing techniques 1979-1980, NIH Publication No. 83-545. Bethesda, MD: US Department of Health and Human Services, Public Health Service, National Institutes of Health, 1982.
2. Hopkins KA. Basic microlymphocytotoxicity test. In: Zachary AA, Teresi GA, eds. ASHI laboratory manual, 2nd ed. Lenexa, KS: American Society of Histocompatibility and Immunogenetics. 1990:195-201.
3. Widmann FK, ed. Standards for blood banks and transfusion services, 15th ed. Bethesda, MD: American Association of Blood Banks, 1993:42.

Method 8.9. HLA Class II (DR) Antigen Typing

Principle

The detection of HLA-DR antigens using purified B-cell preparations is based on antibody-specific, complement-dependent disruption of the cell membrane of the lymphocyte and the demonstration of cell death by penetration of the cell membrane with dye. DR typing is more difficult than HLA-A, -B, -C typing due to the variability of B-cell isolation methods and variability of complement toxicity.

Reagents

1. A purified suspension of B lymphocytes is required. See Method 8.2.
2. Testing trays and complement specifically designed for detection of HLA Class II antigens are used.

Procedure

1. Adjust the B-cell suspension to 2.0-2.5 $\times 10^6$ cells/mL and mix thoroughly.
2. The remainder of the test method is the same as that given for Class I antigen typing except that the incubation of cells and serum is for 1 hour at room temperature and the incubation following the addition of rabbit complement is for 2 hours at room temperature.

Note

When making antigen assignments, each Class II HLA antigen should be defined by at least three antisera if all are operationally monospecific. If multispecific sera must be used, at least five sera should be used to define each HLA Class II antigen.

References

1. Schreuder GMTh. Identification of class II antigens. In: Zachary AA, Teresi GA, eds. ASHI laboratory manual, 2nd edition. Lenexa, KS: American Society for Histocompatibility and Immunogenetics, 1990:178-94.
2. Standards for histocompatibility testing. American Society for Histocompatibility and Immunogenetics. ASHI Quarterly 1992;16:4.
3. Widmann FK, ed. Standards for blood banks and transfusion services, 15th ed. Bethesda, MD: American Association of Blood Banks, 1993:42.

Method 8.10. Mixed Lymphocyte Culture (MLC) Test

Principle

The mixed lymphocyte culture reaction detects the recognition of and response to cellular immune differences between cells from two individuals. Recognition of Class II antigen differences results in T-cell activation and DNA synthesis in responding cells. The degree of DNA synthesis is measured by the ability of the responding cells to incorporate radioactive thymidine into DNA. The MLC test is considered to be an in-vitro model of the afferent limb of an allograft response. The test is used in donor selection for bone marrow and kidney transplantation and in defining Class II antigen differences between different populations of cells.

Samples

1. Blood samples should be collected in heparinized tubes (green-top). All manipulations of blood should be done in the laminar flow hood to minimize contamination.
2. Lymphocytes must be fresh and have excellent viability. Enough heparinized blood is obtained to isolate an adequate number of lymphocytes for each population of cells to be tested as both stimulator cells and responder cells.
3. In addition to mixtures of the two cell populations, there should be a sufficient number of pooled, third-party cells to serve as controls.

Materials

1. Gamma irradiator, cesium-137 (half life of 30.15 ± 0.06 years).
2. Moist air incubator, 37 C with 5% CO_2 and 95% humidity.
3. Cell harvester.
4. Pooled human serum (PHS), sterile: Obtain serum from 10-20 normal untransfused males. Heat-inactivate serum at 56 C for 30 minutes. Screen serum to ensure that it does not contain antilymphocyte antibodies. Pool sera and freeze aliquots at –20 C to –80 C.
5. Complete medium: RPMI-1640 containing 25 mM Hepes buffer, 100 µg/mL penicillin, 100 µg/mL streptomycin and 10-20% PHS.
6. Scintillation counting fluid.
7. ^{3}H-methyl-thymidine (^{3}H-TdR): Specific activity of 6.7 Ci/mmol. Prepare

working solution by diluting 1 mL of 1 mCi/mL stock thymidine with 24 mL of complete culture medium, yielding a working solution of 40 µCi/mL. Store at 4 C.
8. Sterile, round-bottom 96-well tissue culture plates and materials for cell harvesting.
9. Controls
   a. Positive control should be MLC responses from control cells when stimulated by unrelated, irradiated cells. Approximate range is 15,000-75,000 cpm/culture.
   b. Negative control should be MLC responses from control cells when stimulated by irradiated autologous cells. Approximate range is 500-12,500 cpm/culture.
   c. All mononuclear cell (MNC) preparations from Ficoll-Hypaque gradient isolation should be checked for contamination with neutrophils. In case of greater than 20% neutrophil contamination, the test should be repeated.

Procedure

1. Dilute whole blood in HBSS; gently layer on top of the Ficoll-Hypaque gradient in a 5:3 ratio (blood to gradient) in 15-mL sterile, screw-cap tubes and centrifuge at $400 \times g$ for 30 minutes. See Method 8.1.
2. After centrifugation, remove MNC band and dilute at least 1:5 in RPMI-1640.
3. Wash cells twice (in RPMI-1640 supplemented with 5% PHS) at 1000 rpm for 10 minutes. After the second wash, resuspend the cells in 10 mL of culture media (RPMI-1640 plus 5% PHS and 1% penicillin-streptomycin mixture) and count on a hemocytometer slide.
4. Determine the purity of the cell suspension, the viability of the cells and

the lymphocyte concentration. See
Methods 8.3 and 8.4.

5. Adjust the cells from each individual
to 10^7/mL.

6. Transfer a small volume of "responder
cells" to a sterile tube and bring the
volume to at least 2 mL (RPMI 1640 +
20% PHS) so that the final concentration is 5×10^5 *viable cells* per mL. The
viability should be >90%.

7. Transfer a small volume of "stimulator cells" to a sterile tube and bring
the volume to at least 3 mL (RPMI
1640 + 20% PHS) so that the final
concentration is 5×10^5 viable cells
per mL. Viability should be >90%.

8. Irradiate the stimulator cells with a
dose of 30 Gy (3000 rad).

9. Distribute stimulator and responder
cells in triplicate to the wells of
round-bottom microtiter plates using
a repeating pipet. Each well should
receive 100 μL of stimulator cells and
100 μL of responder cells (5×10^4 cells
of each type per well). A sample format is available.[1]

10. Cover the microtiter plates with a
plastic lid and incubate in a 37 C moist
air incubator with 5% CO_2 for 5 days.

11. After incubation, add 25 μL of the
^{3}H-TdR working dilution (1.0 μCi).

12. Incubate as above for 20 hours (overnight).

13. After ^{3}H-TdR pulse, aspirate the cells
onto a glass-fiber filter using the cell
harvester. A variety of automated cell
harvesting machines are commercially available.

14. Mark the filter to identify the relative
positions of the cell harvests on the
filter and dry filters in a dry incubator.

15. Remove the discs from the filter strips
and place in scintillation vials.

16. Add 2.0 mL scintillation fluid to each
vial.

17. Count each vial for at least 2 minutes in a scintillation counter (Beta
counter). Determine the appropriate
counting time depending on the
manufacturer of the counter. Include a ^{3}H standard in each run. Include a vial containing only scintillation fluid as a background in each
run.

Calculations

1. Each combination of stimulator cells
and responder cells is run in triplicate and the counts per minute less
background are averaged.

2. Both stimulation ratio (SR) and percent of relative response (%RR) are
used in the reporting of the results.
The definitions are as follows:

$$SR = RD_x / RR_x$$

$$\%RR = \frac{RD_x - RR_x}{RC_x - RR_x} \times 100, \text{ where}$$

RD_x = the response of lymphocytes from recipient when
stimulated with irradiated
donor cells.

RR_x = the response of lymphocytes of the recipient when
stimulated with irradiated
cells of the recipient (autologous control).

RC_x = the average responses of
recipient when stimulated
with three unrelated, irradiated controls, or two unrelated, irradiated controls
and a pool of unrelated,
irradiated controls.

3. The calculation can be done with a
calculator or with the aid of a computer program developed specifically
for this purpose.

Interpretation

1. %RR values of 20% or less are consistent with compatibility for HLA-D
"identical" types.[1]

2. Bone marrow transplantation MLC response is defined as:
   a. Low response when < 20% RR.
   b. High response when > 20% RR.
3. Renal transplantation MLC response is defined as:
   a. Low response when < 50% RR.
   b. High response when > 50% RR.
4. Plotting a frequency histogram showing the %RR values obtained when testing family member pairs known to differ by 0, 1 or 2 haplotypes provides each laboratory with a standard that can be used to interpret clinical MLC assays when the degree of Class II incompatibility is unknown.

Notes

1. A large number of other technical variables can interfere with the proper performance of the MLC test. These include quality of reagents, bacterial contamination, incubation conditions, activity of the irradiator and of the thymidine, difficulties with harvesting and computational errors.
2. Those doing MLC tests are recommended to consult additional discussions of technical details of this complex test.

Reference

1. Mickelson EM, Hansen JA. The mixed lymphocyte culture (MLC) test. In: Zachary AA, Teresi GA, eds. ASHI laboratory manual, 2nd edition. Lenexa, KS: American Society for Histocompatibility and Immunogenetics, 1990:339-56.

Method 8.11. HLA Antibody Screening

Principle

Patient serum is tested against a panel of known cells. The percentage of panel cells reacting with the patient's serum can be determined and is reported as the panel reactive antibody (PRA). The PRA is a useful index to the degree of HLA alloimmunization of the patient. With more extensive testing the specificity of the patient's HLA antibodies can be assigned.

Reagents

1. Panels of target lymphocytes can be prepared in the laboratory and are also available commercially. Commercially available cell panels are provided with cells at the appropriate concentration frozen in microtiter trays. (See *Standards for Blood Banks and Transfusion Services.*[1])
2. Patient serum.
3. Reagents and materials for the lymphocytotoxicity test. See Methods 8.6 and 8.8.

Procedure[2]

1. Thaw and prepare commercially available panel trays according to the manufacturer's specifications.
2. Fill each well with 10 µL RPMI, centrifuge the trays at 1700 rpm for 30 seconds to collect cells into pellets and remove the DMSO cryoprotectant by flicking the tray.
3. Add 4 µL of mineral oil to each well to prevent evaporation.
4. Add 1-2 µL of test serum to each well. Include a positive control and negative control serum.
5. Incubate the trays at 25 C for 30 minutes.
6. Add 5 µL of rabbit complement and incubate for 1 hour.
7. Stain, fix, read and score reactions for each well. See Methods 8.6 and 8.8.
8. Record the baseline viability from the normal serum control and the positive control. The score of these reactions must meet criteria established in the laboratory for a valid test.

Interpretation

The PRA is expressed as a percentage of total reactivity as follows:

$$\% \text{ PRA} = \frac{\text{No. of positive reactions}}{\text{No. of cells in panel}} \times 100$$

Notes

1. Viable lymphocytes are essential. Decreased cell viability invalidates the test and requires a complete evaluation of reagents and each step of the test.
2. HLA antibody specificities can be determined with more extensive testing against panel cells with known phenotypes. For each possible specificity the number of true positive reactions, false-positive reactions, true negative reactions and false-negative reactions on the panels is recorded. A 2×2 chi square test is then used to calculate the degree of confidence in each proposed specificity. Differentiation between multiple alloantibodies and antibodies with public specificities may require extensive testing.

References

1. Widmann FK, ed. Standards for blood banks and transfusion services. 15th ed. Bethesda, MD: American Association of Blood Banks, 1993:43.
2. Esquenazi V, Gomez C, Gharagozloo H. Screening with frozen cell trays. In: Zachary AA, Teresi GA. ASHI laboratory manual, 2nd ed. Lenexa, KS: American Society of Histocompatibility and Immunogenetics, 1990:263-71.

Infectious Disease Testing

Method 9.1. Hepatitis B Surface Antigen (HBsAg) Testing (RIA/EIA)

Principle

Radioimmunoassay (RIA) and enzyme-linked immunosorbent assay (EIA or ELISA) are two of the widely used types of third-generation tests for hepatitis B surface antigen (HBsAg). Both RIA and EIA employ a solid support (eg, bead, microtiter plate) coated with unlabeled anti-HBs. The reader is referred to the manufacturer's package insert for specific instructions on each commercially available test.

Controls

1. Run replicate known positive and known negative controls supplied by the kit manufacturer with each set of donor and/or patient blood samples. Calculate the cutoff according to the manufacturer's instructions.
2. Check values for the replicate positive control specimens. If the control values do not meet the manufacturer's specifications, repeat the whole run. Validation of a run usually requires that there be a minimum ratio of the mean of the positive control to the mean of the negative control (P:N) and/or a minimum difference between the mean negative and the mean posi-

tive control and/or the readings are within absolute limits.
3. The use of positive controls from another source with counts per minute or absorbance readings close to the cutoff is one additional way to monitor run-to-run variability in the test system or lot-to-lot variation in reagents. If the low level control exceeds acceptance criteria, an investigation should be performed to identify the cause. In such cases, tests with nonreactive results may be reported as the initial test of record; test results that are reactive must be repeated as initially reactive.

Procedure

1. Add the sample to be tested to the coated solid support and incubate at the specified temperature for the time directed by the procedure being used. NOTE: Plasma incubated above 40 C may coagulate.
2. Aspirate the excess sample and wash the solid support. Washing removes extraneous protein and fluid. HBsAg in the test specimen combines specifically with the anti-HBs that has been attached to the solid support and is not removed by washing.
3. Add a specified amount of ^{125}I-labeled or enzyme-linked anti-HBs (the second antibody can be from a different species than the first and may be

monoclonal) and incubate with the solid support. Radiolabeled or enzyme-linked antibody is usually designated anti-HBs*. For some EIA methods the labeled anti-HBs* is added at the same time as the sample and the reaction involves a single incubation step.

4. Aspirate and wash the mixture to remove all labeled anti-HBs* that has not bound to solid phase.
5. Measure the amount of bound anti-HBs* with a gamma counter (or, if enzyme-labeled antibody is used, a spectrophotometer) after incubation with the appropriate substrate.
6. Document review of testing records and interpretation of results prior to release and/or reporting.

Interpretation

For both RIA and EIA a reactive result is a value that exceeds the negative results by more than the level specified by the manufacturer. The lowest value corresponding to a reactive result is referred to as the cutoff.

Notes

1. It is important that *all* reactive donor units and components be removed from inventory. Careful attention must be paid to clerical, labeling, storage and discard steps to prevent accidental release of reactive units.
2. There must be an appropriate and safe method to discard reactive units and components. Autoclaving and incineration are acceptable methods for treatment of "infectious" material. Records of the disposition of all these units must be maintained.

Reference

Hanson MR, Polesky HF. Radioimmunoassay and enzyme immunoassay methods for detecting viral hepatitis markers. Am J Clin Pathol 1983;80:590-3.

Method 9.2. Confirmation Testing for HBsAg

Principle

False-positive reactions for HBsAg are known to occur with RIA and EIA. Before a donor is designated HBsAg-positive (a status that permanently excludes him or her from donating and carries significant clinical and social consequences) it is important to perform repeat testing in duplicate and confirmatory (neutralization) testing on the original specimen. This caution is usually included in the manufacturer's package insert. If repeating the initial test in duplicate reveals a repeatedly reactive result (one or both duplicates reactive), the unit is discarded. A confirmatory neutralization test can be performed, although this is not specifically required by AABB *Standards*. If reactive test result is inhibited by incubation with human serum containing anti-HBs, but not inhibited by incubation with a human serum lacking anti-HBs,[1] the specificity of the result is confirmed. Confirmatory neutralization test reagents are available for all commercial HBsAg tests. The procedure used should be according to the instructions found in the manufacturer's package insert.

Controls

1. Known positive and negative control samples should be tested in the same manner as the donor or patient samples.
2. Check values for positive and negative controls. If the percent neutralization does not meet the specifications stated in the manufacturer's package insert, the run should be repeated.

Procedure

1. Add presumed positive serum to each of four labeled tubes, in the standard manner for the test in use.

2. Add to each of two of the tubes the same volume of a human serum known to contain anti-HBs and to the other two tubes that same volume of a human serum that does not contain anti-HBs.
3. Incubate for 30 minutes at 37 C or as specified in the package insert.
4. Add the incubated serum mixtures to each of four standard supports (bead, microtiter well) with unlabeled anti-HBs.
5. Perform the test as specified in the manufacturer's directions.

Interpretation

1. If incubation with human serum containing anti-HBs reduces the counts or absorbance by more than the amount indicated in the manufacturer's directions (often 50%), when compared to the specimen incubated with human serum lacking anti-HBs, the initial reactive result is considered specific for HBsAg.
2. If the test fails to confirm as positive, the donor may be considered for a reentry protocol.[2] (See Table 4-6.)

References

1. Kahn RA. Donor screening to prevent posttransfusion hepatitis. In: Keating LJ, Silvergleid AJ, eds. Hepatitis. Washington, DC: American Association of Blood Banks, 1981:99-125.
2. Esber EC. Recommendations for the management of donors and units that are initially reactive for hepatitis B surface antigen (HBsAg) (memorandum). Bethesda, MD: FDA Office of Biologics Research and Review, December 2, 1987.

Method 9.3. Anti-HBc Testing

Principle

Testing for antibody to hepatitis B core antigen (anti-HBc) may be part of a di-agnostic workup for patients with suspected HBV infection or part of the routine screening of a blood donor. In the former, differentiation between IgM and IgG antibody can help monitor the course of disease since IgM is usually present during the early and the acute phases, while during and after recovery, IgG anti-HBc is found. In the case of donor screening, anti-HBc may identify cases of asymptomatic or unrecognized (HBsAg nonreactive) infection with HBV.[1] Anti-HBc was recommended as a surrogate marker to identify persons who may have been infected with a NANB agent.[2] In contrast to the assays for HBsAg, most anti-HBc tests are competitive immunoassays in which labeled (isotope or enzyme) antibody competes with antibody in the sample for HBcAg attached to a solid phase. A direct sandwich assay for anti-HBc also is available. See Table 9.3-1 for a summary of the principles of various hepatitis marker tests.

Controls

Run replicate known positive and negative controls supplied by the kit manufacturer with each set of donor and/or patient samples. Calculate the cutoff according to the manufacturer's instructions. See also Method 9.1, Controls, items 2 and 3.

Procedure

1. Add equal volumes of labeled anti-HBc and sample or controls to the test well or bead coated with either naturally or recombinantly derived HBcAg.
2. Incubate at the specified temperature for the time directed by the manufacturer.
3. Wash the solid phase.
4. Measure remaining anti-HBc* in a gamma counter (or, if enzyme-labeled antibody is used, a spectropho-

Table 9.3-1. Principles of Tests for Hepatitis Markers

Test Methods				Positive Result	Test for
DIRECT METHODS (Sandwich)	Antibody-Coated Solid Phase	+ Unknown	+ ^{125}I-labeled antibody (or Enzyme-Antibody Conjugate) ⟶	cpm ↖ (or ABS)	HBsAg HBeAg
	Antigen-Coated Solid Phase	+ Unknown	+ ^{125}I-labeled Antigen (or Enzyme-Antigen Conjugate) ⟶	cpm ↖ (or ABS)	Anti-HBs
(Simultaneous Sandwich)	Antibody-Coated Solid Phase	+ { Unknown + ^{125}I-labeled Antibody (or Enzyme-Antibody Conjugate) }		⟶ cpm ↖ (or ABS)	HBsAg

CAPTURE METHODS

Antigen-Coated Solid Phase + Unknown + Enzyme-labeled Anti-Ig ⟶ ABS ← Anti-HCV

Anti-IgM-Coated Solid Phase + Unknown + Antigen + ^{125}I-labeled Antibody (or Enzyme-Antibody Conjugate) ⟶ cpm (or ABS) ← IgM Anti-HAV / IgM Anti-HBc

INDIRECT METHODS (Competitive)

Antigen-Coated Solid Phase + { Unknown + ^{125}I-labeled Antibody (or Enzyme-Antibody Conjugate) } ⟶ cpm (or ABS) → Anti-HBc / Anti-HAV / Anti-Delta

Antibody-Coated Solid Phase + { Unknown + Antigen } + ^{125}I-labeled Antibody (or Enzyme-Antibody Conjugate) ⟶ cpm → Anti-HBe

tometer) after incubation with the appropriate substrate.
5. Determine reactivity by comparison with the cutoff calculated according to the manufacturer's directions. In competitive assays nonreactive samples have high counts or absorbance readings. In sandwich assays nonreactive samples have low counts or absorbance readings. Validation of the run usually requires that there be either a minimum ratio of the mean of the negative control to the mean of the positive control (N:P) and/or a minimum difference between the mean negative and the mean positive control and/or the readings are within absolute limits.
6. Document review of testing records and interpretation of results prior to release and/or reporting.

Notes

1. The anti-HBc test used for donor screening should detect total anti-HBc (IgG and IgM).
2. As with HBsAg results, initially reactive samples for anti-HBc should be retested in duplicate. If either or both of the duplicates are reactive, the sample is designated as repeatedly reactive for anti-HBc. Results that are ± 10% of the cutoff are often difficult to reproduce. Several studies[2,3] have shown that "borderline" samples in a donor population are probably false positives. Most of these donors fail to have a reactive test when a new sample is drawn and they usually lack other evidence of prior or present HBV infection such as anti-HBs and/or HBsAg.
3. Donors who have a repeatedly reactive anti-HBc test on two donations are to be deferred from further donation of WB and components. Test results exceeding acceptance criteria on any donation is a reason to discard the unit. A blood bank may choose not to notify

donors of their exclusion for the presence of anti-HBc if the plasma is to be used for fractionation and the donor is told that only a portion of his or her donation will be used.

References

1. Zuck TF, Sherwood WC, Bove JR. A review of recent events related to surrogate testing of blood to prevent non-A,non-B posttransfusion hepatitis. Transfusion 1987;27:203-6.
2. Hanson MR, Polesky HF. Evaluation of routine anti-HBc screening of volunteer blood donors: A questionable surrogate test for non-A,non-B hepatitis. Transfusion 1987;27:107-8.
3. Schmidt PJ, Leparc GF, Samia CT. Comparison of assays for anti-HBc in blood donors. Transfusion 1988;28:389-91.

Method 9.4. Alanine Aminotransferase (ALT, ALAT) Testing

Principle

Alanine aminotransferase, previously known as serum glutamic pyruvate transferase (SGPT), is an enzyme found primarily in hepatocytes. It catalyzes the transfer of the amino group from L-alanine to 2-oxoglutarate. In an individual with liver injury or inflammation, ALT is released from the damaged cells into the blood. Elevations can occur early in patients with acute liver disease and may persist in those with chronic liver disease. In addition to viral hepatitis, ALT may be elevated in individuals with drug-induced hepatitis, biliary tract disease, hemochromatosis, Wilson's disease, alpha-1-antitrypsin deficiency, autoimmune disease, hypothyroidism, alcohol ingestion[1] and obesity.[2] Based on information from several prospective studies, donors with ALT levels above normal are more likely to be implicated in transfusion-associated hepatitis cases than donors who have a normal ALT.[3-7] This enzyme also can be transiently elevated because of the variables mentioned above and in some selected donor populations ALT levels may be higher than in others.[8]

Controls

1. Test at least one normal and one abnormal control with each run of donor and/or patient samples.
2. Control samples should have values within the range established by the reagent manufacturer.

Procedure

ALT normally is performed using a standard chemistry analyzer. These instruments vary in their testing characteristics and reagent requirements. The manufacturer's instructions for operation of the instrument and the specific test method recommended by the reagent manufacturer should be followed. The following general method is common to most ALT procedures:

1. Dispense reagent into reaction vessel.
2. Add appropriate volume of sample.
3. Incubate for the appropriate time at the recommended temperature.
4. Compare the ALT level recorded by the instrument with the established cutoff.
5. Document review of testing records and interpretaton of results prior to release and/or reporting.

Interpretation

An ALT level equal to or above the cutoff value[9] indicates that the unit is not ac-

ceptable for transfusion and should be discarded. The cutoff may be defined as two standard deviations above the log mean normal value for a population of otherwise acceptable blood donors, preferably first-time donors. The upper limit of the manufacturer's specified normal range may be used as the cutoff threshold if the institution does not wish to establish its own cutoff.

Notes

1. Most test procedures for ALT are based on measuring kinetics of the conversion of NADH to NAD (see Table 9.4-1). This type of assay requires automation that will precisely time the reaction at a carefully controlled temperature. Multiple spectrophotometric readings are used to determine the rate of change in the absorbance at a specific wavelength (340 nm).
2. Either serum or plasma can be used for ALT testing. The enzyme is labile and should be measured on the day of collection or on samples that have been refrigerated no longer than 7 days before they are tested. Hemolysis can increase the level since ALT is present in red cells. If plasma samples are used, a correction for dilution by the anticoagulant will be necessary.
3. A single ALT value above the cutoff threshold (see Interpretation, above) does not automatically require the donor to be permanently deferred. If the ALT is at or above a value that is

---

Table 9.4-1. Principle of the Alanine Aminotransferase (ALT) Test*

$$\text{1) L-alanine + 2-oxoglutarate} \xrightarrow{\text{ALT}} \text{pyruvate + L-glutamate}$$

$$\text{2) pyruvate + NADH + H}^+ \xrightarrow{\text{LDH}} \text{lactate + NAD}^+$$

*Rate of change of absorbance at 340 nm at a specified pH and temperature is proportional to ALT activity.
(NADH = nicotinamide adenine dinucleotide, reduced; LDH = lactate dehydrogenase)

twice the cutoff threshold, the donor must be permanently deferred and should be notified of the abnormal finding. Donors who, on more than one occasion, have an ALT level above the cutoff but less than twice the cutoff figure must be notified and removed from the list of eligible donors.

References

1. Hanson M, Polesky HF. Factors affecting alanine aminotransferase in blood donors. In: Hopkins R, Field S. Proceedings of the International Hepatitis Workshop. Edinburgh, Scotland: Nuclear Enterprises 1982:93-7.
2. Briere RO. Serum ALT levels: Effect of sex, race, and obesity on unit rejection rate. Transfusion 1988;28:392-3.
3. Hollinger FB. Specific and surrogate screening tests for hepatitis. In: Insalaco SJ, Menitove JE, eds. Transfusion-transmitted viruses: Epidemiology and pathology. Arlington, VA: American Association of Blood Banks, 1987:69-86.
4. Alter HJ. You'll wonder where the yellow went: A 15-year retrospective of posttransfusion hepatitis. In: Moore SB, ed. Transfusion-transmitted viral diseases. Arlington, VA: American Association of Blood Banks, 1987:53-86.
5. Alter HJ, Purcell RH, Feinstone SM, et al. Non-A,non-B hepatitis: A review and interim report of an ongoing prospective study. In: Vyas GN, Cohen SN, Schmid R, eds. Viral hepatitis. Philadelphia: Franklin Institute Press, 1978:359-69.
6. Aach RD, Szmuness W, Mosely JW, et al. Serum alanine aminotransferase of donors in relation to the risk of non-A,non-B hepatitis in recipients: The transfusion-transmitted virus study. N Engl J Med 1981;304:989-94.
7. Stevens CE, Aach RD, Hollinger FB, et al. Hepatitis B virus antibody in blood donors and the occurrence of non-A,non-B hepatitis in transfusion recipients. Ann Intern Med 1984;101:733-8.
8. Shulman I, Saxena S, Nelson J. The impact of alanine aminotransferase testing on Hispanic blood donations. Arch Pathol Lab Med 1987;111:988-9.
9. AuBuchon JP, Wilkinson SJ, Kassapian SJ, Edwards GC. Establishment of a system to standardize acceptability criteria for alanine aminotransferase activity in donor blood. Transfusion 1989;29:17-22.

Method 9.5. Screening Test for Anti-HIV-1, Anti-HIV-2, Anti-HIV-1/2, Anti-HTLV-I and Anti-HCV by Enzyme Immunoassay

Principle

The enzyme-linked immunosorbent assay (EIA or ELISA) method is widely used to screen for the presence of anti-HIV-1, anti-HIV-2, anti-HIV-1/2, anti-HTLV-I and anti-HCV. This method employs a solid phase (bead or microtiter well) coated with the appropriate viral or recombinant proteins or synthetic peptides. Most of the methods are based on detection of bound antibody, using antibody to human IgG. Some use a direct sandwich approach. In the former an initial dilution of the test sample is made, while in the latter the sample is tested undiluted. The following is a general outline of the procedure; the reader is referred to the manufacturer's package insert for specific instructions on commercially available licensed kits.

Materials

1. Sample from donor.
2. Positive and negative control sera supplied with the kit.
3. Diluent for above.
4. Virus-coated solid-phase test assembly.
5. Enzyme-labeled antihuman IgG.
6. Chromogen substrate.
7. Stop solution.
8. Pipets.
9. Incubator.
10. Washing device.
11. Spectrophotometer.

Controls

See Method 9.1.

Procedure

1. Prepare donor or patient sample as specified by the reagent manufacturer and add the prepared sample to a test well or bead coated with virus-specific proteins.
2. Incubate at the temperature specified by the manufacturer.
3. Wash the solid phase and add the specified volume of enzyme-labeled antihuman IgG.
4. Incubate at the temperature specified by the manufacturer.
5. Wash the solid phase and add the specified volume of chromogen substrate.
6. Incubate at the temperature specified by the manufacturer.
7. Add the specified volume of reagent to stop the color development.
8. Measure absorbance in spectrophotometer.
9. Calculate cutoff for test run according to the manufacturer's instructions.
10. Determine reactivity of test samples by comparing sample absorbance with the calculated cutoff. Samples with absorbance readings greater than the cutoff are reactive.
11. Document review of testing records and interpretation of results prior to release and/or reporting.

Notes

1. False-positive reactions with the EIA screening tests are known to occur (see Table 4-5). When a sample from a donor is reactive in screening tests for more than one virus it is possible that he or she has been exposed to multiple viral agents; however, it is also possible that the reactions are false positive. Several donors have been found to react nonspecifically with more than one EIA test system that uses labeled antihuman globulin for detecting the presence of bound antibody. A common feature in many of these donors is recent immunization with influenza vaccine.[1]
2. Prior to designating an individual as anti-HIV, anti-HTLV-I or anti-HCV reactive, it is important to perform further testing. Samples that are reactive on initial screening should be repeated in duplicate by the same method. Any sample reactive in one or both of the repeat tests may be tested by a second and more specific method (eg, Western blot, RIPA, RIBA, PCR) to determine the possible presence of specific viral antibody or viral mRNA.
3. If the kit controls (positive and negative) do not meet the reactivity specified by the manufacturer the entire run is invalid and should be repeated.

Reference

1. Constantine NT, Callahan JD, Watts DM. HIV testing and quality control: A guide for laboratory personnel. Durham, NC: AIDSTECH, Family Health International. 1991.

Method 9.6. Western Blot Test for Anti-HIV-1, Anti-HIV-2 and Anti-HIV-1/2

Principle

The method most widely used as a licensed, more specific test for anti-HIV-1 is Western blot. In this method, viral proteins separated on the basis of molecular weight by electrophoresis are transblotted to nitrocellulose paper. Detection of antibody to specific viral proteins is accomplished by employing an EIA method using the transblotted nitrocellulose as the solid phase. Several commercial kits are available that provide preblotted strips requiring a laboratory to perform only the EIA portion of the method. A general outline of the complete procedure is listed below; specific instructions are provided in the manufacturer's package insert.

Materials

Commercially available kits for Western blot analysis provide nitrocellulose strips that have been preblotted with viral or recombinant proteins. Use the same materials listed in Method 9.5 when using preblotted strips, except that the spectrophotometer is not needed for the Western blot. When using these kits steps 1-5 below are not required.

Procedure

1. Extract virus from cell culture and inactivate, disrupt and disintegrate by treatment with solvent/detergent or other method.
2. Separate viral proteins by electrophoresis on polyacrylamide gel.
3. Transblot separated proteins to nitrocellulose paper.
4. Incubate transblotted nitrocellulose with blocking agent to block sites that nonspecifically bind protein.
5. Cut nitrocellulose into strips containing all viral proteins.
6. Incubate individual nitrocellulose strips with blocking agent in a tube or slotted tray.
7. Add appropriate volume of patient/control sample to blocking agent for each nitrocellulose strip. The sample is added directly to the blocking agent to achieve the appropriate dilution.
8. Incubate diluted sample with nitrocellulose strips containing viral proteins.
9. Remove serum sample and wash nitrocellulose strip.
10. Add the appropriate volume of enzyme-labeled antihuman IgG to nitrocellulose strips and incubate.
11. Remove enzyme-labeled reagent and wash strip.
12. Add the appropriate volume of chromogen substrate to nitrocellulose strips and incubate.
13. Add the appropriate volume of reagent to stop color development.
14. Record and interpret band patterns. (See Fig 4-6.)
15. Document review of testing records and interpretation of results prior to release and/or reporting.

Interpretation

Interpretation of band patterns observed on Western blot is critical to accurate reporting of test results. The recommended criteria for interpretation vary with the kit or method used. For HIV Western blots, the CDC has recommended presence of antibody to at least one envelope protein and one core protein or two envelope proteins for a sample to be interpreted as reactive (see Chapter 4, p 99-101).[1] Samples having reactivity to only one virus-related band or to multiple core bands are usually interpreted as "indeterminate" and additional testing is suggested to determine the individual's HIV status. For HTLV-I, the CDC has recommended that antibodies be demonstrated to both P24 and to a glycoprotein.[2] If the reactive Western blot fails to demonstrate antibodies to a glycoprotein, then a radioimmunoprecipitation assay (RIPA) should be performed to look for such an antibody.

References

1. Centers for Disease Control. Interpretive criteria used to report Western blot results for HIV-1 antibody testing—United States. MMWR 1991;40:692-5.
2. Centers for Disease Control. Licensure of screening tests for antibody to human T-lymphotropic virus type I. MMWR 1988;37:736-40, 745-47.

Method 9.7.
Immunofluorescence Assay (IFA) for Anti-HIV-1

Principle

Cells infected with virus are fixed on a glass slide. Donor or patient serum reactive in the EIA screening tests is incubated with the fixed cells. Antibody in the sample will bind to antigen sites on the viral particles. The reaction mixture is incubated with fluorescent-labeled antihuman IgG. Following incubation and washing, binding of labeled antihuman IgG is read using a fluorescence microscope and the fluorescence pattern is interpreted.

Controls

1. Perform positive and negative controls as recommended by the reagent manufacturer.
2. Test controls and donor/patient samples with cells not infected with virus to control for nonspecific binding.
3. Control samples should be interpreted according to the manufacturer's instructions.

Procedure

1. Add prepared sample to the slide containing fixed virus-infected cells.
2. Incubate according to the test manufacturer's time and temperature recommendations.
3. Wash to remove unbound serum and antibody.
4. Incubate with fluorescent-labeled antihuman IgG.
5. Wash to remove unbound label.
6. Read under a fluorescence microscope and interpret fluorescence pattern.

Interpretation

Follow manufacturer's instructions for interpretation of fluorescence patterns.

References

1. Fluorognost HIV-1 IFA package insert. Vienna, Austria: Waldheim Pharmazeutika, 1992.
2. Use of fluorognost HIV-1 immunofluorescent assay (IFA) (memorandum). Rockville, MD: Food and Drug Administration, April 23, 1992.

Method 9.8. Recombinant Immunoblot Assay (RIBA) for Anti-HCV

Principle

Four recombinant viral proteins representing both structural and nonstructural segments of the HCV viral genome are placed on nitrocellulose strips. (See Fig 4-2.) Detection of antibody to specific viral proteins is accomplished by employing an EIA method using the nitrocellulose strips as the solid phase.

Controls

1. Reactive and nonreactive controls should be run with each batch of donor and/or patient samples.
2. A superoxide dismutase (SOD) band is included on each nitrocellulose strip to identify reactivity to this nonviral component of the recombinant proteins used.

Procedure

1. Incubate nitrocellulose strips with blocking agent.
2. Add donor/patient sample according to manufacturer's package insert.
3. Incubate for the appropriate time at the recommended temperature.
4. Wash strips to remove unbound antibody and serum.
5. Add enzyme-labeled antihuman IgG (conjugate) and incubate for the appropriate time at the temperature recommended.

6. Remove conjugate, wash and add prepared substrate.
7. Stop reaction and read band patterns.

Interpretation

Samples that show reactivity with two or more bands are considered reactive for anti-HCV. Samples that are reactive with only one band or show reactivity with the SOD band are interpreted as indeterminate.[1]

Reference

1. RIBA[tm] HCV test system (package insert). Emeryville, CA: Chiron Corporation, 1990.

Blood Collection, Storage and Component Preparation

Method 10.1. Copper Sulfate Method for Screening Donors for Anemia

Principle

This method is based on specific gravity. A drop of blood dropped into copper sulfate solution of specific gravity 1.053 becomes encased in a sac of copper proteinate, which prevents any change in specific gravity for about 15 seconds. If the drop of blood has a higher specific gravity than the solution, it will sink within 15 seconds. If not, the drop will hesitate, remain suspended or rise to the top of the solution.

This is not a quantitative test; it shows only whether the hemoglobin is below or above acceptable limits. Results indicating satisfactory hemoglobin levels are usually accurate; that is, false-positive reactions are rare. False-negative reactions occur fairly commonly and cause many inappropriate deferrals.[1] Measuring hematocrit or hemoglobin by a colorimetric method often reveals that the prospective donor is, after all, acceptable.

Reagent/Materials

1. Copper sulfate solution at specific gravity 1.053; available commer-

cially. Store in tightly capped containers to prevent evaporation. The solution should be kept at room temperature or brought to room temperature before it is used.
2. Sterile gauze; antiseptic wipes and sterile lancets.
3. Containers for disposing sharps and other biohazardous materials.

Procedure

1. Dispense a sufficient amount (at least 30 mL) of copper sulfate solution to allow the drop to fall approximately 3 inches into appropriately labeled, clean, dry tubes or bottles. Change solution daily or after 25 tests. Be sure the solution is adequately mixed before beginning each day's determinations.
2. Clean the site of skin puncture thoroughly with antiseptic solution and wipe dry with sterile gauze.
3. Using caution, puncture the finger firmly, near the end but slightly to the side, with a sterile, disposable lancet or spring-loaded, disposable needle system. A good free flow of blood is important. Do not squeeze the finger repeatedly, as this may dilute the drop of blood with excess tissue fluid and give falsely low results.

4. Collect blood in an anticoagulated capillary tube without allowing air to enter the tube:
5. Let one drop of blood fall gently from the tube at a height of about 1 cm above the surface of the copper sulfate solution.
6. Observe for 15 seconds.
7. Dispose of needles and blood-contaminated gauze in appropriate containers.

Interpretation

1. If the drop of blood sinks, the donor's hemoglobin is at an acceptable level for blood donation.
2. If the drop of blood does not sink, the donor's hemoglobin is not at an acceptable level for blood donation.

Notes

1. Alternatively, measure hemoglobin by colorimetric method or determine hematocrit.
2. A certificate of analysis from the manufacturer should be obtained with each new lot of copper sulfate solution.
3. Used solution should be disposed of as biohazardous material.

References

1. Lloyd H, Collins A, Walker W, et al. Volunteer blood donors who fail the copper sulfate screening test: What does failure mean, and what should be done? Transfusion 1988;28:467-9.
2. Nelson DA, Morris MW. Basic examination of blood. In: Henry JB, ed. Clinical diagnosis and management by laboratory methods. 18th ed. Philadelphia: WB Saunders, 1991:553-603.

Method 10.2. Preparing the Venipuncture Site

Principle

Iodophor compounds, or other sterilizing compounds, are used to sterilize the venipuncture site prior to blood collection.

Materials

1. Scrub solution: 0.7% aqueous solution of iodophor compound (eg, PVP-iodine or polymer-iodine complex); available in prepackaged single-use form.
2. "Prep" solution: 10% PVP-iodine; available in prepackaged single-use form.
3. Sterile gauze.

Procedure

1. Apply tourniquet or blood pressure cuff and identify venipuncture site; release tourniquet/cuff.
2. Scrub area at least 1.5 inches in all directions from intended site of venipuncture (ie, 3 inches in diameter) for 30 seconds with 0.7% aqueous scrub solution of iodophor compound. Excess foam may be removed, but the arm need not be dry before the next step.
3. Starting at the intended site of venipuncture and moving outward in a concentric spiral, apply "prep" solution; let stand for 30 seconds.
4. Cover the area with dry, sterile gauze if venipuncture will not be done immediately. After the skin has been prepared, it must not be touched again. Do not repalpate the vein at the intended venipuncture site.

Note

For donors sensitive to iodine (tincture or PVP), another method (eg, Exidine scrub; available commercially) should be designated by the blood bank physician.

Reference

Smith LG. Blood collection. In: Green TS, Steckler D, eds. Donor room policies and procedures. Arlington, VA: American Association of Blood Banks, 1985:25-45.

Method 10.3. Phlebotomy and Collection of Samples for Processing and Compatibility Tests

Principle

Blood for transfusion and accompanying samples is obtained from prominent veins on the donor's arm, usually in the area of the antecubital fossa.

Materials

1. Sterile collection bag containing anticoagulant, with integrally attached tubing and needle.
2. Metal clips and hand sealers.
3. Balance system to monitor volume of blood drawn.
4. Sterile gauze and clean instruments (scissors, hemostats, forceps).
5. Test tubes for sample collection.
6. Device for stripping blood in tubing.
7. Dielectric sealer (optional).

Procedure

1. Prepare donor arm as described in Method 10.2.
2. Inspect bag for any defects and discoloration. Apply pressure to check for leaks. The anticoagulant and additive solutions should be inspected.
3. Position bag carefully, being sure it is below the level of the donor's arm.
   a. If balance system is used, be sure counterbalance is level and adjusted for the amount of blood to be drawn. Unless metal clips and a hand sealer are used, make a very loose overhand knot in tubing. Hang the bag and route tubing through the pinch clamp. A hemostat should be placed before the needle is uncapped.
   b. If balance system is not used, be sure there is some way to moni-

tor the volume of blood drawn with a spring scale.
4. Reapply tourniquet or inflate blood pressure cuff. Have donor open and close hand until previously selected vein is again prominent.
5. Uncover sterile needle and do venipuncture immediately. A clean, skillful venipuncture is essential for collection of a full, clot-free unit. Tape the tubing to hold needle in place and cover site with sterile gauze.
6. Open the temporary closure between the interior of the bag and the tubing.
7. Have donor open and close hand slowly every 10-12 seconds during collection.
8. Keep the donor under observation throughout the donation process. The donor should never be left unattended during or immediately after donation.
9. Mix the blood and anticoagulant gently and periodically (approximately every 45 seconds) during collection. Mixing may be done by hand or by placing bag on a mechanical agitator.
10. Be sure blood flow remains fairly brisk, so that coagulation activity is not triggered. Rigid time limits are not warranted if there is continuous, adequate blood flow and constant agitation. Units requiring more than 8 minutes to draw may not be suitable for preparation of platelets, FFP or CRYO. A useful way to monitor the time it takes to collect the unit is to indicate the time of phlebotomy or the maximal allowable time (start time plus 8 minutes) on the bag label.
11. Monitor volume of blood being drawn. If a balance is used, blood flow will stop after the proper amount has been collected. One mL of blood weighs at least 1.053 g, the minimum allowable specific gravity for donors. A convenient figure to use is 1.06 g/mL; a unit containing 405-495 mL should weigh 429-

525 g plus the weight of the container with its anticoagulant.

12. Clamp tubing near venipuncture using a hemostat, metal clip or other temporary clamp. Release blood pressure cuff/tourniquet to 20 mm Hg or less. Next, collect blood processing sample by a method that precludes contamination of the donor unit. There are several ways in which this may be accomplished.

   a. If the blood collection bag contains an in-line needle, make an additional seal with a hemostat, metal clip, hand sealer or a tight knot made from previously prepared loose knot just distal to the in-line needle. Open the connector by separating the needles. Insert the proximal needle into a processing test tube, remove the hemostat, allow the tube to fill and reclamp tubing. Donor needle is now ready for removal.

   b. If the blood collection bag contains an in-line processing tube, be certain that the processing tube, or pouch, is full when the collection is complete and the original clamp is placed near the donor needle. Entire assembly may now be removed from the donor.

   c. If a straight-tubing assembly set is used, the following procedure should be used. Place a hemostat on the tubing allowing about four segments between the hemostat and the needle. Pull tight the loose overhand knot made in step 3. Release the hemostat and strip a segment of the tubing free of blood between the knot and toward the needle (about 1 inch in length). Reapply the hemostat and cut the tubing in the stripped area between the knot and the hemostat. Fill the required tubes by releasing the hemostat. Reclamp the tubing

with the hemostat. Since this system is open, biosafety level 2 precautions should be followed.

13. Deflate and remove tourniquet. Remove needle from arm, if not already removed. Apply pressure over gauze and have donor raise arm (elbow straight) and hold gauze firmly over phlebotomy site with the other hand.

14. Discard needle assembly into biohazard-labeled container designed to prevent accidental injury to and contamination of personnel.

15. Strip donor tubing as completely as possible into the bag, starting at seal. Work quickly, to avoid allowing the blood in the tubing to clot in the tubing. Invert bag several times to mix thoroughly; then allow tubing to refill with anticoagulated blood from the bag. Repeat this procedure a second time.

16. Seal the tubing attached to the collection bag into segments leaving a segment number clearly and completely readable. Attach a whole blood number to one segment to be stored as a retention segment. Knots, metal clips or a dielectric sealer may be used to make segments suitable for compatibility testing. It must be possible to separate segments from the container without breaking sterility of the container. If a dielectric sealer is used, the knot or clip should be removed from the distal end of the tube after a double seal is made.

17. Reinspect container for defects.

18. Recheck numbers on container, processing tubes, donation record and retention segment.

19. Place blood at appropriate temperature. Unless platelets are to be removed, whole blood should be placed at 4 C immediately after collection. If platelets are to be harvested, blood should not be chilled but should be

maintained at 20-24 C until platelets are separated. Platelets must be separated within 8 hours after collection of the unit of whole blood.

Reference

Smith LG. Blood collection. In: Green TS, Steckler D, eds. Donor room policies and procedures. Arlington, VA: American Association of Blood Banks, 1985:25-45.

Method 10.4. Preparation of Red Blood Cells

Principle

RBCs are obtained by removal of supernatant plasma from centrifuged whole blood. This procedure may be modified to prepare RBCs of a desired hematocrit.

Materials

1. Freshly collected Whole Blood, obtained by phlebotomy as described in Method 10.3. Collect blood in a collection unit with integrally attached transfer container(s).
2. Plasma extractor.
3. Metal clips and hand sealer.
4. Clean instruments (scissors, hemostats).
5. Dielectric sealer (optional).
6. Refrigerated centrifuge.

Procedure

1. Centrifuge whole blood using a "heavy" spin, with a temperature setting of 5 C. If rbcs have sedimented, centrifugation is not necessary.
2. Place the primary bag containing centrifuged or sedimented blood on a plasma expressor, and release the spring, allowing the plate of the expressor to contact the bag.
3. Clamp the tubing between the primary and satellite bags with a hemostat or, if a mechanical sealer will not be used, make a loose overhand knot in the tubing.
4. If two or more satellite bags are attached, apply the hemostat to allow plasma to flow into only one of the satellite bags. Penetrate the closure of the primary bag. A scale, such as a dietary scale, may be used to measure the expressed plasma. The specific gravity of plasma is 1.023. The removal of 230-256 g (225-250 mL) of plasma will generally result in residual red cells with a hematocrit between 0.70 and 0.80 (70 and 80%).
5. Reapply the hemostat when the desired amount of supernatant plasma has entered the satellite bag. Seal the tubing between the primary bag and the satellite bag in two places.
6. Check that the satellite bag has the same donor number as that on the primary bag and cut the tubing between the two seals.

Notes

1. If blood is collected in a single bag, modify the above directions as follows: after placing the bag on the expressor, apply a hemostat to the tubing of a sterile transfer bag, aseptically insert the cannula of the transfer bag into the outlet port of the bag of blood, release the hemostat and continue as outlined above.
2. If blood is collected in an additive system, a greater volume of plasma can be removed in step 4. After the plasma is removed the additive is allowed to flow from the attached satellite bag into the red cells. Be sure that an appropriate label and dating period are used.
3. See Table 10.4-1 to prepare RBCs of a specific (desired) hematocrit. (See also Method 11.10.)

Table 10.4-1. Removing Plasma From Units of Whole Blood (To Prepare RBCs With Known Hematocrit)

Hematocrit of Segment From Whole Blood Unit	Volume of Plasma To Be Removed	Final Hematocrit of Red Blood Cell Unit
0.40 (40%)	150 mL	0.56 (56%)
0.39 (39%)	150 mL	0.55 (55%)
0.38 (38%)	160 mL	0.55 (55%)
0.37 (37%)	165 mL	0.54 (54%)
0.36 (36%)	170 mL	0.54 (54%)
0.35 (35%)	180 mL	0.54 (54%)
0.34 (34%)	195 mL	0.55 (55%)
0.33 (33%)	200 mL	0.55 (55%)

Method 10.5. Rejuvenation of Red Blood Cells

Principle

Rejuvenation is a process that is used to restore depleted metabolites and to improve the function and posttransfusion survival of RBCs that have been stored at 4 C for 14 days or longer (the normal outdate plus 3 days).[1,2] After addition of the rejuvenation solution and incubation with the cell concentrate, the component can be prepared for transfusion or for glycerolization and freezing.

Reagents/Materials

1. RBCs obtained from a unit of Whole Blood collected in CPD or CPDA-1.
2. 50 mL Red Blood Cell Processing Solution (Rejuvesol™, Cytosol Laboratories, Braintree, MA), also referred to as rejuvenating solution. It contains pyruvate, inosine, phosphate and adenine.
3. Waterproof plastic bag.

4. Metal clips and hand sealer.
5. Sterile airway.

Method

1. Using aseptic technique, connect the container of rejuvenating solution to the RBCs with a transfer set.
2. By gravity, add 50 mL of rejuvenating solution to the RBCs. Note: A sterile airway is required if the solution is in a bottle. Gently agitate the cell/solution mixture during this addition.
3. Seal the tubing near the blood bag, and incubate the mixture for 1 hour at 37 C. Either a dry incubator or circulating waterbath can be used. If placed in a waterbath, it is essential to protect the RBCs against contamination by using a waterproof overwrap that allows complete submersion of the mixture.
4. If the rejuvenated cells are to be used within 24 hours, wash with saline (2 L unbuffered 0.9% NaCl) by an approved protocol. (Note: The rejuvenating solution is toxic and is not intended for IV administration.) Storage of the washed cells should be at 4 C.
5. If the rejuvenated cells are to be cryopreserved, glycerol can be added to the red cell/rejuvenation solution mixture following the same protocol used for preparing other units for frozen storage.
6. After completion of processing, be sure that units are appropriately labeled and that all applicable records are complete.

References

1. Valeri CR, Zaroules CG. Rejuvenation and freezing of outdated stored human red cells. N Engl J Med 1972;287:1307-13.
2. Brecher ME, Zylstra-Halling VW, Pineda AA. Rejuvenation of erythrocytes preserved with AS-1 and AS-3. Am J Clin Pathol 1991;96:767-9.

Method 10.6. RBC Cryopreservation Using High-Concentration Glycerol—Meryman Method

Principle

Long-term (10 or more years) preservation of RBCs is possible because of the availability of cryoprotective agents. High concentration of glycerol is particularly suitable for this purpose. A practical method is described below.

Materials

1. Donor blood, collected into CPD, CPDA-1.
   a. Complete all blood processing on units intended for freezing.
   b. RBCs can be stored at 1-6 C for up to 6 days before freezing.
   c. RBCs preserved in AS-1 and AS-3 can be stored at 1-6 C for up to 42 days before freezing.
   d. Following rejuvenation, RBCs can be frozen up to 3 days after their expiration date.
   e. Freeze the RBCs within 24 hours of puncturing the seal if a transfer bag and open system have been used.
2. Storage containers—polyvinyl chloride or polyolefin bags (Stericon Inc., Broadview, IL).
3. 6.2 M glycerol lactate solution (400 mL).
4. Cardboard or metal canisters for freezing (Stericon Inc).
5. Hypertonic (12%) sodium chloride solution.
6. 1-6% NaCl, 1 liter for batch wash.
7. Isotonic (0.9%) NaCl with 0.2% dextrose solution.
8. 37 C waterbath or 37 C dry warmer.
9. A commercial instrument for batch or continuous flow washing to de-glycerolize cells frozen in a high glycerol concentration.
10. Freezing tape.
11. Freezer (–65 C or colder).

Procedure

Preparing RBCs for Glycerolization

1. Prepare RBCs from Whole Blood units. Weigh the RBC unit to be frozen. The combined weight of the RBCs and the collection bag should be between 260 g and 400 g.
2. Underweight units can be adjusted to approximately 300 g with the addition of 0.9% NaCl or the plasma need not be removed. Record the weight and, if applicable, document the amount of NaCl added.
3. Document on appropriate record, the whole blood number, ABO group and Rh type, anticoagulant, date of collection, date frozen, expiration time and the initials of the person performing the procedure. If applicable, document lot number of the transfer bag.
4. Warm the RBC unit to at least 25 C, placing the unit in a red cell warmer (dry bath) for 10-15 minutes. The temperature must not exceed 38 C. Alternatively, the RBC unit could be held at room temperature for 1 to 1-½ hours.
5. Place the glycerol bottles in a water-bath at 25-37 C for 15 minutes.
6. Apply a "Red Blood Cells (Human) Frozen" label to the freezing bag in which the RBC unit is to be frozen. Also, label the bag with the following: name of the facility freezing the unit, whole blood number, ABO/Rh label, and date collected, date frozen and expiration date. Also, indicate the cryoprotective agent used.

Glycerolization

1. Document on appropriate form, the lot number of glycerol, freezing bags and 0.9% NaCl (if used).
2. Add approximately 100 mL of glycerol to the RBCs, which are being agitated on a shaker.
3. Allow 5-30 minutes for equilibration without agitation.
4. Allow the partially glycerolized rbcs to flow by gravity into the freezing bag.
5. Add the remaining 300 mL of glycerol (add smaller volumes of glycerol for smaller volumes of rbcs) slowly in a stepwise fashion. Gently mix rbcs during glycerol addition. The final glycerol concentration is 40% w/v.
6. Allow some glycerolized rbcs to flow back into the tubing for segment preparation.
7. Maintain the glycerolized rbcs at room temperature (above 24 C preferred) or warmed to 30-32 C until freezing. The recommended interval between the time the RBCs are removed from the 4 C refrigerator and the time that the unit is placed in the freezer should not exceed 4 hours.

Freezing and Storage

1. Place glycerolized RBCs in a cardboard or metal canister and store in a freezer at –65 C or colder.
2. Label the top edge of the canister with freezing tape marked with the whole blood number, ABO group and Rh type, the date frozen and expiration date.
3. The freezing rate is expected to be less than 10 C/min.
4. Do not bump or handle the frozen RBCs roughly.
5. Store the RBCs at –65 C or colder for up to 10 years. For blood of rare phenotypes, a facility's medical director may wish to extend the storage period. The medical director must document and record the unusual nature of such units and the reason for retaining them past the 10-year storage period prescribed for routine use. If new donor screening tests are being introduced, distribute the frozen rare RBCs not tested for the new markers with a label stating that the unit has been not tested or that the donor was subsequently negative for a given marker. Document the reason for distributing untested products.

Thawing and Deglycerolizing

1. Place the protective canister containing the frozen RBCs in either a 37 C waterbath or 37 C dry warmer.
2. Agitate gently to speed thawing. The thawing process takes at least 10 minutes. Thawed cells should be at 37 C.
3. After RBCs are thawed, use a commercial instrument for batch or continuous flow washing to deglycerolize cells frozen in a high glycerol concentration. Follow individual manufacturer's specific recommendations.
4. Record the lot numbers and manufacturer of all solutions and software used. Label the unit with the "Red Blood Cells (Human), Deglycerolized" label. Also, identify the collecting facility as well as the facility preparing the D-RBCs, ABO group and Rh type, whole blood number, expiration date and time to the transfer pack.
5. Dilute the unit with a quantity of hypertonic (12%) NaCl solution appropriate for the size of the unit. Allow to equilibrate for approximately 5 minutes.
6. Wash with the 1.6% NaCl until deglycerolization is complete. Approximately 2 liters of wash solution are required. To check for residual glycerol, see Method 11.11.

7. Finally, suspend the rbcs in an isotonic (0.9%) solution of NaCl with 0.2% dextrose.

8. After the final component is prepared for issue, fill the integrally attached tubing with an aliquot of rbcs sealed in such a manner that it will be available for subsequent compatibility testing.

9. D-RBCs can be stored for 24 hours at 1-6 C since an open system was used during procedure.

Note

Aliquots of serum or plasma from the donor should be labeled with the unit identification number and date for future use in testing for new disease markers. These aliquots should be stored frozen at <–65 C.

Reference

Meryman HT, Hornblower M. A method for freezing and washing RBCs using a high glycerol concentration. Transfusion 1972;12:145-56.

Method 10.7. RBC Cryopreservation Using High-Concentration Glycerol—Valeri Method

Principle

RBCs collected in 800-mL primary collection bag in CPDA-1 are stored at 4 C for 3-35 days (indated), biochemically modified to rejuvenate and frozen with 40% w/v glycerol in the 800-mL primary container. Outdated RBCs (stored for 36-38 days from collection) are also frozen using this method. The rejuvenation solution contains pyruvate, inosine, phosphate and adenine.

Materials

1. Quadruple plastic bag collection system with 800-mL primary bag. (Fenwal #4R1243 or Cutter #746-74).

2. Hand sealer clips (Fenwal 4R4418).

3. Empty 600-mL polyethylene cryogenic vials (Corning 25702 or Fisher 03-374-6).

4. SCD wafers (Haemon-etics 00325-00).

5. Freezing tape.

6. 600-mL transfer bag.

7. 50 mL Red Blood Cell Processing Solution (Rejuvesol™, Cytosol Laboratories, Braintree, MA).

8. Heat-sealable 8" × 12" plastic bags.

9. Fenwal rejuvenation harness (Fenwal 4C1921).

10. Sterile filtered airway needle (B-D 5200) (for Fenwal rejuvenation harness only).

11. Cutter rejuvenation harness (Cutter 980-52).

12. 500-mL glycerolyte 57 solution (Fenwal 4A7833) or 500-mL solution of 6.2 M glycerolization solution (Cytosol PN-5500).

13. Labels—Red Blood Cells, Frozen, Rejuvenated.

14. Corrugated cardboard storage box (7" × 5.5" × 2" outside dimensions).

Procedure

Preparing RBCs for Glycerolization

1. Collect 450 mL of whole blood in the primary bag. Invert the bag, fold it about 2 inches from the base, secure the fold with tape, and place the bag upright in a centrifuge. Centrifuge and remove the supernatant plasma. The hematocrit of the RBC unit must be 0.75 ± 0.05 (75 ± 5%).

2. Store RBCs in the 800-mL primary bag, along with the adaptor port on the tubing connecting the primary bag and transfer pack, at 1-6 C for

3-35 days (indated) or for 36-38 days (outdated).

3. Prior to rejuvenation, centrifuge stored RBCs to remove all visible plasma. The gross and net weights of the RBCs should not exceed 352 and 280 grams, respectively.

4. Transfer the plasma to the integrally connected transfer pack, fold the integral tubing and replace the hand sealer clip (not crimped).

5. Using a sterile connection device in accordance with the manufacturer's instructions, attach an empty 600-mL transfer pack to the integral tubing of the primary collection bag.

6. Transfer 1 mL of plasma to all three cryogenic vials for future testing.

Biochemical Modification of RBCs

1. Using Fenwal Rejuvenation Harness: Aseptically insert the needle of the Y-type Fenwal Harness into the rubber stopper of a 50-mL Red Blood Cell Processing Solution bottle and the coupler of the set into the adaptor port of the primary collection bag. Insert the filtered airway needle into the rubber stopper of the Red Blood Cell Processing Solution bottle.

2. Using Cutter Rejuvenation Harness: Aseptically insert the *vented white spike with the drip chamber* into the rubber stopper of the Red Blood Cell Processing Solution bottle and the *nonvented spike* into the special adaptor port on the primary collection bag.

3. With gentle manual agitation, allow 50-mL of Red Blood Cell Processing Solution to flow directly into the RBCs.

4. Heat-seal the tubing of the harness set that connects the bottle of Red Blood Cell Processing Solution to the adaptor port. The second tubing of the harness Y-set is used to add glycerol (see below).

5. Completely overwrap the 800-mL primary bag, the integrally connected empty transfer pack and the coupler of the Y-type harness and incubate the RBCs in a 37 C waterbath for 1 hour.

Glycerolization

1. Remove the numbered crossmatch segments, leaving the initial segment and number attached to the collection bag. Weigh the unit.

2. Determine the amount of glycerol to be added based on the gross or net weight of the unit from the values shown in Table 10.7-1. Mark the volume of glycerol to be added on the glycerol bottle for each of the three steps, using the factory graduations on the bottle.

Table 10.7-1. Amount of Glycerol Needed for Different Weights of RBC Units

Gross Weight of Unit (grams)*	Net Weight of Unit (grams)	Initial Addition of Glycerol (mL)	Second Addition of Glycerol (mL)	Third Addition of Glycerol (mL)	Total Glycerol Added (mL)
222–272	150–200	50	50	250	350
273–312	201–240	50	50	350	450
313–402	241–330	50	50	400	500

*Weight of the empty 800-mL primary bag with the integrally attached transfer pack and adaptor port is 72 grams (average).

3. Aseptically insert the coupler of the rejuvenation harness into the outlet port of the rubber stopper on the glycerol solution bottle. For Fenwal harness only, insert a filtered airway needle into the vent portion of the glycerol bottle stopper.

4. Place the RBC bag on a shaker. Add the amount of glycerol shown in Table 10.7-1 for the first volume while the bag is shaking at low speed (180 oscillations/minute).

5. Equilibrate the mixture for 5 minutes without shaking and add the second volume. Equilibrate for 2 minutes. Add the third volume of glycerol, using vigorous manual shaking.

6. Heat-seal the tubing between the empty bottle of glycerol and the tubing proximal to the adaptor port. Ensure that the transfer pack remains integrally attached to the primary collection bag.

7. Centrifuge the RBC-glycerol mixture and transfer all visible supernatant glycerol to the transfer pack, resuspend and mix.

8. Seal the tubing 4 inches from the primary collection bag and detach the transfer pack containing the supernatant fluid and discard.

9. Affix an overlay blood component label, the facility label, and an ABO/Rh label. Record the expiration date on the label.

10. Weigh the unit just prior to freezing and record the weight.

11. Fold over the top portion of the primary bag (approximately 2 inches). Place the primary bag into a plastic bag overwrap and heat-seal the outer bag across the top so that there is as little air as possible.

12. Place one polyethylene cryogenic vial of plasma and the plastic bag containing the glycerolized RBCs in the cardboard box.

13. Affix a "Red Blood Cells, Frozen, Rejuvenated" label, an ABO/Rh label, a facility label and original unit number on the outside of the box. Record or affix collection, freezing and expiration date on the cardboard box.

14. Freeze the unit in a −80 C freezer. No more than 4 hours should be allowed to elapse between the time the RBCs are removed from the 4 C refrigerator and the time they are placed in the −80 C freezer.

Thawing and Deglycerolization

See Method 10.6.

Reference

Valeri CR. SOP red blood cell collected in the CPDA-1 800-mL primary PVC Plastic Bag Collection System and stored for 3-35 days (indated rejuvenated red cells) or for 36-38 days (outdated rejuvenated red cells). Biochemically modified with PIPA solution prior to glycerolization in the primary 800-mL bag with the special adaptor port using 40% w/v glycerol and storage at −80 C, washed in the Haemonetics Blood Processor 115, and stored at 4 C for 24 hours prior to transfusion. Boston, MA: Naval Blood Research Laboratory, Boston University School of Medicine.

Method 10.8. Preparation of Fresh Frozen Plasma

Principle

Plasma is separated from cellular blood elements and frozen to preserve the activity of labile coagulation factors.

Materials

1. Freshly collected Whole Blood, obtained by phlebotomy as described in Method 10.3. Collect blood in a collection unit with integrally attached transfer container(s).

2. Metal clips and hand sealer.
3. Clean instruments (scissors, hemostats).
4. Dielectric sealer (optional).
5. Plasma extractor.

Procedure

1. Centrifuge blood at 4 C using a "heavy" spin within 8 hours after collection, unless also preparing platelets (see Method 10.12).
2. Place primary bag containing centrifuged blood on a plasma extractor and place the attached satellite bag on a dietary scale adjusted to zero. Express the plasma into the satellite bag and weigh the plasma.
3. Seal the transfer tubing with a dielectric sealer or metal clips, but do not obliterate the segment numbers of the tubing. Place another seal nearer the transfer bag.
4. Label the transfer bag with the unit number prior to separation from the original container and record volume of plasma on the label.
5. Cut the tubing between the two seals. The tubing may be coiled and taped against the plasma container; the segments are then available for reverse grouping or other tests, if desired.
6. Place plasma at –18 C or lower within 8 hours of collection of the donor unit.

Method 10.9. Preparation of Cryoprecipitated AHF

Principle

Coagulation Factor VIII (antihemophilia factor, AHF) can be concentrated by cryoprecipitation of freshly collected plasma. Cryoprecipitation is accomplished by rapid freezing of plasma followed by slow thawing at 1-6 C.

Materials

1. Freshly collected Whole Blood, obtained by phlebotomy as described in Method 10.3. Collect blood in a collection unit with two integrally attached transfer container(s).
2. Metal clips and hand sealer.
3. Clean instruments (scissors, hemostats).
4. Dielectric sealer (optional).
5. Plasma extractor.
6. Refrigerated centrifuge.
7. Freezing apparatus: suitable freezing devices include blast freezers or mechanical freezers capable of maintaining temperatures of –18 C or below, dry ice or an ethanol-dry ice bath. In a bath of 95% ethanol and chipped dry ice, freezing will be complete in about 15 minutes.

Procedure

1. Collect blood in a collection unit with two integrally attached transfer containers.
2. Centrifuge blood at 1-6 C using a "heavy" spin. Separate plasma from the RBCs within 8 hours of phlebotomy. Collect at least 200 mL (205 g) of cell-free plasma for processing into cryoprecipitate.
3. Freeze plasma rapidly within 8 hours of phlebotomy. The plasma should become solidly frozen within 1 hour of the time freezing was initiated. Plasma containers immersed in liquid must be protected with a plastic overwrap.
4. Allow the plasma to thaw at 1-6 C by placing the bag in a 4 C shaking waterbath or in a refrigerator. If thawed in a waterbath, use a plastic overwrap (or other means) to keep container ports dry.

5. When the plasma has a slushy consistency, follow either step below:
   a. Centrifuge the plasma at 1-6 C using a "heavy" spin. Hang the bag in an inverted position and allow the supernatant plasma to flow rapidly into the transfer bag, leaving the cryoprecipitate adhering to the sides of the primary bag. Ten to 15 mL of supernatant plasma may be left in the bag to resuspend the cryoprecipitate after thawing. Separate promptly to prevent the cryoprecipitate from redissolving and flowing out of the bag, and then refreeze immediately.
   b. Place the thawing plasma in a plasma expressor when approximately one tenth of the contents is still frozen. With the bag in an upright position, allow the supernatant plasma to flow slowly into the transfer bag, using the ice crystals at the top as a filter. The cryoprecipitate paste will adhere to the sides of the bag or to the ice. Seal the bag when about 90% of the cryoprecipitate-poor plasma has been removed and refreeze the cryoprecipitate immediately.
6. Store at −18 C or lower, preferably −30 C or lower, for up to 12 months from the date of blood collection.

Note

Plasma may be used for cryoprecipitate preparation. The plasma should be stored below −18 C (preferably below −30 C). Cryoprecipitate may be prepared from plasma anytime within 12 months of collection; the expiration date of the cryoprecipitate is 12 months from the date that the original donor blood was collected.

Method 10.10. Thawing and Pooling Cryoprecipitated AHF

Principle

Cryoprecipitated AHF should be rapidly thawed at 30-37 C. The following method permits rapid thawing and pooling of this product.

Materials

1. Circulating waterbath at 37 C (specially designed waterbaths for thawing plasma are available commercially; specially designed dry air heat equipment may be used).
2. Injection ports.
3. Sterile 0.9% sodium chloride for injection.
4. Syringes and needles.

Procedure

1. Cover the container with a plastic overwrap to prevent contaminating the ports with unsterile water, or use a device to keep the containers upright with the ports above water.
2. Resuspend the thawed precipitate carefully and completely, either by kneading it into the residual 10-15 mL of plasma or by adding approximately 10 mL of 0.9% sodium chloride and gently resuspending.
3. Pool by inserting a medication injection site into a port of each bag. Aspirate contents of one bag into a syringe and inject into the next bag. Use the ever-increasing volume to flush each subsequent bag of as much dissolved cryoprecipitate as possible until all contents are in final bag.
4. Maintain thawed product at room temperature. Cryoprecipitate must be administered within 6 hours of thawing and 4 hours of pooling if it is to be used for Factor VIII content. Pools made

from thawed individual units may not be refrozen.

Method 10.11. Preparation of Fibrin Glue

Principle

Fibrinogen contained in a single-donor cryoprecipitate can be clotted by the actions of bovine thrombin and calcium to form a material with adhesive and hemostatic properties. Fibrin glue has many surgical applications and can readily be prepared in the surgical suite.

Materials

1. Cryoprecipitate.
2. Topical bovine thrombin, 1000 units/mL.
3. Sterile 10% (w/v) calcium chloride.
4. Sterile syringe (eg, 20 mL) or container.

Procedure

1. In a sterile syringe/container, mix one volume (approximately 5 mL) of calcium chloride and an equal volume of bovine thrombin.
2. In the same syringe, combine this mixture with two volumes (approximately 10 mL) of thawed cryoprecipitate.

Notes

1. This mixture can be spread immediately over the surgical site or sprayed via syringe.
2. Alternatively, the cryoprecipitate can be placed in one syringe, and the calcium chloride and thrombin in a second syringe. The contents of both syringes can be sprayed simultaneously.
3. After the preparation of fibrin glue, the product should stay within the institution that prepared the fibrin glue and should not be shipped because it is not an FDA-licensed product.

Reference

Gibble JW, Ness PM. Fibrin glue: The perfect operative sealant. Transfusion 1990;30:741-7.

Method 10.12. Preparation of Platelets From Whole Blood

Procedure

Platelets are harvested from Whole Blood following "light-spin" centrifugation. The platelets are concentrated by "heavy-spin" centrifugation with subsequent removal of supernatant plasma.

Materials

1. Freshly collected Whole Blood, obtained by phlebotomy as described in Method 10.3. Collect blood in a collection unit with two integrally attached transfer container(s). The final container must be a plastic approved for platelet storage. Keep blood at room temperature before separating the platelet-rich plasma from the RBCs. This separation must take place within 8 hours.
2. Metal clips and hand sealer.
3. Clean instruments (scissors, hemostats).
4. Plasma extractor.
5. Dielectric sealer (optional).
6. Centrifuge, as calibrated in Method 11.5.

Procedure

1. Do not chill the blood at any time before or during platelet separation. If the temperature of the centrifuge is at 1-6 C, set the temperature control of the refrigerated

centrifuge at 20 C and allow the temperature to rise to approximately 20 C. Centrifuge the blood using a "light"spin. See Method 11.5.

2. Express the supernatant platelet-rich plasma into the transfer bag intended for platelet storage. Seal the tubing twice between the primary bag and Y connector of the two satellite bags and cut between the two seals. Refrigerate the RBCs at 1-6 C.

3. Centrifuge the platelet-rich plasma at 20 C using a "heavy" spin. See Method 11.5.

4. Express the supernatant platelet-poor plasma into the second transfer bag and seal the tubing. Some plasma should remain on the platelet button for storage, but the exact volume is not specified. AABB *Standards* requires that sufficient plasma remains with the platelet concentrate to maintain the pH at 6.0 or higher for the entire storage period, in all the units tested. This usually requires a minimum of 35 mL of plasma when storage is at 20-24 C, but 60-70 mL may be preferable. The platelet-poor plasma may be frozen promptly and stored as FFP, if the separation is completed and freezing initiated within 8 hours of collection of the blood. The volume of FFP prepared after platelet preparation will be substantially less than that prepared from WB.

Method 10.13. Resuspension of Platelets

Principle

Centrifuged platelets aggregate irreversibly if subjected to rough agitation. The procedures described permit resuspension without irreversible aggregation.

Materials

Platelet concentrate, prepared as described in Method 10.12. The container should be left stationary, with the label side down, at room temperature for approximately 1 hour.

Procedure

1. The platelet button may be resuspended in either of two ways:
   a. Manipulate the platelet container gently by hand to allow uniform resuspension.
   b. Place the container on a rotator at room temperature, permitting slow gentle agitation until the platelets are uniformly resuspended. This process may take up to 2 hours.

2. Platelets should be inspected prior to issue to ensure that no platelet aggregates are visible.

Method 10.14. Removing Plasma From Platelet Concentrates

Principle

An adequate volume of plasma is necessary for optimal storage of platelets, but occasional patients receiving the platelets may suffer ill effects if the entire volume is infused. It is permissible to centrifuge stored platelets and remove much of the plasma shortly before transfusion, but appropriate resuspension is necessary. The platelets must remain at room temperature, without agitation, for 20-60 minutes, and then undergo resuspension into the remaining plasma. Transfusion must take place within 4 hours of the time the platelet bag was entered. Volume reduction can be performed on individual units of platelets or on a pool of several units.

There is not full agreement on the optimal centrifugation rate. One study[1] found 35-55% platelet loss in several units centrifuged at $500 \times g$ for 6 minutes, compared with 5-20% loss in units centrifuged at $5000 \times g$ for 6 minutes or $2000 \times g$ for 10 minutes. The authors recommend the lower centrifugal force to avoid damaging the plastic container. A study by Moroff et al[2] found mean platelet loss to be less than 15% in 42 units centrifuged at $580 \times g$ for 20 minutes.

Materials

1. Platelet concentrate, prepared as described in Method 10.12.
2. Metal clips and hand sealer.
3. Clean instruments (scissors, hemostats).
4. Dielectric sealer (optional).
5. Centrifuge, as calibrated in Method 11.5.
6. Plasma extractor.

Procedure

1. Pool platelets into a transfer pack, using standard technique (if desired).
2. Centrifuge at 20-24 C, using one of the following protocols:
   a. $580 \times g$ for 20 minutes.
   b. $2000 \times g$ for 10 minutes.
   c. $5000 \times g$ for 6 minutes.
3. Transfer the bag, without disturbing the contents, to a plasma extractor and remove all but 10-15 mL plasma from single units. Remove somewhat more volume, proportionately, from a pool or from a concentrate prepared by hemapheresis.
4. Mark expiration time on bag as 4 hours after unit was entered, either the time of pooling or the time the seal on the individual unit was broken.
5. Leave bag at 20-24 C, without agitation, for 20 minutes, if centrifuged at

$580 \times g$ or 1 hour if centrifuged at 2000 or $5000 \times g$.
6. Resuspend platelets as described in Method 10.13.

Notes

1. Use of a sterile connecting device permits aseptic plasma removal and eliminates the need to impose a 4-hour limit on the shelf life of the final component. However, see Note 2, below.
2. Reduced volume platelet concentrates, if not transfused within 4 hours of component preparation, may not be distributed outside the processing facility as a licensed product. There are no data to support storage of reduced volume platelet concentrates.

References

1. Simon TL, Sierra ER. Concentration of platelet units into small volumes. Transfusion 1984;24: 173-5.
2. Moroff G, Friedman A, Robkin-Kline L, et al. Reduction of the volume of stored platelet concentrates for use in neonatal patients. Transfusion 1984;24:144-6.

Method 10.15. Removing Leukocytes From Apheresis Platelets

Principle

HLA alloimmunization and associated febrile reactions to platelet transfusions can be reduced in frequency by removal of leukocytes from platelet preparations. The following procedure removes about 96% of the contaminating white cells and about 21% of the platelets. The use of these leukocyte-reduced platelets can diminish undesirable transfusion reactions following incompatible platelet transfusions.

Materials

1. Platelets obtained by apheresis.
2. Plasma extractor.
3. Metal clips and hand sealer.
4. Clean instruments (scissors, hemostats).
5. Dielectric sealer (optional).
6. Centrifuge, calibrated as described in Method 11.5.

Method

1. Maintain apheresis platelets with agitation at room temperature until ready for processing to remove leukocytes.
2. Centrifuge at room temperature at $178 \times g$ for 3 minutes.
3. Express the leukocyte-reduced, platelet-rich supernatant plasma into a transfer pack, being careful not to disturb the leukocyte button.
4. Discard the bag containing the leukocyte button.
5. Mark expiration time on bag as 4 hours after unit was entered.

Notes

1. Use of a sterile connecting device permits aseptic plasma removal and eliminates the need to impose a 4-hour limit on the shelf life of the final component.
2. Filters are now commercially available that provide a superior means for leukocyte removal.

References

1. Herzig RH, Herzig GP, Bull MI, et al. Correction of poor platelet transfusion responses with leukocyte-poor HLA-matched platelet concentrates. Blood 1975;46:743-50.
2. Slichter SJ. Controversies in platelet transfusion therapy. Ann Rev Med 1980;31:509-40.

Method 10.16. Platelet Cryopreservation Using 5% DMSO—Schiffer Method

Principle

Autologous platelets collected from patients with acute leukemia in remission can be cryopreserved and subsequently made available for transfusion support during relapse.[1-4]

Materials

1. Blood freezing bag, Style #2030-2 (Chartermed, Lakewood, NJ).
2. Ultra-low temperature freezer with temperature range down to –140 C.
3. Infusion pump for 60-mL syringe.
4. Platform rocking device.
5. Metal plates with clamps.
6. 10-mL vials of sterile DMSO, Rimso-100. (Tera Pharmaceuticals, Inc., Buena Park, CA. Distributed by Research Industries Corp., Pharmaceutical Division, Salt Lake City, UT).
7. Centrifuge bags.
8. 300 and 600 mL transfer packs with couplers (Baxter Healthcare Corp., Deerfield, IL).
9. Sampling site couplers (Baxter Healthcare Corp., Deerfield, IL).
10. Sterile disposable plastic syringes—3, 10 and 60 mL.
11. 37 C waterbath.
12. 16-gauge butterfly needle with 30" tubing.
13. 18-gauge needles.
14. Blood administration set.

Procedure

Cryopreservation

1. Obtain hemapheresis platelets. Label the bag with the donor's name and the date.

2. Record the net weight of the platelet concentrate (PC).

3. Using a sampling site coupler, add 4.5 mL of additional ACD-A per 100 mL of PC *if* the platelets have been obtained by automated platelet-pheresis. (This additional ACD-A is necessary to prevent platelet clumping following centrifugation since anticoagulant ratios used in automated procedures are lower than when platelets are manually collected from individual blood units).

4. Allow the PC to stand undisturbed at room temperature for 1-2 hours to permit disaggregation of any platelet clumps.

5. Transfer the PC to a labeled 600 mL transfer pack and heat-seal the tubing approximately 6" from the bag. Discard extra tubing.

6. Strip the tubing several times, mixing the PC thoroughly (but gently) in between.

7. Heat seal the tubing 1-2" from the bag. Remove the segment and label it with the donor's name.

8. Perform a platelet count on the segment and weigh the PC; record the information.

9. If gross rbc contamination of the PC is obvious, centrifuge the PC at $65 \times g$ for 12 minutes.

10. Express the platelet-rich plasma supernatant (minus the rbc button) into another labeled 600-mL transfer pack. Obtain a specimen segment as in steps 5-7. Perform a platelet count on the segment; weigh the concentrate and record the net weight and a platelet count on a data sheet.

11. If the initial PC has few or no rbcs, skip steps 9 and 10 and proceed to step 12.

12. Calculate the platelet yield. If it is $>4.4 \times 10^{11}$, split the freeze equally such that each bag contains $\leq 4.4 \times$ 10^{11} platelets. (Example: If platelet yield = 10.5×10^{11}, split the freeze into three bags, each containing 3.5 $\times 10^{11}$ platelets.) Prepare a record for each bag of platelets frozen.

13. Centrifuge the PC at $1250 \times g$ for 15 minutes.

14. Express the platelet-poor plasma (PPP) into another 600-mL transfer pack, leaving behind the undisturbed platelet button and approximately 10 mL of plasma. Clamp the tubing between the two transfer packs; *DO NOT* seal it.

15. Gently mix the platelet button with the 10 mL of plasma.

16. Using a wet folded paper towel, *GENTLY* rub the platelet button until the mixture is homogeneous.

17. If the platelet mixture is still clumped, *STOP*. Allow it to stand undisturbed at room temperature until the clumping has disappeared, usually for 1-2 hours.

18. Using a sampling site coupler, a 60-mL syringe and an 18-gauge needle, withdraw the 10 mL of PC.

19. Unclamp the tubing between the two transfer packs and run 10-15 mL of the PPP into the now empty platelet bag. Reclamp the tubing.

20. Swirl the plasma around inside the platelet bag in order to mix any residual platelets with the plasma.

21. Using the same 60-mL syringe as in step 18, withdraw the residual platelet mixture.

22. Repeat steps 19-21 until all of the platelet mixture is withdrawn and the syringe contains a final volume of 45 mL.

23. Insert a sampling site coupler into one of the ports of a platelet freezing bag and inject the 45 mL of PC. [If performing a split freeze, repeat steps 19-23 until the volume in the platelet freezing bag equals $45 \times$ the number of bags to be frozen. (Exam-

ple: If it was determined in step 12 that the freeze is to be split into three bags, repeat steps 19-23 until the volume in the first platelet freezing bag equals 45 × 3 or 135 mL.) Mix well.

Using the same syringe, withdraw 45 mL of platelet concentrate from the first platelet freezing bag and inject it into a second platelet freezing bag. Repeat until each freeze bag contains 45 mL of platelet concentrate. (Example: There will be three freeze bags, each containing 45 mL of platelet concentrate.)]

24. Using the same syringe, withdraw 40.5 mL of plasma from the PPP bag. Draw up 4.5 mL of DMSO (final syringe volume will now equal 45 mL); gently invert the syringe several times to mix the contents.
25. Disconnect the 18-gauge needle from the syringe and connect a 16-gauge butterfly needle with 30" tubing. Insert the 16-gauge needle into the sampling site coupler already in place in the freezing bag, taking care not to puncture the bag.
26. Place the syringe in an infusion pump set to deliver 3.0 mL/minute.
27. Place the platelets (in the freezing bag) on a rocker so they will be gently mixed while the DMSO mixture is being added. Turn on the rocker and the infusion pump.
28. When all of the DMSO/plasma mixture has been injected into the freezing bag (at a setting of 3.0 mL/minute, the total running time should equal approximately 16 minutes), turn off the infusion pump and remove the syringe from the pump.
29. Turn off the rocker and remove the platelet freezing bag.
30. Withdraw any air in the freezing bag into the now empty 60-mL syringe. Remove the 16-gauge needle from the sampling site coupler in the freezing bag.

31. Clamp the freezing bag port *below* the sampling site coupler (between the bag and the coupler).
32. Remove the sampling site coupler and heat-seal the port, following the directions for the sealer.
33. Place the freezing bag flat and *gently* press it to check for leaks. If there is a leak, reseal the port.
34. Place the bag between two metal plates (to produce a final thickness of approximately 0.5 cm). Clamp the plates together and place them horizontally in the –135 C freezer.
35. For *each bag* of platelets frozen, prepare one transfer pack containing 100 mL of autologous donor plasma and one transfer pack containing 120 mL of autologous donor plasma. Label each bag with the donor's name, the date and the volume.
36. Place the bags of plasma in a freezer at ≤18 C.
37. After 24 hours, the platelets may be removed from the metal plates and filed alphabetically in the freezers.
38. File appropriate records of the cryopreserved platelets alphabetically in a directory.

Thawing

Check the Cryopreserved Platelet Directory to determine what PC units are available for the specific patient.
1. Remove one 100-mL bag and one 120-mL bag of autologous plasma (frozen on the same date as the preselected platelet concentrate) from the ≤18 C freezer. (If autologous plasma is unavailable, use ABO type-specific plasma.)
2. Remove one 10-mL vial of ACD-A from the same freezer.
3. Seal each bag of plasma in a centrifuge bag (in case of breakage) and thaw the bags in a 37 C waterbath, without agitation.

4. Thaw the vial of ACD-A in a rack in the waterbath. Make sure the water level does not reach the cap of the vial so that contamination of the ACD-A is prevented.

5. As soon as the ACD-A and the plasma have thawed, remove them from the waterbath.

6. Remove the preselected bag of frozen platelets from the –135 C freezer.

7. Seal the bag of platelets in a centrifuge bag and thaw it in the 37 C waterbath, without agitation.

8. Remove the platelets from the bath as soon as thawing is complete.

9. Using a 10-mL syringe and an 18-gauge needle, aseptically withdraw the 10 mL of ACD-A from the vial.

10. Insert a sampling site coupler into one port of the 100-mL bag of autologous plasma.

11. Wipe the coupler with an alcohol pad and inject the ACD-A through the coupler into the plasma and gently mix it.

12. Insert one end of a blood administration set into the remaining port of the 100-mL bag of plasma.

13. Insert the other end of the blood administration set into the port of the bag of thawed platelets.

14. Hang the plasma/ACD-A mixture above the platelets.

15. Place the bag of platelets on a rocker (to ensure complete mixing) and adjust the roller clamp on the solution administration set such that the plasma/ACD-A mixture is added to the platelets at a rate of 10 mL per minute (total running time will be 10-15 minutes).

16. When all of the plasma mixture has been added to the platelets, remove the platelets from the rocker.

17. Carefully disconnect the blood administration set from the bag of platelets and transfer the platelet/plasma/ACD-A mixture to a labeled 300-mL transfer pack. (The label should contain the recipient's name, the thaw date and the component type.)

18. When all of the mixture has run into the transfer pack, heat-seal the tubing approximately 1" from the transfer pack. Discard the tubing and the solution administration set.

19. Remove the label from the empty platelet freeze bag, discard the bag and staple the label to the corresponding paper record of the unit.

20. Centrifuge the thawed platelet mixture at $1250 \times g$ for 15 minutes.

21. Carefully remove the platelets from the centrifuge cup and place the bag in the plasma extractor.

22. Express the DMSO-containing supernatant plasma into another 300-mL transfer pack, leaving behind the undisturbed platelet button.

23. Heat-seal the tubing between the two transfer packs and discard the bag containing the supernatant.

24. Insert one end of a double coupler plasma transfer set into one port of the 120-mL bag of autologous plasma; insert the other end into the transfer pack containing the platelets.

25. Open the plasma transfer set roller clamp and allow a small amount (10-15 mL) of autologous plasma to run in with the platelets.

26. Using a wet folded paper towel, GENTLY rub the platelet button until the mixture is homogeneous.

27. While gently agitating the bag of platelets, open the roller clamp on the plasma transfer set and allow the remainder of the plasma to run in with the platelets.

28. Remove the plasma transfer set from the port of the bag of resuspended platelets; discard the set and the empty plasma bag.

29. Insert a sampling site coupler into the open port of the bag containing the platelets.
30. To obtain a sample of the resuspended platelets, wipe the coupler with an alcohol pad and insert a 3-mL syringe and an 18-gauge needle.
31. Withdraw 1-2 mL of platelets into the syringe, but do not remove the syringe from the sampling site coupler. Invert the bag several times so the platelet suspension is thoroughly mixed, then inject the sample in the syringe back into the bag.
32. Repeat step 31 two or three times (so the specimen will be a representative sample) and remove the syringe from the sampling site coupler.
33. Perform a platelet count on the sample and obtain the net weight of the final bag of resuspended platelets. Calculate the platelet yield and the percent recovery. Record the data on the unit record sheet. Record the final platelet volume on the bag label.

References

1. Schiffer CA, Aisner J, Wiernik PH. Frozen autologous platelet transfusion for patients with leukemia. N Engl J Med 1978;299:7-12.
2. Daly PA, Schiffer CA, Aisner J, Wiernik PH. Successful transfusions of platelets cryopreserved for more than 3 years. Blood 1979;54:1023-7.
3. Schiffer CA, Aisner J, Dutcher JP. Platelet cryopreservation using dimethyl sulfoxide. Ann NY Acad Sci 1983;411:161-9.
4. Schiffer CA. Personal communication.

Method 10.17. Platelet Cryopreservation Using 6% DMSO—Valeri Method

Principle

Autologous platelets collected from patients with acute leukemia in remission can be frozen and made available during relapse for transfusion support.[1-3] The procedure may also be used for allogeneic platelets for military use and for alloimmunized patients.

Materials

1. 500-mL polyolefin freezing bag (Biological Storage Bag Style RCM-93, Stericon Inc, Broadview, IL).
2. 1-L polyolefin freezing bag (Biological Storage Bag, Style RCM-3, Stericon Inc).
3. −80 C mechanical freezer.
4. 37 C waterbath.
5. 1 L DMSO (BP 231-1, Fisher Scientific Co., Medford, MA).
6. Wrist action shaker (Burrell Corp., Philadelphia, PA).
7. Acid Citrate Dextrose (ACD), Formula-A (Baxter Healthcare Corp., Fenwal Divison, Deerfield, IL).
8. TA-2 PVC transfer packs (Baxter Healthcare Corp).
9. Aluminum canister [style RCM-3D (14-3/8" × 9-1/8" × 1/2") Stericon Inc]. A larger canister, Style RCM-91D, (11" × 5-5/8" × 3/8") is also available.

Procedure

Cryopreservation

1. Prepare platelets from CPD whole blood or by automated plateletpheresis using ACD-A.
2. Reduce the volume by centrifugation. Resuspend platelets in 30 mL of platelet-poor plasma (PPP) for each unit of platelets (about 7×10^{10} platelets).
3. Save the supernatant PPP in two transfer packs for later use to prepare DMSO in plasma and for washing platelets after thawing (see below).
4. Platelets can be stored at room temperature for up to 4 hours before freezing.
5. Prepare 12% DMSO in PPP by adding 3.6 mL of analytical grade DMSO to 26.4 mL of PPP.

6. Add 30 mL of 12% DMSO to 30 mL of platelets with continuous agitation over 30 minutes. A wrist action shaker at 200 oscillations/minute may be used for this purpose.
7. Place the platelet bag in an aluminum freezing frame and store it in the mid-section of a –80 C mechanical freezer.

Thawing

1. Thaw the platelets for 1-2 minutes in a 37 C waterbath.
2. Dilute the platelets with 100 mL of PPP containing 2% DMSO. Then add 12 mL of ACD-A to the platelets.
3. Centrifuge the platelets at $4500 \times g$ for 5 minutes, remove all the visible supernatant and resuspend in 30 mL of autologous PPP.
4. Store the platelets at room temperature, but transfuse within 4 hours.

Notes

1. This method does not require rate control freezing. With the configuration and the platelet concentrate volume constraints described above, the freezing rate is about 2-3 C/min.
2. The recovery of platelets after transfusion is expected to be about 40% with a normal life span.
3. Platelet loss of 25% is expected during freezing, thawing and processing.
4. The two-step dilution removes approximately 90% of DMSO.
5. The cryopreserved platelets can be stored for at least 8 months at –80 C.
6. Polyolefin plastic bags used to freeze rbcs can be used to freeze a volume of up to 150 mL of a pool of platelet concentrates or an automated plateletpheresis product. In such cases, the plastic bag, which measures 26 × 22 cm, should be folded to reduce its surface by half before placing it in an aluminum container.

References

1. Valeri CR, Feingold H, Marchionni LD. A simple method of freezing platelets using 6% dimethyl-sulfoxide and storage at –80 C. Blood 1974;43:131-6.
2. Valeri CR. Blood banking and the use of frozen blood products. Boca Raton, FL: CRC Press, 1976:297-301.
3. Valeri CR. The current status of platelet and granulocyte cryopreservation. CRC Crit Rev Clin Lab Sci 1981;14:21-74.

Method 10.18. Procedure for Manual 2-Unit Plasmapheresis

Principle

Blood is obtained by phlebotomy using a double-bag collection unit. This is a closed system designed for the uninterrupted collection of two units of Whole Blood (WB). Each primary bag is integrally connected to one or two satellite bags for transfer of plasma and possible further component preparation.

Materials

1. Double-bag collection unit.
2. All other materials described in Method 10.3.

Procedure

1. *Assembling the equipment.* Insert a three-lead recipient set (use spike with integral airway) into a container of normal saline for injection and suspend from an upright pole; if using a rigid container, venting may be required. Remove the sterile cap from the end of the tubing and open the regulator to fill the tubing with saline and eliminate air from the system. Replace the sterile cap.
2. *Preparing the collection bag.* Tie a loose knot in the tubing of each of the primary blood bags below the "Y" connection.

3. *Setting the scale.* Attach bag No. 1 to a device for regulating volume drawn, either a standard phlebotomy monitor or a dietary scale set to zero, to allow observation of volume drawn. Place the three remaining bags on the donor's chair.

4. *Connecting infusion and phlebotomy lines.* Insert a sterile three-way stopcock to the "Y" connection of the blood bag system and attach the saline to it. At the third junction, attach a sterile 10-mL syringe with the stopcock closed at the syringe. Using the stopcock makes it possible to collect blood samples without opening the closed system.

5. *Preparing the donor.* Review the medical history and physical examination. Confirm the donor's identification. Explain the equipment and the procedure to the donor and have the donor sign the Informed Consent Form with you as a witness. Answer all the donor's questions, getting additional explanation and information from a physician or other knowledgeable personnel, if necessary. Ask the donor to empty his or her bladder. Help the donor into a comfortable position in the chair. After having the donor sign the bag labels (see step 6 below), select the vein to be used and place an inverted blood pressure cuff on the arm approximately 4 inches above the site of the venipuncture. Prepare the arm, using a standard procedure; see Method 10.3.

6. *Labeling the bags.* Print the donor's name on each bag. Have the donor sign pressure-sensitive labels and affix one to each bag that will contain components for reinfusion. Before reinfusion of the blood components, ask the donor to identify and initial each bag.

7. *Venipuncture.* Occlude the tubing leading from the needle into the first primary bag with a suitable clamp. Inflate the cuff to 40 mm Hg. Perform the venipuncture; secure the needle with tape; and place sterile 2" × 2" gauze squares over the venipuncture site. Remove the clamp from the tubing into the first collection bag.

8. *Observing the phlebotomy.* Monitor for the presence of continuous blood flow. Gently manipulate the bag at approximately 50-mL collection intervals to ensure adequate mixing with the anticoagulant solution.

9. *Ending the phlebotomy.* After 450 mL has been collected, release the pressure in the blood pressure cuff. Clamp the tubing above the "Y" connection. Tighten the knot in the tubing and apply a clamp approximately 2 inches above the knot. Cut the tubing about an inch above the knot.

10. *Obtaining a laboratory specimen and starting the saline infusion.* Turn the previously closed stopcock toward the donor to allow blood to enter the syringe. Release the clamp between the donor and the stopcock. Withdraw about 10 mL of blood into a syringe. Turn the stopcock to start the saline infusion and adjust the flow regulator. Replace the blood-filled syringe with another sterile syringe, and place the blood into properly labeled tubes for whatever laboratory tests are indicated.

11. *Handling the Whole Blood bag.* Remove the bag from the dietary scale. Strip the tubing from the knot to the bag and seal. Cut and discard the excess tubing.

12. *Balancing blood components for centrifugation.* Place the bag of blood in the centrifuge cup and place it on the balance scale. Place a bag filled with saline in another cup on the opposite side of the scale. To adjust balance, add rubber discs to the lighter cup as needed. Having the centrifuge cups

properly balanced improves separation of the blood components and reduces wear and tear on the centrifuge.

13. *Centrifugation.* Place cups opposite each other in the centrifuge and secure the lid. The temperature inside the centrifuge should be 20 C. Close the centrifuge and set the speed and time as calibrated for platelet-rich plasma. Observe the centrifuge to be sure that this speed is attained. Properly set, the machine will turn off automatically at the set time. Let the rotor come to a complete stop and open the lid. Do not stop the rotor manually and do not disturb the separation of cells and plasma by handling the bags roughly.

14. *Extracting the plasma.* Remove the cups from the centrifuge and place the blood bag in a plasma extractor. Push the spike into the primary bag; this will release the plasma into the transfer bag. After the desired volume of plasma has been obtained, clamp the tubing between the bags. Remove the primary bag from the extractor and heat-seal or double-clip the tubing above the clamp. Cut the tubing at the seal or between the clips. The primary bag now contains red cells to be returned to the donor.

15. *Transfusing RBCs.* Have the donor identify and initial the primary bag. Identify the segment numbers on the primary bag with the segment numbers on the tubing still attached to the donor. Attach the bag to the second lead of the three-way recipient set and suspend from an upright pole. Close off normal saline and open the RBC line. Adjust the flow regulator and infuse the red cells rapidly. If the donor experiences tingling around the mouth or in the fingertips, the infusion should be slowed, since this usually arises from citrate-induced hypocalcemia.

16. *Continuing plasmapheresis.* After the RBCs are returned to the donor, shut off the infusion flow regulator and begin to withdraw the second bag of whole blood. Repeat steps 8 through 15 for the completion of the second unit.

17. *Discontinuing plasmapheresis.* Clamp the tubing above the "Y" connector and remove the blood pressure cuff tape and needle. Apply pressure on the bandage over venipuncture site and have the donor raise the arm straight up and maintain pressure for at least 3 minutes to achieve hemostasis. After the allotted time, inspect the area for hemostasis and allow the donor to lower the arm if there is no bleeding.

18. *Postplasmapheresis instructions.* Apply a sterile bandage over the phlebotomy site. Have the donor leave the dressing exposed while he/she remains at the blood center, so that bleeding will be easily noticed. Observe the donor for any untoward reactions. Inform the donor of possible postphlebotomy complications, as for any other blood donor.

Method 10.19. Processing Marrow With Hydroxyethyl Starch (HES) for Rbc Removal

Principle

This procedure is used to remove red cells from allogeneic marrow that is ABO-incompatible with the recipient's plasma antibodies.

Sample

Marrow should be collected in the operating room using standard procedures. The marrow is anticoagulated with media (eg, minimal essential media with Hank's balanced salt solution) containing heparin.

Typically, 20 mL of medium containing 1000 IU heparin is mixed with each 100 mL of marrow. The marrow is then passed through sterile metal screens or a filter to produce a bone-spicule-free, single cell suspension, which is put into plastic blood transfer bags.

Materials

1. Laminar flow hood.
2. Centrifuge.
3. 1000-mL transfer bags.
4. 600-mL transfer bags.
5. Medication injection sites.
6. Minimal essential media with Hank's balanced salt solution (HBSS).
7. Hetastarch® (average molecular weight 450,000) 6% in 0.9% sodium chloride (HES).

Procedure

1. Pool all marrow in a large transfer bag. Determine total marrow volume. Insert an injection site. Mix bag well. Remove samples for preprocessing tests: nucleated cell count, differential, red cell count, hematocrit, bacterial culture. Divide marrow into transfer bags and record the volume in each bag. The number of bags and bag size is dependent on total marrow volume.
2. Calculate the amount of medium to be added to each bag so that the final hematocrit will be 0.25 (25%). Calculate the amount of HES to add so that the amount of HES in the bag is one part HES to seven parts marrow plus media.
3. Insert an injection site into the middle port of each bag. Add medium and HES. Mix well. Clamp off a coupler/needle transfer tubing with a hemostat. Insert the needle end into the injection site. Insert the coupler end into the side part of a transfer bag.
4. Invert marrow bag. Suspend bag from a hook, and allow rbcs to sediment undisturbed. When plasma-cell interface be-

comes almost clear (after 30-60 minutes), release clamp on transfer tubing, and allow rbcs to flow into attached bag. Drain tubing into red cell bag, and seal tubing close to bag. Weigh all bags. Pool leukocyte-rich plasma into one bag.

5. Remove a sample for nucleated cell count and differential. If the number of nucleated cells collected is not a sufficient dose for the patient protocol, repeat steps 2-4 with the sedimented red cell bags.
6. Centrifuge the nucleated cell rich plasma at 4500 × g for 10 minutes at 20-24 C. Remove plasma into a transfer bag leaving 30-50 mL on the marrow. Pool all marrow into one bag and mix well. Remove samples for post-processing tests: nucleated cell count, differential, red cell count and bacterial culture.

References

1. Thomas ED, Storb R. Technique for human marrow grafting. Blood 1970;36:507-14.
2. Lasky LC, Warkentin PI, Kersey JH, et al. Hemotherapy in patients undergoing blood group incompatible bone marrow transplantation. Transfusion 1983;23:277-85.

Suggested Reading

Areman EM, Deeg HJ, Sacher RA, eds. Bone marrow processing: A manual of current techniques. Philadelphia, PA: FA Davis, 1991.

Method 10.20. Surgical Bone Donor Selection

Principle

Bone can be collected from living donors undergoing orthopedic surgery (eg, total hip replacement). These surgical bones, stored frozen at −65 C or colder are used in patients requiring bone transplants to fill bone defects.

Bone can also be collected from cadavers. However, the collection, preparation and processing is conducted in multipurpose tissue banks.

If these activities are performed in a transfusion service, they must be under the supervision of the medical director.

Materials

1. Surgical bone medical history and consent form.
2. Bone donation information pamphlet.

Procedure

1. Identify patients scheduled for total hip and knee replacement, since they are candidates for femoral head and tibial wedge donations, respectively. This can be done at the time of autologous blood donation or when the surgery is scheduled.
2. For each suitable donor, request that the donor read the facility's bone donation information pamphlet.
3. Complete a health history assessment using the surgical bone medical history form.
4. Inform each donor that repeat testing for anti-HIV-1/HIV-2 and anti-HCV will be required at 6 months or longer following donation.
5. Have the donor sign this form, which also contains consent to donate bone.
6. Apply the same recipient safety criteria for allogeneic blood donation to bone donors. Exclude patients with severe bone disease and those with severe rheumatoid arthritis as bone donors.
7. If the donor is accepted after a health history assessment, record the date of donation (ie, date of surgery) in the department's surgical bone schedule.

References

1. Technical manual for tissue banking. McLean, VA: American Association of Tissue Banks, 1992.
2. Technical manual for surgical bone banking. McLean, VA: American Association of Tissue Banks, 1987.
3. Kakaiya RM, Jackson B. Regional programs for surgical bone banking. Clin Orthop 1990;251: 290-4.

Method 10.21. Surgical Bone Collection

Principle

Advance preparation and a routine protocol are required in order to collect surgical bone from candidate donors.

Materials

1. Single or double (smaller container inside a larger one) collection containers that are either plastic or glass.
2. Impermeable wrapping material.
3. Marking pen.
4. Central supply room (sterilization) facility.
5. Thioglycollate and trypticase soy broth culture media tubes.
6. Collection record form.
7. Disposition record form.

Procedure

1. Prepare glass containers for sterilization. Record the lot number on the lid of each container with a marking pen.
2. Wrap the glass containers in two to three layers of impermeable wrapping material.
3. Submit the containers to central supply room of the hospital for steam sterilization. Use ethylene oxide sterilization for plastic containers.
4. Examine the sterilized containers to make certain that the sterilization indicator strip has changed color appropriately, that the wrapping material is not damaged and that each container package is labeled with an expiration date. The expiration date

is generally 6-60 months. Periodically, containers should be tested to show that the sterility is maintained during storage.

5. Prior to donation, collect 7 mL of EDTA and 7 mL of clotted blood sample for donor testing. The routine screening tests performed within 30 days of bone donations (HBsAg, anti-HIV-1 and -2, anti-HCV, serologic test for syphilis, ALT, anti-HBc, anti-HTLV-I/II, ABO and Rh typing) for blood donation are acceptable as the tests of record for bone donation. Otherwise, a sample at the time of bone donation must be obtained and tested.

6. Surgical bone is collected by the surgeon during surgery. The surgeon or the scrub nurse must also obtain aerobic and anaerobic cultures. Cultures are obtained by swab. Alternatively, two to three small pieces of bone obtained using a rongeur are placed in the culture vessels. After visual inspection of the removed bone, the surgeon may decide that it is not suitable for transplantation.

7. If this is the case, submit the entire bone for routine histologic examination. Those facilities desiring to have a record of the pathologic examination of any tissue removed may submit a small piece of bone for histologic studies. After the appropriate sample is collected, bone is made available for storage and eventual use.

8. The scrub nurse should place collected bone in the container soon after its collection and close the lid securely.

9. The operating room staff should label the container with the patient's name, hospital number, birth date and the date and time of collection. The hospital name may be included if the bone is to be stored in a regional program. Culture tubes are also similarly labeled.

The operating room staff should obtain the completed surgical bone medical history form from patient's chart. Bone container, culture tubes and the above records are forwarded to the blood bank.

10. The operating room staff should complete the following information on the collection record form: expiration dates and lot numbers of collection container and culture tubes, name of the patient, birth date, social security number, hospital number, the name of the surgeon, and the date and time of collection.

11. Instruct the operating room staff to place the collection container on ice if the collected bone is held in the operating room before transport to the blood bank. Bone can be stored at 1-6 C for up to 24-48 hours before it is frozen at −65 C or colder.

Method 10.22. Surgical Bone Processing

Principle

Processing of surgical bone requires inspection of the collected bone, completion of necessary blood tests, proper labeling and quarantine of the collected bone.

Materials

1. Scale to weigh the bone.
2. Plastic adhesive tape.
3. Bone container base label.
4. Unique identification numbers.
5. Test requisition forms.
6. Freezer.
7. Plastic bags.
8. Heat sealer for plastic bags.
9. Autoclave or incinerator.
10. ABO/Rh label.

11. Transplant record form.
12. Disposition record form.

Procedure

1. Visually inspect the bone received from the operating room to determine that the bone graft is not fragmented. Do not open the container.
2. Verify that the information recorded on the container label, culture tubes, collection record form and on the surgical bone medical history form is correct.
3. Check to ensure that the lid of the container is closed tightly.
4. Weigh the container and deduct the weight of the empty container to obtain the weight of the bone. Record this weight on collection record form.
5. Apply a plastic adhesive tape to the lid to ensure further security.
6. Once all of the above information is verified, remove the temporary label that was applied in the operating room from the container and apply a bone container base label.
7. Record the following information on the base label: the type of deposit (femoral head, tibial wedge, femoral head fragmented, ilium block), the unique donor number, weight of the deposit, collection date (optional) and expiration date. The base label should contain the name of the facility processing the bone, the recommended storage conditions and the preservative or antibiotic, if any.
8. Apply the unique identification number to the medical history form, collection record, blood sample tubes, culture tubes and test requisition forms.
9. Place the container into a –65 C or colder freezer and record the time of placement on the collection record form. The bone must be placed in the quarantine section of the freezer.

10. Prepare a test requisition form for routine donor screening and aerobic and anaerobic cultures. Apply the unique donor number to each requisition form.
11. Submit the blood samples for ABO/Rh, anti-HIV-1 and -2, HBsAg, anti-HBc, ALT, anti-HTLV-I/II, anti-HCV and a serologic test for syphilis. Red cell antibody identification is not necessary.
12. Submit the thioglycollate and trypticase soy broth culture tubes for culture for 7-14 days.
13. Processed bones must remain in quarantine until the results of repeat testing for anti-HIV-1 and anti-HCV at 6 months are received and are satisfactory.
14. Review the results of donor blood tests and the cultures. Record them on the collection record form. If the test results indicate that the bone should not be released for transplantation, discard the bone and arrange for autoclaving or incineration for final disposition. Record the discard on the disposition record.
15. If the initial blood tests, culture and the 6-month blood test results show that the bone is suitable for release, review surgical bone medical history form and the collection record form. If all these reviews indicate suitability for release, label the container as described below.
16. Remove the bone from quarantine section of the freezer and remove the outer plastic bag. Record the expiration date on the base label.
17. The container may become frosted with ice. If so, apply warmth with the palm of the hand resting on the container for approximately 1 minute to defrost the area where the label is to be applied. Apply appropriate ABO/Rh label.
18. Place the container into a plastic bag and seal it with heat. Staple the

transplant record form to the outer plastic bag. The transplant record form should be enclosed in a small plastic bag to prevent damage from moisture.

19. Immediately place the container into the section of the freezer designated for bones that are ready for release.

20. The expiration date is 5 years for storage at –65 C or colder. If stored at –18 C or colder, the expiration date should be 6 months.

Notes

1. Bone Inventory
   a. Store bones from donors awaiting 6-month testing in the quarantine section of the freezer. This section should be physically separate from the section containing bones ready for distribution.
   b. A large inventory of ready-to-use bones is possible if a –65 C freezer is available because of the outdating period of several years.
   c. Some transfusion services have –18 C (or lower) freezers for fresh frozen plasma. Surgical bones can be stored with fresh frozen plasma for 6 months.
   d. The size of the inventory depends upon the number of bone transplant surgeries performed, but a minimal inventory may be two to four surgical bones.
   e. An Rh– inventory may be desirable to meet the needs of Rh– patients. If an Rh– patient is transplanted with an Rh+ bone, RhIG prophylaxis may be needed. ABO matching between the recipient and the donor is not necessary. In the absence of surgical bones, other cadaveric bone products can be used. See "Cadaveric Bone" section below.

f. Each bone in quarantine or ready inventory must be recorded in the inventory log. A record of distribution should also be made in the log.

2. Cadaveric Bone
   a. Numerous products, frozen or freeze-dried, prepared from cadaveric donor bones are available.
   b. Frozen cadaveric bone can be quite large and is stored at –65 C or colder.
   c. Large bone grafts such as proximal and distal femur, proximal tibia, hemipelvis and others may be obtained from tissue banks.
   d. Freeze-dried bones are supplied in vacuum-packed glass containers and are stored at room temperatures or colder for 5 years or longer. Storage conditions for albumin are suitable for freeze-dried bone. Freeze-dried small bones include cancellous cubes, tricortical ilium blocks, matchsticks, cancellous or cortical powder and 100-200 other products.
   e. Massive frozen bones (>7 cm) are thawed in the operating room in a sterile basin containing sterile saline at 37 C, but may require 1-4 hours to thaw.
   f. Massive freeze-dried bone should be reconstituted by aseptic introduction of saline into the vacuum packed glass container and placing it in the refrigerator. Reconsitution may require 4-18 hours, depending upon the size and thickness of the graft.
   g. Small freeze-dried bones are reconstituted in the operating room with saline within 15-30 minutes.
   h. The surgeon may add antibiotics to the reconstitution medium.
   i. Depending upon the types of patients receiving bone transplants,

an inventory of small freeze-dried bones may be kept. These may include cancellous cubes and tricortical ilium blocks. Massive bone grafts are generally used in specialized centers. Records for inventory, storage, distribution, discard and transplant are similar to those for surgical bone.

Method 10.23. Surgical Bone Transportation

Principle

Surgical bone should be transported from the operating room on wet ice. Frozen bone should be removed from the inventory and transported on dry ice to the operating room for transplantation.

Materials

1. Blood transport boxes.
2. Plastic bags.
3. Crushed or cubed ice.
4. Dry ice.

Procedure A (at the time of collection)

1. Fill the plastic bag with sufficient wet ice and tie knots to prevent ice spillage.
2. Place the bag into a suitably sized blood transport box.
3. Place the bone container on the top of the ice and pack the empty space with newspaper or other clippings to prevent excessive mobility of the container inside the box. If glass containers are used, sufficient packing to prevent jarring helps to reduce cracking of the containers.

Procedure B (at the time of bone transplantation)

Transport frozen surgical bone using dry ice. The procedure is similar to that for transporting fresh frozen plasma between facilities.

Method 10.24. Surgical Bone Utilization

Principle

Prior to the issue of bone, it is necessary to document the release and recipient data.

Materials

1. Requisition for bone.
2. Order record form.
3. Blood transport boxes.
4. Dry ice.
5. Transplant record.

Procedure

1. Requests are made by the patient's physician.
2. Record the date of order, recipient's name, hospital number, surgeon's name, type of surgery, number and type of surgical bones requested, and the date of transplant surgery.
3. When bone is needed during surgery, transport the bone on dry ice to the operating room. Before use, bone is thawed by allowing the unopened container to remain at room temperature for 15-30 minutes in the operating room.
4. After the thawing interval has elapsed, bone must be removed from the container aseptically. Thawing cannot be assessed until the bone is cut. The surgeon generally removes soft tissues before bone is used. Shaping and cutting

is also performed by the surgeon as needed.

5. Surgical bones are generally used for reconstruction of acetabular and proximal femoral defects. They may also be used to fill a variety of other small bone defects.

6. A transplant record should be completed when bone is used and returned to the facility providing the graft. The following information should be recorded: date of transplant, recipient's name and hospital number, surgeon's name, the type of bone, unique identification number of the graft and any complications.

Quality Control

Method 11.1. Testing Refrigerator Alarms

Principle

The alarm on each blood-storage refrigerator should be checked periodically to be sure that it functions properly. Monthly alarm checks are appropriate until consistent behavior has been demonstrated; quarterly checks are appropriate thereafter. In addition, some alarm systems have a push button to check that the electrical circuits are intact and that the alarm rings. These electrical circuit checks should be performed regularly. The high and low temperatures of activation must be checked and the results recorded. Alarms, according to AABB *Standards*, must be set to activate at a temperature that will allow proper action to be taken before the blood or components reach an undesirable temperature.

Procedure

1. Be sure the alarm circuits are operating and the alarm is switched on. Immerse an easy-to-read mercury thermometer in the container with the alarm thermocouple, and be sure the temperature is between 1-6 C.
2. For low activation: Place the container with the thermocouple and thermometer in a pan containing a slush of ice and water colder than 0 C. To achieve this temperature, add several spoonfuls of table salt to the ice. The temperature should be –4 C or lower.
3. Close the refrigerator door so that the temperature of the interior is not significantly affected.
4. Allow the container to remain in the pan of cold slush, and gently agitate periodically until the alarm sounds. Record this temperature as the low-activation temperature.
5. Remove the container from the slush bath. Allow the fluid to return to normal temperature, and note the temperature at which audible or visible alarm signal stops.
6. For high activation: Place the container with thermocouple and thermometer in a pan containing water at 12-15 C. Keep refrigerator door closed. Allow the fluid in the container to warm slowly with occasional agitation. Record temperature at which alarm sounds as high temperature of activation.
7. Remove container from warm pan, and note temperature at which audible or visible alarm signal ceases.
8. Record the date, the identity of the refrigerator, the low temperature of activation, the high temperature of activation and the name or initials of the person performing the test.
9. Take appropriate corrective actions if temperatures of activation are too low or too high, and record the nature of the correction.

Notes

1. The thermocouple for the alarm should be easily accessible and equipped with a cord long enough so that it can be easily manipulated.
2. The thermocouple for the recording thermometer need not be in the same container as that of the alarm.
3. When the temperatures of activation are checked, the change in temperature should be allowed to occur at a rate that allows slowly responding thermocouples to be accurately measured. Too rapid a change in temperature may give the false impression that the alarm does not sound until a higher temperature is registered.
4. The low temperature of activation should be no lower than 1 C; the high temperature of activation should be no higher than 6 C. Low activation above 1 C and high activation below 6 C do not conflict with the AABB *Standards*.
5. The amount of fluid in which the thermocouple is immersed must be no larger than the volume of the smallest component stored in that refrigerator and should be stored in a container composed of the same material as that holding the component with the smallest volume or, as a minimum, material with similar heat transference characteristics. The thermocouple may be immersed in a smaller volume, but this means the alarm will go off with smaller temperature changes than those registered in a larger volume of fluid. Excessive sensitivity may create a nuisance.
6. With the one-time assistance of a qualified electrician, the required refrigerator and freezer alarm checks of units with virtually inaccessible temperature probes can be performed using an electrical modification cited by Wenz and Owens.[1]
7. Alarms should sound simultaneously at the site of the refrigerator and at the location of the remote alarms, if remote alarms are employed.

Reference

1. Wenz B, Owens RT. A simplified method for monitoring and calibrating refrigerator alarm systems. Transfusion 1980;20:75-8.

Method 11.2. Testing Freezer Alarms

Principle

Freezer temperatures may rise to unacceptable levels for a variety of reasons, some fairly common. It is essential to have a functioning alarm and to have, in a conspicuous place, directions for corrective measures to take if the freezer temperature cannot be corrected rapidly. Common causes of rising temperature include:

1. Freezer door or lid not shut properly.
2. Low level of refrigerant.
3. Compressor failure.
4. Dirty heat exchanger.
5. Loss of electrical power.

Equipment

Freezers must be equipped with a recorder for continuous temperature monitoring, and an audible alarm that sounds at a temperature that will allow appropriate action to be taken to prevent stored components from reaching undesirable temperatures. The diversity of available freezers makes it impossible to give specific instructions applicable to all storage conditions. The SOP manual for each facility must include a detailed description of the methods in local use. If suitable directions for devising a test method are not available in the owner's manual for the freezer/alarm system, the manufacturer or a refrigeration expert should be consulted.

Procedure

1. Test alarms at regular intervals, frequently enough so that personnel are proficient in handling them, and so that malfunctions, should they develop, are likely to be detected.
2. Protect frozen components from exposure to elevated temperatures during the test.
3. Use an independent thermometer that will accurately indicate the temperature of alarm activation and note the temperature registered on the recorder.
4. Warm the alarm probe and thermometer slowly. It is difficult to note the specific temperature of activation during very rapid warming, and the apparent temperature of activation will be too high.
5. Record the temperature at which the alarm sounds, the date of the test, the identity of the person testing and any observations that might suggest impaired activity.
6. Return the freezer and the alarm system to their normal conditions.
7. Take appropriate corrective actions if the alarm sounds at too high a temperature and record the nature of the correction.

Notes

1. Test battery function, electrical circuits and power-off alarms more frequently, perhaps daily, than testing the temperature of activation. Record function, date and identity of person performing the testing.
2. For units with the sensor installed in the wall, apply local warmth to the site, while protecting the contents of the freezer from a rising temperature while the door is open.
3. For units with the sensor installed in the wall or in air, allow the temperature of the entire compartment to

rise to the point at which the alarm sounds; remove the contents or protect frozen contents with insulation during this process.
4. For units with the thermocouple located in antifreeze solution, pull the container and the cables outside the freezer chest for testing, leaving the door shut and the contents protected.
5. For units with a tracking alarm that sounds whenever the temperature reaches a constant interval above the setting on the temperature controller, set the controller to a lower setting and note the temperature interval at which the alarm sounds.
6. Liquid nitrogen freezers must have alarm systems that activate at an unsafe level of contained liquid nitrogen.

Method 11.3. Monitoring Temperature During Shipment

Principle

Some form of temperature indicator or monitoring is desirable when shipping blood over a regular route. An easy method to ascertain, at time of receipt, the temperature of the contents of a shipping box used for WB or liquid-stored RBC components is described below.

Procedure

1. Remove two bags of blood or components.
2. Place the sensing end of a mercury-in-glass or electronic thermometer between the bags (labels facing out) and secure the "sandwich" with two rubber bands.
3. After a few minutes, read the temperature.
4. If the temperature of WB or RBCs exceeds 10 C, quarantine the blood until

appropriate disposition is determined.

Notes

Other suitable methods for monitoring shipments are:
1. Use time/temperature tags (3M Company, St. Paul, MN), one 110 tag per shipping carton. This will record if the temperature has exceeded 10 C.
2. Place a "high-low" mercury thermometer (Taylor Instruments, Rochester, NY) in the shipping box. This simple, reusable thermometer measures and records the highest and lowest temperature during any time period.
3. Place an R&D temperature indicator (Chek Lab Inc, Aurora, IL) in the shipping carton. This reusable device consists of a wax-like material enclosed in a small glass ampule. Small black beads are embedded in the wax. If the temperature exceeds 10 C, the wax will melt, permitting the beads to settle to the bottom.

Method 11.4. Calibrating a Serologic Centrifuge

Principle

Each centrifuge is to be calibrated upon receipt and after adjustments or repairs. Calibrating the centrifuge evaluates the behavior of rbcs in solutions of different viscosity; it does not test the reactivity of different antibodies.

For Immediate Agglutination

Materials

1. Serum containing an antibody that produces 1+ agglutination macroscopically.
2. One sample of rbcs positive for the appropriate antigen and one negative

sample. Prepare a fresh suspension of rbcs in the concentration routinely used in the laboratory (eg, 2-5%).
   a. For saline-active antibodies: Serum from a group A person (anti-B) diluted with 6% albumin to give 1+ macroscopic agglutination (3 mL 22% bovine albumin + 1 mL normal saline = 6% bovine albumin).
      Positive control: Group B rbcs in a 2-5% saline suspension.
      Negative control: Group A rbcs in a 2-5% saline suspension.
   b. For high-protein antibodies: 1 part anti-D diluted with 25-30 parts of 22% or 30% albumin to give 1+ macroscopic agglutination.
      Positive control: D+ rbcs in a 2-5% saline suspension.
      Negative control: D– rbcs in a 2-5% saline suspension.

Procedure

1. For each set of tests, saline and albumin, prepare five 10 × 75-mm or 12 × 75-mm tubes for positive reactions and a duplicate set of tubes for negative reactions. Add the serum and test cells to each tube just before centrifugation.
2. In pairs, one positive and one negative, centrifuge the tubes for different times (eg, 10 seconds, 20 seconds, 30 seconds). Observe each tube for agglutination and record observations. (See example in Table 11.4-1.)

Interpretation

The optimal time of centrifugation is the *least* time required to fulfill these criteria:
1. Agglutination in the positive tubes is as strong as determined in preparing reagents.
2. There is no agglutination or ambiguity in the negative tubes.

Table 11.4-1. Serologic Centrifuge Test Results

Criteria	Time in Seconds				
	10	15	20	30	45
Supernatant fluid clear	No	No	Yes	Yes	Yes
Cell button clearly delineated	No	No	No	Yes	Yes
Cells easily resuspended	Yes	Yes	Yes	Yes	Yes
Agglutination	±	±	1+	1+	1+
Negative tube is negative	Yes	Yes	Yes	Yes	Resuspends roughly

3. The rbc button is clearly delineated and the periphery is sharply defined, not fuzzy.
4. The supernatant fluid is clear.
5. The rbc button is easily resuspended. Since, in the example shown in the table, the 30-second and the 45-second spins fulfill these criteria, the optimal time for this centrifuge is 30 seconds.

For Washing and Antiglobulin Testing

The addition of antihuman globulin (AHG) serum to rbcs may require centrifugation conditions different from those for immediate agglutination because AHG is added to a dry rbc button. The only fluid in the tube is the AHG serum itself. Centrifugation conditions appropriate for both washing and AHG reactions can be determined in one procedure. Note that this procedure does not monitor the completeness of washing; use of globulin-coated cells to control negative AHG reactions provides this check. The procedure described below addresses only the mechanics of centrifugation.

Materials

1. Antihuman globulin (AHG) reagent, unmodified.
2. Positive control: a 2-5% saline suspension of D+ rbcs incubated for 15 minutes at 37 C with anti-D diluted to give 1+ macroscopic agglutination after addition of AHG.
3. Negative control: a 2-5% suspension of D− rbcs, incubated for 15 minutes at 37 C with 6% albumin.
4. Saline, large volumes.

Procedure

1. Prepare five pairs of tubes with positive and negative controls.
2. Fill tubes with saline and centrifuge pairs for different times, eg, 30, 45, 60, 90 and 120 seconds. The rbcs should form a clearly delineated button, with no cells trailing up the side of the tube. After the saline has been decanted, the rbc button should be easily resuspended in the residual fluid. The least time that accomplishes these goals is the optimal time for washing.
3. Repeat washing process on all pairs two more times, using time determined to be optimal.
4. Decant supernatant saline thoroughly and blot rims dry.
5. Add AHG to each of the pairs and centrifuge for different times, eg, 10, 15, 20, 30 and 45 seconds.

Interpretation

Select optimal time according to criteria described in previous procedure.

Method 11.5. Calibrating Centrifuges for Platelet Separation

Principle

Successful platelet preparation is dependent on appropriate calibration of centrifuges. Each centrifuge should be calibrated upon receipt and after adjustment or repair.

Materials

1. Freshly collected Whole Blood, obtained by phlebotomy as described in Method 10.3. Collect blood in a collection unit with two integrally attached transfer containers.
2. An EDTA tube of blood from the donor, in addition to the specimens drawn for routine processing.
3. Metal clips and hand sealer.
4. Clean instruments (scissors, hemostats).
5. Plasma extractor.
6. Dielectric sealer (optional).
7. Centrifuge for calibration. Each centrifuge should be calibrated upon receipt and after adjustment or repair.

Procedure

1. Perform a platelet count on the EDTA specimen. If the donor has a platelet count below 133×10^9/L (133,000/µL), this unit of blood should not be used for calibration.
2. Calculate the number of platelets in the unit of whole blood (WB):
   platelets/µL $\times$ 1000 $\times$ mL of WB = number of platelets in WB.
3. Prepare platelet-rich plasma (PRP) at a selected speed and time (see "light spin," Table 11.5-1).
4. Place a temporary clamp on the tubing so that one satellite bag is closed off. Express the PRP into the other

Table 11.5-1. Centrifugation for Component Preparation

Heavy Spin

Packed red cells Platelet concentrates	$\Big\}$ 5000 $\times$ g, 5 minutes
Cell-free plasma Cryoprecipitate	$\Big\}$ 5000 $\times$ g, 7 minutes

Light Spin

Platelet-rich plasma	2000 $\times$ g, 3 minutes

To calculate relative centrifugal force in g:

$$rcf \text{ (in } g) = 28.38 \text{ R*} \left(\frac{rpm}{1000}\right)^2$$

*R = radius of centrifuge rotor in inches

Times include acceleration but not deceleration times. Times given are approximations only. Each individual centrifuge must be evaluated for the preparation of the various components.

satellite bag. Seal close to primary bag and disconnect the two satellite bags. Do not remove the temporary clamp to the satellite bag until the next step.

5. Strip the tubing several times so the tubing contains a representative sample of PRP.
6. Seal off a segment of the tubing and disconnect so the bag of PRP remains sterile.
7. Perform a platelet count on the sample of PRP in the segment and calculate the number of platelets in the bag of PRP:

platelets/µL $\times$ 1000 $\times$ mL of PRP = number of platelets in PRP

8. Calculate percent yield:

$$\frac{\text{number of platelets in PRP} \times 100}{\text{number of platelets in WB}} = \% \text{ yield}$$

9. Repeat the above process three or four times with different donors, using dif-

ferent centrifuges, different speeds and times of centrifugation.
10. Compare the yields for each set of test conditions.
11. Select the shortest time and lowest speed that result in the highest percent yield of platelets in PRP without unacceptable levels of red cell contamination.
12. Centrifuge the PRP at a selected time and speed to prepare platelet concentrate (PC). (See "heavy spin," Table 11.5-1.)
13. Express the platelet-poor plasma into the second attached satellite bag and seal the tubing, leaving a long section of tubing attached to the platelet bag.
14. Place the platelets on an agitator and leave for at least 1 hour to ensure that the platelets are evenly resuspended. Platelet counts cannot be performed accurately on a component immediately after centrifugation.
15. Strip the tubing several times, mixing its contents well with the contents of the platelet bag. Let the concentrate flow back into the tubing. Seal off a segment of the tubing so that the platelet bag remains sterile.
16. Perform a platelet count.
17. Calculate the number of platelets in the concentrate:

platelets/μL $\times$ 1000 $\times$ mL of PC = number of platelets in PC

18. Calculate percent yield:

$$\frac{\text{number of platelets in PC} \times 100}{\text{number of platelets in PRP}} = \text{\% yield}$$

19. Repeat steps 12 through 18 using different centrifuges, different speeds and times of centrifugation.
20. Compare the yields for each set of centrifuge conditions.
21. Select the shortest time and lowest speed that result in the highest % yield of platelets in the PC.

Note

Once each centrifuge has been calibrated, it is not necessary to recalibrate unless there is a problem with the mechanical functions of the centrifuge.

Method 11.6. Performance Testing of Automatic Cell Washers

Principle

Antihuman globulin (AHG) is inactivated readily by unbound immunoglobulin. Therefore, the antiglobulin test must be done on rbcs washed free of all proteins and suspended in a protein-free medium. Properly functioning cell washers must add large volumes of saline to each tube, resuspend the rbcs adequately, centrifuge cleanly and decant the saline to leave a dry rbc button.

Materials

1. Test tubes (10 $\times$ 75 mm or 12 $\times$ 75 mm).
2. Bovine albumin (or additive routinely used to potentiate antigen-antibody reactions).
3. IgG-coated rbcs (1-2+ reaction in antiglobulin testing).
4. Normal saline.
5. AHG: anti-IgG or polyspecific reagent.

Procedure

1. To each of 12 tubes add two drops of bovine albumin, two or three drops of donor or patient serum, and one drop of sensitized rbcs.
2. Place tubes in centrifuge carrier and seat carrier in the cell washer. Start wash cycle.

3. After addition of saline in second cycle, stop cell washer. Inspect the contents of all tubes. There should be an equal volume of saline in all tubes. (Check manufacturer's directions for correct amount of saline.) Tubes should not be more than 80% full to avoid cross-contamination by splash.
4. Observe all tubes to see that the rbc button has been completely resuspended. Rbcs should not stream up the sides of the test tubes.
5. Continue washing cycle.
6. After third wash and decant cycle, stop rbc washer and inspect all tubes to see that saline has been completely decanted, leaving a dry rbc button. The size of the rbc button should be the same in all tubes and should be the same size as at the start of the wash cycle.
7. Complete wash cycle. Add AHG according to manufacturer's directions, centrifuge and read all tubes for agglutination. If the rbc washer is functioning properly, all tubes should show agglutination.

Notes

1. Further investigation is needed if:
   a. There is variation in the amount of saline.
   b. The rbc button is not resuspended completely.
   c. There is no agglutination in the antiglobulin phase.
   d. There is a significant decrease in the size of the rbc button.
2. Rbc washers that automatically add AHG should be checked further to be sure that they are adding AHG. In step 7 above, the AHG would be added automatically, and failure of addition would be apparent by absence of agglutination. The volume of AHG should be inspected and found to be equal in all tubes. Many manufacturers market AHG colored with green dye for use in these rbc washers so that it will

be immediately obvious if the reagent has not been added. The volume of AHG delivered by these rbc washers must be checked monthly to see that the volume delivered is that specified in the manufacturer's directions and that delivery is uniform in all tubes.

Method 11.7. Standardization and Calibration of Thermometers

Principle

Standardization and calibration of thermometers ensure appropriate temperature reading of the equipment used during collection, processing and storage of blood and blood components.

Method 11.7.1. Liquid-in-Glass Laboratory Thermometers

Principle

Liquid-in-glass thermometers are widely used to ensure that blood bank equipment is able to maintain desired temperatures. Standardization and calibration of these thermometers should be performed at a temperature close to the temperature the equipment is intended to maintain. This procedure must be performed prior to initial use and subsequently if there is reason to suspect change or damage.

Materials

1. National Institute of Standards and Technology (NIST) certified thermometer or thermometer with NIST-traceable calibration certificate.
2. Liquid-in-glass (often referred to as equipment) thermometer.
3. Suitable water container(s).
4. Crushed ice.
5. Record form.

Procedure

1. Before choosing a thermometer for a particular application, consider all the governing factors; be sure that the thermometer will be used for its proper immersion; and follow the manufacturer's instructions. When using a certified thermometer, always read and follow the applicable notes.
2. Categorize the thermometers. Test in groups, comparing similar thermometers. Do not compare dissimilar thermometers.
3. Place a numbered piece of tape around the top of each thermometer to be tested.
4. Fill a suitable container with water that has a temperature close to the temperature the thermometer will monitor. To calibrate at 37 C, insert the NIST thermometer and thermometers to be tested in a waterbath. To calibrate at lower temperatures (ie, 0 C or 4 C) fill a suitable container with an appropriate mixture of water and crushed ice. Make sure the tips of all devices are at the same level. Keep the ends of the sensors in the liquid, not in the upper ice.
5. Stir constantly in a random motion until the desired temperature is reached. Allow the thermometers to equilibrate for 5 minutes.
6. Observe and record the temperature of each thermometer. Note any split in the column. Split columns cause inaccurate readings.
7. On appropriate form, document the date of testing, the thermometer identification number, the temperature reading and the initials of the person who performed the test. A result is acceptable if the reading on a thermometer agrees with the NIST thermometer within 1 C. If expected result is not achieved, the thermometer should be returned to the distributor (if newly purchased), or labeled

with the correction factor and used in noncritical work, or discarded. When reuniting a separated mercury column, try the cooling method first.[1] Document corrective action.

Reference

1. Ween S. Care and use of liquid-in-glass laboratory thermometers. ISA Transactions 1968;7:93-100.

Method 11.7.2. Electronic Oral Thermometers

Principle

All electronic thermometers must have their calibration verified, even those that are defined as "self-calibrating." Calibration must be performed prior to the initial use and periodically thereafter.

Procedure

1. Verify thermometer calibration utilizing any of the following methods:
   a. Use of manufacturer's instructions: Follow the procedures developed by the manufacturer as part of the manufacturer's labeling to verify thermometer calibration.
   b. Use of a calibration device: If using a device that elicits a series of responses from the thermometer to verify calibration, follow procedures developed by the manufacturer of the device.
   c. Use of a waterbath: Calibrate the thermometer by inserting the probe in a waterbath that has been standardized with a NIST thermometer. A result is acceptable if the reading on the thermometer agrees with the NIST thermometer within 0.1 F.
2. On appropriate form, document the date of testing, thermometer identifi-

cation number, temperature reading and the initials of the person performing the test. If expected result is not achieved, the thermometer should be returned to the distributor. Document corrective action.

Method 11.8. Quality Control for the Copper Sulfate Solution Used for Hemoglobin Determination of Blood Donors

Principle

Copper sulfate solution is used for screening blood donors for a semi-quantitative estimation of donor's hemoglobin concentration.

Either of the two methods presented below are considered acceptable for quality control of copper sulfate solution.

Method 11.8.1. Functional Measurement of Copper Sulfate Solution

Principle

Copper sulfate solution can be checked to ensure that appropriate behavior (sinking or floating) of a drop of blood sample containing the predetermined amount of hemoglobin occurs.

Procedure

1. Before using a new lot of copper sulfate solution, obtain several blood samples with known hemoglobin levels. A range around a concentration of 125 g/L (12.5 g/dL) is preferred.
2. Gently, place a drop of each blood sample into a vial of copper sulfate solution with a specific gravity of 1.053.

3. Blood samples with Hb levels >125 g/L must sink and those with Hb levels <125 g/L must float.
4. Document on appropriate form the date of testing, the name of the manufacturer, the lot number, the expiration date, the results and the initials of the person performing the test. Document corrective action when the desired results are not achieved.

Method 11.8.2. Measurement of Specific Gravity of Copper Sulfate Solution

Principle

Copper sulfate solution's specific gravity is measured and compared to the stated value of the manufacturer.

Procedure

1. The specific gravity of the solution may be measured before its use, with a calibrated hydrometer. A specific gravity of 1.053 ± 0.0003 is acceptable.
2. Document on appropriate form the date of testing, the name of the manufacturer, the lot number, the expiration date and the initials of the person performing the test. Document corrective action when the desired results are not achieved.

Method 11.9. Monitoring Cell Counts of Hemapheresis Components

Principle

Aliquots of components prepared by hemapheresis can be utilized to determine their cellular content.

Materials

1. Apheresis component.
2. Metal clips and hand sealer.
3. Clean instruments (scissors, hemostats).
4. Dielectric sealer (optional).
5. Cell counting equipment.

Procedure

1. Strip tubing attached to the well-mixed component bag four times, to ensure that contents of tubing are representative of component in bag.
2. Seal a 5-8 cm (2-3 inch) segment distal to the collection bag. There should be approximately 2 mL of fluid in the segment. Double-seal end of tubing next to component bag and detach segment.
3. Empty contents of segment into a suitably labeled tube.
4. Determine cell counts; change values to cells/mL [multiply by 1000 (or 10^3) if using device that reports cells/µL].
5. Multiply cells/mL by the volume of the component, in mL, to obtain total cell count in the component.

Method 11.10. Determinating the Hematocrit of RBC Units

Principle

For packed RBCs preserved in CPDA-1, maximal viability during storage requires an appropriate ratio of cells to the preservative. An 0.80 (80%) hematocrit or less ensures there is adequate glucose for red cell metabolism and enough citrate to maintain acceptable pH levels during storage up to 35 days. For CPDA-1 packed RBCs, four or more units should be tested each month, and at least 90% of the units tested should have a hematocrit of 0.80 (80%) or less.

For CPD, AS-1 and AS-3 preservatives, the scientific data do not indicate

that viability is compromised with high hematocrits for the allowable storage intervals. Therefore, for these preservatives, there is no need to measure the hematocrits of packed RBCs.

Method 11.11. Checking the Adequacy of Deglycerolization of RBCSs

Principle

The osmolality or refractive index of the final wash, or an attempt to perform a crossmatch with the D-RBCs, will indicate if the glycerol was adequately removed.

The osmolality of the supernatant fluid from the deglycerolized unit should not be greater than 500 mOsm/kg. When the deglycerolization process is inadequate, the rbcs will lyse when mixed with recipient serum or plasma during the crossmatch. Comparing the supernatant fluid from the final wash with a commercially prepared color standard is a simple method to detect excessive free hemoglobin.

Residual glycerol should be monitored as part of a periodic QA program, whenever a problem occurs in the processing of a unit or if the amount of hemolysis appears excessive.

Materials

1. Deglycerolized rbcs, 0.5 mL.
2. Normal saline.
3. Color comparator (available commercially).

Procedure

1. Add 0.5 mL of deglycerolized rbcs to 10 mL of normal saline.
2. Mix well and centrifuge for 1 minute at $1000 \times g$.

3. Estimate level of hemolysis by comparing the specimen with a known control or by comparison with a commercially available color comparator. There should be no more than 3% hemolysis.
4. On appropriate form, document the date of testing, the blood unit number, the results and the initials of the person performing the test. Document corrective action when the desired result is not achieved.

References

1. Jones FS, ed. Accreditation requirements manual, 4th ed. Bethesda, MD: American Association of Blood Banks, 1992:103-20.
2. Meryman HT, Hornblower M. Quality control for deglycerolized red blood cells. Transfusion 1981;21:235-40.
3. Silver H, Umlas J, Kenney P, et al. A simplified method for quality control of deglycerolized erythrocytes. Transfusion 1982;22:254-6.

Method 11.12. Counting Residual White Blood Cells in Leukocyte-Reduced Red Cell Concentrates

Principle

The residual white blood cell (wbc) content of leukocyte-reduced RBCs or WB can be determined using a large volume hemocytometer. The rbcs are first lysed and then the wbc nuclei are stained with a crystal violet stain.

Materials

1. Hemocytometer chamber with 50 µL counting volume (eg, Nageotte Brite Line Chamber®, Hausser Scientific, Horsham, PA).
2. Crystal violet stain made of 0.01% w/v crystal violet in 1% v/v acetic acid (eg, Turks solution, Columbia Diagnostics, Springfield, VA).
3. Red cell lysing agent (eg, Zapoglobin®, Coulter Diagnostics, Miami, FL).
4. Pipettor with disposable tips accurate to 40 µL.
5. Talc-free gloves, clean plastic test tubes, plastic petri dish, filter paper.
6. Light microscope with 10× ocular lens and 20× objective.

Procedure

1. Pipet 40 µL of lysing agent into a clean test tube.
2. Place a representative sample of the RBCs or WB to be tested in a clean test tube. The hematocrit of the sample to be tested should not exceed 0.60 (60%).
3. Pipet 100 µL of the RBC or WB sample into the tube containing 40 µL of lysing agent. Pipet up and down several times in order to mix the two fluids until the pipet tip is no longer coated with intact red cells.
4. Pipet 360 µL of crystal violet stain into the mixture. Pipet up and down to mix the fluids. The final volume is now 500 µL.
5. Using a pipet, load the mixture onto the hemocytometer, which has been fitted with a coverslip, until the counting area is completely covered but not overflowing.
6. Cover the hemocytometer with a moist lid to prevent evaporation. (A plastic petri dish into which a piece of damp filter paper has been placed works well.)
7. Allow the hemocytometer to rest undisturbed for 20 minutes during which time the wbcs will settle to the counting area of the chamber.
8. Remove the moist cover, place the hemocytometer on the microscope and count the wbcs present in the entire 50 µL volume using a 20× objective.

9. Calculations:
   a. The wbc concentration in the original sample expressed in wbcs/μL equals the number of observed wbcs divided by 10. (The correction factor of 10 is needed since the 50 μL sample was diluted 5 fold by lysing agent and stain.)
   b. The residual wbc content of the original unit is determined as: wbcs/unit = wbcs/μL × 10^3 (μL/mL) × Unit's Volume (mL)

Notes

1. Talc-free gloves are recommended since talc particles in gloves can be misread as wbcs.
2. Experience identifying wbcs stained in crystal violet can be obtained by examining samples from RBCs that have not been leukocyte-reduced.
3. The morphology of wbcs deteriorates during refrigerated storage and may result in inaccurate results when counting stored blood.
4. The accuracy of the counting method can be validated from a reference sample with a high wbc content in which the wbc concentration has been determined by another means. Serial dilutions of this reference sample are then prepared using blood that has been rendered extremely leukocyte-reduced by two filtrations through a leukocyte-reduction filter. The observed wbc concentration of the serially diluted samples can then be compared to the expected wbc concentration.
5. The technique is not known to be accurate at wbc concentrations < 1 wbc/μL.

Reference

Dzik WH, Szuflad P. Method for counting white cells in white cell-reduced red cell concentrates (letter). Transfusion 1993;33:272.

Method 11.13. Counting Residual White Blood Cells in Leukocyte-Reduced Platelets

Principle

The residual white blood cell (wbc) content of leukocyte-reduced platelets can be determined using a large-volume hemocytometer. The wbc nuclei are stained with a crystal violet stain.

Materials

1. Hemocytometer chamber with 50 μL counting volume (eg, Nageotte Brite Line Chamber®, Hausser Scientific, Horsham, PA).
2. Crystal violet stain made of 0.01% w/v crystal violet in 1% v/v acetic acid (eg, Turks solution, Columbia Diagnostics, Springfield, VA).
3. Pipettor with disposable tips accurate to 40 μL.
4. Talc free gloves, clean plastic test tubes, plastic petri dish, filter paper.
5. Light microscope with 10X ocular lens and 20X objective.

Procedure

1. Place a representative sample of platelets to be counted in a clean test tube.
2. Pipet 100 μL of the platelet sample into a clean test tube.
3. Pipet 400 μL of crystal violet stain into the 100 μL of platelets. Pipet up and down to mix the fluids. The final volume is now 500 μL.
4. Using a pipet, load the mixture onto the hemocytometer, which has been fitted with a coverslip, until the counting area is completely covered but not overflowing.
5. Cover the hemocytometer with a moist lid to prevent evaporation. (A plastic petri dish into which a piece

of damp filter paper has been placed works well.)

6. Allow the hemocytometer to rest undisturbed for 10 minutes during which time the wbcs will settle to the counting area of the chamber.

7. Remove the moist cover, place the hemocytometer on the microscope, and count the wbcs present in the entire 50 µL volume using a 20× objective.

8. Calculations:

   a. The wbc concentration in the original sample expressed in wbcs/µL equals the number of observed wbcs divided by 10. (The correction factor of 10 is needed since the 50 µL sample was diluted 5-fold by stain.)

   b. The residual wbc content of the original unit is determined as:
   wbcs/unit = wbcs/µL × 10^3 (µL/mL) × Unit's Volume (mL).

Notes

1. Talc-free gloves are recommended since talc particles in gloves can be misread as wbcs.

2. Experience identifying wbcs stained in crystal violet can be obtained by examining samples from platelets that have not been leukocyte-reduced.

3. The accuracy of the counting method can be validated from a reference sample with a high wbc content in which the wbc concentration has been determined by another means. Serial dilutions of this reference sample are then prepared using platelets that have been rendered extremely leukocyte-reduced by two filtrations through a leukocyte-reduction filter. The observed wbc concentration of the serially diluted samples can then be compared to the expected wbc concentration.

4. The technique is not known to be accurate at wbc concentrations of < 1 wbc/µL.

Reference

Lutz P, Dzik WH. Large-volume hemocytometer chamber for accurate counting of white cells (wbcs) in wbc-reduced platelets: Validation and application for quality control of wbc-reduced platelets prepared by apheresis and filtration. Transfusion 1993;33:409-12.

Appendices

Appendices

Appendix 1. Normal Values in Adults

Determination	SI Units	Conventional Units
Alanine amino-transferase (ALT)	4–36 U/L at 37 C	4–36 U/L at 37 C
Bilirubin, total		
Adult	2–21 μmol/L	0.1–1.2 mg/dL
Newborn	17–205 μmol/L	1–12 mg/dL
Haptoglobin	0.6–2.7 g/L	60–270 mg/dL
Hematocrit		
Males	0.40–0.54	40–54%
Females	0.38–0.47	38–47%
Hemoglobin		
Males	135–180 g/L	13.5–18.0 g/dL
Females	120–160 g/L	12.0–16.0 g/dL
Hemoglobin A_2	0.015–0.035 total Hb	1.5–3.5% total Hb
Hemoglobin F	0–0.01 total Hb	<1% total Hb
Hemoglobin (plasma)	5–50 mg/L	0.5–5.0 mg/dL
Immunoglobulins		
IgG	8.0–18.0 g/L	800–1801 mg/dL
IgA	1.1–5.6 g/L	113–563 mg/dL
IgM	0.5–2.2 g/L	54–222 mg/dL
IgD	5.0–30 mg/L	0.5–3.0 mg/dL
IgE	0.1–0.4 mg/L	0.01–0.04 mg/dL
Methemoglobin	<0.01 total Hb	<1% total Hb
Platelet count	$150–450 \times 10^9$/L	$150–450 \times 10^3$/mm^3
Red Blood Cells		
Males	$4.6–6.2 \times 10^{12}$/L	$4.6–6.2 \times 10^6$/mm^3
Females	$4.2–5.4 \times 10^{12}$/L	$4.2–5.4 \times 10^6$/mm^3
Reticulocyte count	$25–75 \times 10^9$/L	$25–75 \times 10^3$/mm^3
Vicosity, relative	$1.4–1.8 \times$ water	$1.4–1.8 \times$ water
White Blood Cells	$4.5–11.0 \times 10^9$/L	$4.5–11.0 \times 10^3$/mm^3

Henry JB. Clinical diagnosis and management by laboratory methods. 18th ed. Philadelphia: WB Saunders, 1991.

Appendix 2. Coagulation Factors*

International Designation	Common Name	% of Normal Needed for Hemostasis	% In Vivo Recovery	Stability in Stored Blood	Biologic Half-Life
Factor I	Fibrinogen	12–50	50–70	Stable	3–6 days
Factor II	Prothrombin	10–25	50	Stable	2–5 days
Factor V	Proaccelerin	10–30	~80	Labile	4.5–36 hours
Factor VII	Proconvertin	>10	100	Stable	2–5 hours
Factor VIII	Antihemophilic factor	30–40	60–70	Labile	8–12 hours
Factor IX	Christmas factor	15–40	20	Stable	18–24 hours
Factor X	Stuart-Prower factor	10–40	50–95	Stable	20–42 hours
Factor XI	PTA	20–30	90	?Stable	40–80 hours
Factor XIII	Fibrin stabilizing factor	<5	50–100	Stable	12 days

*Composite data from the following references:
Henry JB. Clinical diagnosis and management by laboratory methods. 18th ed. Philadelphia: WB Saunders, 1991.
Williams WJ, Beutler E, Erslev AJ, Lichtman MA. Hematology. 4th ed. New York: McGraw Hill, 1990.
Mollison PL, Engelfreit CP, Contreras M. Blood transfusion in clinical medicine. 9th ed. Oxford: Blackwell Scientific Publications, 1993.

Appendix 3. Approximate Normal Values for Red Cell, Plasma and Blood Volumes

	Infant[1]		Adult[2]	
	Premature	Term Birth at 72 hours	Male	Female
Red Cell				
Volume mL/kg	50	40	26	24
Plasma				
Volume mL/kg	58	47	40	36
Blood				
Volume mL/kg	108	87	66	60

The adult values should be modified to correct for:

1. Below age 18: Values are increased by 10%.
2. Weight loss:
   a. Marked weight loss within 6 months—calculations made at original weight.
   b. Gradual weight loss over a longer period of time—calculations made at present weight and raised 10-15%.
3. Obese and short: values are reduced by 10%.
4. Elderly patient: values are reduced by 10%.
5. Pregnancy[3]:

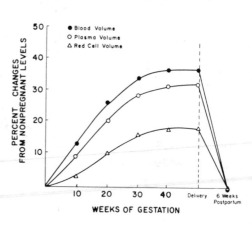

Estimation of Body Surface Area[4]:

$$BSA(m^2) = \sqrt{\frac{Ht(cm) \times Wt(kg)}{3600}} \text{ or } \sqrt{\frac{Ht(in) \times Wt(lb)}{3131}}$$

Blood Volume (BV)[5]:

BV = 2740 mL/m^2—males
BV = 2370 mL/m^2—females

Hematocrit[6]:

Venous hematocrit = H_v (blood obtained by vein or finger puncture)

Whole–body hematocrit= H_B
$$H_B = (H_v) \times (0.91)$$

References

1. Miller D. Normal values and examination of the blood: perinatal period, infancy, childhood and adolescence. In: Miller DR, Baehner RL, McMillan CW, Miller LP, eds. Blood diseases of infancy and childhood. St. Louis: C.V. Mosby, 1984:21,22.
2. Albert SN. Blood volume. Springfield: Charles C. Thomas, 1963:26.
3. Peck TM, Arias F. Hematologic changes associated with pregnancy. Clin Obstet Gynecol 1979; 22:788.
4. Mosteller RD. Simplified calculation of body-surface area. N Engl J Med 1987;317:1098.
5. Shoemaker WC. Fluids and electrolytes in the acutely ill adult. In: Shoemaker WC, Ayres S, Grenvik A, et al, eds. Textbook of critical care. 2nd ed. Philadelphia: WB Saunders Co., 1989: 1130.
6. Mollison PL, Engelfreit CP, Contreras M. Blood transfusion in clinical medicine. 9th edition. Oxford: Blackwell Scientific Publications, 1993.

Appendix 4. Typical Normal Values in Tests of Hemostasis and Coagulation (Adults)

Test	Normal Value
Activated partial thrombo-plastin time	25–35 seconds
Bleeding time	2–8 minutes
Coagulation factors	500–1500 U/L
Fibrin degradation products	<10 mg/L
Fibrinogen	2.0–4.0 g/L
Plasma D-dimers	<200 mg/L
Protein C	70–1400 U/L
Protein S (total)	70–1400 U/L
Prothrombin time	10–13 seconds
Thrombin time	17–25 seconds

Henry JB. Clinical diagnosis and management by laboratory methods. 18th ed. Philadelphia: WB Saunders, 1991.

Appendix 5. Countries With Significant Malaria Risk*

AFRICA	AFRICA CONT.	ASIA
Algeria[1]	Sierra Leone	Afghanistan
Angola	Somalia	Bangladesh[34]
Benin (Dahomey)	South Africa[12]	Bhutan[35]
Botswana[2]	Sudan	China[36]
Burkina Faso (Upper Volta)	Swaziland[13]	India
Burundi	Tanzania, United Rep.	Indonesia[37]
Cameroon	Togo	Iran, Islamic Republic of[38]
Central African Republic	Uganda	Iraq[39]
Chad	Zaire	Kampuchea, Democratic
Comoros	Zambia	(Cambodia)
Congo	Zimbabwe (Rhodesia)[14]	Laos, People's Democratic
Cote d'Ivoire (Ivory Coast)		Republic[40]
Djibouti	**AMERICAS**	Malaysia[41]
Egypt[3]		Myanmar (Burma)[42]
Equatorial Guinea	Argentina[15]	Nepal[43]
Ethiopia[4]	Belize (Br. Honduras)[16]	Oman
Gabon	Bolivia[17]	Pakistan
Gambia	Brazil[18]	Philippines[44]
Ghana	Colombia[19]	Saudi Arabia[45]
Guinea	Costa Rica[20]	Sri Lanka (Ceylon)[46]
Guinea-Bissau	Ecuador[21]	Syrian Arab Republic[47]
Kenya[5]	El Salvador[22]	Thailand[48]
Liberia	French Guiana	Turkey[49]
Libyan Arab Jamahiriya[6]	Guatemala[23]	United Arab Emirates[50]
Madagascar[7]	Guyana[24]	Viet Nam[51]
Malawi	Honduras[25]	Yemen[52]
Mali	Mexico[26]	
Mauritania[8]	Nicaragua[27]	
Mauritius[9]	Panama[28]	**OCEANIA**
Morocco[10]	Paraguay[29]	
Mozambique	Peru[30]	Papua New Guinea
Namibia[11]	Suriname[31]	Solomon Islands
Niger	Venezuela[32]	Vanuatu (New Hebrides)[53]
Nigeria		
Rwanda	**CARIBBEAN**	
Sao Tome & Principe		
Senegal	Dominican Republic[33]	
	Haiti	

*Health information for international travel, 1992. US Dept. of Health and Human Services, Centers for Disease Control, Atlanta. HHS Publication No. (CDC) 92-8280. For countries listed without a footnote, the whole country has a malaria risk.

Notes

1. Very limited risk in Sahara Region.
2. Northern part of country (north of 21° S).
3. Rural areas of Nile Delta, El Faiyum area, the oases and part of southern (upper) Egypt.
4. All areas except no risk in Addis Ababa and above 2000 meters.
5. All areas (including game parks) except no risk in Nairobi and areas above 2500 meters.
6. Very limited risk in two small foci in southwest of country.
7. All; highest risk in coastal areas.
8. All areas, except no risk in northern region; ie, Dakhlet-Nouadhibou, Inchiri, Adrar and Tiris-Zemour.
9. Rural areas only, except no risk on Rodriguez Island.
10. Very limited risk in rural areas of coastal provinces.
11. All areas of Ovamboland and Caprivi Strip.
12. Rural areas (including games parks) in the north, east, and western low altitude areas of Transvaal and in the Natal coastal areas north of 28° S.
13. All lowland areas.
14. All areas, except no risk in city of Harare.
15. Rural areas near Bolivian border, ie, Salta and Jujuy Provinces.
16. Rural areas, except no risk in central coastal District of Belize.
17. Rural areas only, except no risk in highland areas; ie, Oruro Dept., and Prov. of Ingavi, Los Andes, Omasuyos and Pacajes, (La Paz Dept.) and southern and central Potosi Department.
18. Acre and Rondonia States, Terr. of Amapa and Roraima, and in part of rural areas of Amazonas, Goias, Maranhao, Mato Grosso and Para States (travelers who will only visit the coastal states from the horn to the Uruguay border are not at risk).
19. Rural areas only, except no risk in Bogota and vicinity.
20. Limited risk in rural areas except there is no risk in central highlands; ie, Cartago and San Jose Provinces.
21. All areas in the provinces along the eastern border and Pacific coast; ie, Esmeraldas, El Oro, Guayas (including Guayaquil), Los Rios, Manabi, Morona-Santiago, Napo, Pastaza, Pichincha and Zamora-Chinchipe provinces. Travelers who only visit Quito and vicinity, the central highland tourist areas or the Galapagos Islands are not at risk.
22. Rural areas only.
23. Rural areas only, except no risk in central highlands.
24. Rural areas in the southern interior and northwest coast; ie, Rupununi and north west regions.
25. Rural areas only.
26. Rural areas of the following states: Oaxaca, Chiapas, Guerrero, Campeche, Quintana Roo, Sinaloa, Michoacan, Nayarit, Colima, Tabasco. Major resort areas on the Pacific and Gulf coasts are not at risk.
27. Rural areas only; however, risk exists in outskirts of Chinandega, Leon, Granada, Managua, Nandaime and Tipitapa.
28. Rural areas of the eastern provinces (Darien and San Blas) and the northwestern provinces (Boca del Toro and Veraguas). There is no risk in the Canal Zone or in Panama City and vicinity.
29. Rural areas bordering Brazil.
30. Rural areas. No risk in Lima and vicinity, coastal area south of Lima or the highland tourist areas (Cuzco, Machu Picchu, Lake Titicaca). Risk exists in rural areas of Departments of Amazonas, Cajamarca (except Hualgayoc Province), La Libertad (except Otuzco, Santiago de Chuco Provinces), Lambayeque, Loreto, Piura (except Talara province), San Martin and Tumbes; Provinces of Santa (Ancash Dept.), parts of La Convencion (Cuzco Dept.), Tayacaja (Huancavelica Dept.), Satipo (Junin Dept.).
31. Rural areas only, except no risk in Paramaribo District and coastal areas north of 5° N.
32. Rural areas of all border states and territories and the southeastern states of Barinas, Merida and Portuguesa.
33. All rural areas except no risk in tourist resorts. Highest risk in provinces bordering Haiti.
34. All areas except no risk in city of Dhaka.
35. Rural areas in districts bordering India.
36. Travelers visiting cities and popular rural sites on usual tourist routes are generally not at risk. Rural areas only except no risk in northern provinces bordering Mongolia and in the western provinces of Heilungkiang, Kirin, Ningsia Hui Tibet and Tsinghai. North of 33° N latitude, transmission occurs July to November; between 33° N and 25° N latitude transmission occurs May to December; south of 25° N latitude transmission occurs year-round.
37. In general, rural areas only, except high risk in all areas of Irian Jaya (western half of island of New Guinea). No risk in resort areas of Bali and Java. Malaria transmission in Indonesia (except for Irian Jaya) is largely

confined to rural areas not visited by most travelers; most travel to rural areas of Indonesia is during daytime hours when there is minimal risk of exposure.

38. Rural areas only in the provinces of Sistan-Baluchestan and Hormozgan, the southern parts of Fars, Kohgiluyeh-Boyar, Lorestan, and Chahar Mahal-Bakhtiari, and the north of Khuzestan.

39. All areas in northern region; ie, Duhok, Erbil, Kirkuk, Ninawa, Sulaimaniya Provinces.

40. All areas, except no risk in city of Vientiane.

41. In peninsular Malaysia and Sarawak (NW Borneo) malaria is limited to the rural hinterland; urban and coastal areas are malaria free. Sabah (NE Borneo) has malaria throughout. Malaria transmission in Malaysia (except Sabah) is largely confined to rural areas not visited by most travelers; most travel to rural areas is during daytime hours when there is minimal risk of exposure.

42. Rural areas only. Malaria transmission in Myanmar (Burma) is largely confined to rural areas not visited by most travelers; most travel to rural areas of Myanmar (Burma) is during daytime hours when there is minimal risk of exposure.

43. Rural areas in Terai Dist. and Hill districts below 1,200 meters. There is no risk in Katmandu.

44. Rural areas only except there is no risk in Provinces of Bohol, Catanduanes, Cebu, and Leyte. Malaria transmission in the Philippines is largely confined to rural areas not visited by most travelers; most travel to rural areas in the Philippines is during daytime

hours when there is minimal risk of exposure.

45. All areas in western provinces except no risk in the high altitude areas of Asir Province (Yemen border) and the urban areas of Jeddah, Mecca, Medina and Taif.

46. All areas except Colombo. Risk exists in districts of Amparai, Anuradhapura, Badulla (part), Batticaloa, Hambantota, Jaffna, Kardy, Kegalle, Kurungala, Mannar, Matale, Matara, Moneragala, Polonnaruwa, Puttalam, Ratnapura, Trincomalee and Vavuniya.

47. Rural areas only, except no risk in southern and western Districts of Deir-es-zor and Sweida.

48. Rural areas only. Malaria transmission in Thailand is largely confined to forested rural areas principally along the borders with Kampuchea (Cambodia) and Myanmar (Burma) not visited by most travelers; most travel to rural areas in Thailand is during daytime hours when there is minimal risk of exposure.

49. Southeast Anatolia from coastal city of Mersin to the Iraqi border (Cukorova/Amikova areas).

50. Northern Emirates, except no risk in cities of Dubai, Sharjah, Ajman, Umm al Qaiwan and Emirate of Abu Dhabi.

51. Rural areas only, except no risk in the Red and Mekong Deltas.

52. All areas, except no risk in two northwestern provinces; ie, Sada and Hajja and in the City of Aden or airport perimeter.

53. All areas, except no risk on Fortuna Island.

Appendix 6. Blood Donor Immunization Deferral Schedule

Immunizations	Disposition
Cholera	No deferral if symptom-free and afebrile
Diphtheria	
Hepatitis B—Heptavax-B® Engerix-B® Recombivax-Hb®	
Influenza	
Paratyphoid	
Pertussis	
Plague	
Polio (injection, Salk)	
Rabies (unless given following an animal bite)	
Rocky Mountain spotted fever	
Tetanus	
Typhoid	
Typhus	
Measles (Rubeola)	2-week deferral
Mumps	
Polio (oral, Sabin)	
Smallpox (after scab has fallen off or 2 weeks after injection)	
Yellow fever	
German Measles (rubella)	4-week deferral
Rh Immune Globulin	6-week deferral
Rabies (following an animal bite)	1-year deferral
Hepatitis B Immune Globulin (HBIG)	

Appendix 7. Generally Acceptable Physical Findings in Prospective Blood Donors

Physical Findings	Acceptable, if
Weight	50 kg (110 lb) or more
Temperature	37.5 C (99.6 F) or below
Pulse	50–100 beats per minute
Blood Pressure	180/100 mm Hg or below
Hemoglobin	125 g/L (12.5 g/dL) or above (finger, vein or earlobe)

Appendix 8. Frequencies (%) of Selected Rh Antigens

Antigen	Whites	Blacks
D	85	93
C	70	30
E	30	20
c	80	96
e	98	99

Appendix 9. Directory of Organizations

American Association of Blood Banks (AABB)
8101 Glenbrook Road
Bethesda, MD 20814-2749
(301) 907-6977
FAX: (301) 907-6895

American Association of Tissue Banks (AATB)
1350 Beverly Road, Suite 220A
McLean, VA 22101
(703) 827-9582
FAX: (703) 356-2918

American Blood Resources Association (ABRA)
P.O. Box 669
Annapolis, MD 21404-0669
(410) 263-8296
FAX: (410) 263-2298

American Medical Association (AMA)
515 N. State Street
Chicago, IL 60610
(312) 464-5000 (call for specific dept.)
FAX: (312) 464-4184

American Red Cross (ARC) Blood Services
1750 New York Avenue
Washington, DC 20006
(202) 737-8300

American Society of Anesthesiologists (ASA)
520 N. Northwest Highway
Park Ridge, IL 60068-2573
(708) 825-5586

American Society of Clinical Pathologists (ASCP)
2100 West Harrison Street
Chicago, IL 60612-3798
(312) 738-1336
FAX: (312) 738-1619

American Society for Apheresis (ASFA)
3900 East Timrod St.
Tucson, AZ 85711
(602) 327-8584
FAX: (602) 322-6778

American Society for Histocompatibility and
   Immunogenetics (ASHI)
P.O. Box 15804
Lenexa, KS 66285-5804
(913) 541-0009
FAX: (913) 541-0156

Armed Services Blood Program Office (ASBPO)
5109 Leesburg Pike
Falls Church, VA 22041-3258
(703) 756-8010
FAX: (703) 756-0243

Centers for Disease Control and Prevention (CDC)
1600 Clifton Road, NE
Atlanta, GA 30333
(404) 639-3311
FAX: (404) 639-3296

College of American Pathologists (CAP)
325 Waukegan Road
Northfield, IL 60093-2750
(708) 446-8800
FAX: (708) 446-8807

Council of Community Blood Centers (CCBC)
Suite 700, The Folger Building
725 15th Street, N.W.
Washington, DC 20005
(202) 393-5725
FAX: (202) 393-1282

Food and Drug Administration (FDA)
Center for Biologics Evaluation
   and Research (CBER)
1401 Rockville Pike, HFB1
Bethesda, MD 20852-1448
(301) 496-3556
FAX: (301) 402-0763

International Society of Blood Transfusion (ISBT)
c/o National Directorate of NBTS, NWRHA
Gateway House
Picadilly South
Manchester
M60 7LP England
061-236-2263
FAX: 061-236-0519

Joint Commission on Accreditation of
   Healthcare Organizations (JCAHO)
1 Renaissance Boulevard
Oakbrook Terrace, IL 60181
(708) 916-5600
FAX: (708) 916-5644

National Bone Marrow Donor Registry (NBMDR)
3433 Broadway Street NE, 400
Minneapolis, MN 55413
(800) 654-1247
FAX: (612) 627-5899

National Committee for Clinical
   Laboratory Standards (NCCLS)
771 E. Lancaster Avenue
Villanova, PA 19085
(215) 525-2435
FAX: (215) 527-8399

National Hemophilia Foundation (NHF)
110 Greene Street, Suite 303
New York, NY 10012
(800) 424-2634
(212) 219-8180
FAX: (212) 431-0906

United Network for Organ Sharing (UNOS)
1100 Boulders Parkway, Suite 500
P.O. Box 13770
Richmond, VA 23225-8770
(804) 330-8500
FAX: (804) 330-8507

Index

Index

volume drawn, 552
venipuncture site, 12-13, 16, 718
crossmatched, labeling and release of, 328-329
identification, 15-16
inventory management, 591-596
loss, in neonates, 451
orders, routine surgical, 329-330, 491, 594
recovery, *See* Blood, collection, IBC, PBC
reissuing, 68, 419
release, urgent, *See* Emergency issue
type and screen, 315
unit selection, 315-316
ABO, 315
Rh, 315-316
usage considerations, 593
outdate rate, 584, 591
volume, 764
exchange transfusion, 458-459
newborn, 437
normal values, 766-767
volume drawn, 552
See also Donor blood; Whole blood
Blood centers, regional, 595
Blood derivatives, hepatitis risk, 84
Blood filters, 420, 450
Blood groups, 259-282
changing one type to another, 316, 416
nomenclature and genetics, 195-197
terminology, 189
Blood pressure, donors, 12
Blood vessels, transplantation, 127
Blood warmers, 419, 548
Bombay phenotype, 220
Bone, storage, 126
Bone banking, 125-126, 741-747
Bone marrow
ABO incompatible, 135
donor registry, 137
freezing, 134
harvesting, 133
processing, 133
rbc removal with HES, 740-741
storage, 134
transplantation, 302
autologous, 132

C

Cabinets, biological safety, 515-517
Cancer, in donor, 6
Capillary testing, 630-631
Cardiac difficulties
donor reactions, 19
performance, 390
Cardiac output, 389-392
C3b inactivation, 160
Cell grouping, *See* RBCs
Cell-mediated lympholysis (CML) test, 298
Cell suspension, 318

Cell washers, 180
performance testing, 755-756
Centrifugation, separation of autologous from transfused rbcs, 637-638
Centrifuges
calibrating for platelet separation, 754-755
component preparation, 57-58, 547
microhematocrit, 551-552
microplate tests, 613
serologic testing, 546-547, 601-602, 752-753
Cephalothin, drug positive DAT, 375
Ch antigen, 278
Chagas' disease, 8, 485
Chemical hazards, 509, 525-529, 535, 537
data sheets, 535
disposal, 526
protective equipment, 525
CHD, *See* Anemia, cold autoimmune hemolytic
Chimerism, bone marrow transplant, 137
Chloroquine, IgG dissociation, 635-636
Chromium label, and in-vivo crossmatch, 678-680
Circulatory effects, hemapheresis, 44-45
Circulatory overload, 482-483
Cis-product antigens, *See* Rh blood group
Citrate toxicity, hemapheresis, 44
Class I antigens, MHC, 289, 291-292
crossmatch, 693, 695-696
typing, 697-700
Class II antigens, MHC, 289, 292
crossmatch, 693, 696-697
typing, 700-703
Class III antigens, MHC, 290
Clean up, 516, 521, 532
Clothing, biosafety, 515, 520
Clotting promotion in incompletely clotted specimens, 606
Coagulation
deficiencies, 403-407
hemorrhagic disease of the newborn, 461
hemolytic transfusion reactions, 478
massive transfusion, in, 416-417
normal values, 766-767
Codominant inheritance, 193, 195
autosomal, 193
sex-linked, 195
Collection facilities, mobile, 69
Compatibility testing, 639-642
neonatal, 449-450
records, 569
streamlining tests, 356
Complement
addition of, 366
AHG reactions, 365, 184-185
alternative pathway, 159-160
anti-Jk, 182, 185
binding, antibody-mediated, 184-185
Class II antigens, MHC, 290
classical pathway, 156-159
coating globulin, sole, 182, 185